Clinical Immunology: A Case-Based Approach

Clinical Immunology: A Case-Based Approach

Editor: Ashley Crawford

MURPHY & MOORE
www.murphy-moorepublishing.com

www.murphy-moorepublishing.com

MURPHY & MOORE

Cataloging-in-Publication Data

Clinical immunology : a case-based approach / edited by Ashley Crawford.
p. cm.
Includes bibliographical references and index.
ISBN 978-1-63987-113-1
1. Clinical immunology. 2. Clinical immunology--Case studies. 3. Immunology. 4. Immunodiagnosis.
5. Immunotherapy. I. Crawford, Ashley.
RC582 .C55 2022
616.079--dc23

Murphy & Moore Publishing,
1 Rockefeller Plaza,
New York City, NY 10020, USA

ISBN 978-1-63987-113-1 (Hardback)

Contents

Preface

The network of biological processes which protect an organism from diseases is termed as the immune system. The branch of medicine which deals with the study of the diseases which are caused by problems in the immune system is known as clinical immunology. It encompasses the failure, divergent action, and malignant growth of the cellular components of the immune system. The diseases studied within this field can be classified into immunodeficiency and autoimmunity. Immunodeficiency involves the immune system being unable to provide adequate response. Autoimmunity refers to the situation wherein the immune system attacks the body of the host. The book aims to shed light on some of the unexplored aspects of clinical immunology and the recent researches in this field. It elucidates the concepts and innovative models through a case based approach. Those with an interest in this field would find this book helpful.

Significant researches are present in this book. Intensive efforts have been employed by authors to make this book an outstanding discourse. This book contains the enlightening chapters which have been written on the basis of significant researches done by the experts.

Finally, I would also like to thank all the members involved in this book for being a team and meeting all the deadlines for the submission of their respective works. I would also like to thank my friends and family for being supportive in my efforts.

Editor

1

Evolving strategies for cancer and autoimmunity: back to the future

Peter J. L. Lane*, Fiona M. McConnell, Graham Anderson, Maher G. Nawaf, Fabrina M. Gaspal and David R. Withers

MRC Centre for immune Regulation, Birmingham Medical School, Birmingham, UK

Edited by:
Fang-Ping Huang, Imperial College London, UK

Reviewed by:
Julian Dyson, Imperial College London, UK
Mohey Eldin El Shikh, Queen Mary University of London, UK

***Correspondence:**
Peter J. L. Lane, MRC Centre for immune Regulation, Birmingham Medical School, Vincent Drive, Birmingham B15 2T, UK
e-mail: p.j.l.lane@bham.ac.uk

Although current thinking has focused on genetic variation between individuals and environmental influences as underpinning susceptibility to both autoimmunity and cancer, an alternative view is that human susceptibility to these diseases is a consequence of the way the immune system evolved. It is important to remember that the immunological genes that we inherit and the systems that they control were shaped by the drive for reproductive success rather than for individual survival. It is our view that human susceptibility to autoimmunity and cancer is the evolutionarily acceptable side effect of the immune adaptations that evolved in early placental mammals to accommodate a fundamental change in reproductive strategy. Studies of immune function in mammals show that high affinity antibodies and CD4 memory, along with its regulation, co-evolved with placentation. By dissection of the immunologically active genes and proteins that evolved to regulate this step change in the mammalian immune system, clues have emerged that may reveal ways of de-tuning both effector and regulatory arms of the immune system to abrogate autoimmune responses whilst preserving protection against infection. Paradoxically, it appears that such a detuned and deregulated immune system is much better equipped to mount anti-tumor immune responses against cancers.

Keywords: CD4 T cell, autoimmunity, tolerance mechanisms, cancer, regulation, memory, keyword

INTRODUCTION

In our society today, cancer and autoimmunity are major causes of suffering and death, and a huge financial burden on health services worldwide. The strongest genetic link with autoimmunity is to major histocompatibility (MHC) class II genes, implicating CD4 T cells in autoimmune pathogenesis. Less obviously, CD4 T cells are also implicated in defective immunity to tumors, as CD4 regulatory T cells (Tregs) limit effector responses to tumor antigens.

Our studies have centered on CD4 immunity and its regulation, and have been informed by the striking observation that the key features of the CD4 immune system – high affinity antibody responses, memory, and CD4 regulation – co-evolved with placentation in mammals (1–3). A simple comparison of the numbers of species in different mammalian groups – monotremes, 2; marsupials, ~400; placentals, ~5000 – illustrates the reproductive advantage conferred by placentation. The contribution of the immune system to this advantage is threefold: the bringing of unborn young to immunocompetence at birth; protection after birth by maternal transfer of high affinity IgG; and reduction in exposure of offspring to disease epidemics due to memory responses in the community, the latter two being CD4 T cell dependent functions. Note that the pressure on the immune defenses due to the physical frailty of the placental newborn is enormous, as demonstrated by the fact that even with the immune protections described, mortality is exponentially higher in infants than in adults (4). The high potency of effector immune responses demanded by placentation carries high risk of pathological autoimmunity, which has been substantially addressed by the co-evolution of T regulatory mechanisms. But because Darwinian selection favors reproductive success rather than individual survival, the protection of the developing fetus takes precedence over the risk of personal suffering and even death in post-reproductive adults. And we believe that the less than complete limitation of autoimmunity by T regulation already carries its own risk, also consequent on the stringent necessity of reproductive success. Before placentation, protection of the self from effector responses required tolerance to tissue specific self-antigens; the evolution of placentation required this tolerance to extend to placenta- and fetus-specific antigens as well. Additionally, we think that the intermittent nature of pregnancy fosters the selection of dominant forms of tolerance (see Evolution of the Placenta – A New Organ). Our view is supported by two lines of evidence: – the wide expression of fetus- and placenta-specific antigens by human cancers in both males and females (5), reflecting selection of cancer cells that can gain advantage from the immune regulation protecting the developing embryo and fetally derived placenta; – recent identification of memory Tregs induced specifically by fetally derived antigens (6). Although deletional tolerance no doubt also operates to maintain tolerance to fetally derived antigens, the particular advantage of dominant tolerance to fetal antigens expressed in the placental trophoblast is that it could also confer bystander tolerance to fetal alloantigens at the feto-maternal interface, to which there is no opportunity for maternal thymic tolerance, particularly during first time pregnancies before there is priming to induce Tregs specific for alloantigens (6).

In this article, we start by reviewing the fundamental changes that occurred in mammals over the last 200 million years [see **Figure 1** Ref. (7)] and that form the context of the sequential genetic changes that enabled new immunological structures and functions to evolve. We then review the evidence that the resulting "modern" mammalian immune system can be detuned to give a minimal essential immune system for health: a system that, without compromising immunity to infection, can both abrogate pathogenic CD4 driven autoimmune responses and augment anti-tumor immunity.

BRIEF HISTORY OF MAMMALS FROM AN IMMUNOLOGICAL PERSPECTIVE

Comparative genomics and the fossil record have been used as a timeline for the evolution of mammals from the common reptilian ancestor [**Figure 1** Ref. (7)]. This timeline highlights the major physiological changes that emerged: the evolution of homeothermy, of hair (insulation), and of lactation (an effective strategy to nourish homeothermic offspring). All mammals, including the egg laying monotremes, have these characteristics, which distinguish them from the cold-blooded common ancestor they share with reptiles and birds.

ORIGINS OF LYMPH NODES

The development of these characteristic mammalian attributes was accompanied by changes in the immune system, both anatomically and functionally. The most striking gross anatomical change is the emergence of intra-lymphatic lymphoid aggregates (the ancestors of lymph nodes) in the common mammalian ancestor. All jawed vertebrates have a spleen and lymphoid aggregates in the mucosal associated lymphoid tissues, but only mammals have lymphoid structures that are intra-lymphatic as opposed to lymphatic-associated. In chickens, lymphoid aggregates are found in the wall but not the lumen of lymphatics (8), which is a similar arrangement to the so called isolated lymphoid follicles (ILFs) found at mucosal sites in all vertebrates, and associated with

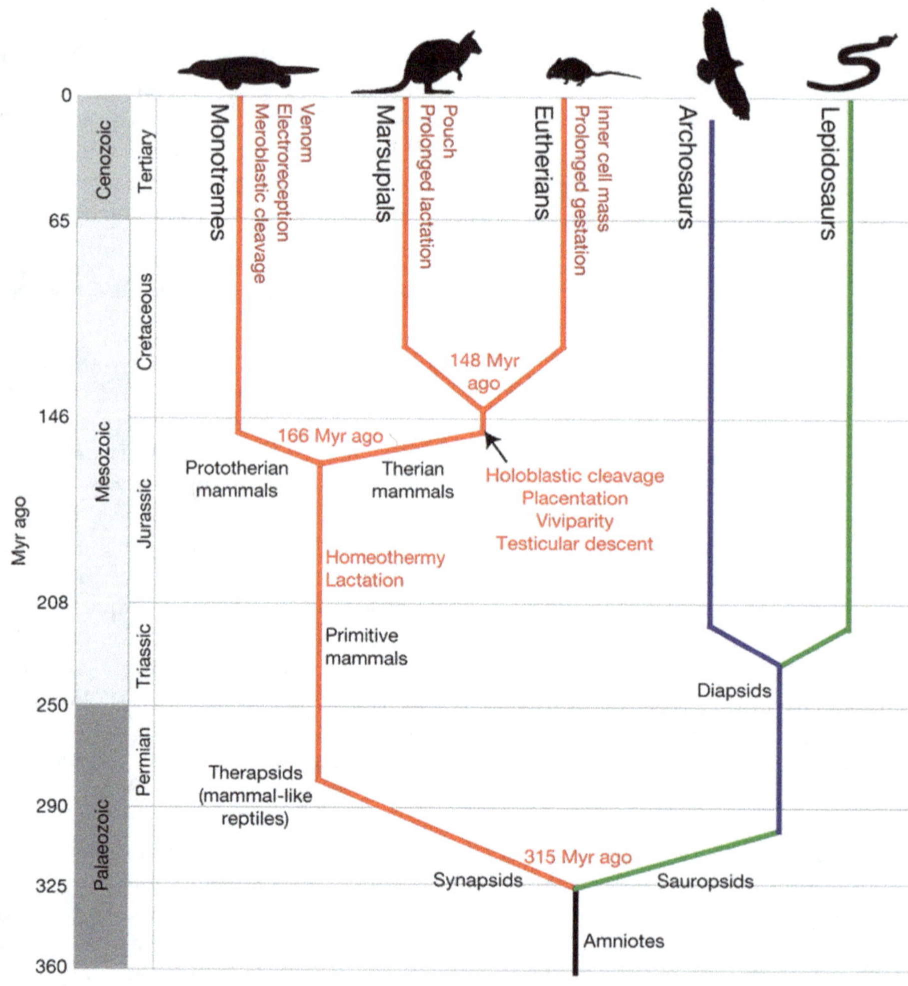

FIGURE 1 | Emergence of traits along the mammalian lineage. Amniotes split into the sauropsids (leading to birds and reptiles) and synapsids (leading to mammal-like reptiles). These small early mammals developed hair, homeothermy, and lactation (red lines). Monotremes diverged from the therian mammal lineage ~166 Myr ago and developed a unique suit of character (dark-red text). Therian mammals with common characters split into marsupials and eutherians around 148 Myr ago (dark-red text). Geological eras and periods with relative times (million years ago) are indicated on the left. Mammal lineages are in red; diapsid reptiles, shown as archosaurs (birds, crocodilians, and dinosaurs), are in blue; and lepidosaurs (snakes, lizards, and relatives) are in green.

but not inside lymphatics (e.g., the lacteals in the gut). In contrast, vascularized intra-lymphatic ILF-like structures are found in both of the extant monotremes (9, 10). Why did these intra-lymphatic structures, which are the precursors of mammalian lymph nodes, evolve? Possible explanations in our view are linked to the evolution of homeothermy in mammals, with the consequent increased demand for nutrients. The mucosal system of mammals has a much more extensive surface area for absorption of food than reptiles, and consequently has increased exposure to bacteria, both commensal and non-commensal, in the gut. One view therefore, is that these intra-lymphatic lymphoid structures evolved in the mesentery of the gut as a "firewall" to block the entry of gut bacteria into the systemic circulation (11). In any case, comparative genomics supports the view that intra-lymphatic lymphoid structures evolved in the common mammalian ancestor, as the L-selectin gene (SELL) first appears in monotremes (www.ensembl.org). This molecule occurs on lymphocytes and directs their exit from blood vessels into lymphatics (as lymph nodes are essentially intra-lymphatic structures), and is not present in reptiles or birds, which however do have genes for the inflammatory selectins present on endothelium, E-(SELE), and P-selectin (SELP). SELE and SELP are chromosomally co-located in mammals with L-selectin, indicating that SELL is likely to have arisen by gene duplication in the common mammalian ancestor.

Microscopically, the ILFs found inside the lymphatics of monotremes contain B cell germinal center (GC)-like structures with follicular CD4 T cells (10), but they do not contribute to affinity maturation of the B cell response or to memory; secondary antibody responses in monotremes are very similar to primary ones (2). In the absence of a link to affinity maturation, it seems probable that these GC-like inclusions mediated the diversification of the B cell repertoire, after the fashion of the GC-like structures seen to develop in the Bursa of Fabricius in chickens, where the B cell repertoire is diversified by activation induced cytosine deaminase (AID)-dependent gene conversion of immunoglobulin variable region genes (12). In placental animals like sheep, primary diversification of the B cell repertoire through gene conversion and somatic hypermutation also occurs in the gut associated lymphoid tissues (13), so it is quite plausible that this is the function first appearing inside intra-lymphatic nodules in monotremes. Orthologs of IgE and IgG also evolved in the common mammalian ancestor; in monotremes (14), unlike placental animals, switched immunoglobulin isotypes are produced in primary immune responses, and it is possible that the sites of AID-dependent class switching, to not only IgE and IgG, but also IgA, are the intra-lymphatic ILFs.

IgA CONTROL OF ANTI-INFLAMMATORY AND RESPONSES TO GUT MICROBIOTA

IgA is the most abundant immunoglobulin, and secreted IgA is the main immunoglobulin at mucosal surfaces. Orthologs of IgA are present in reptiles, birds, and mammals but not amphibians and fish, indicating that this immunoglobulin class evolved in the common amniotic ancestor of land animals. The evolution of the amniotic egg was critical to the capacity of vertebrates to colonize non-aquatic habitats, as it freed their reproduction from the dependency on access to water retained by amphibian species. However, terrestrial habitats brought new challenges in the form of different food sources and different microbiota colonizing the gut. In this context, the anti-inflammatory properties of IgA are likely to have been crucial. Tsuji et al. (15) present several pieces of evidence pointing to the importance of IgA in maintaining a normal gut flora. AID-deficient mice developed abnormal gut flora, which was associated with impaired switching to IgA in ILFs in the mucosa. This IgA-dependent class switching was shown to be T cell independent, but dependent on AID expression in ILF GC-like structures.

ORIGIN OF CD4 IMMUNITY

Modern mammals share a 450-Myr-old common ancestor with cartilaginous fish, and indeed all jawed vertebrates have RAG-dependent adaptive immune systems. However, recent sequencing of the elephant shark genome has revealed no evidence for the CD4 gene, and indeed no evidence of either FoxP3, the gene linked to evolution of CD4 regulation (16), or ROR-gamma (RORc), the transcription factor required for the development of Th17 CD4 T cells (17). This suggests that CD4 T cells were not part of the ancestral RAG-dependent adaptive immune system, but evolved later. Recent data have implicated both CD4 Th17 cells and Tregs in IgA immunity.

FoxP3$^+$ AND Th17 CD4 T CELLS ARE INVOLVED IN IgA PRODUCTION IN THE GUT

The FoxP3 gene is highly conserved in all placental mammals (www.ensembl.org). Given that members of the FoxP gene family are consistently highly conserved across all animal groups, this would not be surprising, except that by comparison, FoxP3 orthologs in marsupials, marsupials, reptiles, monotremes, fish, and amphibians show much reduced conservation. The step gain in conservation of FoxP3 in placental mammals is consistent with a gain of function specific to placentation (18). Similarly, IL17a, the principle IL17 cytokine secreted by Th17 T cells, is exclusive to mammalian genomes, and therefore evolved in the common mammalian ancestor.

The conventional view of FoxP3$^+$ Tregs is that their primary role is to suppress or modulate CD4 dependent immune responses (19), but there is evidence that they also function in the T cell dependent switching to IgA in the gut: Foxp3 expressing Tregs were potent inducers of IgA after transfer in T cell deficient mice (20); Tregs were found to be important mediators of induction of IgA to flagellin, a molecule common to commensal and pathogenic bacteria (21). The latter result raised the very interesting idea that a key function of Tregs is to promote the generation of IgA antibodies to commensal bacteria in the gut, so maintaining homeostasis of gut microbiota and preventing inappropriate inflammatory immune responses. A possible role for the ancestral FoxP3-dependent Tregs could therefore be to moderate immune responses to commensal bacteria by effectively providing help for B cells.

This suggestion is somewhat controversial, as recent studies have implicated Th17 cells rather than Tregs in the induction of IgA in the gut (22, 23). Cao et al. implicated the mammalian specific cytokine IL17a in the production of IgA to flagellin. The available data are however not necessarily contradictory, as in humans at least a significant fraction of Tregs isolated from mucosal surfaces co-express FoxP3 and RORγt, the key Th17 transcription factor (24), in addition to producing IL17a. A scenario compatible with the evidence is that there was co-evolution of Th17 and $FoxP3^+$ T cells in the common mammalian ancestor, at least in part to promote IgA antibody production in the gut, and in any case to act synergistically to promote integrity at mucosal surfaces.

EVOLUTION OF HIGH AFFINITY ANTIBODIES AND MEMORY IN THE COMMON PLACENTAL ANCESTOR

As discussed earlier (see "Origins of Lymph Nodes" above), despite having intra-lymphatic lymphoid follicles containing GCs, monotremes do not make high affinity antibody responses or demonstrate CD4 memory (2, 9, 10). They do not have true lymph nodes with segregated B and T cell areas, but these structures evolved in the common placental ancestor; all marsupials and placental mammals have lymph nodes, and demonstrate the capacity to make high affinity antibodies and memory (1, 3, 25, 26). These advances are linked to the evolution of new genes, notably the lymphotoxin βreceptor (LTβR) and its ligands, which are not only essential for lymph node development but also for making high affinity antibodies and memory.

LYMPHOID TISSUE INDUCER CELLS: Rorγ DEPENDENT, AND LINKED WITH BOTH LYMPH NODE AND CD4 MEMORY DEVELOPMENT

Reina Mebius was the first to characterize murine lymphoid tissue inducer cells (LTi) (27). Their function in the development of lymphoid tissues was revealed when it was found that mice deficient in the orphan retinoic acid receptor gamma (RORγ) lacked both this $CD4^+CD3^-$ LTi population and lymph nodes (28, 29). These studies link LTi unequivocally with the development of lymph nodes, cryptopatches, and ILFs through their expression of the tumor necrosis superfamily members (TNFSF) for the lymphotoxin beta receptor (LTβR), $LT\alpha_1\beta_2$ (30), and TRANCE (31); more recent studies have also shown that LTi are rich sources of the cytokine, interleukin 22 (IL22) (32), which is associated with the promotion of defenses at epithelial sites (33–35). This would permit the LTi a function in the promotion of innate immunity that is distinct from the induction of lymphoid tissues.

Additionally, our work has shown that LTi persist in adult lymphoid tissues in both mouse (36) and man (37), but are distinguished from the neonatal population by their expression of high levels of OX40-ligand (OX40L)(TNFSF4) (36, 37) and in mouse, CD30L(TNFSF8) (36). Our studies have found that CD4 T cell memory function is highly dependent on signaling through both OX40 and CD30 (38), suggesting additional roles for LTi in the mediation of adaptive CD4 dependent immune responses.

IMPORTANCE OF THE IMMUNE CONTRIBUTION TO PLACENTATION

It is difficult to refute the significance of the co-evolution of high affinity antibodies and lymph nodes with placentation. Zinkernagel (39) takes the view that memory and high affinity antibodies are chiefly relevant because they protect offspring via maternal transfer of high affinity antibodies, and the way in which immunological functions have evolved during placentation broadly supports his perception. We know that orthologs of IgG first appeared in the common mammalian ancestor because monotremes have them (14). The neonatal Fc receptor (FCGRT), however, which is the gene that enables the crucial transfer of IgG from mother to offspring as well prolonging the beneficial effects of IgG by increasing its half-life (40), is only present in marsupial and placental genomes. Studies of human infant mortality to most common infections show an exponential decline with the age (4) with exception of the first year of life where transfer of maternal IgG plays a crucial role in infant survival through protective immunity. Indeed in many placental animals failure to transfer maternal IgG is fatal. Comparative genomics therefore supports the idea that the development of the capacity to make high affinity antibodies and transfer them to offspring is an integral component of the evolution of a fundamental change in reproductive strategy.

CO-EVOLUTION OF HIGH AFFINITY ANTIBODIES WITH FoxP3-DEPENDENT REGULATION

In placentals, GCs in B follicles are the locations where T cell dependent B cell selection drives the generation of high affinity antibodies (41), but there must exist mechanisms to edit self-reactive GC B cells that acquire self-reactivity. This can occur because self-proteins can be inadvertently conjugated to foreign proteins (e.g., apoptotic virally infected cells), and therefore GC B cells that acquire self-reactivity by chance have the capacity to get help from GC follicular T helper cells. Indeed, it is very common in viral infections in humans to get transient low affinity autoantibody production, but this does not usually go on to generate high affinity class switched autoantibodies.

Recent studies have shown that Tregs are also present in normal GC (42, 43) and the fact that high affinity IgG autoantibodies to a wide variety of tissue-restricted antigens are found in FoxP3-deficient mice indicates that Tregs must be pivotal in preventing the generation of these autoantibodies. Although it is by no means clear how Tregs in GC prevent autoantibodies being generated, there is better evidence for how self-specific Tregs are selected. Recent work has shown the critical role of the thymic medulla in the selection of thymic derived regulatory but not conventional T cells (44). The gene AIRE, expressed in the thymic medulla, controls the expression of many tissue-restricted antigens (45, 46). Intrathymic deletion of self-specific T cells is substantially AIRE-dependent (47), but the process of selection against tissue-restricted antigens is also a plausible mechanism by which Tregs specific for self-antigen could be selected in thymus and go on to exert their effects in the periphery.

When considering the origin of the requirement for regulation of immune effectors, it is clear that, in the absence of memory and high affinity IgG, the consequences for monotremes of inadvertently making anti-self antibody responses are mild; all their antibodies are low-titer, low affinity, and transiently produced, so one would surmise that the requirement for regulation is limited. Substantial changes in the FoxP3 gene occurred during the evolution of placentation (18), and the relevance of this is further demonstrated by the failure of regulation in placental animals having mutant forms of FoxP3 lacking critical domains (18).

EVOLUTION OF THE PLACENTA – A NEW ORGAN

The major advantage of placentation over oviparous forms of reproduction is that it greatly increases the chances of reproductive success by prolonging the parental protection of the developing offspring, including increasing the chance of surviving infection courtesy of a more mature immune system, initially supported by high affinity maternal IgG antibodies. A recent detailed study of placental fossils combined with comparative genomic data concluded that all modern placentals (Eutherians) are derived from a common placental ancestor that survived the mass extinction 65 Myr ago that eliminated terrestrial dinosaurs (48). Inferences from this study are that this common Eutherian ancestor had a hemochorial placenta with the fetal and maternal blood circulations in intimate contact. Marsupials represent an intermediate step toward this state; they are born very immature and before their immune system develops, but nevertheless get the benefit of protection from predation by *ex utero* occupation of the maternal pouch, where lactation provides the added advantage of maternally transferred antibodies. Marsupials have a yolk sac (Metatherian) placenta, which is simple and relatively impervious to feto-maternal exchange, thus dodging the issue of maternal recognition of fetal and placental antigens. In Eutherian mammals, however, the placenta is fully adapted to cope with a fetus that develops to maturity. There are many new genes that arose during the evolution of placentation to program the development of the placenta (a fetally derived organ) (49), and in addition there are genes essential for survival of the fetus itself *in utero*. The common ancestor of marsupials and placentals, in which these new genes were evolving, had the capacity to make high affinity antibodies; for the hemochorial placenta with its proximity of maternal and fetal circulations, the selective drive for immune regulation capable of protecting the fetus from rejection by its own mother was clearly decisive.

Two facts need to be remembered concerning the placenta:

- Morphologically it is very diverse in different classes of mammal, reflecting the strong evolutionary pressure for mammals with different lifestyles to adapt reproductively to different external conditions. This is reflected in the evolution of new genes and new gene families in different mammalian classes and is particularly evident on the X chromosome, where many of the placental genes are concentrated and which also evolved from an autosomal chromosome in placentals (5).
- Placentation is an intermittent phenomenon, so maintaining T cell tolerance to the rapidly evolving new proteins that are not present in mammalian females post birth, but to which T cell tolerance will be essential if they are to be reproductively successful is a real challenge. From an evolutionary perspective, it is therefore not difficult to understand why the adaptation to placentation might select for mechanisms of dominant tolerance mediated by Tregs, i.e., where Tregs specific for some of the newly evolving placental and fetal-restricted antigens could suppress maternal effector responses against them, whereas other, maybe less abundant or otherwise less conspicuous, neo-antigens would escape without significant Treg reaction. A further point is that this dominant regulation against thymic expressed placental antigens expressed at the feto-maternal interface could also suppress allorecognition of paternal MHC.

EVOLVING MATERNAL TOLERANCE TO FETUS AND PLACENTA

Because it seems very likely that the problem of maternal tolerance to fetal and placental proteins had already been solved in the common eutherian placental ancestor, we looked for genetic differences between marsupials and eutherian placental mammals in the genes linked to induction and selection of Tregs in mTECs in thymus. The T cell costimulatory molecule CD28 is vital for Treg selection (50), and CD28 ligands, particularly CD80, are expressed on AIRE^{+} mTECs. In all eutherian placental genomes examined, AIRE, the gene associated with selection of antigen-specific Tregs is chromosomally co-located with the CD28 paralog, ICOS-ligand. The ICOS signaling pathway is crucial for the generation of high affinity antibodies in GCs (51); particularly pertinent to the genetic association between ICOSL and AIRE, it is also required for the effective Treg suppressive function (52). Thus the ICOS gene is a pivot between high affinity antibody production and effective Treg function against immune responses to self, raising the very interesting possibility that the expression of this gene facilitated the selection of self-antigen-specific Tregs found in GCs (43), which then edit self-reactive B cells in GCs driven by ICOS signaling interactions.

The comparative genomics of these interactions is instructive. In all marsupial genomes examined, AIRE and ICOSL are not co-located, but are on separate chromosomes, as is also the case in reptiles and birds. Maybe the genetic translocation that brought AIRE and ICOSL together in the common placental ancestor also mediated the co-expression of AIRE with ICOSL on mTECs. We think that this co-expression was likely to have facilitated development of the process of selecting antigen-specific Tregs, and see it as an illustration of how mutually beneficial processes could serve as selective advantages for one another: here the genetic mechanism for improving antibody affinity (ICOS signaling) co-evolved with the genetic mechanism maintaining tolerance to self (selection of antigen-specific Tregs via AIRE) to modify the generation of high affinity antibodies to tissue-restricted antigens – in this case those expressed in the placenta and fetus. This allows antibodies to pathogens to be transferred to offspring, protecting them from infection without causing autoimmunity, which is a genuine risk, as there are many examples of passive maternal transfer of IgG autoantibodies causing disease in the neonate. In FoxP3^{KO}OX40CD30^{KO} mice where not only affinity maturation, but also autoantibody production is impaired, the requirement for Tregs is obviated.

Other studies have linked Tregs specifically with the maintenance of allotolerance at the feto-maternal interface (53–55). However, our data from the FoxP3^{KO}OX40CD30^{KO} mice do not support this interpretation. Our data show that FoxP3^{KO}OX40CD30^{KO} mice are fully able to reject allografts (data not shown) but we found no evidence that female FoxP3^{KO}OX40CD30^{KO} mice rejected allogeneic fetuses. Recent data suggest that immunosuppression in the fetal circulation need not be cell-mediated and implicates the expression of arginase by fetal blood cells (56). Because the fetus is normally sterile, such a global suppression of immune responses in the fetal circulation, and therefore by definition also at the fetal/maternal interface in the placenta, is in our view, a potential mechanism to prevent maternal lymphocytes that enter the fetal circulation inducing rejection. The selective expression of immunosuppressive arginase in the fetal red blood cells in the fetal circulation also helps to explain why lymphocytes in the maternal compartment are still able to respond. For example, although in pregnancy there is susceptibility to some infections, notably influenza, pregnant women make good antibody responses after vaccination (57). We think, therefore that the requirement for regulation in the form of Tregs is more relevant in the context of the mother, to allow antibody responses in particular to foreign proteins derived from infectious pathogens (maternal IgG then passively protects offspring after birth) to go ahead, but to head off responses to fetal or placental antigens that enter the maternal circulation.

MINIMAL IMMUNE SYSTEM FOR MAMMALIAN HEALTH

Our studies had shown that the TNF-family members, OX40 and CD30-ligand were crucial for the development of high affinity antibodies and memory (38). Although CD30 and its ligand were present in the common amniotic ancestor, true orthologs of OX40-ligand, which plays the dominant role in both affinity maturation and memory, are only present in the mammalian lineage (www.ensembl.org). To ask the question of whether CD4 regulation and memory could have co-evolved in the common placental ancestor we reasoned that mice deficient in FoxP3 (no Tregs) and also deficient in OX40 and CD30 (no high affinity antibodies and memory) would mimic at least to some extent the immune system of the common mammalian ancestral immune system seen in monotremes, and would not exhibit autoimmunity. This was the case (58).

Our mice are interesting in several respects. First, the generation of autoantibodies is abrogated in these mice and they fail to develop the widespread autoimmunity seen in mice and men. The development of FoxP3^{KO} disease is CD4 dependent (19) but the FoxP3^{KO}CD30OX40^{KO} mice do not behave as CD4-deficient as they do generate GCs and switched antibody not dissimilar to that observed in monotreme responses. Furthermore, they control many herpes viruses (CD8 immunity is preserved) as well as bacteria. The behavior of the immune responses in the CD30OX40^{KO} mice is mirrored in a single reported case of OX40-deficiency in humans (59). Although the individual did suffer from Kaposi's sarcoma, she controlled common Herpes virus infections, and was not unduly susceptible to bacterial infections, despite the absence of recall CD4 memory responses.

If one accepts Zinkernagel's view that the development of memory and high affinity antibodies is a strategy optimized for reproductive success rather than individual survival, then the Foxp3^{KO}OX40CD30^{KO} immune system in our view represents the "minimal immune system for health," the necessary and sufficient platform that had evolved in the common mammalian ancestor before the evolution of high affinity antibodies and memory induced a compromise in the form of susceptibility to autoimmunity.

HUMAN AUTOIMMUNITY AND BLOCKADE OF OX40 AND CD30 SIGNALING PATHWAYS

In human genome wide association studies (GWAS) class II polymorphisms are the strongest genetic link, highlighting the role of CD4 T cells in immunopathology, either due to failure to select antigen-specific Tregs in thymus that subsequently protect, or because CD4 effector T cells drive pathology. The significance of the Foxp3^{KO}OX40CD30^{KO} mice with a global defect in Tregs is that it suggests that blocking OX40 alone, or in combination with CD30, would be very effective treatment for wide number of CD4 driven autoimmune diseases without rendering patients susceptible to infection. This is further supported by evidence that shows that FoxP3^{KO} disease can also be blocked by co-injection of antibodies that block OX40 and CD30 signaling pathways (58).

CANCERS MIMIC THE IMMUNE EVASION STRATEGY OF PREGNANCY

The link between placentation and cancer is hardly new (60). From our perspective, a substantial role for dominant FoxP3-dependent regulation was to facilitate the growth of the fetus and placenta, both expressing many neo-antigens, while at the same time being permissive particularly for the generation of antibodies to pathogens. Recent whole exome sequencing of human cancers has also revealed their enormous heterogeneity (61). Although in theory this should render tumors immunogenic to the CD8 immune system in particular, it is clear that dominant Treg tolerance is a major stumbling block to the development of effective anti-tumor immune responses if Tregs specific for self-antigens can suppress immune responses to tumor-specific antigens.

Two gene examples illustrate the point. The first is the gene alpha-fetoprotein (AFP), the fetal albumin adapted to *in utero* survival, an autosomal gene. The second is the gene PLAC1 expressed in the trophoblast of the placenta of all placental animals, and exclusive to placental animals. Both of these genes are part of the genetic adaption to placental reproduction, but they are also widely expressed in human cancers. This fact suggests that the suppressive effect of fetal and placental antigens on immune responses might have led to the success of cancers that express them. As stated earlier, medullary epithelium in thymus (mTEC) is crucial for the selection of Tregs but not conventional T cells (44). Both PLAC1 and AFP are over-expressed in mTECs [compared to cortical epithelium (cTECs)] (our own data and also www.immgen.org), so it is quite plausible that Tregs specific for these proteins could be selected in thymus. Support for this type of dominant tolerance preventing immune responses to cancer is also provided by the following study (62).

In this study, T cell receptors (TCRs) from tumor infiltrating Tregs found in a murine model of prostate cancer were cloned. TCR transgenic mice positively selected Tregs in thymus in both male and female mice, indicating that they were not tumor-specific Tregs, and as they were found in female mice, were not selected in prostate! Their mTEC thymic derivation was further supported by the observation that selection was dependent on AIRE, the gene that controls expression of many tissue-restricted antigens in the thymus (45).

DE-TUNING THE IMMUNE SYSTEM TO UNBLOCK CD8 ANTI-CANCER IMMUNE RESPONSES

Strategies that suppress Treg function [CTLA4 blockade (63, 64) and PD-1 (65)] have been effective in releasing CD8 anti-tumor immune responses, particularly when used in combination (66). Because Tregs suppress CD4 driven autoimmunity, autoimmunity is a major cause of morbidity and mortality in these treatments. Like Foxp3^{KO} mice, CTLA4^{KO} mice die of CD4 driven autoimmunity (67) so in reality CTLA4 blockade can only be partial in human patients.

However, our studies in FoxP3^{KO}OX40CD30^{KO} mice suggest that that CD4 mediated immunity can be obviated in FoxP3^{KO} without seriously compromising autoimmunity. To test whether these mice were capable of mounting anti-tumor immune responses we used the well established murine melanoma line B16 (68). This tumor grows rapidly in syngeneic B16 mice but tumor growth is virtually abrogated in FoxP3^{KO}OX40CD30^{KO} mice (our unpublished observations). To us this observation has potential important implications for the treatment of human cancers as it offers the option of permitting effective CD8 anti-tumor responses while preventing the unpleasant CD4 driven autoimmune side effects.

SUMMARY

In this perspective we outline a strategy for attenuating CD4 driven immunopathology by blockade of the TNF super family members, OX40L (in particular), and CD30L (synergistic with OX40L). Studies of immune function in mice deficient in OX40 and CD30 reveal that although CD4 immunity is reduced, deficient mice are able to deal with the common viral and bacterial infections that can be associated with conventional immunosuppressive strategies. We suggest that antibodies that block these pathways may have therapeutic benefit in human autoimmune diseases mediated by CD4 T cells without compromising resistance to infection.

Recent work has shown that blockade of regulatory T cell function with CTLA4-blocking antibodies has revealed impressive "repressed" CD8 immune responses to neo-antigens expressed by human cancers, particular melanoma, but also some other solid tumors. However, this has been at the expense of CD4 driven autoimmunity that can have considerable morbidity and even mortality. Our work indicates that in the absence of OX40 and CD30, FoxP3-dependent Tregs are dispensable, and mice deficient in OX40, CD30, and FoxP3 mount excellent CD8-dependent anti-tumor immune responses.

As stated above, it is our view that human susceptibility to autoimmunity and cancer are the evolutionarily acceptable side effects of the immune adaptations that evolved in early placental mammals to accommodate a fundamental change in reproductive strategy, and by reversing this process, a detuned and deregulated immune system is much better equipped to mount anti-tumor immune responses against cancers but is also resistant to chronic CD4 driven autoimmune disease.

ACKNOWLEDGMENTS

This work was funded by Program Grant support for the Medical Research Council, UK to Graham Anderson and Peter J. L. Lane.

REFERENCES

1. Shearer MH, Robinson ES, Vandeberg JL, Kennedy RC. Humoral immune response in a marsupial *Monodelphis domestica*: anti-isotypic and anti-idiotypic responses detected by species-specific monoclonal anti-immunoglobulin reagents. *Dev Comp Immunol* (1995) **19**:237–46. doi:10.1016/0145-305X(95)00001-A
2. Wronski EV, Woods GM, Munday BL. Antibody response to sheep red blood cells in platypus and echidna. *Comp Biochem Physiol A Mol Integr Physiol* (2003) **136**:957–63. doi:10.1016/S1095-6433(03)00325-8
3. Kreiss A, Wells B, Woods GM. The humoral immune response of the Tasmanian devil (*Sarcophilus harrisii*) against horse red blood cells. *Vet Immunol Immunopathol* (2009) **130**:135–7. doi:10.1016/j.vetimm.2009.02.003
4. Martin WJ. Mortality in childhood during 1920-38. *Br Med J* (1945) **1**:363–5. doi:10.1136/bmj.1.4393.363
5. Simpson AJ, Caballero OL, Jungbluth A, Chen YT, Old LJ. Cancer/testis antigens, gametogenesis and cancer. *Nat Rev Cancer* (2005) **5**:615–25. doi:10.1038/nrc1669
6. Rowe JH, Ertelt JM, Xin L, Way SS. Pregnancy imprints regulatory memory that sustains anergy to fetal antigen. *Nature* (2012) **490**:102–6. doi:10.1038/nature11462
7. Warren WC, Hillier LW, Marshall Graves JA, Birney E, Ponting CP, Grutzner F, et al. Genome analysis of the platypus reveals unique signatures of evolution. *Nature* (2008) **453**:175–83. doi:10.1038/nature06936
8. Biggs PM. The association of lymphoid tissue with the lymph vessels in the domestic chicken (*Gallus domesticus*). *Acta Anat (Basel)* (1957) **29**:36–47. doi:10.1159/000141159
9. Diener E, Ealey EH. Immune system in a monotreme: studies on the Australian echidna (*Tachyglossus aculeatus*). *Nature* (1965) **208**:950–3. doi:10.1038/208950a0
10. Connolly JH, Canfield PJ, McClure SJ, Whittington RJ. Histological and immunohistological investigation of lymphoid tissue in the platypus (*Ornithorhynchus anatinus*). *J Anat* (1999) **195**(Pt 2):161–71. doi:10.1046/j.1469-7580.1999.19520161.x
11. Macpherson AJ, Smith K. Mesenteric lymph nodes at the center of immune anatomy. *J Exp Med* (2006) **203**:497–500. doi:10.1084/jem.20060227
12. Reynaud CA, Dahan A, Anquez V, Weill JC. Somatic hyperconversion diversifies the single Vh gene of the chicken with a high incidence in the D region. *Cell* (1989) **59**:171–83. doi:10.1016/0092-8674(89)90879-9
13. Reynaud CA, Garcia C, Hein WR, Weill JC. Hypermutation generating the sheep immunoglobulin repertoire is an antigen-independent process. *Cell* (1995) **80**:115–25. doi:10.1016/0092-8674(95)90456-5
14. Zhao Y, Cui H, Whittington CM, Wei Z, Zhang X, Zhang Z, et al. *Ornithorhynchus anatinus* (platypus) links the evolution of immunoglobulin genes in eutherian mammals and nonmammalian tetrapods. *J Immunol* (2009) **183**:3285–93. doi:10.4049/jimmunol.0900469
15. Tsuji M, Suzuki K, Kitamura H, Maruya M, Kinoshita K, Ivanov II, et al. Requirement for lymphoid tissue-inducer cells in isolated follicle formation and T cell-independent immunoglobulin A generation in the gut. *Immunity* (2008) **29**:261–71. doi:10.1016/j.immuni.2008.05.014
16. Fontenot JD, Gavin MA, Rudensky AY. Foxp3 programs the development and function of CD4+CD25+ regulatory T cells. *Nat Immunol* (2003) **4**:330–6. doi:10.1038/ni904
17. Ivanov II, McKenzie BS, Zhou L, Tadokoro CE, Lepelley A, Lafaille JJ, et al. The orphan nuclear receptor RORgammat directs the differentiation program of proinflammatory IL-17+ T helper cells. *Cell* (2006) **126**:1121–33. doi:10.1016/j.cell.2006.07.035
18. Andersen KG, Nissen JK, Betz AG. Comparative genomics reveals key gain-of-function events in Foxp3 during regulatory T cell evolution. *Front Immunol* (2012) **3**:113. doi:10.3389/fimmu.2012.00113
19. Blair PJ, Bultman SJ, Haas JC, Rouse BT, Wilkinson JE, Godfrey VL. CD4+CD8- T cells are the effector cells in disease pathogenesis in the scurfy (sf) mouse. *J Immunol* (1994) **153**:3764–74.
20. Tsuji M, Komatsu N, Kawamoto S, Suzuki K, Kanagawa O, Honjo T, et al. Preferential generation of follicular B helper T cells from Foxp3+ T cells in gut Peyer's patches. *Science* (2009) **323**:1488–92. doi:10.1126/science.1169152
21. Cong Y, Feng T, Fujihashi K, Schoeb TR, Elson CO. A dominant, coordinated T regulatory cell-IgA response to the intestinal microbiota. *Proc Natl Acad Sci U S A* (2009) **106**:19256–61. doi:10.1073/pnas.0812681106
22. Cao AT, Yao S, Gong B, Elson CO, Cong Y. Th17 cells upregulate polymeric Ig receptor and intestinal IgA and contribute to intestinal homeostasis. *J Immunol* (2012) **189**:4666–73. doi:10.4049/jimmunol.1200955

23. Hirota K, Turner JE, Villa M, Duarte JH, Demengeot J, Steinmetz OM, et al. Plasticity of Th17 cells in Peyer's patches is responsible for the induction of T cell-dependent IgA responses. *Nat Immunol* (2013) **14**:372–9. doi:10.1038/ni.2552
24. Voo KS, Wang YH, Santori FR, Boggiano C, Wang YH, Arima K, et al. Identification of IL-17-producing FOXP3+ regulatory T cells in humans. *Proc Natl Acad Sci U S A* (2009) **106**:4793–8. doi:10.1073/pnas.0900408106
25. Canfield PJ, Hemsley S. The roles of histology and immunohistology in the investigation of marsupial disease and normal lymphoid tissue. *Dev Comp Immunol* (2000) **24**:455–71. doi:10.1016/S0145-305X(00)00009-4
26. Kreiss A, Obendorf DL, Hemsley S, Canfield PJ, Woods GM. A histological and immunohistochemical analysis of lymphoid tissues of the Tasmanian devil. *Anat Rec (Hoboken)* (2009) **292**:611–20. doi:10.1002/ar.20896
27. Mebius RE, Rennert P, Weissman IL. Developing lymph nodes collect CD4+CD3- LTbeta+ cells that can differentiate to APC, NK cells, and follicular cells but not T or B cells. *Immunity* (1997) **7**:493–504. doi:10.1016/S1074-7613(00)80371-4
28. Kurebayashi S, Ueda E, Sakaue M, Patel DD, Medvedev A, Zhang F, et al. Retinoid-related orphan receptor gamma (RORgamma) is essential for lymphoid organogenesis and controls apoptosis during thymopoiesis. *Proc Natl Acad Sci U S A* (2000) **97**:10132–7. doi:10.1073/pnas.97.18.10132
29. Sun Z, Unutmaz D, Zou YR, Sunshine MJ, Pierani A, Brenner-Morton S, et al. Requirement for RORgamma in thymocyte survival and lymphoid organ development. *Science* (2000) **288**:2369–73. doi:10.1126/science.288.5475.2369
30. Futterer A, Mink K, Luz A, Kosco-Vilbois MH, Pfeffer K. The lymphotoxin beta receptor controls organogenesis and affinity maturation in peripheral lymphoid tissues. *Immunity* (1998) **9**:59–70. doi:10.1016/S1074-7613(00)80588-9
31. Kong YY, Yoshida H, Sarosi I, Tan HL, Timms E, Capparelli C, et al. OPGL is a key regulator of osteoclastogenesis, lymphocyte development and lymph-node organogenesis. *Nature* (1999) **397**:315–23. doi:10.1038/16852
32. Takatori H, Kanno Y, Watford WT, Tato CM, Weiss G, Ivanov II, et al. Lymphoid tissue inducer-like cells are an innate source of IL-17 and IL-22. *J Exp Med* (2009) **206**:35–41. doi:10.1084/jem.20072713
33. Wolk K, Kunz S, Witte E, Friedrich M, Asadullah K, Sabat R. IL-22 increases the innate immunity of tissues. *Immunity* (2004) **21**:241–54. doi:10.1016/j.immuni.2004.07.007
34. Aujla SJ, Chan YR, Zheng M, Fei M, Askew DJ, Pociask DA, et al. IL-22 mediates mucosal host defense against Gram-negative bacterial pneumonia. *Nat Med* (2008) **14**:275–81. doi:10.1038/nm1710
35. Satoh-Takayama N, Vosshenrich CA, Lesjean-Pottier S, Sawa S, Lochner M, Rattis F, et al. Microbial flora drives interleukin 22 production in intestinal NKp46+ cells that provide innate mucosal immune defense. *Immunity* (2008) **29**:958–70. doi:10.1016/j.immuni.2008.11.001
36. Kim MY, Gaspal FM, Wiggett HE, McConnell FM, Gulbranson-Judge A, Raykundalia C, et al. CD4(+)CD3(-) accessory cells costimulate primed CD4 T cells through OX40 and CD30 at sites where T cells collaborate with B cells. *Immunity* (2003) **18**:643–54. doi:10.1016/S1074-7613(03)00110-9
37. Kim S, Han S, Withers DR, Gaspal F, Bae J, Baik S, et al. CD117(+) CD3(-) CD56(-) OX40L(high) cells express IL-22 and display an LTi phenotype in human secondary lymphoid tissues. *Eur J Immunol* (2011) **41**:1563–72. doi:10.1002/eji.201040915
38. Gaspal FM, Kim MY, McConnell FM, Raykundalia C, Bekiaris V, Lane PJ. Mice deficient in OX40 and CD30 signals lack memory antibody responses because of deficient CD4 T cell memory. *J Immunol* (2005) **174**:3891–6.
39. Zinkernagel RM, Hengartner H. Protective 'immunity' by pre-existent neutralizing antibody titers and preactivated T cells but not by so-called 'immunological memory'. *Immunol Rev* (2006) **211**:310–9. doi:10.1111/j.0105-2896.2006.00402.x
40. Raghavan M, Bjorkman PJ. Fc receptors and their interactions with immunoglobulins. *Annu Rev Cell Dev Biol* (1996) **12**:181–220. doi:10.1146/annurev.cellbio.12.1.181
41. MacLennan ICM. Germinal centers. *Annu Rev Immunol* (1994) **12**:117–39. doi:10.1146/annurev.iy.12.040194.001001
42. Chung Y, Tanaka S, Chu F, Nurieva RI, Martinez GJ, Rawal S, et al. Follicular regulatory T cells expressing Foxp3 and Bcl-6 suppress germinal center reactions. *Nat Med* (2011) **17**:983–8. doi:10.1038/nm.2426
43. Linterman MA, Pierson W, Lee SK, Kallies A, Kawamoto S, Rayner TF, et al. Foxp3+ follicular regulatory T cells control the germinal center response. *Nat Med* (2011) **17**:975–82. doi:10.1038/nm.2425
44. Cowan JE, Parnell SM, Nakamura K, Caamano JH, Lane PJ, Jenkinson EJ, et al. The thymic medulla is required for Foxp3+ regulatory but not conventional CD4+ thymocyte development. *J Exp Med* (2013) **210**:675–81. doi:10.1084/jem.20122070
45. Derbinski J, Schulte A, Kyewski B, Klein L. Promiscuous gene expression in medullary thymic epithelial cells mirrors the peripheral self. *Nat Immunol* (2001) **2**:1032–9. doi:10.1038/ni723
46. Gotter J, Brors B, Hergenhahn M, Kyewski B. Medullary epithelial cells of the human thymus express a highly diverse selection of tissue-specific genes colocalized in chromosomal clusters. *J Exp Med* (2004) **199**:155–66. doi:10.1084/jem.20031677
47. Mathis D, Benoist C. A decade of AIRE. *Nat Rev Immunol* (2007) **7**:645–50. doi:10.1038/nri2136
48. O'Leary MA, Bloch JI, Flynn JJ, Gaudin TJ, Giallombardo A, Giannini NP, et al. The placental mammal ancestor and the post-K-Pg radiation of placentals. *Science* (2013) **339**:662–7. doi:10.1126/science.1229237
49. Rawn SM, Cross JC. The evolution, regulation, and function of placenta-specific genes. *Annu Rev Cell Dev Biol* (2008) **24**:159–81. doi:10.1146/annurev.cellbio.24.110707.175418
50. Tai X, Cowan M, Feigenbaum L, Singer A. CD28 costimulation of developing thymocytes induces Foxp3 expression and regulatory T cell differentiation independently of interleukin 2. *Nat Immunol* (2005) **6**:152–62. doi:10.1038/ni1160
51. McAdam AJ, Greenwald RJ, Levin MA, Chernova T, Malenkovich N, Ling V, et al. ICOS is critical for CD40-mediated antibody class switching. *Nature* (2001) **409**:102–5. doi:10.1038/35051107
52. Herman AE, Freeman GJ, Mathis D, Benoist C. CD4+CD25+ T regulatory cells dependent on ICOS promote regulation of effector cells in the prediabetic lesion. *J Exp Med* (2004) **199**:1479–89. doi:10.1084/jem.20040179
53. Aluvihare VR, Kallikourdis M, Betz AG. Regulatory T cells mediate maternal tolerance to the fetus. *Nat Immunol* (2004) **5**:266–71. doi:10.1038/ni1037
54. Rowe JH, Ertelt JM, Aguilera MN, Farrar MA, Way SS. Foxp3(+) regulatory T cell expansion required for sustaining pregnancy compromises host defense against prenatal bacterial pathogens. *Cell Host Microbe* (2011) **10**:54–64. doi:10.1016/j.chom.2011.06.005
55. Samstein RM, Josefowicz SZ, Arvey A, Treuting PM, Rudensky AY. Extrathymic generation of regulatory T cells in placental mammals mitigates maternal-fetal conflict. *Cell* (2012) **150**:29–38. doi:10.1016/j.cell.2012.05.031
56. Elahi S, Ertelt JM, Kinder JM, Jiang TT, Zhang X, Xin L, et al. Immunosuppressive CD71+ erythroid cells compromise neonatal host defence against infection. *Nature* (2013) **504**:158–62. doi:10.1038/nature12675
57. Steinhoff MC, Omer SB, Roy E, Arifeen SE, Raqib R, Altaye M, et al. Influenza immunization in pregnancy – antibody responses in mothers and infants. *N Engl J Med* (2010) **362**:1644–6. doi:10.1056/NEJMc0912599
58. Gaspal F, Withers D, Saini M, Bekiaris V, McConnell FM, White A, et al. Abrogation of CD30 and OX40 signals prevents autoimmune disease in FoxP3-deficient mice. *J Exp Med* (2011) **208**:1579–84. doi:10.1084/jem.20101484
59. Byun M, Ma CS, Akcay A, Pedergnana V, Palendira U, Myoung J, et al. Inherited human OX40 deficiency underlying classic Kaposi sarcoma of childhood. *J Exp Med* (2013) **210**(9):1743–59. doi:10.1084/jem.20130592
60. Beard J. Embryological aspects and etiology of carcinoma. *Lancet* (1902) **159**:1758–61. doi:10.1016/S0140-6736(01)89936-0
61. Watson IR, Takahashi K, Futreal PA, Chin L. Emerging patterns of somatic mutations in cancer. *Nat Rev Genet* (2013) **14**:703–18. doi:10.1038/nrg3539
62. Malchow S, Leventhal DS, Nishi S, Fischer BI, Shen L, Paner GP, et al. Aire-dependent thymic development of tumor-associated regulatory T cells. *Science* (2013) **339**:1219–24. doi:10.1126/science.1233913
63. Hodi FS, O'Day SJ, McDermott DF, Weber RW, Sosman JA, Haanen JB, et al. Improved survival with ipilimumab in patients with metastatic melanoma. *N Engl J Med* (2010) **363**:711–23. doi:10.1056/NEJMoa1003466
64. Robert C, Thomas L, Bondarenko I, O'Day S, Jw MD, Garbe C, et al. Ipilimumab plus dacarbazine for previously untreated metastatic melanoma. *N Engl J Med* (2011) **364**:2517–26. doi:10.1056/NEJMoa1104621
65. Topalian SL, Hodi FS, Brahmer JR, Gettinger SN, Smith DC, McDermott DF, et al. Safety, activity, and immune correlates of anti-PD-1 antibody in cancer. *N Engl J Med* (2012) **366**:2443–54. doi:10.1056/NEJMoa1200690

66. Wolchok JD, Kluger H, Callahan MK, Postow MA, Rizvi NA, Lesokhin AM, et al. Nivolumab plus ipilimumab in advanced melanoma. *N Engl J Med* (2013) **369**:122–33. doi:10.1056/NEJMoa1302369
67. Tivol EA, Borriello F, Schweitzer AN, Lynch WP, Bluestone JA, Sharpe AH. Loss of CTLA-4 leads to massive lymphoproliferation and multiorgan tissue destruction, revealing a critical negative regulatory role of CTLA-4. *Immunity* (1995) **3**:541–7. doi:10.1016/1074-7613(95)90125-6
68. Overwijk WW, Restifo NP. B16 as a mouse model for human melanoma. *Curr Protoc Immunol* (2001) **Chapter 20**(Unit 20):21. doi:10.1002/0471142735.im2001s39

2

Asymmetry in erythroid-myeloid differentiation switch and the role of timing in a binary cell-fate decision

Afnan Alagha[1] and Alexey Zaikin[2]*

[1] Nonlinear Analysis and Applied Mathematics Research Group (NAAM), Department of Mathematics, King Abdulaziz University, Jeddah, Saudi Arabia
[2] Department of Mathematics and Institute for Women's Health, University College London, London, UK

Edited by:
Carmen Molina-Paris, University of Leeds, UK

Reviewed by:
Koji Yasutomo, University of Tokushima, Japan
Maria L. Toribio, Spanish Research Council (CSIC), Spain

***Correspondence:**
Alexey Zaikin, Department of Mathematics and Institute for Women's Health, University College London, Gower Street, London WC1E 6BT, UK
e-mail: alexey.zaikin@ucl.ac.uk

GATA1-PU.1 genetic switch is a paradigmatic genetic switch that governs the differentiation of progenitor cells into two different fates, erythroid and myeloid fates. In terms of dynamical model representation of these fates or lineages corresponds to stable attractor and choosing between the attractors. Small asymmetries and stochasticity intrinsically present in all genetic switches lead to the effect of delayed bifurcation which will change the differentiation result according to the timing of the process and affect the proportion of erythroid versus myeloid cells. We consider the differentiation bifurcation scenario in which there is a symmetry-breaking in the bifurcation diagrams as a result of asymmetry in external signaling. We show that the decision between two alternative cell fates in this structurally symmetric decision circuit can be biased depending on the speed at which the system is forced to go through the decision point. The parameter sweeping speed can also reduce the effect of asymmetry and produce symmetric choice between attractors, or convert the favorable attractor. This conversion may have important contributions to the immune system when the bias is in favor of the attractor which gives rise to non-immune cells.

Keywords: GATA1-PU.1 switch, differentiation, immune cells, pluripotent cells

1. INTRODUCTION

The importance of studying the immune system has attracted mathematicians and biologists to discover more of its features in recent years. One of the mechanisms is to study the genetic networks that control the lineage commitment of hematopoietic stem cells, which produce the full range of blood cells, including the immune cells (1). Many mathematical models have been used to study the differentiation of progenitor cell into erythroid and myeloid lineages based on the expression of lineage-specific transcription factors GATA1 and PU.1, respectively (2, 3). An important question arises in these models about the causes of bifurcation and symmetry-breaking and whether they occur in response to intrinsic cues or extrinsic signals. In fact, the integration of both intrinsic and extrinsic factors has received an extensive attention to elucidate the roles of external signals in cell-fate decision processes, and most importantly its relationship to the production of immune cells (3–6). Another important and interesting factor that can affect the decision of the cell is the speed of external signals or the speed of crossing the critical region (7–9). Remarkably, varying control parameter with time has been studied in many other systems. Ashwin et al. (10) have investigated how the rate of change of a parameter (or input) imposes significant changes in the climate system. It is found that rapid change may force the system to move away from a branch of attractors. This dependence on the rate was referred to as R-tipping. Another more recent study (11) has discovered how the stress response in bacteria is determined by the rate of environmental change. An increase in environmental stress leads to a single uniform pulse of alternative sigma factor σ^B activation, a general stress response pathway, with amplitude depending on the rate at which the stress increased. It is found that faster stresses lead to larger and sharper activation of σ^B, reflecting the fact that the activation process is rate-dependent. A question naturally arises how rate dependent signaling will affect the immune cell-fate selection via a differentiation of progenitor cells. We have studied these phenomena in the most paradigmatic switch responsible for the differentiation of immune cells, the GATA1-PU.1 switch. Moreover, we have considered how the shape of external signals may have an impact in decision-making process. The paper is structured as follows, we review the model of Huang et al. (2) and investigate, in addition to the symmetric scenario, the asymmetric scenario in two ways: (i) under the effect of asymmetric change of parameters; and (ii) under the effect of external signals, using two kinds of signals (see Materials and Methods). Furthermore, we will test the effect of parameter sweeping speed on the distribution of trajectories in the attractors of the dynamical system.

2. MATERIALS AND METHODS

2.1. THE GATA1-PU.1 GENE REGULATORY CIRCUIT

The model of the genetic switch responsible for differentiation contains mutual inhibition and is shown in (**Figure 1A**). The regulatory dynamics can be described by the following form (2):

$$\frac{dX_1}{dt} = \frac{a_1 X_1^n}{r_{a_1}^n + X_1^n} + \frac{b_1 r_{b_1}^n}{r_{b_1}^n + X_2^n} - k_1 X_1 + \sigma_{X_1}\xi_{X_1} \quad (1)$$

$$\frac{dX_2}{dt} = \frac{a_2 X_2^n}{r_{a_2}^n + X_2^n} + \frac{b_2 r_{b_2}^n}{r_{b_2}^n + X_1^n} - k_2 X_2 + \sigma_{X_2}\xi_{X_2} \quad (2)$$

where X_1 and X_2 are the concentrations of two transcription factors GATA1 and PU.1, respectively. These equations model the dynamics of self-activation and cross-inhibition with Hill functions (12). The parameters a_1, a_2 represent self-activation rates, the parameters b_1, b_2 are basal expression rates, k_1, k_2 are deactivation rates, the parameters r's are thresholds at which the inflection point in the Hill function occurs, and n is the Hill coefficient. The first terms of equations (1) and (2) give the contribution from self-activation, while the second terms measure the effect of cross-inhibition on basal activation rates, and the third terms the degradation. To take account of intrinsic gene expression stochasticity, we consider the differential equations (1) and (2) in the Langevin form by adding multiplicative noise terms (the last ones) where ξ_{X_1} and ξ_{X_2} stand for a Gaussian noise and $\sigma_{X_{1,2}}$ depend on $X_{1,2}$ as suggested in Ref. (13). These noise terms model the contribution of intrinsic noise which is unavoidable in biological systems. External cell signaling can be included in the model as follows

$$\frac{dX_1}{dt} = \frac{a_1 S_1 X_1^n}{r_{a_1}^n + X_1^n} + \frac{b_1 r_{b_1}^n}{r_{b_1}^n + X_2^n} - k_1 X_1 \quad (3)$$

$$\frac{dX_2}{dt} = \frac{a_2 S_2 X_2^n}{r_{a_2}^n + X_2^n} + \frac{b_2 r_{b_2}^n}{r_{b_2}^n + X_1^n} - k_2 X_2 \quad (4)$$

where S_1 and S_2 represent external signals to the genetic switch. Here, we are interested in two generic forms of signals:

- *Linear signals*: In this form (7) the external signals may have different rising times but they are equal in the steady state at $S_{max} = 10$ (see **Figure 2A**). For the sake of simplicity we assume that S_1 reaches to the steady state faster than S_2, and thus the rising time T_1 of S_1 is smaller than the rising time T_2 of S_2. They both increase linearly with time according to

$$S_1(t) = \begin{cases} \frac{S_{max}}{T_1} t & if \quad t \leq T_1 \\ S_{max} & if \quad t > T_1 \end{cases} \quad (5)$$

$$S_2(t) = \begin{cases} \frac{S_{max}}{T_2} t & if \quad t \leq T_2 \\ S_{max} & if \quad t > T_2 \end{cases} \quad (6)$$

The difference between S_1 and S_2 and the maximal difference A (**Figure 2B**) are defined as follows

$$\Delta S(t) = S_1(t) - S_2(t),\ A = max(\Delta S(t)) = S_{max}\left(1 - \frac{T_1}{T_2}\right) \quad (7)$$

- *Adaptation form of signals*: As suggested in Ref. (14) to achieve biochemical adaptation the signals have transient growth stage where they reach to their maxima, and decay stage where they decay and saturate to their steady states (see **Figure 3**). As for the first form, S_1 has a rising time, θ_1, smaller than S_2, θ_2, and the

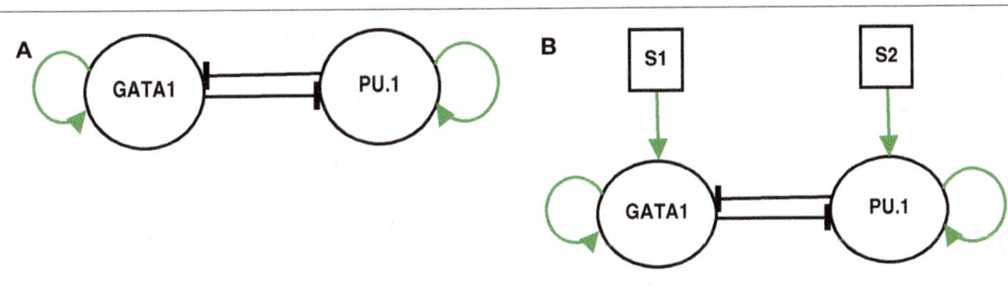

FIGURE 1 | GATA1-PU.1 genetic switch with and without external signals. (A) The isolated switch consists of two transcription factors GATA1 and PU.1 that activate themselves while inhibit each other's expression. **(B)** The exposure of the same switch in **(A)** to two external signals S_1 and S_2.

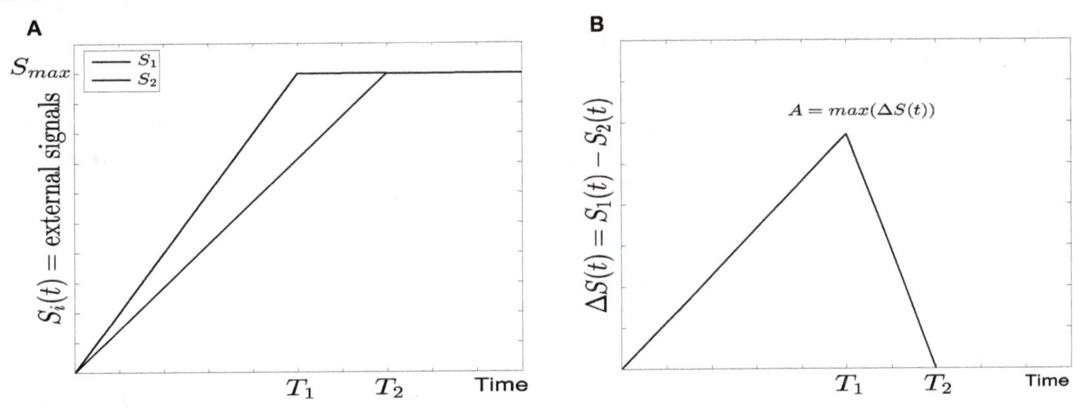

FIGURE 2 | Linear form of external signals in GATA1-PU.1 genetic switch. (A) Two external signals S_1 and S_2 with different rising times but equal steady states at $S_{max} = 10$. **(B)** The difference between the external signals with maximal asymmetry at A.

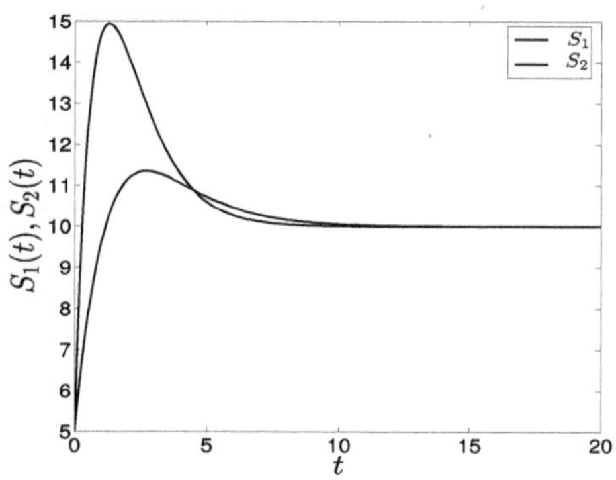

FIGURE 3 | Adaptation form of external signals in GATA1-PU.1 genetic switch. The external signals S_1 and S_2 have different rising times but equal steady states at $v = 10$. Note that at the end of the signaling the system is structurally symmetric.

value of saturation is 10. They have the following form

$$S_1(t) = \frac{h_1}{\theta_1^2} t e^{-\frac{t}{\theta_1}} + \frac{v}{1+e^{-t}} \tag{8}$$

$$S_2(t) = \frac{h_2}{\theta_2^2} t e^{-\frac{t}{\theta_2}} + \frac{v}{1+e^{-t}} \tag{9}$$

where h_1, h_2 control the amplitude of signals, and θ_1, θ_2 are scale parameters. The second terms control the saturation of the signals to the value $v = 10$ (selected value). The maxima occur at $t_{max} = \theta_{1,2}$. Consequently, we have chosen θ (θ_1 or θ_2) to be the value which determines the speed since as we increase θ, which represents the rising time, we increase the time at which the maximum occurs. In other words, we decrease the speed of the signal variation.

2.2. TESTING OF THE PARAMETER SWEEPING SPEED

To test the effect of speed, we compute the ratio R numerically using

$$R = \frac{N_u}{N_t} \tag{10}$$

It represents the ratio between trajectories or cells which go to the top (or to the upper branch) of the bifurcation diagram, and trajectories that go to both upper and lower branches during simulation. Obviously, $R = 1$ if all cells choose the upper branch in the decision of their fate, $R = 0.5$ if the proportions of cells between two branches are equal, and $R = 0$ if all cells prefer the lower branch.

Heun's method is used for solving the differential equations. In simulation of stochastic differential equations we have used Matlab, and all bifurcation diagrams and nullclines were generated in XPPAUT. $\delta(t)$ is an integration step size.

3. RESULTS

3.1. GATA1-PU.1 GENETIC SWITCH WITHOUT EXTERNAL SIGNALS

This switch (**Figure 1A**) represents a paradigm for gene regulatory networks that govern the differentiation (2). It consists of two transcription factors GATA1 and PU.1 with self-stimulation and cross-inhibition. GATA1 is a master regulator of the erythroid lineage, and PU.1 is a master regulator of the myeloid lineage, and the two lineages arise from a common myeloid progenitor cell (1, 15).

3.1.1. *Bifurcation analysis for symmetric scenario*

In the symmetric scenario, the parameters of the model are changed symmetrically with respect to X_1 and X_2. Hence, the rates of self-activation, cross-inhibition, deactivation, and thresholds are equal for both transcription factors (see Materials and Methods). Then, this scenario is divided into two parts depending on the kind of bifurcation which results in during a change of the parameters.

- *Supercritical pitchfork bifurcation*: This type of bifurcation can occur when b is increased from 0.5 to 1 (**Figure 4A**), or when r is decreased from 1.8 to 1.2 (**Figure 5C**). In this kind of bifurcation, a transition occurs from monostability to bistability. The monostable state represents progenitor cell in undifferentiated state and has the ability to differentiate into two different fates. At this state, both transcription factors in the network are produced at approximately equal levels as it can be seen from the intersection point of nullclines in (**Figure 4B**). At the differentiation process, the progenitor cell is destabilized and two new attractors appear with equal basins of attraction (**Figure 4C**).
- *Subcritical pitchfork bifurcation*: This type of bifurcation occurs for many parameter changes. It can happen when k is changed from 1 to 1.5 (**Figure 5A**), when a is decreased from 1 to 0.5 (**Figure 5B**), when b is increased from 0.3 to 0.4 (**Figure 5D**), and when r is increased from 0.5 to 1 (**Figure 5C**). In this kind of bifurcation, a transition occurs from tristability to bistability (**Figures 5E,F**). In this situation, the progenitor cell (metastable state) coexists with the two fates, and the two transcription factors are expressed at equal or low levels. At the bifurcation process, it becomes unstable and makes discontinuous transition to either erythroid or myeloid fates with equal basins of attraction.

3.1.2. *Bifurcation analysis for asymmetric scenario*

Here, the parameters of the model are changed asymmetrically with respect to X_1 and X_2. For example, we can increase one of the parameters and keep the other constant, or decrease one of the parameters and keep the other constant, or both. This asymmetric change will cause symmetry-breaking in the bifurcation diagrams and makes one of the attractors more favorable than the other. Similarly, we note two types of bifurcation:

- *Supercritical pitchfork bifurcation*: In order to get this kind of bifurcation with symmetry-breaking, we increase a_1 and k_2 (see Materials and Methods for their definitions) and as a result, X_1 is increased. Then, the bifurcation occurs when b is changed from 0.6 to 1 (**Figures 6A–C**). Now, the uncommitted progenitor cell represented by monostability is not in the middle but at the point where X_1 is higher. After bifurcation, the erythroid fate becomes dominant since it has a larger basin of attraction to the right of the separatrix (**Figure 6C**).

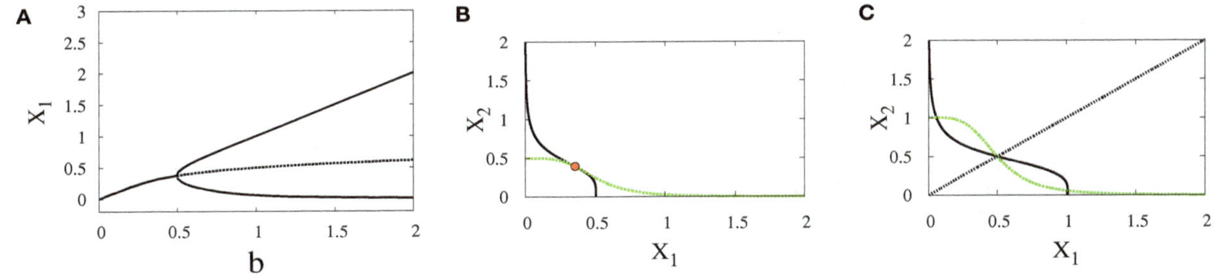

FIGURE 4 | Supercritical pitchfork bifurcation diagrams for symmetric scenario. Bifurcation diagram **(A)** and nullclines at the beginning **(B)** and end **(C)** of the bifurcation. For all diagrams, $n = 4$, $r = 0.5$, $a_1 = a_2 = 0.01$, $k_1 = k_2 = 1$. The solid lines indicate stability, while dashed lines indicate unstable branches.

- *Subcritical pitchfork bifurcation*: The bifurcation occurs when b is varied from 0.3 to 0.4. This gives imperfect subcritical pitchfork bifurcation (**Figure 7A**). The change in system behavior from tristability to bistability is depicted in (**Figures 7B,C**). At the progenitor cell, both transcription factors have low levels but the progenitor cell is not exactly in the middle. After bifurcation, one of the attractors corresponding to erythroid lineage becomes dominant as a result of increasing self-activation of GATA1.

3.1.3. Trajectories and the effect of parameter sweeping speed

To investigate the effect of the different speeds of the parameter sweeping we concentrate on the asymmetric supercritical pitchfork bifurcation, and similar results can be seen in the other kind of bifurcation. The graphical solutions of X_1 and X_2 after solving the differential equations (see equations (1) and (2) in Materials and Methods) are shown in (**Figure 8A**). As the time increases, the values of X_1 increase and the values of X_2 decrease. In fact, for small values of noise, this is the expected behavior from the dominance of the erythroid attractor.

To examine the effect of the speed with which the system crosses the critical region, we vary b linearly with time according to $b(t) = \alpha t$, where α is the slope, and compute the ratio R (see Materials and Methods). The result is shown in (**Figure 8B**). For low speeds, the ratio R is high which means that most of the cells choose the erythroid lineage due to the produced asymmetry, and this lineage leads to and include red blood cells. On the other hand, as we increase the speed, this ratio tends to zero. Two conclusions follow from this behavior. First, large speeds reduce the effect of asymmetry gradually and convert the favorable attractor completely when the ratio tends to zero. Second, $R = 0$ means that the myeloid fate becomes more favorable by cells. The myeloid fate leads to the immune cells of the immune system (16).

3.2. GATA1-PU.1 GENETIC SWITCH UNDER EXTERNAL SIGNALING

To elucidate the effect of external signals on the dynamics of the switch, we consider external signals acting upon the switch (**Figure 1B**), see also equations (3) and (4). The external signals enhance the activation of X_1 and X_2. **Figure 9** highlights the bifurcation in the parameter space (S_1, S_2) for the chosen set of parameters. The borders separate between the regions of monostability and the region of bistability, and this indicates to the existence of supercritical pitchfork bifurcation under the two following scenarios.

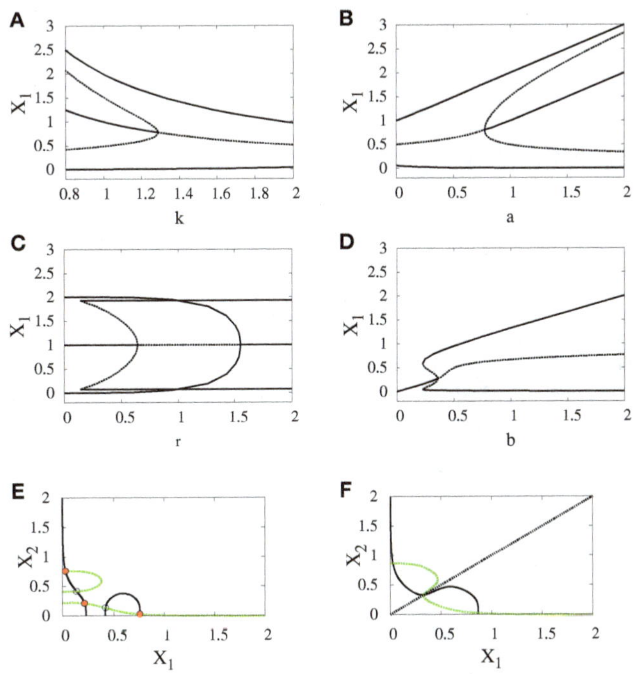

FIGURE 5 | Subcritical pitchfork bifurcation diagrams for symmetric scenario. Bifurcation diagrams **(A–D)** and nullclines at the beginning **(E)** and end **(F)** of the bifurcation diagram **(D)**. For all $n = 4$. For **(A)** $a = 1$, $b = 1$, $r = 0.5$, **(B)** $b = 1$, $k = 1$, $r = 0.5$, **(C)** $a = 1$, $b = 1$, $k = 1$, **(D–F)** $a_1 = a_2 = 1$, $k_1 = k_2 = 1.5$. In **(C)** there is also supercritical pitchfork bifurcation.

3.2.1. Bifurcation analysis for symmetric scenario

Under this scenario, both signals S_1 and S_2 are equal. The nullclines in (**Figures 10A,B**) exhibit the bifurcation from monostability to bistability. This symmetry will give us near-symmetric bifurcation diagram (**Figure 10C**) with progenitor cell located in the middle and have equal probabilities to choose between erythroid (upper attractor) and myeloid (lower attractor) fates.

3.2.2. Bifurcation analysis for asymmetric scenario

In contrary to the above scenario, now the signals have different parameters. As a result, the monostable state (**Figure 10D**) is at the point where X_1 is higher since S_1 which acts on X_1 is larger. After bifurcation, the attractor at which X_1 is high has a larger

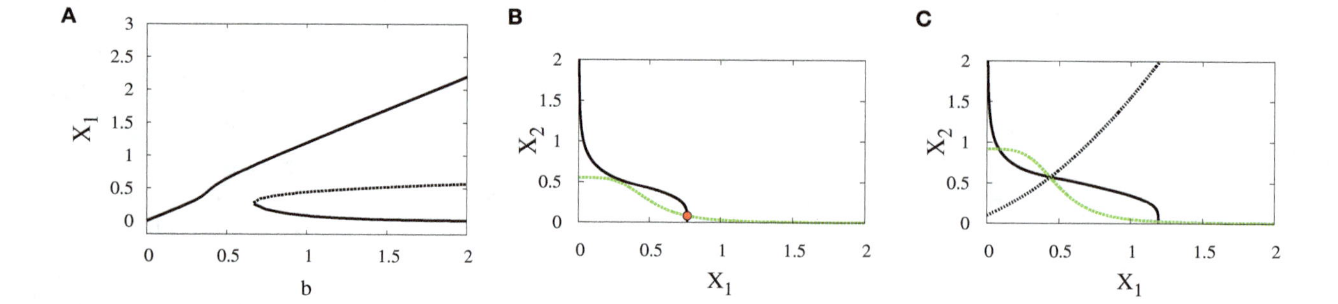

FIGURE 6 | Asymmetric scenario. Supercritical pitchfork bifurcation diagrams. Bifurcation diagram **(A)** and nullclines at the beginning **(B)** and end **(C)** of the bifurcation. The parameters are $n=4$, $r=0.5$, $a_1=0.2$, $a_2=0.01$, $k_1=1$, $k_2=1.1$.

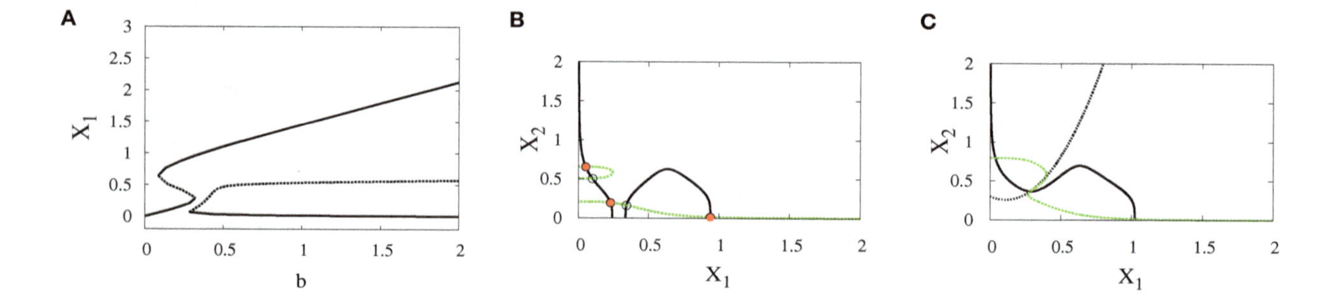

FIGURE 7 | Asymmetric scenario. Subcritical pitchfork bifurcation diagrams. Bifurcation diagram **(A)** and nullclines at the beginning **(B)** and end **(C)** of the bifurcation. The parameters are $n=4$, $r=0.5$, $a_1=1.2$, $a_2=1$, $k_1=1.5$, $k_2=1.6$.

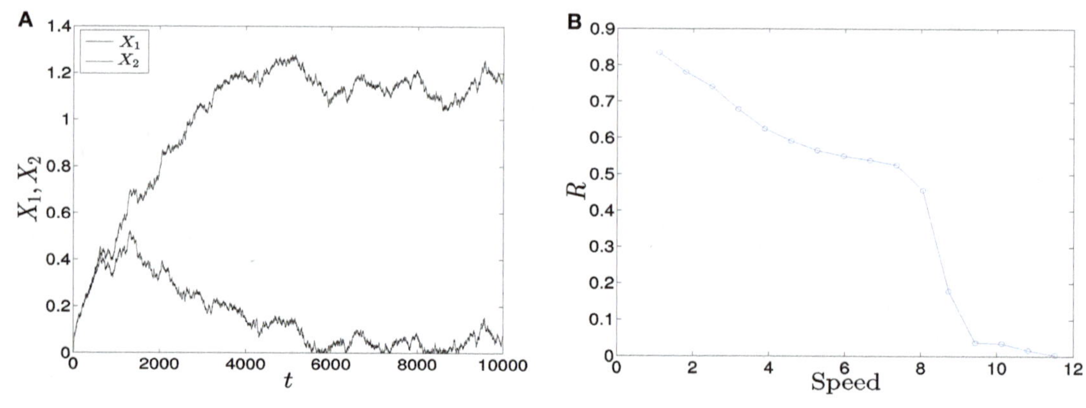

FIGURE 8 | Trajectories and parameter sweeping speed. **(A)** Time evolution of X_1 and X_2 in the asymmetric supercritical pitchfork bifurcation. **(B)** The effect of increasing the speed of crossing the critical region on the distribution of trajectories in the attractors for 10000 iterations. As the speed is increased, the ratio R changes from 1 to 0. Hence, increasing the speed causes a large switch from the favorable attractor to the other one. Parameters are $a_1=0.2$, $a_2=0.01$, $k_1=1$, $k_2=1.1$, $n=4$, $r=0.5$. Also, in **(A)** $\sigma^2=0.01$, **(B)** $\sigma^2=0.5$.

basin of attraction (**Figure 10E**). We can note in (**Figure 10F**) how this asymmetry produces symmetry-breaking in the bifurcation diagram and so the decision of the cell will be biased.

3.2.3. Trajectories and speed-dependent cellular decision making

To study how signal asymmetry, noise, and decision making will result in the dependence of the parameter sweeping speed we have considered with two kinds of signals (See Materials and Methods):

- *Linear signals*: The signals are shown in (**Figure 2A**). The asymmetry between the two signals is transient and the symmetry is retained after some time (**Figure 2B**). The behavior of trajectories of X_1 and X_2 under the influence of this form of signals is shown in (**Figure 11A**). As the time increases, the values of X_1 increase and the values of X_2 decrease. Hence, trajectories of X_1 and X_2 choose the attractor at which X_1 is higher since S_1 is faster. Next, to test the effect of increasing the speed on choosing the attractors (stable steady states) of genetic switch in the presence of noise and transient asymmetry A, we vary T_1 in $S_1(t) = \frac{S_{max}}{T_1} t$ with constant values of A and S_{max}, and T_2 will be changed according to the formula $T_2 = \frac{S_{max}}{S_{max}-A} T_1$ (7). With increasing the speed (**Figure 11B**), the ratio R tends to 0.5. Thus, increasing the speed increases the symmetry between erythroid and myeloid lineages and reduce the effect of asymmetry which is produced by external signals.

- *Adaptation form of signals*: The signals take the non-linear form shown in (**Figure 3**) and as for the linear form, S_1 is faster than S_2. The trajectories in this form behave almost like the first form (**Figure 11C**). To study the effect of the speed, we vary θ_1 and θ_2 such that θ_1 is smaller than θ_2. Then, we compute the ratio R and the result is depicted in (**Figure 11D**). It shows ratio tending to 0.5 as θ is increased. But increasing θ decreases the speed, so, surprisingly, now we regain the symmetry in the switch by decreasing the speed of external signals.

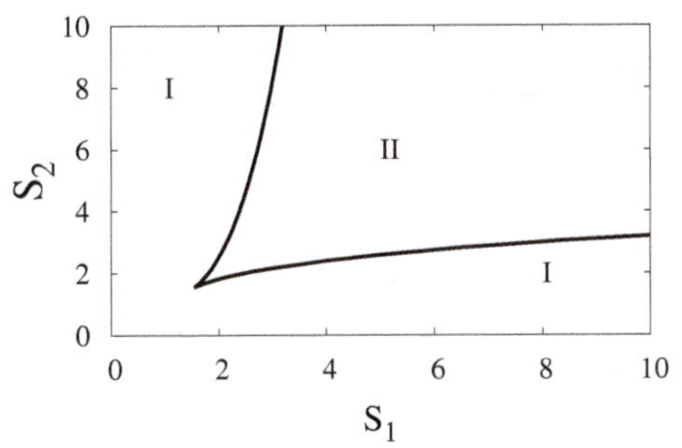

FIGURE 9 | Two-parameter bifurcation diagram. The bifurcation in the parameter space (S_1, S_2), where S_1 and S_2 are external signals in the genetic switch. The borders separate between the regions of monostability *I* and the region of bistability *II*. Parameters are $a_1 = a_2 = 0.05$, $b_1 = b_2 = 0.45$, $r = 0.5$, $k_1 = k_2 = 1$.

4. DISCUSSION

We have shown the importance of parameter sweeping speed when the gene regulatory circuit of immune cell differentiation is exposed to external factors that cause symmetry-breaking and make one of the attractors or fates more favorable than the other. In our study, symmetry-breaking is caused by three factors. The first factor is the asymmetric change of parameters which gives ratio tends to zero as the speed is increased (**Figure 8B**). This means we get large conversion from the favorite attractor, the erythroid lineage, to the myeloid lineage. The importance of this effect may appear in cases where the person has a problem with immunity due to the decrease in the production of immune cells, so even when there is a bias in the cell and this bias has the effect of choosing the attractor where GATA1 is upregulated, the cell can be forced to

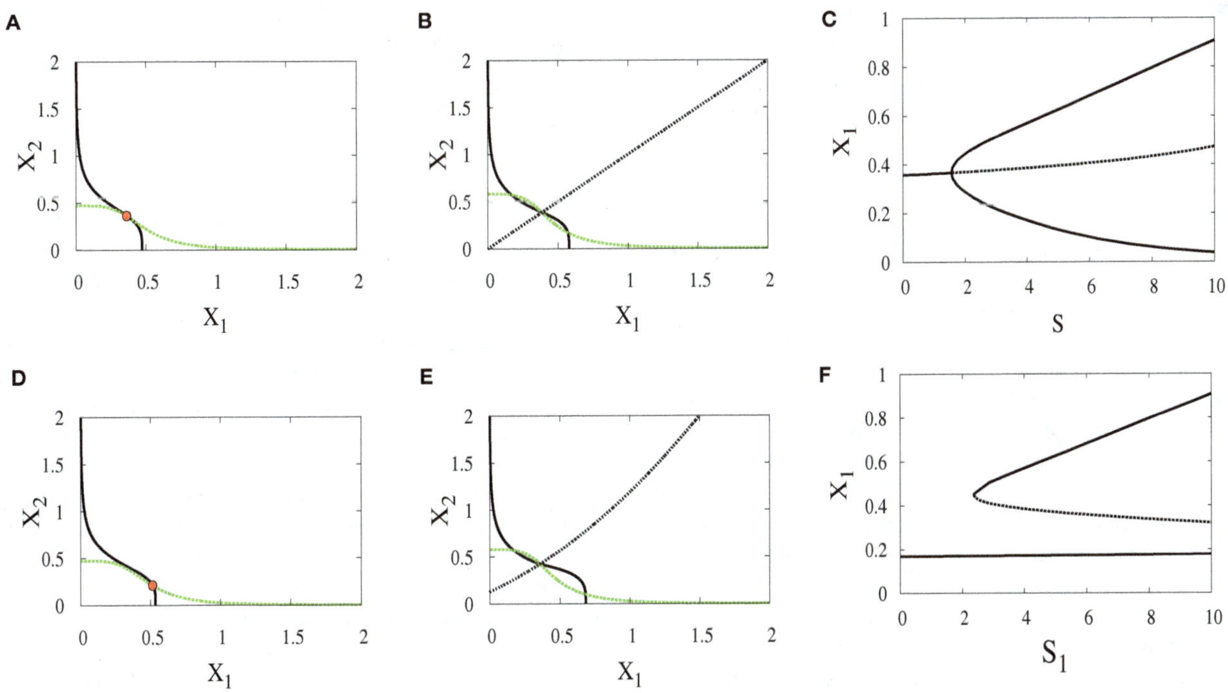

FIGURE 10 | Nullclines and bifurcation diagrams with symmetric and asymmetric external signals. For all figures, $a_1 = a_2 = 0.05$, $b_1 = b_2 = 0.45$, $r = 0.5$, $k_1 = k_2 = 1$, $n = 4$. **(A)** Nullclines for $S_1 = S_2 = 1$ show one stable steady state, **(B)** nullclines for $S_1 = S_2 = 4$ show bistability, **(C)** near-symmetric supercritical pitchfork bifurcation, **(D)** nullclines for $S_1 = 3$, $S_2 = 1$ show one stable steady state shifted to the right, **(E)** nullclines for $S_1 = 6$, $S_2 = 4$ show bistability with larger basin of attraction to the right of the separatrix (almost diagonal line), **(F)** imperfect supercritical pitchfork bifurcation due to the asymmetry between the external signals.

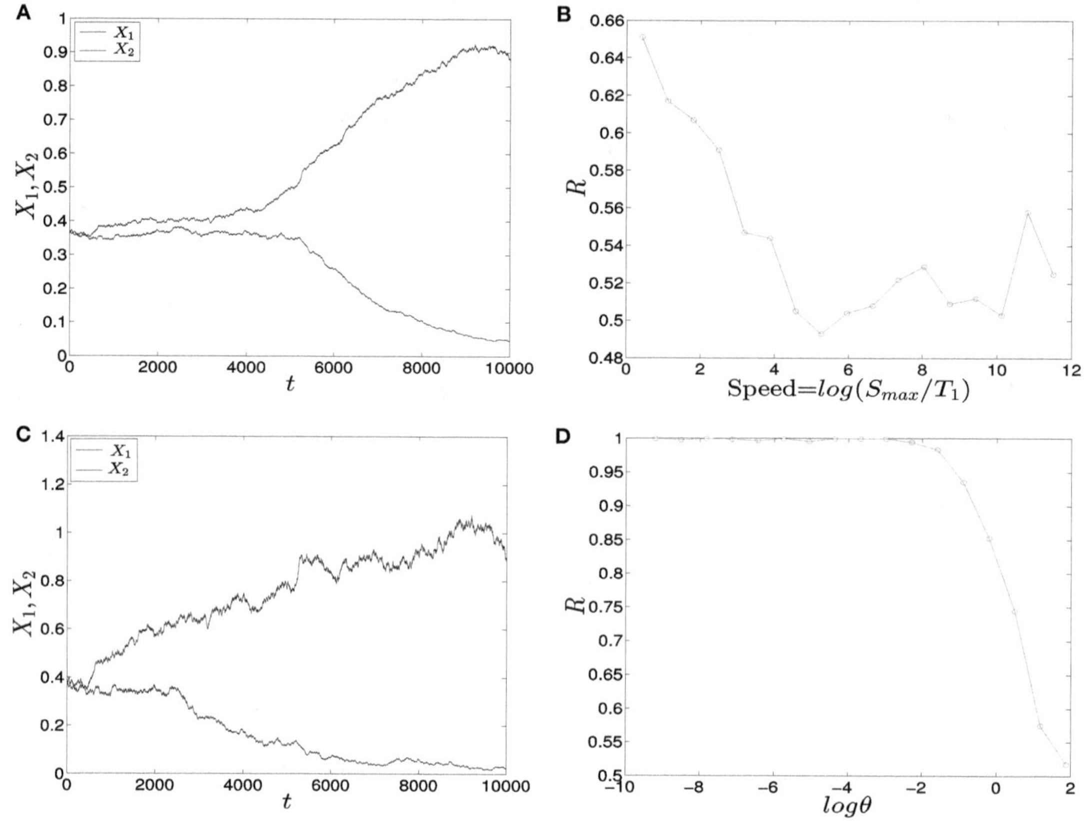

FIGURE 11 | Trajectories and effect of the external signaling speed. In **(A,C)** the time evolution of X_1 and X_2 under the effect of linear and adaptation form of signals is shown, respectively. The values of X_1 increase and the values of X_2 decrease because S_1 is chosen to be faster than S_2. Hence, trajectories choose the attractor which has a larger value of X_1. **(B)** The effect of increasing the speed of linear form of signals for 1000 iterations. As the speed is increased, the ratio R tends to 0.5. Thus, increasing the speed increases the symmetry in the switch. **(D)** The effect of speed with the adaptation form of signals. Decreasing the speed gives ratio R tending to 0.5. Surprisingly, now decreasing the speed increases the symmetry in the switch. Parameters in **(A)**, **(B)** are $A = 2.5$, $S_{max} = 10$, **(C,D)** $h_1 = h_2 = 10$, $v = 10$, and for all we have $a_1 = a_2 = 0.05$, $b_1 = b_2 = 0.45$, $r = 0.5$, $k_1 = k_2 = 1$.

choose the attractor where PU.1 is upregulated by increasing the speed of crossing the critical region and so enhancing the production of immune cells. The second factor is linear form of signals (**Figure 2A**) and in this case we get ratio tends to 0.5 with increasing the speed (**Figure 11B**). This result may be important in situations that need symmetry between erythroid and myeloid cells, or when decreasing the probability of choosing the erythroid lineage is required. The third factor is represented by non-linear form of signals, i.e., signals describing biochemical adaptation (**Figure 3**). Here, decreasing the speed blinds the asymmetry and produce symmetry between the two lineages (**Figure 11D**). Taken together, the external signals, its shape, and its speed may have critical effects on choosing the attractors and affect the cell-fate determination.

Notably, we followed the model of Huang et al. (2) to study the differentiation into erythroid and myeloid fates. On the other hand, there is a scheme in Ref. (1, 17) that gives additional kinds of cells or lineages under each transcription factor. In this scheme, GATA1 is responsible for differentiation into erythroid or megakaryocyte cells, and PU.1 leads to either lymphoid lineage (B and T cells) which gives the *Adaptive Immune Cells*, or myeloid lineage (macrophages and granulocytes) that produces the *Innate Immune Cells*. So for this scheme, the importance of parameter sweeping speed is increased as the fate corresponding to high concentration of PU.1 is able to produce the different types of immune cells.

Of particular interest and agreement with our conclusions about the importance of external signals, Heuser et al. (6) have showed the crucial role of external signals in MN1 leukemia. They have investigated the requirement of FLT3 and c-Kit signals for MN1 leukemia. Overexpression of MN1 induces myeloid leukemia and blocks erythroid differentiation. FLT3 and c-Kit signaling direct MN1-expressing cells toward the myeloid lineage, so disruption of these signals may prevent leukemia. Interestingly, the disruption of these external signals doesn't delay the disease latency but induces a switch from myeloid to erythroid lineage. Thus, the external signals can alter leukemia stem cell differentiation fates.

Many models have focused on the role of external signals in the differentiation process (3, 5) but they haven't given any attention to the shape of signals or to the speed of these signals. Additionally, many works have made their studies limited to the symmetric scenario for the sake of simplicity (2, 18). But in this paper, we have studied the asymmetric scenarios and investigated the effect of external signaling speed on the system's dynamics. As a prospect, it would be specially interesting to study the effect of speed on more complicated models and including other factors that may have a role in the differentiation process of hematopoietic stem cells, which can lead to better understanding of the immune system. Furthermore, an experimental evidence is needed to support the predictions from the mathematical models.

ACKNOWLEDGMENTS

This project was supported by the Deanship of Scientific Research (DSR), King Abdulaziz University (KAU), Jeddah, under grant No. (20/34/Gr). Alexey Zaikin acknowledges support from CR-UK and Eve Appeal (PROMISE-2016).

REFERENCES

1. Laslo P, Pongubala JMR, Lancki DW, Singh H. Gene regulatory networks directing myeloid and lymphoid cell fates within the immune system. *Semin Immunol* (2008) **20**:228–35. doi:10.1016/j.smim.2008.08.003
2. Huang S, Guo Y, May G, Enver T. Bifurcation dynamics in lineage-commitment in bipotent progenitor cells. *Dev Biol* (2007) **305**:695–713. doi:10.1016/j.ydbio.2007.02.036
3. Chickarmane V, Enver T, Peterson C. Computational modeling of the hematopoietic erythroid-myeloid switch reveals insight into cooperativity, priming, and irreversibility. *PLoS Comput Biol* (2009) **5**(1):e1000268. doi:10.1371/journal.pcbi.1000268
4. Palani S, Sarkar CA. Positive receptor feedback during lineage commitment can generate ultrasensitivity to ligand and confer robustness to a bistable switch. *Biophys J* (2008) **95**:1575–89. doi:10.1529/biophysj.107.120600
5. Palani S, Sarkar CA. Integrating extrinsic and intrinsic cues into a minimal model of lineage commitment for hematopoietic progenitors. *PLoS Comput Biol* (2009) **5**(9):e1000518. doi:10.1371/journal.pcbi.1000518
6. Heuser M, Park G, Moon Y, Berg T, Xiang P, Kuchenbauer F. Extrinsic signals determine myeloid-erythroid lineage switch in MN1 leukemia. *Exp Hematol* (2010) **38**:174–9. doi:10.1016/j.exphem.2010.01.003
7. Nene NR, Garca-Ojalvo J, Zaikin A. Speed-dependent cellular decision making in nonequilibrium genetic circuits. *PLoS One* (2012) **7**(3):e32779. doi:10.1371/journal.pone.0032779
8. Nene NR, Zaikin A. Interplay between path and speed in decision making by high-dimensional stochastic gene regulatory networks. *PLoS One* (2012) **7**(7):e40085. doi:10.1371/journal.pone.0040085
9. Nene NR, Zaikin A. Decision making in noisy bistable systems with time-dependent asymmetry. *Phys Rev E Stat Nonlin Soft Matter Phys* (2013) **87**:012715. doi:10.1103/PhysRevE.87.012715
10. Ashwin P, Wieczorek S, Vitolo R, Cox P. Tipping points in open systems: bifurcation, noise-induced and rate-dependent examples in the climate system. *Philos Trans A Math Phys Eng Sci* (2012) **370**:1166–84. doi:10.1098/rsta.2011.0306
11. Young JW, Locke JCW, Elowitz MB. Rate of environmental change determines stress response specificity. *Proc Natl Acad Sci U S A* (2013) **110**:4140–5. doi:10.1073/pnas.1213060110
12. Weiss JN. The Hill equation revisited: uses and misuses. *FASEB J* (1997) **11**:835–41.
13. Gillespie DT. The chemical Langevin equation. *J Chem Phys* (2000) **113**:297–306. doi:10.1063/1.481811
14. Ma W, Trusina A, El-Samad H, Lim WA, Tang C. Defining network topologies that can achieve biochemical adaptation. *Cell* (2009) **138**:760–73. doi:10.1016/j.cell.2009.06.013
15. Cinquin O, Demongeot J. High-dimensional switches and the modelling of cellular differentiation. *J Theor Biol* (2005) **233**:391–411. doi:10.1016/j.jtbi.2004.10.027
16. Kawamoto H, Katsura Y. A new paradigm for hematopoietic cell lineages: revision of the classical concept of the myeloid-lymphoid dichotomy. *Cell* (2009) **30**:193–200. doi:10.1016/j.it.2009.03.001
17. Adolfsson J, Mansson R, Buza-Vidas N, Hultquist A, Liuba K, Jensen CT, et al. Identification of *Flt3*$^{+}$ lympho-myeloid stem cells lacking erythro-megakaryocytic potential: a revised road map for adult blood lineage commitment. *Cell* (2005) **121**:295–306. doi:10.1016/j.cell.2005.02.013
18. Foster DV, Foster JG, Huang S, Kauffman SA. A model of sequential branching in hierarchical cell fate determination. *J Theor Biol* (2009) **260**:589–97. doi:10.1016/j.jtbi.2009.07.005

3

Induced pluripotent stem cells: challenges and opportunities for cancer immunotherapy

Patty Sachamitr[†], Simon Hackett[†] and Paul Jonathan Fairchild[*]

Sir William Dunn School of Pathology, University of Oxford, Oxford, UK

Edited by:
Fang-Ping Huang, Imperial College London, UK

Reviewed by:
Angel Porgador, Ben-Gurion University of the Negev, Israel
Kerry Campbell, Fox Chase Cancer Center, USA

***Correspondence:**
Paul Jonathan Fairchild, Sir William Dunn School of Pathology, University of Oxford, South Parks Road, Oxford OX1 3RE, UK
e-mail: paul.fairchild@path.ox.ac.uk

[†] Patty Sachamitr and Simon Hackett have contributed equally to this work.

Despite recent advances in cancer treatment over the past 30 years, therapeutic options remain limited and do not always offer a cure for malignancy. Given that tumor-associated antigens (TAA) are, by definition, self-proteins, the need to productively engage autoreactive T cells remains at the heart of strategies for cancer immunotherapy. These have traditionally focused on the administration of autologous monocyte-derived dendritic cells (moDC) pulsed with TAA, or the *ex vivo* expansion and adoptive transfer of tumor-infiltrating lymphocytes (TIL) as a source of TAA-specific cytotoxic T cells (CTL). Although such approaches have shown some efficacy, success has been limited by the poor capacity of moDC to cross present exogenous TAA to the CD8$^+$ T-cell repertoire and the potential for exhaustion of CTL expanded *ex vivo*. Recent advances in induced pluripotency offer opportunities to generate patient-specific stem cell lines with the potential to differentiate *in vitro* into cell types whose properties may help address these issues. Here, we review recent success in the differentiation of NK cells from human induced pluripotent stem (iPS) cells as well as minor subsets of dendritic cells (DCs) with therapeutic potential, including CD141$^+$XCR1$^+$ DC, capable of cross presenting TAA to naïve CD8$^+$ T cells. Furthermore, we review recent progress in the use of TIL as the starting material for the derivation of iPSC lines, thereby capturing their antigen specificity in a self-renewing stem cell line, from which potentially unlimited numbers of naïve TAA-specific T cells may be differentiated, free of the risks of exhaustion.

Keywords: cancer, immunotherapy, dendritic cell, cytotoxic T cell, NK cell, pluripotency, iPS cell

CANCER AND THE IMMUNE SYSTEM: A HISTORICAL PERSPECTIVE

Although it was Paul Ehrlich who, in 1909, first introduced the concept of the immune system as a means of controlling the incidence of cancer, it was 50 years later, with development of the field of cellular immunology and discovery of the role of the immune system in allograft rejection (1), that this notion first gained traction. In 1970, Burnet and Thomas introduced the concept of immunological surveillance and postulated that the immune system had a mechanism for eliminating potentially dangerous mutated cells and speculated that lymphocytes were actively involved in the process by the recognition of neo-antigens, either unique to the tumor (tumor-specific antigens; TSAs) or shared by other somatic cells (tumor-associated antigens; TAAs) (2, 3). This theory was met with skepticism, due in part, to the observation that the incidence of tumors in immune compromised *nude* mice did not differ substantially from their wild type counterparts (4, 5). These observations were, however, counter-balanced by the discovery that tumors may lack immunogenicity, not due to the absence of TAAs *per se* but rather their inability to activate the immune system (6). This subsequently gave rise to the modified concept of cancer immunoediting (7), which postulates that a developing tumor is under a constant immunological selection pressure, leading either to its elimination, the establishment of a dynamic equilibrium between the tumor and the immune system, or its escape from immune surveillance, resulting in unopposed growth. It is now accepted that one of the hallmarks of cancer is the lack of immune regulation (8) and that certain cancers therefore have the propensity to induce a state of autoimmunity in some individuals. While the underlying mechanisms remain to be clarified, mutations in specific TAAs may increase their immunogenicity, eliciting T and B cell responses that readily cross-react with the wild type protein, expressed in other cell types or anatomical locations. Indeed, a recent study has shown that certain cancer patients develop the chronic autoimmune rheumatic disease, systemic sclerosis (9), illustrating the important concept that immune surveillance harnesses elements of the autoreactive T-cell repertoire to elicit anti-tumor responses, sometimes at the cost of collateral damage to self-tissues: it is the same autoreactive repertoire that cancer immunotherapy seeks to recruit.

APPROACHES TO CANCER IMMUNOTHERAPY

Radiation, chemotherapy, and surgery are the three traditional methods for controlling the spread of cancer, which, although effective, may fail to completely eliminate neoplastic cells or the cancer stem cells that sustain a developing tumor. Additionally, the lack of specificity of these approaches and the damage to otherwise healthy tissues may lead to severe morbidity and, in extreme cases, mortality. Given its inherent specificity, adaptability, and capacity to generate a memory response, cancer immunotherapy promises to be more effective and durable than classical treatment modalities (10).

Cytokines, such as interleukin-2 (IL-2), interferon-α (IFN-α), and tumor necrosis factor-α (TNF-α) have been used non-specifically to stimulate an anti-tumor response. These cytokines act either by directly inhibiting growth of the tumor cells or by promoting proliferation and sustained cytokine production by T cells and NK cells, thereby increasing their ability to target tumor cells. Some cytokines, such as granulocyte-macrophage colony-stimulating factor (GM-CSF), act on antigen-presenting cells (APCs), inducing upregulation of MHC and co-stimulatory molecules, which promote their capacity to activate lymphocytes. A number of cytokines, used singly or in combination, have proven effective in increasing the anti-tumor immune response and have, in recent years, entered clinical trials for the treatment of advanced cancer (11). IL-2 has, for instance, been approved by the US Food and Drug Administration (FDA) for the treatment of metastatic melanoma and renal-cell carcinoma (12). However, given the non-specificity of the approach, low response rates, and toxic side effects, additional understanding of cytokine signaling pathways and their function *in vivo* are still required (11).

The identification of a number of well-defined TAAs and Tissue Specific Antigens (TSAs), along with the development of hybridoma technology (13), has facilitated the production of monoclonal antibodies (mAbs) that either directly target these antigens or block central pathways involved in tumor function. mAbs have, for instance, been used to inhibit molecules such as CTLA-4 and PD-1, since upregulation of their ligands by tumor cells may inhibit T-cell function, enhancing their ability to evade immune surveillance (14, 15). In recent clinical trials of the PD-1-specific mAb, BMS-936558, objective and durable responses were observed in approximately one in four to one in five patients with non-small cell lung cancer, melanoma, or renal-cell cancer. Immunohistochemical staining of tumor specimens prior to the onset of treatment, revealed that intra-tumoral expression of PD-1 ligand (PD-L1) correlated with the induction of anti-tumor responses, providing a means of stratifying patients in order to identify those most likely to respond to treatment and greatly increasing the likely future clinical impact of mAb therapy (16). Although it was the exquisite specificity of mAbs that first earned them the name "magic bullets," response rates remain disappointingly low when used as a single therapy (17–19). One reason for this poor performance may lie in the fact that administration of therapeutic mAbs is inherently passive, failing to generate a memory response. Furthermore, the repeated administration required as a result, may elicit neutralizing anti-idiotypic responses, which greatly limit efficacy.

In contrast, the ultimate aim of cancer immunotherapy is to activate the immune system to recognize the tumor, thereby generating a specific and durable effector T-cell response. In order to achieve this goal, adoptive transfer of TAA-specific T cells has been explored, involving their expansion *ex vivo* and re-administration to the same patients from whom they were originally derived (20). Alternatively, the ability of DCs to present TAAs to T cells has been harnessed to generate an immune response against tumor cells. Whereas adoptive T-cell transfer may generate a burst of T-cell immunity that is short-lived, DC-based vaccines have the potential to induce a sustained immune response with the capacity for subsequent recall (21). It has been shown that DC vaccination, following adoptive T-cell transfer, may further boost anti-tumor responses, suggesting a rationale for combining the two therapeutic strategies (21). In this review, we shall discuss recent experience of harnessing DCs and T cells for cancer immunotherapy and obstacles hindering their success. We shall also focus on the emerging use of patient-specific induced pluripotent stem cells (iPSCs) for the differentiation of DCs, T cells, and NK cells and discuss how this novel source holds promise for overcoming some of the shortfalls of conventional cancer immunotherapy.

CELL-BASED IMMUNOTHERAPIES AND THEIR OBSTACLES

As sentinels of the immune system, DCs play a pivotal role in eliciting the primary immune response to antigen. The ability of DCs to process and present protein antigens via the canonical endocytic pathway is crucial to this process (22). However, some subsets of DCs also possess the ability to capture exogenous antigens and cross present them via MHC class I direct to $CD8^+$ T cells, thereby eliciting a cytotoxic T-cell response (23–25). Since cancer cells are poor APCs due to constitutively low expression of MHC class I and II determinants, the generation of protective anti-tumor immunity depends upon the cross presentation of tumor antigens by DCs (22–24). Although various DC-based cancer vaccines have been exploited in the past and the properties, advantages, and disadvantages of each extensively reviewed (20, 26, 27), it is most commonly DCs cultured *ex vivo* from peripheral blood monocytes (monocyte-derived dendritic cells, moDCs) that have shown the greatest clinical benefit. Indeed, one such vaccine, Provenge, has entered the market for the routine treatment of prostate cancer and involves the co-culture of moDCs obtained by leukapheresis, with the TSA, prostatic acid phosphatase (PAP), to which T-cell responses have been detected following their reinfusion into patients (28).

The majority of the clinical trials involving cancer vaccination have used autologous moDCs cultured *ex vivo* and pulsed with soluble TAA before re-administration to patients with the hope of inducing a tumor-specific immune response (29). Although many of these trials have shown that immunotherapy based on the use of mature moDC is safe, well-tolerated, and able to elicit an immune response against the tumor (27), the overall results have been disappointing, showing significant inter-trial variability between outcomes (30–32). This may be due, in no small part, to the donor-to-donor variability in yield and quality of moDCs, which is further compounded by long-term exposure to chemotherapeutic agents. Furthermore, the poor capacity of moDCs to cross present exogenous TAAs to CTLs, limits the magnitude of the cell-mediated immunity required to clear established tumors.

The recent identification of cross presenting DCs in man, equivalent to the $CD8\alpha^+$ subset that has long been recognized in the mouse, has rejuvenated interest in the use of DCs in cancer immunotherapy (33, 34). These cells are defined by their expression of the surface marker CD141 and the chemokine receptor XCR1 and are found in the peripheral blood, tonsils, and bone marrow (35). They display an unrivaled capacity to cross present exogenous antigen to $CD8^+$ T cells, and hence to elicit effective cell-mediated immunity. While the properties of $CD141^+$ $XCR1^+$

DCs make them ideal candidates for immunotherapy against cancer, their trace numbers in peripheral blood (<0.1%) limit their therapeutic exploitation (25). Alternative sources of cross presenting DCs, including their isolation from the spleen or *in vitro* differentiation from hematopoietic progenitor cells, have so far failed to overcome these obstacles (36).

Since the holy grail of cancer immunotherapy is to stimulate tumor-specific T cells that will elicit a cytotoxic response with high specificity and minimal toxicity, adoptive transfer of TAA-specific T cells has gained popularity over the past few years (37, 38). Adoptive T-cell transfer involves the isolation of T lymphocytes from the patients and their reinfusion to treat disease. The adoptive transfer of T cells was first documented in rodents in 1955, where it was noted that T cells obtained from lymph nodes draining a tumor were able to confer immunity when transferred into the peritoneum of a secondary host, bearing a similar tumor (39). Almost three decades later, it was observed that the incubation of murine splenocytes with IL-2 generated large numbers of cells, called lymphokine-activated killer (LAK) cells, which were capable of lysing tumor cells with little effect on other somatic cells (40). These LAK cells were later shown to decrease tumor number and size in humans in a wide variety of tumors including pulmonary and hepatic metastases (41, 42). This work served as the basis for the use of tumor-infiltrating lymphocytes (TILs) in immunotherapy (43, 44). The combination of a lymphodepleting preparative regimen with adoptive transfer of TILs and administration of IL-2 has been shown to promote cancer regression in patients with metastatic melanoma, leukemias, and other types of tumor (44, 45).

The possibility of genetic modification of the T cells to overcome the immunosuppressive environment created by the tumor may lead to more effective therapies in the future, although current strategies for genetic modification are limited (46) and T cells are known to constitute particularly intractable targets. Nevertheless, the possibility of genetically engineering T cells to recognize specific TAAs makes it possible to target potentially any tumor using adoptive T-cell transfer (47), while leaving other tissues intact. The majority of clinical approaches use virus-based transduction of tumor antigen-specific T-cell receptor (TCRs) or chimeric antigen receptors (CARs) to generate T cells stably expressing tumor-specific transgenes which, although efficient, is expensive and risks insertional mutagenesis. Non-viral approaches to genetically engineer T cells have so far utilized transposon elements such as piggyback or zinc finger nucleases (46). TALEN and CRISPR/Cas-9-based-approaches, which allow for the insertion of transgenes into defined chromosomal loci, are, however, currently being actively explored (48, 49). Despite the attractiveness of using CAR technology to target cancer, only the treatment of B cell leukemia has so far proven successful using this approach. Furthermore, recent work has shown that the treatment of patients with myeloma or melanoma using T cells engineered to express affinity-enhanced TCRs for an HLA-A*01-restricted epitope of MAGE-A3 resulted in severe myocardial damage secondary to widespread T-cell infiltration leading ultimately to fatal cardiogenic shock. These findings have clearly shown how even altering the affinity of the TCR for its ligand may introduce unanticipated cross-reactivity with potentially fatal off-target toxicity (50).

Although much effort has been invested into the adoptive transfer of unmodified T cells in the treatment of cancer, outcomes have been disappointing. It is, for instance, sometimes challenging to identify tumor-specific T cells in patients with non-solid tumors. TILs can also be difficult to isolate from biopsies of most melanomas. *Ex vivo* expansion of tumor-specific CTLs can also prove difficult: in the case of EBV-specific CTLs, for instance, 3 months is required for the production of sufficient CTLs for re-administration to the patient, with obvious implications for disease progression. Often, reinfusion of T cells is required following adoptive transfer for the induction of a durable response due to the exhaustion of the expanded CTLs.

NK cells have likewise been used for adoptive transfer, due to their innate ability to recognize tumor cells deficient in MHC class I. NK cells have been isolated form peripheral blood, expanded *ex vivo*, activated using IL-2 or, more recently, the combination of IL-12, IL-15, and IL-18 (51), and re-administered to patients (52). Interestingly, although the use of autologous cells is normally preferred, several studies have demonstrated that the use of allogeneic NK cells is significantly more effective (53, 54). Accordingly, the results of several studies have shown NK cells to be well-tolerated following adoptive transfer with encouraging results of up to 20 months' survival following their administration (55). Nevertheless, low circulating numbers of NK cells in peripheral blood, coupled with the difficulty in their expansion and their inability to stimulate a robust response *in vivo*, limits their use in immunotherapy.

Given the difficulty of obtaining sufficient numbers of cells to target tumors *in vivo*, the advent of induced pluripotency offers unrivaled opportunities. The proven ability to produce iPS cells from individuals in a patient-specific manner with the capacity for indefinite self-renewal and unrestricted differentiation potential, may facilitate the scale-up in production of critical hematopoietic cell types, for many of which, protocols have already been optimized. Below, we outline the history of induced pluripotency and discuss the properties that make them attractive candidates for use in immunotherapy.

BRIEF HISTORY OF PLURIPOTENCY

Since their first description, embryonic stem (ES) cells have been regarded as the "gold standard" for pluripotency, displaying the capacity for indefinite self-renewal and differentiation into any somatic cell type, irrespective of its embryonic germ-layer of origin. Mouse ES cells were first isolated in 1981 by Martin Evans (56), work which later earned him the 2007 Nobel Prize for Physiology or Medicine. Nevertheless, it was not until 1998 that Thomson and colleagues succeeded in deriving ES cells from the inner cell mass of human blastocysts that were surplus to requirements following *in vitro* fertilization (57). Human ES cell lines, like their mouse counterparts, were found to be pluripotent, expressing embryonic markers such as SSEA-3, SSEA-4, TRA-1–60, and alkaline phosphatase and, following injection into immune compromised mice, forming teratomas containing cell types and tissues from all three embryonic germ layers.

Since their first derivation, there has been much interest in the use of human ES cells as a source of diverse cell types for drug discovery, regenerative medicine, and immunotherapy. However, their use has been highly controversial due to the ethical sensitivities surrounding their derivation from human blastocysts, as well as the inevitable scientific constraints of using an allogeneic source of cells. In 2006, Yamanaka and colleagues demonstrated the feasibility of deriving pluripotent stem cells from adult mouse fibroblasts by retroviral transduction with genes encoding Oct3/4, Sox2, c-Myc, and Klf4 (58). These so-called iPS cells are indistinguishable at the cellular level from conventional ES cells, acquiring the capacity for indefinite self-renewal, unrestricted differentiation potential and, following injection into mouse blastocysts, the ability to generate germline-competent chimeras. These findings were subsequently translated to human dermal fibroblasts in 2007 by two independent groups (59, 60), showing, in principle, the feasibility of generating iPS cells on an individual basis. This seminal work offered a means of "personalizing" pluripotency in a manner free of the ethical concerns, while simultaneously addressing the immunological issues that limit the effectiveness of allogeneic therapies. Indeed, the production of iPS cells in an autologous fashion has paved the way for harnessing the potential of pluripotency for immunotherapeutic intervention in the pursuit of treatments for numerous indications.

Given the broad clinical applicability that iPS cells may enjoy in the future, there have been many efforts to develop and optimize the re-programming process to increase the safety profile of the resulting cell lines (**Table 1**). Protocols based on retroviral transduction may result in insertional mutagenesis while inducing the ectopic upregulation of developmental genes, which may subsequently render cells immunogenic (61). The direct delivery of re-programming proteins into somatic cells (62) and transfection with synthetic mRNA (63) have both proven successful, albeit yielding iPS cells at very low efficiency. Interestingly, small molecules, such as the histone deacetylase inhibitor, valproic acid, have been demonstrated to increase this efficiency by up to 100-fold (64). More importantly, recent work has shown that full re-programming may be achieved with a combination of seven small molecules alone, suggesting that induced pluripotency may not be dependent on the use of virus-based delivery systems (65). To achieve this, the authors screened 10,000 small molecules in order to find suitable replacements for each transcription factor. Three molecules, forskolin, 2-methyl-5-hydroxytryptamine, and D4476 were, for instance, identified as chemical substitutes for Oct3/4.

Perhaps the most dramatic advance in this rapidly evolving field has, however, been the recent description of stimulus-triggered fate conversion of cells (66), in which transient exposure of terminally differentiated cells to adverse conditions such as low pH, induces the upregulation of pluripotency genes. This approach has been shown to confer on cells such as murine lymphocytes, the capacity to form germline-competent chimeras following injection into recipient blastocysts, or the formation of entire offspring in tetraploid complementation assays. However, this method has yet to be verified independently and further characterization of the iPS cell lines produced in this way must be conducted and the translation of protocols to adult human cells has yet to be achieved, this approach may one day allow the generation of iPS cells lines with minimal intervention, compatible with downstream clinical applications.

Although traditionally much of the interest in iPS cells has focused on applications in regenerative medicine, other indications include their use as a novel source of hematopoietic cell types for cancer immunotherapy (**Figure 1**). The opportunity to derive iPS cells in a patient-specific manner, together with their tractability for genome editing using newly developed technologies such as the CRISPR–Cas-9 system (67) make them attractive

Table 1 | Methods of reprogramming and complications associated with derived iPS cell lines.

	Advantages	Disadvantages
Forced expression of genes via retrovirus	Well-characterized method, long history of use, arguably a simple approach and low cost, relatively high reprogramming rates of 0.01–0.02%	Integration into the genome may generate immunogenic cells, virus will only enter cells in mitosis, use of oncogenes such as c-Myc
Small molecules	Low cost of compounds, increases the efficiency of reprogramming	Only recent reports of full reprogramming achievable with small molecules alone: further characterization of lines generated needed
Synthetic miRNA	No integration within the genome	Very low reprogramming efficiency, miRNA degrades rapidly, modification of miRNA complicated, and time-consuming
Forced expression of genes via Sendai virus	No integration into the genome, higher efficiency of reprogramming than using retrovirus, diluted out of culture upon passage rapidly, high reprogramming rate of 0.1%	Difficult to work with, therefore most commonly used as pre-packaged "kits," which are expensive compared to other viral methods of reprogramming
Episomal plasmid vector system	No genomic footprint	Very low efficiency of reprogramming (0.0002%), loss of episomal plasmid
Stimulus-triggered acquisition of pluripotency (STAP)	No nuclear transfer or introduction of transcription factors	Limited capacity for self-renewal when compared to ES cells. Reports have yet to be independently verified

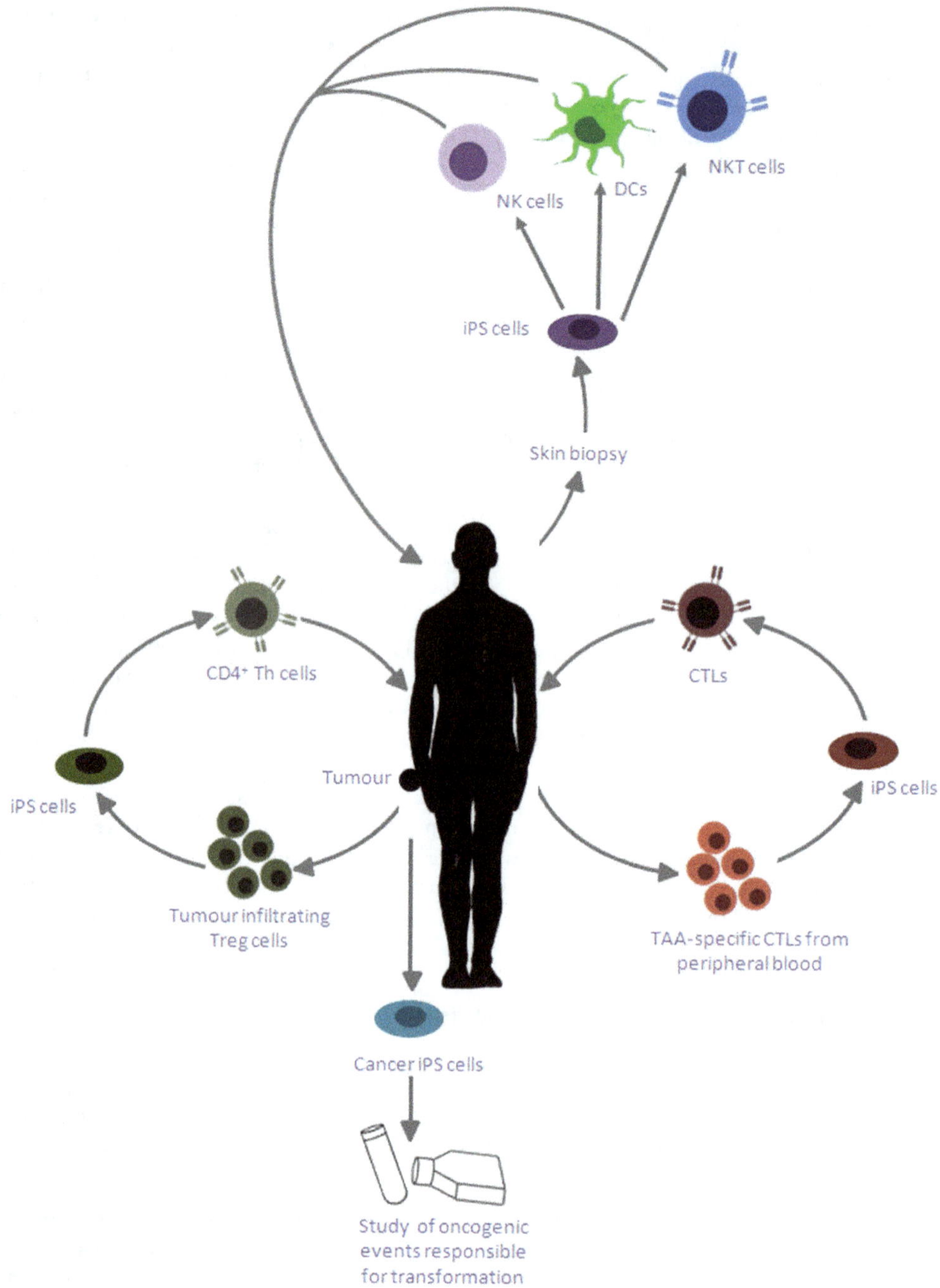

FIGURE 1 | Applications of iPS cells for cancer immunotherapy. iPS cells reprogramed from skin biopsies of cancer patients can be differentiated into DCs, which can be reintroduced into patients to cross present TAA. These iPS cells can also be differentiated into NK cells and NKT cells, which can be adoptively transferred into the patient to target cancer cells; iPS cells can be generated by reprogramming tumor-specific CTLs, which can provide an unlimited source of naïve $CD8^+$ T cells with the desired specificity; tumor-infiltrating Treg cells may likewise be reprogramed into iPS cells and redifferentiated into $CD4^+$ Th cells, which are capable of providing help to the CTLs to target cancerous cells; these iPS cells can also be exploited to study the genetic basis of transformation and its influence of primary cell types.

candidates for such applications. Furthermore, their indefinite capacity for self-renewal may greatly facilitate the scale-up of cell production, offering unrivaled opportunities for overcoming many of the obstacles encountered using conventional sources of cells.

EXPLOITING INDUCED PLURIPOTENCY FOR THE STUDY AND TREATMENT OF CANCER

CANCER iPS CELLS AS MODELS OF DISEASE PROGRESSION

The use of iPS cell lines to model *in vitro* a broad range of human disease states has already begun to yield important advances in our understanding of their pathogenesis and progression. Nevertheless, the generation of iPS cells from primary cancer cells has remained a significant challenge, proving successful for only a limited number of cancers due, most likely, to the associated genetic or chromosomal abnormalities introducing a state of genetic instability (68). Although reprogramming of gastrointestinal cancer cells to a pluripotent state has been achieved by careful modification of culture conditions and reprogramming factors (69), it has proven necessary to use retroviral vectors to introduce the necessary transgenes, which risks the introduction of confounding mutations that may interfere with the phenotype of cells differentiated from the resulting iPS cell lines. Application of the latest non-viral reprogramming technologies to primary cancer cells is, therefore, paramount for gaining insight into the impact that oncogenic events may have on a range of primary cell types. The potential that such an approach offers for drug discovery and toxicity screening may facilitate the future identification of therapeutic targets as well as novel neo-antigens that may be exploited for vaccination purposes.

CANCER VACCINATION USING iPS CELL-DERIVED DCs

Given the significant donor-to-donor variability encountered in the use of moDCs for cancer immunotherapy, early research focused on the potential of pluripotency to provide a more homogenous source of DCs amenable to scale-up. Accordingly, several groups reported the successful differentiation of functional DCs from both mouse and human ES cells (70, 71). Since the use of animal products for their differentiation made them unsuitable for clinical applications, Tseng and colleagues succeeded in developing protocols for their differentiation in an animal product-free manner, compatible with their downstream use *in vivo* (72). Although these DCs were shown to be functional, possessing the ability to endocytose, process, and present foreign antigen to naïve CD4$^+$ T cells, their clinical utility was restricted both by their limited capacity for cross presentation of antigen to MHC class I-restricted CD8$^+$ T cells and their differentiation from allogeneic sources, requiring matching at certain HLA loci. Recent work in our laboratory has, however, demonstrated that CD141$^+$XCR1$^+$ DCs can be successfully derived from human iPS cells using a cocktail of GM-CSF, stem cell factor (SCF), vascular endothelial growth factor (VEGF), and bone morphogenetic protein-4 (BMP4). This protocol was found to be compatible with the exclusion of all animal products, ensuring the downstream clinical compliance of the DCs obtained (73). Unlike moDCs used for comparison, these DCs were shown to efficiently cross present the TAA, Melan A, supplied exogenously in recombinant form, to naïve CD8$^+$ T cells *in vitro*, stimulating a primary Melan A-specific immune response that could be tracked using tetramer technology (73). Since iPS cells have indefinite capacity for self-renewal *in vitro*, this approach provides a potentially unlimited source of autologous DCs that might bypass the issue of patient-to-patient variability and the confounding effects of long-term chemotherapy that impacts adversely on the circulating monocytes from which conventional moDCs are derived.

DIFFERENTIATION OF T CELLS FOR ADOPTIVE TRANSFER

While the use of DCs to stimulate TAA-specific immune responses *in vivo* offers the prospect of establishing durable immunological memory, an alternative strategy for cancer immunotherapy has been the adoptive transfer of antigen-specific T cells, expanded *ex vivo*. Since such expansion regimes risk the functional exhaustion of the resulting cells, the differentiation of potentially unlimited numbers of primary T cells from pluripotent stem cells has proven an attractive goal. The co-culture of mouse ES cells with the OP9 stromal cell line constitutively expressing delta-like ligand 1 (OP9-DL1), has been shown to successfully support their differentiation into T-cell progenitors (74, 75). Nevertheless, their final commitment to the T-cell lineage requires their introduction into fetal thymus organ cultures, so as to provide a microenvironment conducive to TCR gene rearrangement and subsequent positive selection of a diverse CD4$^+$ and CD8$^+$ T-cell repertoire. On transferring these ES cell-derived T cells into RAG2$^{-/-}$ mice, immune reconstitution was readily observed, strongly suggesting that T cells generated in this way were functionally mature. Although these findings suggest that pluripotent stem cells may serve as a potentially unlimited source of naïve T cells for adoptive transfer, the requirement for an appropriate thymic microenvironment to support V(D)J recombination and positive selection poses significant ethical and pragmatic barriers to the translation of protocols to the human.

A logical way to overcome this hurdle might be to harness induced pluripotency to generate iPS cells from T cells that have already undergone V(D)J recombination and are known to exhibit a desirable antigen specificity. Any T cells differentiated from the parent iPS cell line would maintain the original antigen specificity of the parent cells, and may, therefore, differentiate *in vitro* in a thymus-independent manner. Recent studies have reported the successful differentiation of antigen-specific T cells from an iPS cell line itself generated from CTL specific for an epitope from the melanoma antigen MART-1 (76). These cells were expanded by stimulation with anti-CD3 mAbs, thereby generating CD8$^+$ T cells, which were shown to respond to MART-1, demonstrating retention of their original antigen specificity.

Given the low frequency of tumor-specific T cells in the periphery of individuals and difficulties surrounding their identification, Themeli and colleagues exploited the tractability of iPS cells for genetic modification to introduce a bicistronic lentiviral vector encoding 19–28z, a CAR specific for CD19, expressed by the majority of leukemias and lymphomas. The authors were able to optimize differentiation conditions to allow for serum and feeder free generation of hematopoietic progenitor cells which, when co-cultured with OP9-DL1 stromal cells in the presence of SCF, Flt3L, and interleukin-7 (IL-7), differentiated into T cells expressing the CD19-specific CAR. T cells produced in this way were activated by CD19$^+$ APCs and, upon infusion into mice, potently inhibited tumor progression (77).

While the use of CARs may circumvent the requirement for the identification of antigen-specific T cells, an alternative method of capturing desirable antigen specificities might be to exploit TILs whose presence within a developing tumor provides compelling evidence for their specificity. Whereas CD8$^+$ CTL are readily obtained from tumor biopsies and lend themselves to reprogramming, other T-cell subsets are also evident including regulatory T (Treg) cells. The presence of these Treg cells is known to negatively correlate with survival rates (78), due to their capacity to suppress anti-tumor immune responses and facilitate evasion of the developing tumor from the host immune system. If tumor-specific Treg cells could likewise be reprogramed to pluripotency, their redifferentiation along the T-cell lineage might provide opportunities for their phenotypic reassignment into effector T cells, providing a valuable source of $CD4^{+}$ T-cell help for endogenous CTL responses in danger of exhaustion.

One of the major hurdles to harnessing this approach is defining extracellular Treg-specific markers. Currently, the most widely used marker for Treg cells is Foxp3 among $CD4^{+}CD25^{+}$ cells (79). As this transcription factor is expressed solely in the nucleus, however, sorting of cells based on its expression is not feasible. Nevertheless, recent work has demonstrated that CD127 expression inversely correlates with Foxp3 and hence the suppressive function of human $CD4^{+}$ Treg cells (80). In addition to low CD127 expression, expression of CD45RA is also apparent in human $CD4^{+}$ Treg cells (81): sorting cells based on a $CD4^{+}CD25^{+}$ $CD127^{low}CD45RA^{+}$ phenotype would, therefore, represent the most effective strategy currently available for isolating antigen-specific Treg cells infiltrating the tumor microenvironment.

NK CELL-BASED IMMUNOTHERAPY

Although much interest has focused on the use of NK cells in cancer immunotherapy, obtaining sufficient numbers for administration to patients remains a significant limitation. In 2005, Woll and colleagues used a two-step process to differentiate human ES cells into NK cells *in vitro*. These cells had the ability to lyse human tumor cells deficient in MHC class I expression and up-regulate cytokine production (82). Subsequently, NK cells were successfully differentiated from human iPS cells, using a similar two-stage culture system (83), the cells obtained representing a pure population that did not require cell sorting or co-culture with xenogeneic stromal cells. Moreover, sufficient cytotoxic NK cells could be differentiated from 250,000 iPS cells to treat a single patient, suggesting that iPS cells provide a scalable platform for the clinical implementation of such an approach.

In addition to *bona fide* NK cells, it has recently proven possible to derive NKT cells from iPS cells. NKT cells are characterized by the expression of an invariant TCR encoded by $V\alpha24$–$J\alpha18$ in humans and $V\alpha14$–$J\alpha18$ in mice (84). These cells share the properties of both NK cells and T cells and are thought to play an important role in cancer immune surveillance (85). Indeed, NKT cells differentiated from mouse iPS cells were shown to secrete large quantities of IFNγ and actively suppress tumor growth *in vivo* (86). The differentiation of NKT cells from iPS cells may, therefore, make this elusive cell type readily accessible for cancer immunotherapy in the future.

CONCLUSION

Although significant advances have been made in cancer immunotherapy over the past decade with the discovery of human cross presenting DCs and the use of CARs and TCR transfer for the generation of more effective T-cell therapy, the requirements for high specificity, minimal toxicity, and the capacity for immunological memory have yet to be achieved. It has been suggested that since no single therapy is likely to fulfill all these criteria, adoptive transfer of tumor-specific T cells might be combined with DC vaccination to generate a durable immune response (87). Given the unrestricted differentiation potential of iPS cells, prospects for the differentiation of either cell type from the same patient-specific cell line provide a comprehensive approach. Furthermore, their potential for the efficient scale-up of cell production and tractability for new generation genome engineering tools, such as the CRISPR/Cas-9 system and transcription activator-like effector nucleases (TALENs) (48, 49) may herald a new era in cancer immunotherapy, in which treatments are exquisitely tailored to the individual needs of the patient.

ACKNOWLEDGMENTS

We are grateful to Tim Davies and Alison Leishman for helpful discussions and suggestions. Work on induced pluripotency in the authors' laboratory is supported by the Regenerative Medicine Initiative of the Britain-Israel Research and Academic Exchange Partnership (BIRAX).

REFERENCES

1. Old LJ, Boyse EA. Immunology of experimental tumors. *Annu Rev Med* (1964) **15**:167–86. doi:10.1146/annurev.me.15.020164.001123
2. Burnet FM. The concept of immunological surveillance. *Prog Exp Tumor Res* (1970) **13**:1–27.
3. Burnet M. Immunological factors in the process of carcinogenesis. *Br Med Bull* (1964) **20**:154–8.
4. Stutman O. Chemical carcinogenesis in nude mice: comparison between nude mice from homozygous matings and heterozygous matings and effect of age and carcinogen dose. *J Natl Cancer Inst* (1979) **62**:353–8.
5. Rygaard J, Povlsen CO. The mouse mutant nude does not develop spontaneous tumours. An argument against immunological surveillance. *Acta Pathol Microbiol Scand B Microbiol Immunol* (1974) **82**:99–106.
6. Van Pel A, Boon T. Protection against a nonimmunogenic mouse leukemia by an immunogenic variant obtained by mutagenesis. *Proc Natl Acad Sci U S A* (1982) **79**:4718–22. doi:10.1073/pnas.79.15.4718
7. Dunn GP, Bruce AT, Ikeda H, Old LJ, Schreiber RD. Cancer immunoediting: from immunosurveillance to tumor escape. *Nat Immunol* (2002) **3**:991–8. doi:10.1038/ni1102-991
8. Hanahan D, Weinberg RA. Hallmarks of cancer: the next generation. *Cell* (2011) **144**:646–74. doi:10.1016/j.cell.2011.02.013
9. Joseph CG, Darrah E, Shah AA, Skora AD, Casciola-Rosen LA, Wigley FM, et al. Association of the autoimmune disease scleroderma with an immunologic response to cancer. *Science* (2013) **343**:152–7. doi:10.1126/science.1246886
10. Klebanoff CA, Gattinoni L, Restifo NP. CD8+ T-cell memory in tumor immunology and immunotherapy. *Immunol Rev* (2006) **211**:214–24. doi:10.1111/j.0105-2896.2006.00391.x
11. Lee S, Margolin K. Cytokines in cancer immunotherapy. *Cancers (Basel)* (2011) **3**:3856–93. doi:10.3390/cancers3043856
12. Dutcher J. Current status of interleukin-2 therapy for metastatic renal cell carcinoma and metastatic melanoma. *Oncology (Williston Park)* (2002) **16**:4–10.
13. Kohler G, Milstein C. Continuous cultures of fused cells secreting antibody of predefined specificity. *Nature* (1975) **256**:495–7. doi:10.1038/256495a0
14. Pardoll DM. The blockade of immune checkpoints in cancer immunotherapy. *Nat Rev Cancer* (2012) **12**:252–64. doi:10.1038/nrc3239
15. Sharma P, Wagner K, Wolchok JD, Allison JP. Novel cancer immunotherapy agents with survival benefit: recent successes and next steps. *Nat Rev Cancer* (2011) **11**:805–12. doi:10.1038/nrc3153
16. Topalian SL, Hodi FS, Brahmer JR, Gettinger SN, Smith DC, McDermott DF, et al. Safety, activity, and immune correlates of anti-PD-1 antibody in cancer. *N Engl J Med* (2012) **366**:2443–54. doi:10.1056/NEJMoa1200690

17. Rasul KI, Kerr DJ. Targeted therapies: cetuximab plus chemotherapy in patients with advanced NSCLC. *Nat Rev Clin Oncol* (2009) **6**:499–500. doi:10.1038/nrclinonc.2009.108
18. Adams GP, Weiner LM. Monoclonal antibody therapy of cancer. *Nat Biotechnol* (2005) **23**:1147–57. doi:10.1038/nbt1137
19. Winter MC, Hancock BW. Ten years of rituximab in NHL. *Expert Opin Drug Saf* (2009) **8**:223–35. doi:10.1517/14740330902750114
20. Palucka K, Banchereau J. Cancer immunotherapy via dendritic cells. *Nat Rev Cancer* (2012) **12**:265–77. doi:10.1038/nrc3258
21. Park MY, Kim CH, Sohn HJ, Oh ST, Kim SG, Kim TG. The optimal interval for dendritic cell vaccination following adoptive T cell transfer is important for boosting potent anti-tumor immunity. *Vaccine* (2007) **25**:7322–30. doi:10.1016/j.vaccine.2007.08.037
22. Kurts C, Robinson BW, Knolle PA. Cross-priming in health and disease. *Nat Rev Immunol* (2010) **10**:403–14. doi:10.1038/nri2780
23. Bevan MJ. Minor H antigens introduced on H-2 different stimulating cells cross-react at the cytotoxic T cell level during in vivo priming. *J Immunol* (1976) **117**:2233–8.
24. Bevan MJ. Cross-priming for a secondary cytotoxic response to minor H antigens with H-2 congenic cells which do not cross-react in the cytotoxic assay. *J Exp Med* (1976) **143**:1283–8. doi:10.1084/jem.143.5.1283
25. Sachamitr P, Fairchild PJ. Cross presentation of antigen by dendritic cells: mechanisms and implications for immunotherapy. *Expert Rev Clin Immunol* (2012) **8**:547–55. doi:10.1586/eci.12.45
26. Banchereau J, Fay J, Pascual V, Palucka AK. Dendritic cells: controllers of the immune system and a new promise for immunotherapy. *Novartis Found Symp* (2003) **252**:226–35. doi:10.1002/0470871628.ch17 discussion 235–228, 257–267,
27. Palucka K, Banchereau J, Mellman I. Designing vaccines based on biology of human dendritic cell subsets. *Immunity* (2010) **33**:464–78. doi:10.1016/j.immuni.2010.10.007
28. Kantoff PW, Higano CS, Shore ND, Berger ER, Small EJ, Penson DF, et al. Sipuleucel-T immunotherapy for castration-resistant prostate cancer. *N Engl J Med* (2010) **363**:411–22. doi:10.1056/NEJMoa1001294
29. Lesterhuis WJ, de Vries IJ, Adema GJ, Punt CJ. Dendritic cell-based vaccines in cancer immunotherapy: an update on clinical and immunological results. *Ann Oncol* (2004) **15**(Suppl 4):iv145–51. doi:10.1093/annonc/mdh919
30. Robson NC, Hoves S, Maraskovsky E, Schnurr M. Presentation of tumour antigens by dendritic cells and challenges faced. *Curr Opin Immunol* (2010) **22**:137–44. doi:10.1016/j.coi.2010.01.002
31. Sorensen RB, Andersen RS, Svane IM, Engell-Noerregaard L, Hadrup SR, Balslev E, et al. Thor Straten P: CD8 T-cell responses against cyclin B1 in breast cancer patients with tumors overexpressing p53. *Clin Cancer Res* (2009) **15**:1543–9. doi:10.1158/1078-0432.CCR-08-1412
32. Engell-Noerregaard L, Hansen TH, Andersen MH, Thor Straten P, Svane IM. Review of clinical studies on dendritic cell-based vaccination of patients with malignant melanoma: assessment of correlation between clinical response and vaccine parameters. *Cancer Immunol Immunother* (2009) **58**:1–14. doi:10.1007/s00262-008-0568-4
33. Bachem A, Guttler S, Hartung E, Ebstein F, Schaefer M, Tannert A, et al. Superior antigen cross-presentation and XCR1 expression define human CD11c+CD141+ cells as homologues of mouse CD8+ dendritic cells. *J Exp Med* (2010) **207**:1273–81. doi:10.1084/jem.20100348
34. Jongbloed SL, Kassianos AJ, McDonald KJ, Clark GJ, Ju X, Angel CE, et al. Human CD141+ (BDCA-3)+ dendritic cells (DCs) represent a unique myeloid DC subset that cross-presents necrotic cell antigens. *J Exp Med* (2010) **207**:1247–60. doi:10.1084/jem.20092140
35. Segura E, Durand M, Amigorena S. Similar antigen cross-presentation capacity and phagocytic functions in all freshly isolated human lymphoid organ-resident dendritic cells. *J Exp Med* (2013) **210**:1035–47. doi:10.1084/jem.20121103
36. Poulin LF, Salio M, Griessinger E, Anjos-Afonso F, Craciun L, Chen JL, et al. Characterization of human DNGR-1+ BDCA3+ leukocytes as putative equivalents of mouse CD8alpha+ dendritic cells. *J Exp Med* (2010) **207**:1261–71. doi:10.1084/jem.20092618
37. Varela-Rohena A, Carpenito C, Perez EE, Richardson M, Parry RV, Milone M, et al. Genetic engineering of T cells for adoptive immunotherapy. *Immunol Res* (2008) **42**:166–81. doi:10.1007/s12026-008-8057-6
38. Rosenberg SA, Yannelli JR, Yang JC, Topalian SL, Schwartzentruber DJ, Weber JS, et al. Treatment of patients with metastatic melanoma with autologous tumor-infiltrating lymphocytes and interleukin 2. *J Natl Cancer Inst* (1994) **86**:1159–66. doi:10.1093/jnci/86.15.1159
39. Mitchison NA. Studies on the immunological response to foreign tumor transplants in the mouse. I. The role of lymph node cells in conferring immunity by adoptive transfer. *J Exp Med* (1955) **102**:157–77. doi:10.1084/jem.102.2.157
40. Mule JJ, Shu S, Schwarz SL, Rosenberg SA. Adoptive immunotherapy of established pulmonary metastases with LAK cells and recombinant interleukin-2. *Science* (1984) **225**:1487–9. doi:10.1126/science.6332379
41. Mazumder A, Rosenberg SA. Successful immunotherapy of natural killer-resistant established pulmonary melanoma metastases by the intravenous adoptive transfer of syngeneic lymphocytes activated in vitro by interleukin 2. *J Exp Med* (1984) **159**:495–507. doi:10.1084/jem.159.2.495
42. Rosenberg SA. Immunotherapy of cancer by systemic administration of lymphoid cells plus interleukin-2. *J Biol Response Mod* (1984) **3**:501–11.
43. Rosenberg SA, Packard BS, Aebersold PM, Solomon D, Topalian SL, Toy ST, et al. Use of tumor-infiltrating lymphocytes and interleukin-2 in the immunotherapy of patients with metastatic melanoma. A preliminary report. *N Engl J Med* (1988) **319**:1676–80. doi:10.1056/NEJM198812223192527
44. Dudley ME, Wunderlich JR, Robbins PF, Yang JC, Hwu P, Schwartzentruber DJ, et al. Cancer regression and autoimmunity in patients after clonal repopulation with antitumor lymphocytes. *Science* (2002) **298**:850–4. doi:10.1126/science.1076514
45. Dudley ME, Wunderlich JR, Yang JC, Sherry RM, Topalian SL, Restifo NP, et al. Adoptive cell transfer therapy following non-myeloablative but lymphodepleting chemotherapy for the treatment of patients with refractory metastatic melanoma. *J Clin Oncol* (2005) **23**:2346–57. doi:10.1200/JCO.2005.00.240
46. Kalos M, June CH. Adoptive T cell transfer for cancer immunotherapy in the era of synthetic biology. *Immunity* (2013) **39**:49–60. doi:10.1016/j.immuni.2013.07.002
47. Morgan RA, Dudley ME, Wunderlich JR, Hughes MS, Yang JC, Sherry RM, et al. Cancer regression in patients after transfer of genetically engineered lymphocytes. *Science* (2006) **314**:126–9. doi:10.1126/science.1129003
48. Schwank G, Koo BK, Sasselli V, Dekkers JF, Heo I, Demircan T, et al. Functional repair of CFTR by CRISPR/Cas9 in intestinal stem cell organoids of cystic fibrosis patients. *Cell Stem Cell* (2013) **13**:653–8. doi:10.1016/j.stem.2013.11.002
49. Hockemeyer D, Wang H, Kiani S, Lai CS, Gao Q, Cassady JP, et al. Genetic engineering of human pluripotent cells using TALE nucleases. *Nat Biotechnol* (2011) **29**:731–4. doi:10.1038/nbt.1927
50. Linette GP, Stadtmauer EA, Maus MV, Rapoport AP, Levine BL, Emery L, et al. Cardiovascular toxicity and titin cross-reactivity of affinity-enhanced T cells in myeloma and melanoma. *Blood* (2013) **122**:863–71. doi:10.1182/blood-2013-03-490565
51. Ni J, Miller M, Stojanovic A, Garbi N, Cerwenka A. Sustained effector function of IL-12/15/18-preactivated NK cells against established tumors. *J Exp Med* (2012) **209**:2351–65. doi:10.1084/jem.20120944
52. Fujisaki H, Kakuda H, Shimasaki N, Imai C, Ma J, Lockey T, et al. Expansion of highly cytotoxic human natural killer cells for cancer cell therapy. *Cancer Res* (2009) **69**:4010–7. doi:10.1158/0008-5472.CAN-08-3712
53. Ruggeri L, Mancusi A, Capanni M, Martelli MF, Velardi A. Exploitation of alloreactive NK cells in adoptive immunotherapy of cancer. *Curr Opin Immunol* (2005) **17**:211–7. doi:10.1016/j.coi.2005.01.007
54. Miller JS, Soignier Y, Panoskaltsis-Mortari A, McNearney SA, Yun GH, Fautsch SK, et al. Successful adoptive transfer and in vivo expansion of human haploidentical NK cells in patients with cancer. *Blood* (2005) **105**:3051–7. doi:10.1182/blood-2004-07-2974
55. Dillman RO, Duma CM, Ellis RA, Cornforth AN, Schiltz PM, Sharp SL, et al. Intralesional lymphokine-activated killer cells as adjuvant therapy for primary glioblastoma. *J Immunother* (2009) **32**:914–9. doi:10.1097/CJI.0b013e3181b2910f
56. Evans MJ, Kaufman MH. Establishment in culture of pluripotential cells from mouse embryos. *Nature* (1981) **292**:154–6. doi:10.1038/292154a0
57. Thomson JA, Itskovitz-Eldor J, Shapiro SS, Waknitz MA, Swiergiel JJ, Marshall VS, et al. Embryonic stem cell lines derived from human blastocysts. *Science* (1998) **282**:1145–7. doi:10.1126/science.282.5391.1145
58. Takahashi K, Yamanaka S. Induction of pluripotent stem cells from mouse embryonic and adult fibroblast cultures by defined factors. *Cell* (2006) **126**:663–76. doi:10.1016/j.cell.2006.07.024

59. Takahashi K, Tanabe K, Ohnuki M, Narita M, Ichisaka T, Tomoda K, et al. Induction of pluripotent stem cells from adult human fibroblasts by defined factors. *Cell* (2007) **131**:861–72. doi:10.1016/j.cell.2007.11.019
60. Nakagawa M, Koyanagi M, Tanabe K, Takahashi K, Ichisaka T, Aoi T, et al. Generation of induced pluripotent stem cells without Myc from mouse and human fibroblasts. *Nat Biotechnol* (2008) **26**:101–6. doi:10.1038/nbt1374
61. Zhao T, Zhang ZN, Rong Z, Xu Y. Immunogenicity of induced pluripotent stem cells. *Nature* (2011) **474**:212–5. doi:10.1038/nature10135
62. Kim D, Kim CH, Moon JI, Chung YG, Chang MY, Han BS, et al. Generation of human induced pluripotent stem cells by direct delivery of reprogramming proteins. *Cell Stem Cell* (2009) **4**:472–6. doi:10.1016/j.stem.2009.05.005
63. Warren L, Manos PD, Ahfeldt T, Loh YH, Li H, Lau F, et al. Highly efficient reprogramming to pluripotency and directed differentiation of human cells with synthetic modified mRNA. *Cell Stem Cell* (2010) **7**:618–30. doi:10.1016/j.stem.2010.08.012
64. Huangfu D, Maehr R, Guo W, Eijkelenboom A, Snitow M, Chen AE, et al. Induction of pluripotent stem cells by defined factors is greatly improved by small-molecule compounds. *Nat Biotechnol* (2008) **26**:795–7. doi:10.1038/nbt1418
65. Hou P, Li Y, Zhang X, Liu C, Guan J, Li H, et al. Pluripotent stem cells induced from mouse somatic cells by small-molecule compounds. *Science* (2013) **341**:651–4. doi:10.1126/science.1239278
66. Obokata H, Wakayama T, Sasai Y, Kojima K, Vacanti MP, Niwa H, et al. Stimulus-triggered fate conversion of somatic cells into pluripotency. *Nature* (2014) **505**:641–7. doi:10.1038/nature12968
67. Mali P, Yang L, Esvelt KM, Aach J, Guell M, DiCarlo JE, et al. RNA-guided human genome engineering via Cas9. *Science* (2012) **339**:823–6. doi:10.1126/science.1232033
68. Ramos-Mejia V, Fraga MF, Menendez P. iPSCs from cancer cells: challenges and opportunities. *Trends Mol Med* (2012) **18**:245–7. doi:10.1016/j.molmed.2012.04.001
69. Miyoshi N, Ishii H, Nagai K, Hoshino H, Mimori K, Tanaka F, et al. Defined factors induce reprogramming of gastrointestinal cancer cells. *Proc Natl Acad Sci U S A* (2009) **107**:40–5. doi:10.1073/pnas.0912407107
70. Zhan X, Dravid G, Ye Z, Hammond H, Shamblott M, Gearhart J, et al. Functional antigen-presenting leucocytes derived from human embryonic stem cells in vitro. *Lancet* (2004) **364**:163–71. doi:10.1016/S0140-6736(04)16629-4
71. Fairchild PJ, Brook FA, Gardner RL, Graca L, Strong V, Tone Y, et al. Directed differentiation of dendritic cells from mouse embryonic stem cells. *Curr Biol* (2000) **10**:1515–8. doi:10.1016/S0960-9822(00)00824-1
72. Tseng SY, Nishimoto KP, Silk KM, Majumdar AS, Dawes GN, Waldmann H, et al. Generation of immunogenic dendritic cells from human embryonic stem cells without serum and feeder cells. *Regen Med* (2009) **4**:513–26. doi:10.2217/rme.09.25
73. Silk KM, Silk JD, Ichiryu N, Davies TJ, Nolan KF, Leishman AJ, et al. Cross-presentation of tumour antigens by human induced pluripotent stem cell-derived CD141(+)XCR1(+) dendritic cells. *Gene Ther* (2012) **19**:1035–40. doi:10.1038/gt.2011.177
74. Schmitt TM, de Pooter RF, Gronski MA, Cho SK, Ohashi PS, Zuniga-Pflucker JC. Induction of T cell development and establishment of T cell competence from embryonic stem cells differentiated in vitro. *Nat Immunol* (2004) **5**:410–7. doi:10.1038/ni1055
75. Schmitt TM, Zuniga-Pflucker JC. Induction of T cell development from hematopoietic progenitor cells by delta-like-1 in vitro. *Immunity* (2002) **17**:749–56. doi:10.1016/S1074-7613(02)00474-0
76. Vizcardo R, Masuda K, Yamada D, Ikawa T, Shimizu K, Fujii S, et al. Regeneration of human tumor antigen-specific T cells from iPSCs derived from mature CD8(+) T cells. *Cell Stem Cell* (2013) **12**:31–6. doi:10.1016/j.stem.2012.12.006
77. Themeli M, Kloss CC, Ciriello G, Fedorov VD, Perna F, Gonen M, et al. Generation of tumor-targeted human T lymphocytes from induced pluripotent stem cells for cancer therapy. *Nat Biotechnol* (2013) **31**:928–33. doi:10.1038/nbt.2678
78. Huang Y, Wang FM, Wang T, Wang YJ, Zhu ZY, Gao YT, et al. Tumor-infiltrating FoxP3+ Tregs and CD8+ T cells affect the prognosis of hepatocellular carcinoma patients. *Digestion* (2012) **86**:329–37. doi:10.1159/000342801
79. Bilate AM, Lafaille JJ. Induced CD4+Foxp3+ regulatory T cells in immune tolerance. *Annu Rev Immunol* (2012) **30**:733–58. doi:10.1146/annurev-immunol-020711-075043
80. Liu W, Putnam AL, Xu-Yu Z, Szot GL, Lee MR, Zhu S, et al. CD127 expression inversely correlates with FoxP3 and suppressive function of human CD4+ T reg cells. *J Exp Med* (2006) **203**:1701–11. doi:10.1084/jem.20051745
81. Hoffmann P, Eder R, Boeld TJ, Doser K, Piseshka B, Andreesen R, et al. Only the CD45RA+ subpopulation of CD4+CD25high T cells gives rise to homogeneous regulatory T-cell lines upon in vitro expansion. *Blood* (2006) **108**:4260–7. doi:10.1182/blood-2006-06-027409
82. Woll PS, Martin CH, Miller JS, Kaufman DS. Human embryonic stem cell-derived NK cells acquire functional receptors and cytolytic activity. *J Immunol* (2005) **175**:5095–103.
83. Knorr DA, Ni Z, Hermanson D, Hexum MK, Bendzick L, Cooper LJ, et al. Clinical-scale derivation of natural killer cells from human pluripotent stem cells for cancer therapy. *Stem Cells Transl Med* (2013) **2**:274–83. doi:10.5966/sctm.2012-0084
84. Stanic AK, De Silva AD, Park JJ, Sriram V, Ichikawa S, Hirabyashi Y, et al. Defective presentation of the CD1d1-restricted natural Va14Ja18 NKT lymphocyte antigen caused by beta-D-glucosylceramide synthase deficiency. *Proc Natl Acad Sci U S A* (2003) **100**:1849–54. doi:10.1073/pnas.0430327100
85. Fujii SI, Shimizu K, Okamoto Y, Kunii N, Nakayama T, Motohashi S, et al. NKT cells as an ideal anti-tumor immunotherapeutic. *Front Immunol* (2013) **4**:409. doi:10.3389/fimmu.2013.00409
86. Watarai H, Fujii S, Yamada D, Rybouchkin A, Sakata S, Nagata Y, et al. Murine induced pluripotent stem cells can be derived from and differentiate into natural killer T cells. *J Clin Invest* (2010) **120**:2610–8. doi:10.1172/JCI42027
87. Schattenberg AV, Dolstra H. Cellular adoptive immunotherapy after allogeneic stem cell transplantation. *Curr Opin Oncol* (2005) **17**:617–21. doi:10.1097/01.cco.0000181405.60213.1c

4

Therapeutic use of dendritic cells to promote the extranodal priming of anti-tumor immunity

Lu Chen[1], Kellsye L. Fabian[1], Jennifer L. Taylor[2] and Walter J. Storkus[1,2,3]*

[1] Department of Immunology, University of Pittsburgh School of Medicine, Pittsburgh, PA, USA
[2] Department of Dermatology, University of Pittsburgh School of Medicine, Pittsburgh, PA, USA
[3] University of Pittsburgh Cancer Institute, Pittsburgh, PA, USA

Edited by:
Lisa Helene Butterfield, University of Pittsburgh, USA

Reviewed by:
James Harold Finke, Cleveland Clinic, USA
James Joseph Mulé, Moffitt Cancer Center, USA

***Correspondence:**
Walter J. Storkus, Departments of Dermatology and Immunology, University of Pittsburgh, W10041.2 BST, 200 Lothrop Street, Pittsburgh, PA 15213, USA
e-mail: storkuswj@upmc.edu

Ectopic lymphoid tissue, also known as tertiary lymphoid organs (TLO) develop adaptively within sites of chronic tissue inflammation, thereby allowing the host to efficiently crossprime specific immune effector cells within sites of disease. Recent evidence suggests that the presence of TLO in the tumor microenvironment (TME) predicts better overall survival. We will discuss the relevance of extranodal T cell priming within the TME as a means to effectively promote anti-tumor immunity and the strategic use of dendritic cell (DC)-based therapies to reinforce this clinically preferred process in the cancer-bearing host.

Keywords: dendritic cells, extranodal, cross-priming, therapy, cancer

INTRODUCTION

In the classical model of peripheral T cell activation, tissue-resident dendritic cells (DCs) capture antigens (such as foreign pathogens, tumor cell debris, etc.) in an inflammatory microenvironment, leading to the migration of antigen-laden CCR7$^+$ DC to regional draining lymph nodes [LN; aka secondary lymphoid organs (SLO)], where activation of cognate T cells occurs (1–3). After appropriate proliferative expansion and maturation, T effector cells may then enter the blood circulation and be recruited into tissue sites where they are competent to recognize and react against relevant antigen-presenting cells, such as virally infected host cells or tumor cells (4). Recent evidence obtained in a range of translational and clinical models suggests, however, that this classical/conventional paradigm may be operationally overly simplistic, and that extranodal (cross)priming of antigen-specific T cells can occur in peripheral tissues, often times in conditionally established tertiary lymphoid organs (TLO) (5–9).

SLO/TLO DEVELOPMENT: NATURAL AND INDUCED

The developmental formation of SLO is believed to require the interaction of so-called lymphoid tissue inducer cells (LTi) bearing a CD3$^-$CD4$^+$CD45$^+$IL-7R$^+$c-Kit$^+$ phenotype that produce lymphotoxin α/β [LTα/β; Ref. (10, 11)] with LTβR$^+$ stromal "organizer" cell populations that may derive from adipocyte precursors (12), leading to corollary stromal cell elaboration of the SLO homeostatic chemokines CCL19, CCL21, and CXCL13 (8, 9, 13–15). These chemokines sustain recruitment of LTi and other lymphocytes into SLO, resulting in the development of a mature lymphoid organ architecture [i.e., based on the formation of follicular structures containing B cells and surrounding "cortical" zones that are diffusely populated by CD4$^+$ and CD8$^+$ T cells, antigen-presenting cells (including CD11c$^+$ DC), and PNAd$^+$ high-endothelial venules (HEV; (8, 15–19))].

Naive (CD62L$^+$CCR7$^+$) T cells enter SLO via interaction with PNAd$^+$ HEV which are "decorated" with the CCR7 ligand chemokines CCL19 and CCL21 on their luminal surface, thereby facilitating lymphocyte extravasation/directed motility from the blood into the lymph node (20). Of these two chemokines, CCL21 may play the more dominant role in recruiting naïve lymphocytes into SLO, while CCL19 may be differentially cytoprotective in sustaining nodal populations of lymphocytes (20–22). Prolonged CCR7-mediated signaling into recruited T cells, leads to intrinsic upregulation of the sphingosine-1 phosphate receptor 1, EDG1 (23), which is involved in the ultimate departure of primed T cell populations from SLO into the peripheral blood circulation (24, 25).

While classical SLO are encapsulated structures that develop in predictable locations as a consequence of normal immune system development, under pathologic conditions, ectopic lymphoid tissues (aka TLO) may develop in peripheral tissue sites of chronic inflammation (13, 26). TLO formation has been reported within inflamed organs of patients with rheumatoid arthritis (27–29), psoriatic arthritis (30), diabetes mellitus (31–33), autoimmune gastritis [AIG; Ref. (32)], juvenile dermatomyositis (34), and Sjögren's syndrome (35), among others. TLO formation has also been identified in the lungs of influenza virus-infected mice (36), the livers of hepatitis C virus (HCV)-infected patients (37) and in the stomachs of patients infected with *Helicobacter pylori* (38). "Dysfunctional" human lung allografts exhibiting chronic inflammatory responses have also been found to commonly contain TLO (17).

Furthermore, a burgeoning literature supports tumor-associated TLO as important sites of extranodal T cell priming and epitope spreading in the responder T cell repertoire (13, 39). TLO have been identified in a subset of human melanoma lesions, in which mature DC were found to maintain intimate contact with recruited T cell populations, consistent with the notion of operational extranodal (cross)priming within the tumor microenvironment (TME) (40, 41). Similar results have been reported for murine melanoma models (7, 8). In line with this model, naïve lymphocytes have been identified in TLO within pulmonary lesions of patients with lung cancer, making it likely that these immune cells encounter their cognate antigen for the first time and develop into antigen-specific T effector cells within the TME *in vivo* (16, 42). TLO featuring DC/Type-1 T cell clusters proximal to B cell "nests" have also been identified in human non-small-cell lung cancer specimens (43). In such instances, the density of mature DC found in TLO appeared to be associated with improved long term survival (6, 43). In a subset of patients with breast cancer, HEV have been found in close proximity to $LT\beta^{+}LAMP^{+}$ DC in association with profound B/T cell infiltrates in the TME and a more favorable clinical outcome (44). Furthermore, Mulé and colleagues have recently performed a metagene analysis on human (Stage IV, non-locoregional) melanoma metastases and identified a 12-chemokine gene signature (i.e., CCL2, CCL3, CCL4, CCL5, CCL8, CCL18, CCL19, CCL21, CXCL9, CXCL10, CXCL11, CXCL13) correlating with the presence of TLO (containing $CD20^{+}$ B cell follicles with prominent areas of $CD4^{+}$ and $CD8^{+}$ T cells, but not $FoxP3^{+}$ T_{reg} cells), with better overall survival noted in the TLO^{+} subset of patients (41). In a similar vein, Gu-Trantien et al. (45) have also recently observed that the presence of breast cancer infiltrating follicular $CD4^{+}$ T helper cells (Tfh; expressing CD200, FBLN7, ICOS, SGPP2, SH2D1A, TIGIT, and PDCD1/PD-1, and producing the CXCL13 chemokine) may be directly correlated with; (i) the degree of tumor-infiltrating lymphocytes (TIL), (ii) the formation of TLO-like structures in cancer tissue, and (iii) improved patient clinical response to pre-operative chemotherapy and/or post-surgical disease-free survival.

The conditional formation of TLO in peripheral tissues appears to require the coordinate participation of a similar cast of cellular participants, soluble mediators, and signaling pathways associated with the orchestration of SLO development (14, 15). Ectopic delivery of $LT\alpha/\beta$ or LIGHT (aka TNFSF-14 or CD258) promotes $PNAd^{+}$ HEV, CCL19/CCL21 production, massive naïve T cell infiltration, and (tumor-specific) cross-priming in the context of TLO structures (9, 18, 36, 46–49). For example, targeted therapeutic delivery of $LT\alpha$ into the TME via the administration of a fusion protein encompassing the $LT\alpha$ molecule linked to an antibody recognizing a tumor plasma membrane-associated disialoganglioside GD2 (i.e., ch14.18-$LT\alpha$) resulted in slowed tumor progression and the establishment of mature TLO structures within 9 days of treatment initiation (8). The $LT\beta R$ ligands $LT\alpha/\beta$ and LIGHT appear to act directly on endothelial cells and DC in activating NFκB and promoting the expression of adhesion molecules, such as PNAd, VCAM-1, E-selectin, and ICAM-1 by HEV and IL-12p70 production from DC (50–52). In particular, LIGHT is essential for DC-mediated cross-priming of antigen-specific Type-1 T cells (53). Indeed, ectopic expression of LIGHT in the TME elicits profound infiltration and cross-priming of naïve anti-tumor T cells in concert with upregulated stromal cell production of TLO-associated chemokines (CCL21, CXCL9, CXCL10, and CXCL13), increased expression of vascular adhesion molecules (MAdCAM-1, VCAM-1, PNAd), and the presence of mature DC within the TME (9). Interestingly, DC, natural killer (NK) cells, and even B cells can serve as $LT\alpha/\beta$ producers in pro-inflammatory environments, allowing for the establishment of an autocrine feed-forward loop promoting TLO development in peripheral tissues (36, 54–59). Consistent with these findings noted for pro-TLO immunobiology of $LT\beta R$ ligands, blockade of the $LT\beta R$ precludes formation of TLO *in vivo* (60).

In a similar manner, induced expression or ectopic delivery of $LT\beta R$ downstream mediators, CCL19 or CCL21, in the TME results in inhibition of tumor growth or complete rejection of established tumors associated with increased infiltration by $CD3^{+}CCR7^{+}$ T cells and/or DCs in a range of cancer models (32, 61–70). Interestingly, these interventional maneuvers may also reduce frequencies of tumor-associated immunosuppressive T_{reg} cells and MDSC (61).

During the ontogeny of TLO in peripheral tissues, lymphatic vessels (i.e., $PNAd^{+}$, MAdCAM-1^{+}, LYVE-1^{+}, and/or Prox-1^{+} HEV) and disorganized clusters of APC and infiltrating lymphocytes appear in advance of canonical mature lymphoid organ architecture characterized by B cell follicular regions (19, 71). Signals that instigate the diffuse-to-organized structural transition of TLO may be provided by cognate T cell recognition of relevant target cell populations within nascent TLO (15, 72). It is important to note, however, that immature TLO have been oft-associated with locoregional immune sequelae including manifestations of autoimmunity and anti-tumor efficacy (5, 32, 71). Hence, while mature TLO may ultimately develop in the chronic disease setting, clinical meaningful immunobiology occurs in advance of such structural developments.

THERAPEUTIC PROMOTION OF TLO

If the formation of TLO allows for extranodal (cross)priming of antigen-specific T cells that are linked to disease pathogenesis (i.e., autoimmunity) or resolution (i.e., infectious disease, cancer), then means by which to prevent or enhance TLO development, respectively, in affected tissues would be anticipated to impact clinical outcome. Perhaps the most strategically simple means by which to apply this paradigm in the cancer setting reflects the implantation of SLO/TLO directly into the TME. Recently, scaffold-based lymphoid tissue engineering has been developed as a means to transplant "intact" TLO directly into tumors in order to affect clinical benefit (73). A previously mentioned alternative to this strategy is clearly the delivery of the $LT\beta R$ ligands $LT\alpha$, $LT\beta$, or LIGHT, agonist anti-$LT\beta R$ antibodies or downstream TLO-associated chemokines (CCL19, CCL21, CXCL13) via protein-based or genetic therapy in order to instigate the locoregional development of TLO in the TME leading to inhibition of tumor growth *in vivo* and extended overall survival (8, 9, 48, 74, 75).

USE OF DC-BASED THERAPY TO PROMOTE EXTRANODAL PRIMING OF ANTI-TUMOR T CELLS

It also appears that the administration of appropriately activated/engineered DC is sufficient to nucleate and/or maintain the development of TLO *in vivo* (36, 72). For instance, mice vaccinated sub-cutaneously with syngenic DC loaded with apoptotic/necrotic B16 melanoma cell debris develop operational TLO [pseudocapsule; PNAd$^+$ vascular endothelial cells (VEC), T cell/DC infiltrates] at sites of injection, leading to the activation of protective anti-tumor immunity (72). DC genetically engineered to secrete high-levels of CCL21 (DC.CCL21) and injected directly into B16 murine melanomas promote strong extranodal T cell cross-priming/recruitment into the TME, even in LTα −/− mice that lack SLO (8, 68). The superiority of DC.CCL21 in enhancing the cross-priming of protective Type-1 anti-tumor T cell responses has also been confirmed in alternate murine models (76, 77).

In our recent paper (5), we noted that DC engineered to express the Type-1 transactivator protein T-bet (DC.Tbet) and injected directly into sarcomas growing progressively in C57BL/6 mice, led to the cross-priming of protective immunity that was independent of host CD11c$^+$ or BATF3$^+$ DC or the ability of the injected DC.Tbet to migrate to SLO. Instead, we detected the rapid recruitment of NK cells and naïve T cells into the TME within 48 h of DC.Tbet administration, and the differentiation of these TIL into Type-1 effector cells *in situ* within the TME. As shown in **Figure 1**, we observed a diffuse but interactive collection of CD11c$^+$ DC and Tbet$^+$ cells [including both T cells (5) and B220$^+$ B cells] within the TME of MCA205 sarcomas by 48 h post-treatment with DC.Tbet, but not control DC. PNAd$^+$ HEV were not evident at this early time point, but were readily imaged in proximity to large DC-Tbet$^+$ lymphocyte clusters by 5 days post-treatment with DC.Tbet (but not control DC). These data suggest that extranodal priming of protective immunity using therapeutic DC delivery occurs in advance of the formal adoption of classical TLO anatomic structures within the TME (**Figure 2**), and that indeed, the development of such Type-1 cognate immunity (and its pro-inflammatory signals) in the TME may be required for subsequent evolution of mature TLO formatting, as described by Schrama et al. (8). Interestingly, a gene array analysis of DC.Tbet versus control DC did not reveal any striking differences in expression of LTA, LTB, LIGHT, CCL19, CCL21, or CXCL13 mRNA transcripts, suggesting a potentially novel mechanism associated with early TLO development triggered by this DC-based therapy [(5) and Chen, unpublished data]. In this regard, we noted a striking enhancement in DC.Tbet production of IL-36γ/IL-1F9 (>34-fold; Chen, unpublished data). IL-36γ is a novel IL-1 family member cytokine that has been previously reported to be a potent recruiter and activator of naïve T cells that develop strong Type-1 functional polarity (78, 79). As in the case of LTβR ligands, IL-36 also triggers NFκB activation in IL-36R$^+$ DC (79–82), which may prove pivotal for autocrine potentiation of Type-1 DC function and a pro-TLO TME. Whether tumor-associated VEC express IL-36R and activated NFκb in response to IL-36 remains an unanswered question. We are currently evaluating the impact of IL-36γ knock-down in DC.Tbet in order to determine the direct relevance of IL-36γ in the development of TLO and protective immunity in the TME of mice treated with intratumoral administration of DC.Tbet.

SUMMARY AND FUTURE PERSPECTIVES

In the cancer setting, the ability of the host to develop ectopic lymphoid organs (TLO) within or proximal to sites of active disease appears to represent a positive prognostic factor for overall patient survival. TLO represent a regional "factory" in which naïve T cells (and B cells) may be cross-primed by tumor-resident antigen-presenting cells, such as DC, leading to poly-specific adaptive immunity that may limit disease progression and conceivably metastatic spread. By limiting the need for antigen-loaded DC to

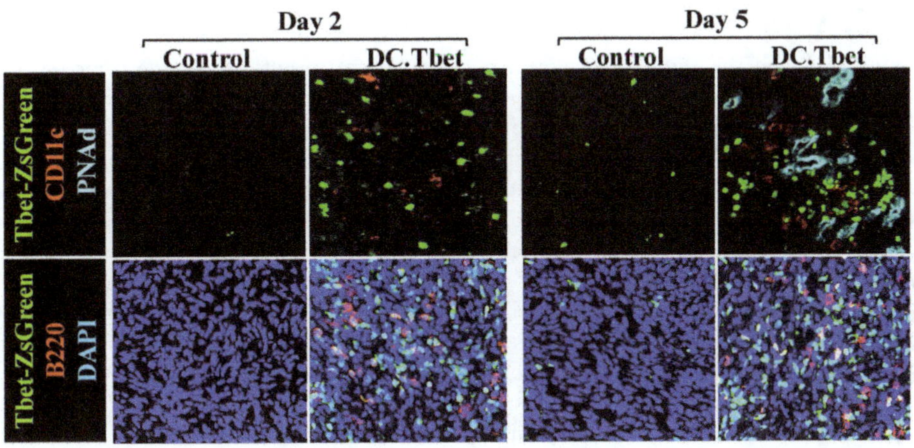

FIGURE 1 | Intratumoral administration of dendritic cells engineered to express T-bet/TBX21 (DC.Tbet) promote the rapid infiltration of Type-1-polarized lymphocytes and dendritic cells and the development of PNAd$^+$ endothelial cells (i.e., HEV). Tbet-ZsGreen Tg mice were injected sub-cutaneously with syngenic MCA205 sarcoma cells and tumors allowed to progressively grow for 7 days, at which time control DC (Control) or DC engineered with recombinant adenovirus to express murine T-bet cDNA were inoculated directly into tumors, as previously described (5). Two or 5 days after DC injection, the mice were euthanized and tumor sections evaluated by fluorescence microscopy for expression of Tbet-ZsGreen protein, CD11c (a marker of DC), B220 (a B cell marker), and PNAd (i.e., Peripheral lymph Node Addressin; a high endothelial venule (HEV) cell marker). PNAd$^+$ HEV were not observed by 2 days post-treatment, but became prevalent by 5 days post-injection of DC.Tbet cells. B, T, and NK cell infiltrates into DC.Tbet [Figure 1 and (5)] exhibited a diffuse distribution pattern in day 2 and day 5 DC.Tbet-treated tumors. Type-1 polarity in infiltrating cells is denoted by nuclear expression of Tbet-ZsGreen. Data are representative of images obtained in three independent experiments performed.

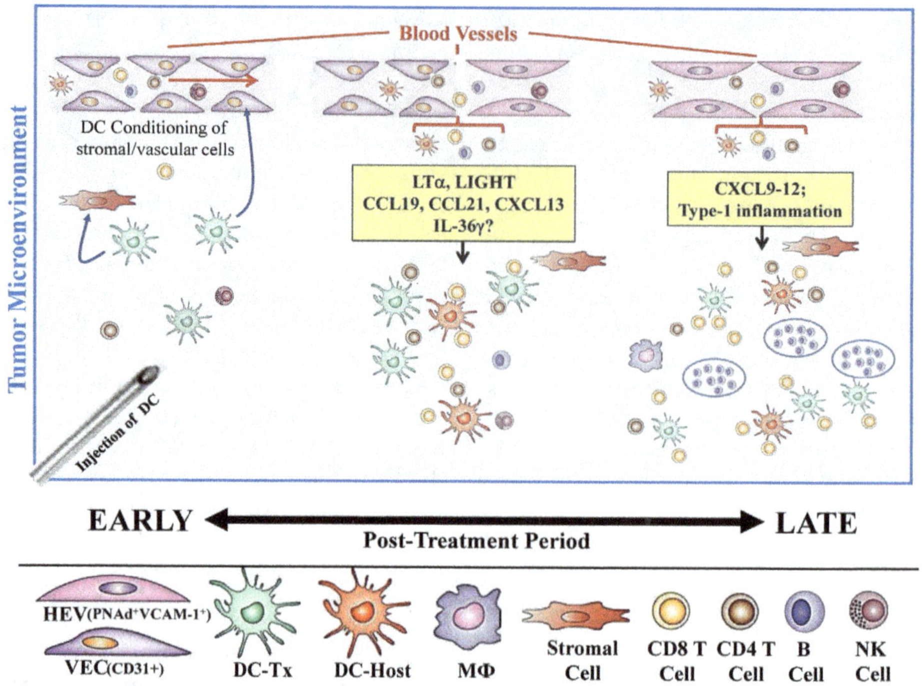

FIGURE 2 | Hypothetical paradigm for extranodal priming of T cells after intratumoral administration of DC.Tbet cells. Injection of DC.Tbet (but not control DC) into the TME leads to the conditioning of tumor-associated stromal cells and vascular endothelial cells (VEC), resulting in stromal cell production of chemokines recruiting naïve leukocytes (B, T, NK cells) and VEC expression of adhesion molecules, such as VCAM-1, as early as day 2 post-treatment [Figure 1 and (5)]. Recruited lymphocytes are assembled in diffuse patterns around CD11c$^+$ (both injected and host) DC and have already acquired Type-1 functional polarization, based on expression of the Tbet reporter protein (Tbet-ZsGreen) *in vivo*. PNAd$^+$ HEV are not formally required for early recruitment of naïve T cells into the TME since these structures do not become discernible until later time points [i.e., day 5; Figure 1 and (5)]. B220$^+$ B cells recruited into the TME as a consequence of treatment with DC.Tbet cells are not organized into follicle-like structures during the day 2–5 time period, but may become organized in this manner at even later time points (i.e., ≥day 9 post-therapy), based on previous reports employing alternate immunotherapeutic interventions, such as ch14.18-LTα (8). While therapeutic benefits in our model were largely T cell-dependent and detectable prior to the establishment of formal TLO structures (based on the development of B cell follicles), the presence of "mature" TLO in human tumors has been associated with better clinical prognosis.

migrate to tumor-draining SLO, and the corollary requirement of SLO-primed T cells to be recruited back into tumor sites, TLO may operationally increase the efficiency of anti-tumor T cell cross-priming and the therapeutic action of such T effector cells in the TME. Translational studies clearly suggest that TLO formation in the TME may be therapeutically fostered by the directed delivery of LTβR ligands in both protein- and gene-based formats. At present, LTβR agonist-based therapies are in their infancy with only rhLTα thus far evaluated in phase I clinical trials, where minimal anti-tumor efficacy was observed in patients with melanoma or renal cell carcinoma (83). The inability to focus this potent TLO induction agent in appropriate sites of disease in order to most effectively recruit and activate protective immunity in treated patients must be considered a possible limitation to the current treatment strategy. The ligation of rhLTα to a cancer-specific antibody or the intratumoral administration of this agent could improve anti-tumor efficacy and coordinately reduce current off-target toxicities [i.e., grade III chill, grade III fever, and grade III dyspnea; Ref. (83)].

Improved targeted delivery of LTβR ligand or downstream chemokine gene therapies is conceptually attractive given pre-clinical results in murine tumor models. To date, however, only a recombinant adenovirus encoding hCCL21 has been developed for phase I clinical application, with the intent to deliver rAd.CCL21-infected patient DC directly into tumors in patients with late stage human lung cancer (84) or in vaccine formulations applied to patients with melanoma (85). Although this approach requires further optimization of the clinical vector based on low levels of CCL21 produced by engineered DC, melanoma patients treated at the lowest dose tier of DC.CCL21 did develop lymph node-like structures based on immunohistochemical analysis of vaccination site biopsies (James Mulé, personal communication). Our own pre-clinical data would support the clinical application of DC.Tbet directly into accessible tumor lesions as a means to drive TLO development and protective immunity in the TME. Motivation for the development of prospective phase I trials using DC.Tbet cells will be intensified when the underlying mechanism of action for this treatment modality has been defined.

Finally, in a related note, antagonists of LTβR ligands (such as BTLA and CD160) have been shown to be immunosuppressive molecules in inhibiting DC homeostasis as well as the protective effector functions mediated by T cells and NK cells (74, 86–90).

It is therefore conceivable that endogenous levels of TLO development and corollary anti-tumor immunity may be bolstered therapeutically as a consequence of administering agents (i.e., antagonist antibodies or DC genetically engineered to produce specific inhibitors locoregionally in the TME) that are capable of blocking the action of BTLA or CD160 *in vivo*.

ACKNOWLEDGMENTS

This work was supported by NIH R01 grant CA169118 (Walter J. Storkus). This project used the University of Pittburgh Cancer Institute's Vector Core Facility supported by the NIH CCSG award P30 CA047904.

REFERENCES

1. Nierkens S, Tel J, Janssen E, Adema GJ. Antigen cross-presentation by dendritic cell subsets: one general or all sergeants? *Trends Immunol* (2013) **34**:361–70. doi:10.1016/j.it.2013.02.007
2. Apetoh L, Locher C, Ghiringhelli F, Kroemer G, Zitvogel L. Harnessing dendritic cells in cancer. *Semin Immunol* (2011) **23**:42–9. doi:10.1016/j.smim.2011.01.003
3. Melief CJ. Cancer immunotherapy by dendritic cells. *Immunity* (2008) **29**:372–83. doi:10.1016/j.immuni.2008.08.004
4. Mueller SN, Gebhardt T, Carbone FR, Heath WR. Memory T cell subsets, migration patterns, and tissue residence. *Annu Rev Immunol* (2013) **31**:137–61. doi:10.1146/annurev-immunol-032712-095954
5. Chen L, Taylor JL, Sabins NC, Lowe DB, Qu Y, You Z, et al. Extranodal induction of therapeutic immunity in the tumor microenvironment after intratumoral delivery of Tbet gene-modified dendritic cells. *Cancer Gene Ther* (2013) **20**:469–77. doi:10.1038/cgt.2013.42
6. Fridman WH, Dieu-Nosjean MC, Pagès F, Cremer I, Damotte D, Sautès-Fridman C, et al. The immune microenvironment of human tumors: general significance and clinical impact. *Cancer Microenviron* (2013) **6**:117–22. doi:10.1007/s12307-012-0124-9
7. Thompson ED, Enriquez HL, Fu YX, Engelhard VH. Tumor masses support naive T cell infiltration, activation, and differentiation into effectors. *J Exp Med* (2010) **207**:1791–804. doi:10.1084/jem.20092454
8. Schrama D, Voigt H, Eggert AO, Xiang R, Zhou H, Schumacher TN, et al. Immunological tumor destruction in a murine melanoma model by targeted LTα independent of secondary lymphoid tissue. *Cancer Immunol Immunother* (2008) **57**:85–95. doi:10.1007/s00262-007-0352-x
9. Yu P, Lee Y, Liu W, Chin RK, Wang J, Wang Y, et al. Priming of naive T cells inside tumors leads to eradication of established tumors. *Nat Immunol* (2004) **5**:141–9. doi:10.1038/ni1029
10. Carragher DM, Rangel-Moreno J, Randall TD. Ectopic lymphoid tissues and local immunity. *Semin Immunol* (2008) **20**:26–42. doi:10.1016/j.smim.2007.12.004
11. Mebius RE, Rennert P, Weissman IL. Developing lymph nodes collect $CD4^+CD3^-LT\beta^+$ cells that can differentiate to APC, NK cells, and follicular cells but not T or B cells. *Immunity* (1997) **7**:493–504. doi:10.1016/S1074-7613(00)80371-4
12. Bénézech C, Mader E, Desanti G, Khan M, Nakamura K, White A, et al. Lymphotoxin-β receptor signaling through NF-κB2-RelB pathway reprograms adipocyte precursors as lymph node stromal cells. *Immunity* (2012) **37**:721–34. doi:10.1016/j.immuni.2012.06.010
13. Stranford S, Ruddle NH. Follicular dendritic cells, conduits, lymphatic vessels, and high endothelial venules in tertiary lymphoid organs: parallels with lymph node stroma. *Front Immunol* (2012) **3**:350. doi:10.3389/fimmu.2012.00350
14. Randall TD, Carragher DM, Rangel-Moreno J. Development of secondary lymphoid organs. *Annu Rev Immunol* (2008) **26**:627–50. doi:10.1146/annurev.immunol.26.021607.090257
15. Cupedo T, Jansen W, Kraal G, Mebius RE. Induction of secondary and tertiary lymphoid structures in the skin. *Immunity* (2004) **21**:655–67. doi:10.1016/j.immuni.2004.09.006
16. de Chaisemartin L, Goc J, Damotte D, Validire P, Magdeleinat P, Alifano M, et al. Characterization of chemokines and adhesion molecules associated with T cell presence in tertiary lymphoid structures in human lung cancer. *Cancer Res* (2011) **71**:6391–9. doi:10.1158/0008-5472.CAN-11-0952
17. Sato M, Hirayama S, Matsuda Y, Wagnetz D, Hwang DM, Guan Z, et al. Stromal activation and formation of lymphoid-like stroma in chronic lung allograft dysfunction. *Transplantation* (2011) **91**:1398–405. doi:10.1097/TP.0b013e31821b2f7a
18. Drayton DL, Ying X, Lee J, Lesslauer W, Ruddle NH. Ectopic LTα/β directs lymphoid organ neogenesis with concomitant expression of peripheral node addressin and a HEV-restricted sulfotransferase. *J Exp Med* (2003) **197**:1153–63. doi:10.1084/jem.20021761
19. Ruddle NH. Lymphoid neo-organogenesis: lymphotoxin's role in inflammation and development. *Immunol Res* (1999) **19**:119–25. doi:10.1007/BF02786481
20. Comerford I, Harata-Lee Y, Bunting MD, Gregor C, Kara EE, McColl SR. A myriad of functions and complex regulation of the CCR7/CCL19/CCL21 chemokine axis in the adaptive immune system. *Cytokine Growth Factor Rev* (2013) **24**:269–83. doi:10.1016/j.cytogfr.2013.03.001
21. Link A, Vogt TK, Favre S, Britschgi MR, Acha-Orbea H, Hinz B. Fibroblastic reticular cells in lymph nodes regulate the homeostasis of naive T cells. *Nat Immunol* (2007) **8**:1255–65. doi:10.1038/ni1513
22. Luther SA, Tang HL, Hyman PL, Farr AG, Cyster JG. Coexpression of the chemokines ELC and SLC by T zone stromal cells and deletion of the ELC gene in the plt/plt mouse. *Proc Natl Acad Sci U S A* (2000) **97**:12694–9. doi:10.1073/pnas.97.23.12694
23. Shannon LA, McBurney TM, Wells MA, Roth ME, Calloway PA, Bill CA, et al. CCR7/CCL19 controls expression of EDG-1 in T cells. *J Biol Chem* (2012) **287**:11656–64. doi:10.1074/jbc.M111.310045
24. Britschgi MR, Link A, Lissandrin TK, Luther SA. Dynamic modulation of CCR7 expression and function on naive T lymphocytes *in vivo*. *J Immunol* (2008) **181**:7681–8.
25. Pham TH, Okada T, Matloubian M, Lo CG, Cyster JG. S1P1 receptor signaling overrides retention mediated by G alpha I-coupled receptors to promote T cell egress. *Immunity* (2007) **28**:122–33. doi:10.1016/j.immuni.2007.11.017
26. Pabst O, Herbrand H, Bernhardt G, Förster R. Elucidating the functional anatomy of secondary lymphoid organs. *Curr Opin Immunol* (2004) **16**:394–9. doi:10.1016/j.coi.2004.05.014
27. Weyand CM, Goronzy JJ. Ectopic germinal center formation in rheumatoid synovitis. *Ann N Y Acad Sci* (2003) **987**:140–9. doi:10.1111/j.1749-6632.2003.tb06042.x
28. Kim EA, Lee KS, Johkoh T, Kim TS, Suh GY, Kwon OJ, et al. Interstitial lung diseases associated with collagen vascular diseases: radiologic and histopathologic findings. *Radiographics* (2002) **22**:S151–65. doi:10.1148/radiographics.22.suppl_1.g02oc04s151
29. Rangel-Moreno J, Hartson L, Navarro C, Gaxiola M, Selman M, Randall TD. Inducible bronchus-associated lymphoid tissue (iBALT) in patients with pulmonary complications of rheumatoid arthritis. *J Clin Invest* (2006) **116**:3183–94. doi:10.1172/JCI28756
30. Cañete JD, Santiago B, Cantaert T, Sanmartí R, Palacin A, Celis R, et al. Ectopic lymphoid neogenesis in psoriatic arthritis. *Ann Rheum Dis* (2007) **66**:720–6. doi:10.1136/ard.2006.062042
31. Dresch C, Leverrier Y, Marvel J, Shortman K. Development of antigen cross-presentation capacity in dendritic cells. *Trends Immunol* (2012) **33**:381–8. doi:10.1016/j.it.2012.04.009
32. Winter S, Rehm A, Wichner K, Scheel T, Batra A, Siegmund B, et al. Manifestation of spontaneous and early autoimmune gastritis in CCR7-deficient mice. *Am J Pathol* (2011) **179**:754–65. doi:10.1016/j.ajpath.2011.04.012
33. Heath WR, Belz GT, Behrens GM, Smith CM, Forehan SP, Parish IA, et al. Cross-presentation, dendritic cell subsets, and the generation of immunity to cellular antigens. *Immunol Rev* (2004) **199**:9–26. doi:10.1111/j.0105-2896.2004.00142.x
34. López De Padilla CM, Vallejo AN, Lacomis D, McNallan K, Reed AM. Extranodal lymphoid microstructures in inflamed muscle and disease severity of new-onset juvenile dermatomyositis. *Arthritis Rheum* (2009) **60**:1160–72. doi:10.1002/art.24411
35. Bombardieri M, Pitzalis C. Ectopic lymphoid neogenesis and lymphoid chemokines in Sjogren's syndrome: at the interplay between chronic inflammation, autoimmunity and lymphomagenesis. *Curr Pharm Biotechnol* (2012) **13**:1989–96. doi:10.2174/138920112802273209
36. GeurtsvanKessel CH, Willart MA, Bergen IM, van Rijt LS, Muskens F, Elewaut D, et al. Dendritic cells are crucial for maintenance of tertiary lymphoid structures

in the lung of influenza virus-infected mice. *J Exp Med* (2009) **206**:2339–49. doi:10.1084/jem.20090410

37. Mosnier JF, Degott C, Marcellin P, Hénin D, Erlinger S, Benhamou JP. The intraportal lymphoid nodule and its environment in chronic active hepatitis C: an immunohistochemical study. *Hepatology* (1993) **17**:366–71. doi:10.1002/hep.1840170304
38. Mazzucchelli L, Blaser A, Kappeler A, Schärli P, Laissue JA, Baggiolini M, et al. BCA-1 is highly expressed in *Helicobacter pylori*-induced mucosa-associated lymphoid tissue and gastric lymphoma. *J Clin Invest* (1999) **104**:R49–54. doi:10.1172/JCI7830
39. McMahon EJ, Bailey SL, Castenada CV, Waldner H, Miller SD. Epitope spreading initiates in the CNS in two mouse models of multiple sclerosis. *Nat Med* (2005) **11**:335–9. doi:10.1038/nm1202
40. van Baren N, Coulie PG. Ongoing adaptive immune responses in the microenvironment of melanoma metastases. *Ann N Y Acad Sci* (2013) **1284**:62–5. doi:10.1111/nyas.12093
41. Messina JL, Fenstermacher DA, Eschrich S, Qu X, Berglund AE, Lloyd MC, et al. 12-Chemokine gene signature identifies lymph node-like structures in melanoma: potential for patient selection for immunotherapy? *Sci Rep* (2012) **2**:765. doi:10.1038/srep00765
42. Pagès F, Galon J, Dieu-Nosjean MC, Tartour E, Sautès-Fridman C, Fridman WH. Immune infiltration in human tumors: a prognostic factor that should not be ignored. *Oncogene* (2010) **29**:1093–102. doi:10.1038/onc.2009.416
43. Dieu-Nosjean MC, Antoine M, Danel C, Heudes D, Wislez M, Poulot V, et al. Long-term survival for patients with non-small-cell lung cancer with intratumoral lymphoid structures. *J Clin Oncol* (2008) **26**:4410–7. doi:10.1200/JCO.2007.15.0284
44. Martinet L, Filleron T, Le Guellec S, Rochaix P, Garrido I, Girard JP. High endothelial venule blood vessels for tumor-infiltrating lymphocytes are associated with lymphotoxin β-producing dendritic cells in human breast cancer. *J Immunol* (2013) **19**:2001–8. doi:10.4049/jimmunol.1300872
45. Gu-Trantien C, Loi S, Garaud S, Equeter C, Libin M, de Wind A, et al. $CD4^+$ follicular helper T cell infiltration predicts breast cancer survival. *J Clin Invest* (2013) **123**:2873–92. doi:10.1172/JCI67428
46. Onder L, Danuser R, Scandella E, Firner S, Chai Q, Hehlgans T, et al. Endothelial cell-specific lymphotoxin-β receptor signaling is critical for lymph node and high endothelial venule formation. *J Exp Med* (2013) **210**:465–73. doi:10.1084/jem.20121462
47. Kanodia S, Da Silva DM, Karamanukyan T, Bogaert L, Fu YX, Kast WM. Expression of LIGHT/TNFSF14 combined with vaccination against human papillomavirus Type 16 E7 induces significant tumor regression. *Cancer Res* (2010) **70**:3955–64. doi:10.1158/0008-5472.CAN-09-3773
48. Loeffler M, Le'Negrate G, Krajewska M, Reed JC. Attenuated *Salmonella* engineered to produce human cytokine LIGHT inhibit tumor growth. *Proc Natl Acad Sci U S A* (2007) **104**:12879–83. doi:10.1073/pnas.0701959104
49. Lee Y, Chin RK, Christiansen P, Sun Y, Tumanov AV, Wang J, et al. Recruitment and activation of naive T cells in the islets by lymphotoxin beta receptor-dependent tertiary lymphoid structure. *Immunity* (2006) **25**:499–509. doi:10.1016/j.immuni.2006.06.016
50. Suna S, Sakata Y, Sato H, Mizuno H, Nakatani D, Shimizu M, et al. Up-regulation of cell adhesion molecule genes in human endothelial cells stimulated by lymphotoxin-α: DNA microarray analysis. *J Atheroscler Thromb* (2008) **15**:160–5. doi:10.5551/jat.E553
51. Madge LA, Kluger MS, Orange JS, May MJ. Lymphotoxin-α1/β2 and LIGHT induce classical and noncanonical NF-κB-dependent pro-inflammatory gene expression in vascular endothelial cells. *J Immunol* (2008) **180**:3467–77.
52. Morel Y, Truneh A, Costello RT, Olive D. LIGHT, a new TNF superfamily member, is essential for memory T helper cell-mediated activation of dendritic cells. *Eur J Immunol* (2003) **33**:3213–9. doi:10.1002/eji.200324410
53. Xu G, Liu D, Okwor I, Wang Y, Korner H, Kung SK, et al. LIGHT is critical for IL-12 production by dendritic cells, optimal CD4+ Th1 cell response, and resistance to *Leishmania major*. *J Immunol* (2007) **179**:6901–9.
54. Nielsen JS, Nelson BH. Tumor-infiltrating B cells and T cells: working together to promote patient survival. *Oncoimmunology* (2012) **1**:1623–5. doi:10.4161/onci.21650
55. Moussion C, Girard JP. Dendritic cells control lymphocyte entry to lymph nodes through high endothelial venules. *Nature* (2011) **479**:542–6. doi:10.1038/nature10540
56. Muniz LR, Pacer ME, Lira SA, Furtado GC. A critical role for dendritic cells in the formation of lymphatic vessels within tertiary lymphoid structures. *J Immunol* (2011) **187**:828–34. doi:10.4049/jimmunol.1004233
57. Wendland M, Willenzon S, Kocks J, Davalos-Misslitz AC, Hammerschmidt SI, Schumann K, et al. Lymph node T cell homeostasis relies on steady state homing of dendritic cells. *Immunity* (2011) **35**:945–57. doi:10.1016/j.immuni.2011.10.017
58. Lo JC, Chin RK, Lee Y, Kang HS, Wang Y, Weinstock JV, et al. Differential regulation of CCL21 in lymphoid/nonlymphoid tissues for effectively attracting T cells to peripheral tissues. *J Clin Invest* (2003) **112**:1495–505. doi:10.1172/JCI200319188
59. Paya CV, Kenmotsu N, Schoon RA, Leibson PJ. Tumor necrosis factor and lymphotoxin secretion by human natural killer cells leads to antiviral cytotoxicity. *J Immunol* (1988) **141**:1989–95.
60. Pablos JL, Santiago B, Tsay D, Singer MS, Palao G, Galindo M, et al. A HEV-restricted sulfotransferase is expressed in rheumatoid arthritis synovium and is induced by lymphotoxin-α/β and TNF-α in cultured endothelial cells. *BMC Immunol* (2005) **6**:6. doi:10.1186/1471-2172-6-6
61. Kar UK, Srivastava MK, Andersson A, Baratelli F, Huang M, Kickhoefer VA, et al. Novel CCL21-vault nanocapsule intratumoral delivery inhibits lung cancer growth. *PLoS One* (2011) **6**:e18758. doi:10.1371/journal.pone.0018758
62. Kanagawa N, Niwa M, Hatanaka Y, Tani Y, Nakagawa S, Fujita T, et al. CC-chemokine ligand 17 gene therapy induces tumor regression through augmentation of tumor-infiltrating immune cells in a murine model of preexisting CT26 colon carcinoma. *Int J Cancer* (2007) **121**:2013–22. doi:10.1002/ijc.22908
63. Marinkovic T, Garin A, Yokota Y, Fu YX, Ruddle NH, Furtado GC, et al. Interaction of mature $CD3^+CD4^+$ T cells with dendritic cells triggers the development of tertiary lymphoid structures in the thyroid. *J Clin Invest* (2006) **116**:2622–32. doi:10.1172/JCI28993
64. Yang SC, Batra RK, Hillinger S, Reckamp KL, Strieter RM, Dubinett SM, et al. Intrapulmonary administration of CCL21 gene-modified dendritic cells reduces tumor burden in spontaneous murine bronchoalveolar cell carcinoma. *Cancer Res* (2006) **66**:3205–13. doi:10.1158/0008-5472.CAN-05-3619
65. Yang SC, Hillinger S, Riedl K, Zhang L, Zhu L, Huang M, et al. Intratumoral administration of dendritic cells overexpressing CCL21 generates systemic antitumor responses and confers tumor immunity. *Clin Cancer Res* (2004) **10**:2891–901. doi:10.1158/1078-0432.CCR-03-0380
66. Hillinger S, Yang SC, Zhu L, Huang M, Duckett R, Atianzar K, et al. EBV-induced molecule 1 ligand chemokine (ELC/CCL19) promotes IFN-gamma-dependent antitumor responses in a lung cancer model. *J Immunol* (2003) **171**:6457–65.
67. Nomura T, Hasegawa H, Kohno M, Sasaki M, Fujita S. Enhancement of anti-tumor immunity by tumor cells transfected with the secondary lymphoid tissue chemokine EBI-1-ligand chemokine and stromal cell-derived factor-1α chemokine genes. *Int J Cancer* (2001) **91**:597–606. doi:10.1002/1097-0215(200002)9999:9999<::AID-IJC1107<3.0.CO;2-J
68. Kirk CJ, Hartigan-O'Connor D, Nickoloff BJ, Chamberlain JS, Giedlin M, Aukerman L, et al. T cell-dependent antitumor immunity mediated by secondary lymphoid tissue chemokine: augmentation of dendritic cell-based immunotherapy. *Cancer Res* (2001) **61**:2062–70.
69. Sharma S, Stolina M, Zhu L, Lin Y, Batra R, Huang M, et al. Secondary lymphoid organ chemokine reduces pulmonary tumor burden in spontaneous murine bronchoalveolar cell carcinoma. *Cancer Res* (2001) **61**:6406–12.
70. Sharma S, Stolina M, Luo J, Strieter RM, Burdick M, Zhu LX, et al. Secondary lymphoid tissue chemokine mediates T cell-dependent antitumor responses *in vivo*. *J Immunol* (2000) **164**:4558–63.
71. Mounzer RH, Svendsen OS, Baluk P, Bergman CM, Padera TP, Wiig H, et al. Lymphotoxin-α contributes to lymphangiogenesis. *Blood* (2010) **116**:2173–82. doi:10.1182/blood-2009-12-256065
72. Mac Keon S, Gazzaniga S, Mallerman J, Bravo AI, Mordoh J, Wainstok R. Vaccination with dendritic cells charged with apoptotic/necrotic B16 melanoma induces the formation of subcutaneous lymphoid tissue. *Vaccine* (2010) **28**:8162–8. doi:10.1016/j.vaccine.2010.09.095
73. Kobayashi Y, Kato K, Watanabe T. Synthesis of functional artificial lymphoid tissues. *Discov Med* (2011) **12**:351–62.
74. Ware CF. Targeting lymphocyte activation through the lymphotoxin and LIGHT pathways. *Immunol Rev* (2008) **223**:186–201. doi:10.1111/j.1600-065X.2008.00629.x

75. Lukashev M, LePage D, Wilson C, Bailly V, Garber E, Lukashin A, et al. Targeting the lymphotoxin-β receptor with agonist antibodies as a potential cancer therapy. *Cancer Res* (2006) **66**:9617–24. doi:10.1158/0008-5472.CAN-06-0217
76. Liang CM, Ye SL, Zhong CP, Zheng N, Bian W, Sun RX, et al. More than chemotaxis: a new anti-tumor DC vaccine modified by rAAV2-SLC. *Mol Immunol* (2007) **44**:3797–804. doi:10.1016/j.molimm.2007.03.026
77. Terando A, Roessler B, Mulé JJ. Chemokine gene modification of human dendritic cell-based tumor vaccines using a recombinant adenoviral vector. *Cancer Gene Ther* (2004) **11**:165–73. doi:10.1038/sj.cgt.7700671
78. Tripodi D, Conti F, Rosati M, Maccauro G, Saggini A, Cianchetti E, et al. IL-36 a new member of the IL-1 family cytokines. *J Biol Regul Homeost Agents* (2012) **26**:7–14.
79. Vigne S, Palmer G, Martin P, Lamacchia C, Strebel D, Rodriguez E, et al. IL-36 signaling amplifies Th1 responses by enhancing proliferation and Th1 polarization of naive $CD4^+$ T cells. *Blood* (2012) **120**:3478–87. doi:10.1182/blood-2012-06-439026
80. Frey S, Derer A, Messbacher ME, Baeten DL, Bugatti S, Montecucco C, et al. The novel cytokine interleukin-36 is expressed in psoriatic and rheumatoid arthritis synovium. *Ann Rheum Dis* (2013) **72**:1569–74. doi:10.1136/annrheumdis-2012-202264
81. Shaik Y, Sabatino G, Maccauro G, Varvara G, Murmura G, Saggini A, et al. IL-36 receptor antagonist with special emphasis on IL-38. *Int J Immunopathol Pharmacol* (2013) **26**:27–36.
82. Vigne S, Palmer G, Lamacchia C, Martin P, Talabot-Ayer D, Rodriguez E, et al. IL-36R ligands are potent regulators of dendritic and T cells. *Blood* (2011) **118**:5813–23. doi:10.1182/blood-2011-05-356873
83. Wang FH, Li YH, Li S, Jiang WQ, Guan ZZ. [Phase I clinical trial of intravenous recombinant human lymphotoxin-alpha derivative]. *Ai Zheng* (2006) **25**: 501–4.
84. Baratelli F, Takedatsu H, Hazra S, Peebles K, Luo J, Kurimoto PS, et al. Preclinical characterization of GMP grade CCL21-gene modified dendritic cells for application in a phase I trial in non-small cell lung cancer. *J Transl Med* (2008) **6**:38. doi:10.1186/1479-5876-6-38
85. Mulé JJ. Dendritic cell-based vaccines for pancreatic cancer and melanoma. *Ann N Y Acad Sci* (2009) **1174**:33–40. doi:10.1111/j.1749-6632.2009.04936.x
86. Pasero C, Speiser DE, Derré L, Olive D. The HVEM network: new directions in targeting novel costimulatory/co-inhibitory molecules for cancer therapy. *Curr Opin Pharmacol* (2012) **12**:478–85. doi:10.1016/j.coph.2012.03.001
87. Steinberg MW, Cheung TC, Ware CF. The signaling networks of the herpesvirus entry mediator (TNFRSF14) in immune regulation. *Immunol Rev* (2011) **244**:169–87. doi:10.1111/j.1600-065X.2011.01064.x
88. Cai G, Freeman GJ. The CD160, BTLA, LIGHT/HVEM pathway: a bidirectional switch regulating T-cell activation. *Immunol Rev* (2009) **229**:244–58. doi:10.1111/j.1600-065X.2009.00783.x
89. De Trez C, Schneider K, Potter K, Droin N, Fulton J, Norris PS, et al. The inhibitory HVEM-BTLA pathway counter regulates lymphotoxin receptor signaling to achieve homeostasis of dendritic cells. *J Immunol* (2008) **180**:238–48.
90. Granger SW, Rickert S. LIGHT-HVEM signaling and the regulation of T cell-mediated immunity. *Cytokine Growth Factor Rev* (2003) **14**:289–96. doi:10.1016/S1359-6101(03)00031-5

5

Pre-clustering of the B cell antigen receptor demonstrated by mathematically extended electron microscopy

Gina J. Fiala[1,2,3†], **Daniel Kaschek**[4†], **Britta Blumenthal**[1,5], **Michael Reth**[1,3,6], **Jens Timmer**[3,4] **and Wolfgang W. A. Schamel**[1,3,5 *]

[1] *Faculty of Biology, Department of Molecular Immunology, Albert Ludwigs University Freiburg, Freiburg, Germany*
[2] *Spemann Graduate School of Biology and Medicine (SGBM), Albert Ludwigs University Freiburg, Freiburg, Germany*
[3] *Centre for Biological Signalling Studies BIOSS, Albert Ludwigs University Freiburg, Freiburg, Germany*
[4] *Institute of Physics, Albert Ludwigs University Freiburg, Freiburg, Germany*
[5] *Medical Faculty, Centre for Chronic Immunodeficiency CCI, University Clinics Freiburg, Albert Ludwigs University Freiburg, Freiburg, Germany*
[6] *Max Planck-Institute of Immunobiology and Epigenetics, Freiburg, Germany*

Edited by:
Carmen Molina-Paris, University of Leeds, UK

Reviewed by:
Shiv Pillai, Harvard Medical School, USA
To-Ha Thai, Beth Deaconess Israel Medical Center, USA

***Correspondence:**
Wolfgang W. A. Schamel, Faculty of Biology, Department of Molecular Immunology, Albert Ludwigs University Freiburg, Schänzle Straße 18, Freiburg 79104, Germany
e-mail: wolfgang.schamel@biologie.uni-freiburg.de

[†] *Gina J. Fiala and Daniel Kaschek have contributed equally to this work.*

The B cell antigen receptor (BCR) plays a crucial role in adaptive immunity, since antigen-induced signaling by the BCR leads to the activation of the B cell and production of antibodies during an immune response. However, the spatial nano-scale organization of the BCR on the cell surface prior to antigen encounter is still controversial. Here, we fixed murine B cells, stained the BCRs on the cell surface with immuno-gold and visualized the distribution of the gold particles by transmission electron microscopy. Approximately 30% of the gold particles were clustered. However the low staining efficiency of 15% precluded a quantitative conclusion concerning the oligomerization state of the BCRs. To overcome this limitation, we used Monte-Carlo simulations to include or to exclude possible distributions of the BCRs. Our combined experimental-modeling approach assuming the lowest number of different BCR sizes to explain the observed gold distribution suggests that 40% of the surface IgD-BCR was present in dimers and 60% formed large laminar clusters of about 18 receptors. In contrast, a transmembrane mutant of the mIgD molecule only formed IgD-BCR dimers. Our approach complements high resolution fluorescence imaging and clearly demonstrates the existence of pre-formed BCR clusters on resting B cells, questioning the classical cross-linking model of BCR activation.

Keywords: BCR, oligomerization, electron microscopy, immuno-gold-labeling, Monte Carlo simulation, maximum-likelihood method

1. INTRODUCTION

Cells communicate with each other and with their surroundings through transmembrane receptors that are embedded in the plasma membrane. Thus, it is of high interest to understand how these receptors and other cell surface proteins, such as adhesion molecules or channels, are organized on the membrane. Initially it was thought that proteins and lipids freely diffuse in membranes and that they are randomly distributed (1). With the concept of lipid rafts it was noted that specialized microdomains on the cell surface exist, where some proteins are concentrated and others are excluded (2). Although the raft concept had to be modified, since in biological membranes they are smaller and more transient than in artificial model membranes (3), it is clear that proteins are not randomly distributed on the cell surface. One example of the immune system is the T cell antigen receptor that can form pre-clustered oligomers, called nanoclusters, on T cells (4–7). Nanoclusters form before and independently of any ligand encounter. Interestingly, T cells can control the degree of TCR nanoclustering, in order to regulate their avidity toward multivalent ligands and thus their sensitivity (8–10). This indicates that studying the nano-scale distribution of a receptor contributes to the understanding of the function of the receptor. Less well understood is a potential pre-clustering of the B cell antigen receptor (BCR). The BCR is expressed on B cells and controls the development of these cells and their activation upon contact with the BCR's ligand, called antigen. The BCR is composed of the membrane-bound immunoglobulin (mIg) molecule and a heterodimer of the Igα (mb-1) and Igβ (B29) proteins (11). The mIg molecule binds to the antigen and exists in different isotypes, of which the mIgD form is the most abundant one on resting mature B cells (12, 13). The Igα/Igβ dimer contains phosphorylatable tyrosines in the cytoplasmic tails (14) and transmits the signal of antigen-binding to the cytoplasmic signaling machinery. The first evidence for BCR pre-clustering, i.e., the existence of BCR oligomers, was obtained by Blue Native gel electrophoresis (15–17). Upon extraction of the IgD- and IgM-BCRs from the cell membrane of resting B cells using low concentrations of detergent, the BCRs were found in oligomers. Importantly, a mutant mIgD molecule, in which the transmembrane region was mutated (called mIgD-hSbap), only formed dimers (16). Thus, in the BCR as well as in the TCR (10), the transmembrane region of the ligand-binding subunits is involved in the pre-clustering. Later, three approaches were used to investigate whether the BCR forms oligomers in living cells. Firstly, a FRET approach was used, and oligomers were not detected (18). Secondly, a bifluorescence complementation approach was used, and BCR oligomers were detected (19). The differences in these two procedures and possible functional implications of pre-clustered BCR oligomers were recently discussed (20). Thirdly, the superresolution microscopy method direct stochastic optical reconstruction microscopy (dSTORM) was used to show that BCRs were organized as pre-clusters on the surface of resting primary B cells (21). Here, we used a validated technique, that we had previously used to study TCR pre-clustering (6, 8), in order to answer the question of whether BCR oligomers exist and if yes what their sizes are. To this end, we used fixed B cells and labeled the BCRs with specific antibodies that were bound to gold particles (immuno-gold-staining), prepared cell surface replicas and analyzed the nano-scale distribution of the gold particles by transmission electron microscopy (TEM). This approach allowed visualization of BCRs on cell surface areas that do not adhere to any experimental support, giving the opportunity to analyze untouched (and non-modified) receptors. A general challenge of immuno-gold-labeling is its low staining efficiency, which is compensated by mathematical modeling and statistical methods, allowing solid conclusions to be drawn from the experimental data.

2. MATERIALS AND METHODS

2.1. EXPERIMENTAL PROCEDURES

2.1.1. *Cell culture and cell fixation*

The murine B cell lines J558L (not expressing any BCR) and J558Lδm/mb-1flN (expressing an IgD-BCR) were previously described (16). We also used a J558L line that expressed a mutant IgD-BCR, in which the transmembrane region of the mIgD molecule was mutated (mIgD-hSbap) (16). Cells were cultured in RPMI 1640 complete medium supplemented with 10% fetal calf serum, 2 mM L-glutamine, 100 U/ml penicillin/streptomycin, 10 mM HEPES, and 50 mM 2-mercaptoethanol and grown at 37°C in a humidified atmosphere with 5% CO2. Cells were fixed with freshly prepared, ice-cold 4% paraformaldehyde in PBS for 20 min at 4°C at a cell density of 10×10^6 cells/ml. After fixing, cells were washed twice with cold PBS.

2.1.2. *Immuno-gold-staining and analysis of gold-reagent*

Unstimulated PFA-fixed cells were stained with the primary anti-idiotypic antibody Ac146 (22) at saturating concentration of 20 mg/ml in PBS with 1% BSA for 1 h on ice. This antibody binds to the variable regions of the BCR used in this study. Staining with a secondary anti-mouse IgG antibody conjugated to 10 nm gold (Aurion) was performed for 1 h on ice. Prior to cell staining, the aggregation state of the gold-reagent was tested by adsorbing diluted suspensions of the gold-reagent onto collodion/carbon-coated EM grids, which were analyzed in transmission electron microscopy (TEM, **Figure 2**).

2.1.3. *Surface replica preparation*

Labeled cells were adsorbed to L-poly-lysine-treated micas, followed by a second fixation with 0.1% glutaraldehyde on ice for 30 min. Micas containing stained cells were covered with an untreated piece of mica and fast-frozen in a Reichert-Jung (now Leica) KF-80 plunge freezing unit using the secondary cryogen liquid ethane. Metal replicas were prepared in a freeze fracture unit (BAF 060; BAL-TEC) where the cell-containing mica slide was freeze-etched at −150°C for 12 min to sublime surface ice. Frozen cells were then shadowed with 2 nm of evaporated platinum at an angle of 45°C and strengthened by a uniformly thick 20 nm electron-translucent carbon layer evaporated perpendicular to the mica surface plane. The metal replica of the surface was released from the mica by floating it on commercial bleach where it remained over night for digestion of the organic material. The floating replica was washed three times in distilled water to remove attached organic material and chemicals and then picked up on uncoated copper EM grids. For a detailed protocol see Ref. (23).

2.1.4. *Analysis of metal replicas by TEM*

Replicas mounted on EM grids were examined in a transmission electron microscope (1200-EX II; JOEL) operating at 100 kV. Gold particle numbers and the gold cluster size distribution were counted and analyzed for at least 3 cells per sample at an augmentation of 25000. Gold particles were considered to be part of the same cluster when they were adjacent or less distant than 10 nm (the diameter of a single gold particle), taking into account that the diameter of the BCR is around 10 nm (24). Pictures were taken at augmentations of 5000 (cell overview), 120000, and 300000 (gold-labeling).

2.1.5. *Quantification of the number of BCRs per cell*

The number of BCRs per cell was determined based on a saturation binding assay. About 1×10^6 J558Lδm/mb-1flN cells were stained for 30 min at 4°C with increasing concentrations of an FITC-coupled anti-IgD antibody (BD Pharmingen, clone 11-26c.2a). Following 5 extensive washing steps, the fluorescence signal was measured in duplicates using a SpectraMax 190 Absorbance Microplate Reader. In order to convert the fluorescence signal intensity into the number of antibodies, a calibration of the antibody was performed by fitting the model $y = mx + b$ to the standard concentrations x and fluorescence signals y. Here m denotes the slope and b denotes the intercept of the calibration curve. In order to infer the number of receptors on the cells, antibody was spotted in different concentrations. The saturation model $y = y_0 + \frac{ax}{b+x}$ was fitted to the sample data. Here, x denotes the antibody concentration and y denotes the fluorescence signal after washing. The parameter y_0 was measured explicitly. The remaining parameters, i.e., the maximal fluorescence signal gain a and the saturation constant b were estimated from the data. From the maximum signal gain a, the corresponding concentration of bound antibody was computed from the calibration curve, i.e., $\Delta x = \frac{a}{m}$. Finally, the number of receptors per cell was computed by the formula $n = \frac{\Delta x \cdot N_A \cdot V}{k \cdot N_{\text{cells}} \cdot M}$, where $N_A = 6.022 \times 10^{23}$ 1/mol, $V = 50\ \mu$l, $k = 2$, $N_{\text{cells}} = 5 \times 10^5$, and $M = 146.389 \times 10^3$ g/mol denote Avogadros constant, the volume per well, the number antibody binding sites per receptor, the number of cells, and the molecular weight of the antibody. From the parameters obtained by the calibration and saturation curve, we get $n = 122400 \pm 7500$. The uncertainty of the number of receptors per cell is dominated by the uncertainty of a, the maximum signal gain. The uncertainty of a is propagated to the error of n by Gaussian error propagation.

2.2. MONTE-CARLO SIMULATION OF OBSERVED GOLD CLUSTER SIZE DISTRIBUTION

The immuno-gold-staining and counting process was simulated by a Monte-Carlo approach. It is assumed that the observed gold cluster size distribution is a superposition of distributions generated by single size oligomers. Each oligomer size produces a characteristic distribution of observed gold cluster sizes that depends on the staining efficiency. The characteristic distribution ranges from exclusively monomeric observation to exclusively single size oligomeric observation for staining probabilities zero and one, respectively. The distributions in between zero and one depend on the oligomer geometry, which is reflected by the number of next neighbors of an average receptor. This number is at least 2, i.e., for linear arrangement of the receptors. For other cases, like dense circle packing resulting in a triangular geometry it is 6 and for a quadratic grid it is 8. Simulations have been performed for linear arrangements and quadratic grids which reflect different extremes. An additional factor for the observed size distribution is the gold-reagent itself, which is potentially pre-clustered. Further, the staining efficiency, i.e., the number of receptors that are stained; the geometry, i.e., the receptor positions within the oligomers being stained; and potential unspecific stainings, i.e., presence of gold particles that are not bound to any BCR, have to be considered. For given oligomer size, staining efficiency, geometry, and gold distribution, the observed gold cluster size distribution is obtained by repeated random number generation for the number of stained receptors, their positions and the number of gold particles per staining spot. For each set of random numbers, the resulting representation of the gold particle pattern is evaluated by the simulation program and the number of counted monomers, dimers, etc., is collected. This procedure was performed 10^5 times for 10 staining probabilities between 2 and 40%, underlying BCR oligomer sizes from 1 to 40 and three geometries, i.e., linear, triangular, and quadratic. In addition, the simulation approach has been adapted to explain the observation of the gold-reagent control experiment.

2.3. STATISTICAL INFERENCE

The result of each gold-staining experiment is a distribution of gold cluster sizes determined from gold particle counting in the microscope. These experimental data are compared to the simulated data and by means of statistical methods it is decided whether simulation and experiment are in accordance. We tested four major hypotheses: receptors are organized as:

1. BCR oligomers of a unique fixed size s,
2. BCR monomers and oligomers of a unique fixed size s,
3. BCR dimers and oligomers of a unique fixed size s,
4. BCR monomers, dimers, and oligomers of a unique fixed size s.

For each hypothesis, a likelihood function is derived based on the assumption of Poisson statistics for the counted gold oligomers. The corresponding log-likelihood reads

$$l(\theta) = \sum_i m_i(\theta) - N_i \log(m_i(\theta)) + \sum_{k=1}^{N_i} \log k, \qquad (1)$$

where m_i is the number of expected BCR oligomers of size i predicted by the simulation and N_i is the number of gold oligomers counted in the experiment. Minimization is performed with respect to the parameter vector θ which is defined differently for each hypothesis. This is explicitly

$$m_i^{(1)}(\theta) = \theta \cdot n_{i,sim}(s), \qquad (2)$$

$$m_i^{(2)}(\theta) = \theta_1 \cdot n_{i,sim}(1) + \theta_2 \cdot n_{i,sim}(s), \qquad (3)$$

$$m_i^{(3)}(\theta) = \theta_1 \cdot n_{i,sim}(2) + \theta_2 \cdot n_{i,sim}(s), \qquad (4)$$

$$m_i^{(4)}(\theta) = \theta_1 \cdot n_{i,sim}(1) + \theta_2 \cdot n_{i,sim}(2) + \theta_3 \cdot n_{i,sim}(s), \qquad (5)$$

where $n_{i,sim}(s)$ denotes the simulated observed gold cluster size distribution given the underlying BCR oligomer size. I.e., the parameter vector θ reflects the composition of BCR oligomers on the surface. For each simulated data set, i.e., for each triplet (staining efficiency p, underlying cluster size s, geometry g), the maximization of the log-likelihood results in an estimate for the parameter vector θ, denoted by $\hat{\theta}$, that explains the experimental data best. In addition, to test if the log-likelihood value $l(\hat{\theta})$ is in accordance with the data, parametric bootstrapping is employed. In parametric bootstrapping, the model prediction $m_i(\hat{\theta})$ is used to generate *de novo* observation data. In our case, 10^3 random samples have been drawn from a Poisson distribution with mean $m_i(\hat{\theta})$ and have been treated like gold particle observations. For each sample, the log-likelihood is maximized again and the values are collected in a histogram approximating the asymptotic log-likelihood distribution. The original value $l(\hat{\theta})$ is compared to different statistics of the sampled distribution, among these p-value and weighted distance to the mean $\Delta = \frac{l(\hat{\theta}) - \langle l(\theta) \rangle}{\sigma_{l(\theta)}}$. The hypotheses are rejected based on these values for $p < 0.01$ and $\Delta > 3$, respectively.

3. RESULTS

3.1. THE WORKFLOW

Here we derived the size distribution of the IgD-BCRs on the cell surface of J558L transfectants from the measured distribution of gold particles after staining the BCRs with immuno-gold. "Size distribution of the BCRs" is defined as the percentage of BCRs in a given cluster size, such as 5% of the BCRs are in BCR monomers, 45% are in BCR dimers, and 50% are in BCR trimers. Our workflow consists of two phases. The first is carried out in the wet lab and comprises immuno-gold-labeling of the BCRs on untreated and PFA-fixed cells, followed by cell surface replica preparation and the quantification of the gold particle cluster size distribution on the replicated cell surface area by TEM (**Figure 1**, steps 1 and 2). As the staining efficiency reached by immuno-gold-labeling is low, the obtained immuno-gold data cannot directly be converted into the distribution of the BCRs. Thus, in the second phase mathematical modeling is used to derive the BCR distribution from the gold particle data. To do so, we assume a large number of different BCR distributions, such as only one defined size (only monomers, or only dimers, or only trimers, etc.) or a combination of sizes (for example, dimers and trimers). The observed gold particle size distributions are then stochastically simulated using a Monte-Carlo simulation of the staining process, and the likelihood that the gold size distribution represents a given BCR size distribution is

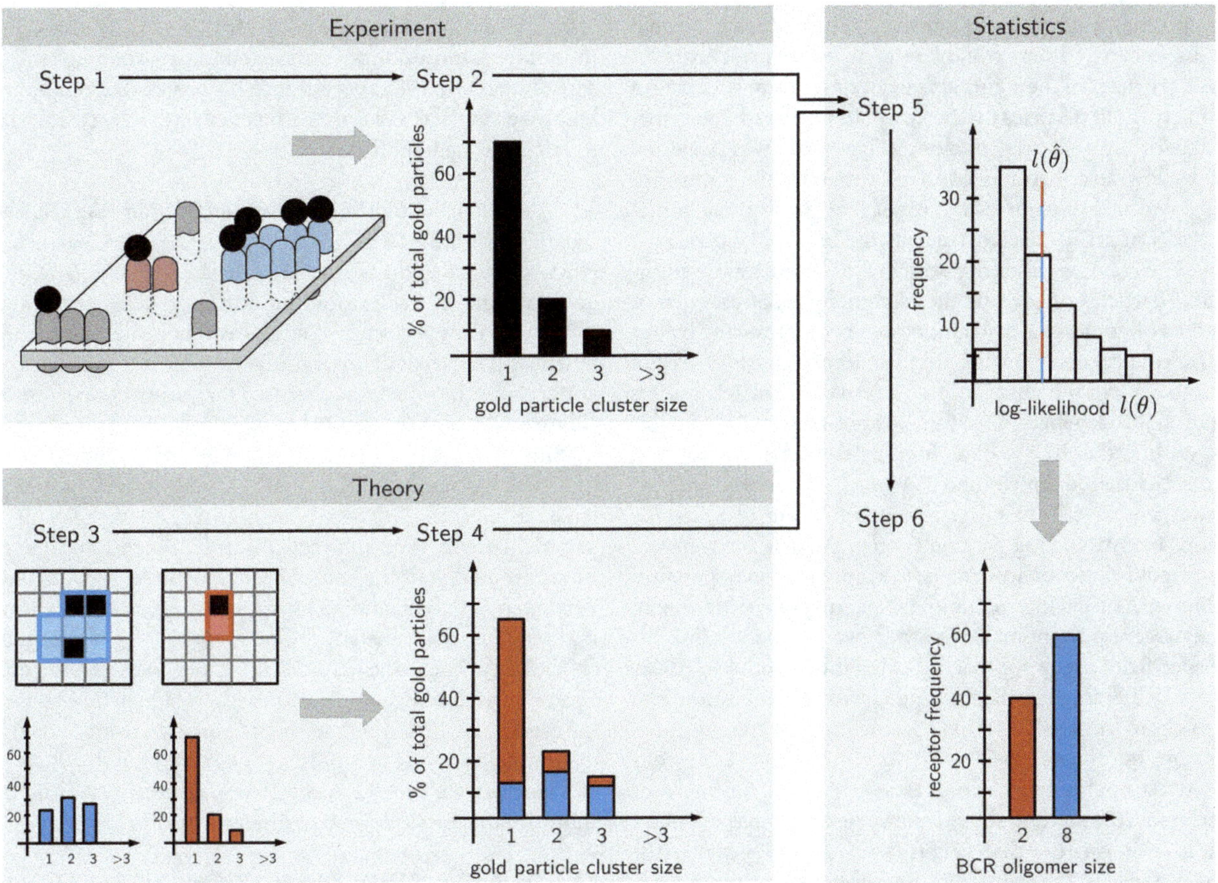

FIGURE 1 | Scheme of the workflow. The approach is divided into six steps partitioned into experimental (steps 1 and 2), theoretical (steps 3 and 4), and statistical parts (steps 5 and 6). In step 1, the IgD-BCRs on the surface of resting and fixed B cells are stained with immuno-gold and the gold particles visualized by TEM. In step 2, the gold particles are counted, generating an observed gold cluster size distribution. In step 3, the staining process is simulated by Monte-Carlo procedures based on hypothetical BCR nanocluster size distributions, generating characteristic gold particle cluster distributions for the observed gold-labeling. Gold particles are shown in black and BCRs in blue or red (each BCR occupies one square, thus showing a blue 8 mer and a red dimer). In step 4, superposition parameters are estimated based on the observed gold particle distributions by maximum-likelihood estimation. In step 5 based on the estimated parameters, *de novo*, *in silico* cluster size distributions are repeatedly generated and the corresponding log-likelihood is re-optimized, providing a histogram of log-likelihood values. Step 6; if in accordance with the data, the theory makes a valid prediction for the underlying BCR nanocluster distribution and the relative amounts of the nanocluster sizes is calculated.

calculated. Each single BCR oligomer size produces a characteristic distribution of observed gold cluster sizes that depends on (1) the pre-clustering of the gold-reagent, i.e., presence of monomeric, dimeric, or trimeric gold particles in the staining reagent, (2) the immuno-gold-staining efficiency, i.e., the percentage of BCRs that are labeled by gold particles, (3) unspecific binding of the gold-reagent to the B cell, independent of any BCR, (4) the oligomer geometry which is reflected by the number of next neighbors of an average receptor within the BCR oligomer, this number is at least 2, i.e., for linear chains of receptors, or up to 8 for a quadratic grid (**Figure 3A**). The Monte-Carlo simulation provides information on the staining patterns and thus, the visible gold cluster size distribution (step 3). To match the data, several such gold cluster distributions are superposed with different strengths. These strengths, called the superposition parameters, are estimated from the data and give rise to a hypothesized underlying BCR size distribution (step 4). Based on the estimated superposition parameters the gold particle observation data is repeatedly generated and the parameters are re-estimated. This process results in a distribution of log-likelihood values which, in case of good agreement between model and data, contains the original log-likelihood value $l(\hat{\theta})$ (step 5). For the log-likelihood value, the threshold corresponding to a p-value of 0.01 can be computed which when being exceeded allows to reject the model. Otherwise, for a model log-likelihood value in the interior of the distribution, the model makes a valid prediction for the underlying BCR oligomer size distribution (step 6). This means that the observed gold cluster distribution can be fully explained by the predicted BCR oligomer distribution.

3.2. ESTIMATION OF THE DEGREE OF PRE-CLUSTERING OF THE GOLD-REAGENT

To address a possible pre-clustering of the gold-reagent used for the BCR immuno-gold-labeling, the gold-reagent alone was adsorbed onto collodion/carbon-coated EM grids, i.e., without receptor binding, and analyzed by TEM (**Figure 2A**). The few observed gold particle dimers and trimers could be due to either pre-clustering of the gold particles in the staining reagent or random collocation of monomeric gold particles on the grid. The observed size distribution data of the gold-reagent alone (**Figure 2B**) was subjected to our workflow described above and interpreted as the staining of one huge quadratic oligomer. The size of this quadratic oligomer is the number of image pixels divided by the number of pixels per gold dot. The staining efficiency was first assessed by the number of gold particles divided by the oligomer size. Subsequently, the observed oligomer size distribution has been simulated by our Monte-Carlo approach showing that random collocation is not sufficient to explain the number of observed gold particle dimers but that the gold-reagent is indeed already pre-clustered. From this analysis, we find that 92.8% of all gold particles are monomeric, 6.5% are pre-clustered dimers, and 0.7% are pre-clustered trimers. These numbers have been taken into account for all following simulations by introducing parameters representing the inherent fraction of gold dimers and trimers. A complementary perspective on **Figure 2A** is its interpretation as staining of a surface with exclusively receptor monomers. This perspective enables insights into the specificity of the approach. Testing the hypothesis "100% monomers," differences in the staining efficiency should not lead to differences in the log-likelihood because only the total number of counts but not the observed size distribution changes. In contrast, when testing alternative hypotheses such as "100% dimers" or "100% trimers," the method should allow rejecting those hypotheses. Indeed, this was the case (**Figure 2C**). The plot shows the weighted distance to the mean and the p-value based on the log-likelihood. These values were computed for different hypothetical staining efficiencies, represented by different colors, and dominant oligomer sizes, represented by the x-axis. Already for hypothetical staining efficiencies larger than 3% all tested hypotheses other than "100% monomers" can be rejected with $p \leq 0.001$. Conversely, the monomer assumption is not rejected for any staining efficiency, in accordance with the expectation. This proofs that our approach is highly sensitive as a staining efficiency of 3% is already sufficient to reject wrong hypotheses.

3.3. CALCULATION OF THE IMMUNO-GOLD-STAINING EFFICIENCY FOR THE IgD-BCR

Next, we calculated the staining efficiency of the BCR immuno-gold-labeling process, using the murine B cell line J558Lm/mb-1flN (16). These cells express IgD-BCRs on their surface, as seen by a flow cytometric analysis using the same monoclonal anti-BCR antibody (Ac146) that was also used for the immuno-gold-labeling (**Figure 3B**). The total number of IgD-BCRs per cell was experimentally determined to be 122400 ± 7500 BCRs (described in the Methods section). The total cell surface area of a J558L cell is $782 \pm 25\,\mu m^2$ (25) resulting in an expected mean density of 156 BCRs/μm^2. We analyzed three J558Lδm/mb-1flN cells by immuno-gold-staining and TEM. The three areas analyzed by TEM were 101, 183, and 152 μm^2 and the expected BCR number in those areas was calculated to be 15600, 28080, and 23400 BCRs, respectively. The achieved BCR immuno-gold-labeling efficiency was calculated based on the number of gold particles observed in the areas (2192, 3577, and 3876 gold particles, respectively) assuming one gold particle to represent one BCR. Thus, the BCR labeling efficiencies were 14.1, 12.7, and 16.6%, respectively. Thus, the BCR staining efficiency in our experiment was approximately 15%.

3.4. THE ANTI-BCR IMMUNO-GOLD-STAINING IS SPECIFIC FOR THE BCR

To prove that the anti-BCR immuno-gold-labeling protocol only stained BCRs, we compared J558L cells that lack BCR expression

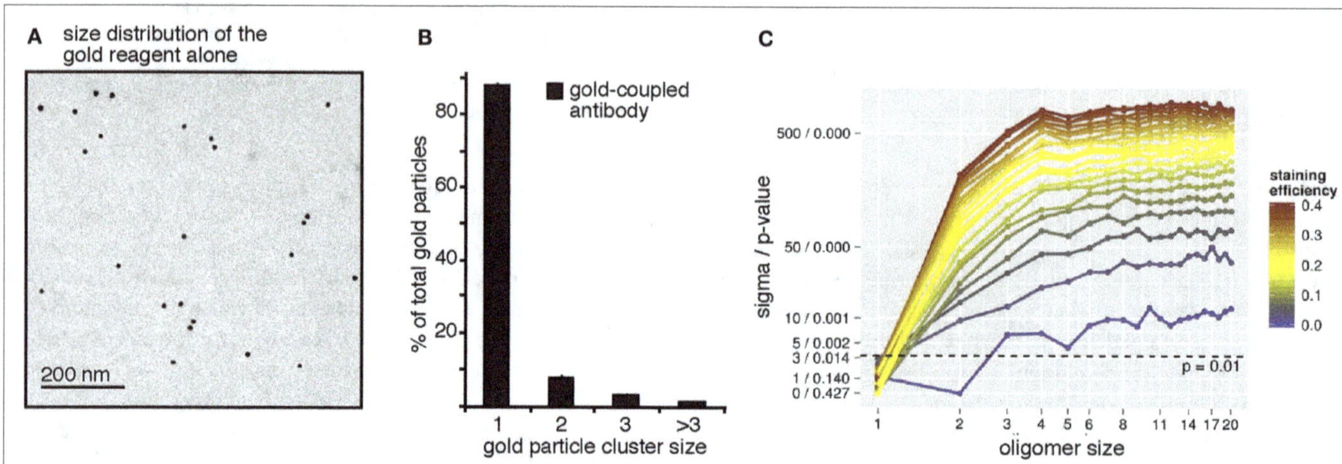

FIGURE 2 | The antibody-coupled gold-reagent is mainly monomeric. **(A)** The gold-reagent alone was adsorbed onto collodion/carbon-coated EM grids and analyzed by TEM. **(B)** Analysis of the clustering of 2041 gold particles alone showed 88% monomeric gold particles, 8% of gold particles as close as dimers, 3% were counted as trimers, and 1% as clusters of larger sizes. **(C)** The gold-reagent cluster size distribution was re-evaluated by our workflow, interpreting the cluster counts as receptor staining. Pre-clustering of the gold-reagent was taken into account. For different assumed receptor oligomer sizes (x-axis) and staining efficiencies (color scale), significance level and p-value were computed (y-axis). Models are rejected above the dashed line corresponding to a p-value of 0.01. The analysis confirms the monomer hypothesis and rejects other hypotheses with $p < 0.01$ (above the dashed line) for staining efficiencies larger 3%.

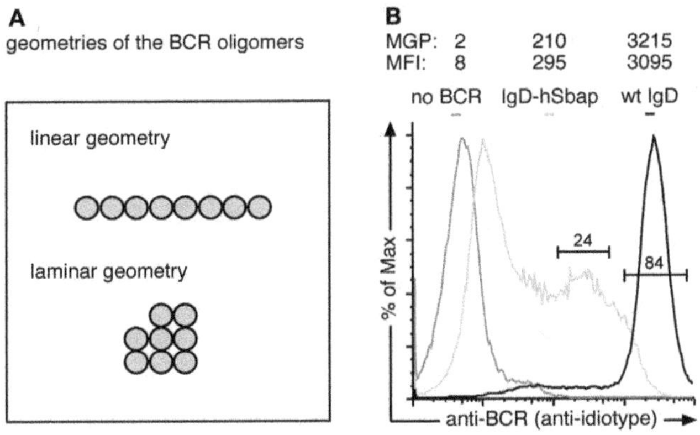

FIGURE 3 | The anti-BCR immuno-gold-labeling is specific. (A) The Monte-Carlo simulations were performed for two possible BCR oligomer geometries: a linear and a laminar geometry. **(B)** J558Lδm/mb-1flN cells expressing the wt IgD-BCR (black line), J558L cells without any BCR (dark gray line) or IgD-hSbap BCR-expressing J558L (light gray line) were labeled with the anti-BCR antibody Ac146 and subsequently stained with FITC-labeled anti-mouse IgG or gold-coupled anti-mouse IgG antibodies. Fluorescently labeled cells were analyzed by flow cytometry, and mean fluorescent intensities (MFI) of the gated populations are given. Gold labeled cells were subjected to replica preparation and analyzed by TEM. The mean gold particle (MGP) number detected on the cell replicas confirms specific labeling of the BCR on wt and IgD-hSbap expressing J558L cells, while immuno-gold-labeling of J558L not expressing BCR does not result in significant gold particle detection on surface replicas.

and the J558Lδm/mb-1flN cells (**Figure 3A**). Flow cytometry analysis confirmed no BCR expression on J558L cells. Immuno-gold-labeling of the J558L cells resulted in 2 gold particles per observed area, while J558Lδm/mb-1flN cells were stained with 3215 gold particles on average (**Figure 3A**). Thus (nearly) each gold particle is representing a BCR.

3.5. DETERMINATION OF THE SIZE DISTRIBUTION OF WT IgD-BCR OLIGOMERS

For our simulations to determine the size distribution of the wt IgD-BCR, we have used the immuno-gold data from J558Lδm/mb-1flN cells (**Figure 4A**) and the corresponding size distribution of the gold particles (**Figure 4B**). The quantification of gold clusters by TEM revealed 66% gold monomers, 21% gold in dimers, 7.5% gold in trimers, and a fraction of 5.5% gold particles were part of oligomers of four or more gold particles. To account for different possible geometries of each individual BCR cluster, simulations have been performed for linear and laminar BCR arrangements (**Figure 3B**). Firstly, we have assumed a linear arrangement of the BCRs (**Figure 4C**). Assuming the presence of one defined BCR oligomer size, labeled by x, we have performed simulations for BCR monomers (1), BCR dimers (2), BCR trimers (3), etc. (**Figure 4C**, top, left panel). The different staining probabilities are denoted by the color coding being centered around the experimentally measured value of 15%. All curves outside a range of ±5% were shaded. For the single size assumption none of the assumed BCR cluster sizes is in agreement with the data (below the dotted line). The discrepancy between data and model does not change any more as soon as the assumed BCR oligomer size is larger than 6 because the observed size distribution produced by them is almost identical. In particular, this means that linear BCR oligomers larger than 6 or even a mixture of large BCR oligomers is not in accordance with the experimental data at the given staining efficiency. Also a mixture of small and large BCR oligomer sizes, e.g., $1 + x$ (BCR monomers and one BCR cluster size of x, upper, right panel), $2 + x$ (BCR dimers and one BCR cluster size of x, lower, left panel), or $1 + 2 + x$ (BCR monomers, dimers, and one BCR cluster size of x, lower, right panel), is unable to explain the observed data by linearly arranged receptor oligomers, thus, leading to a full rejection of this geometry hypothesis. Secondly, we have assumed a laminar arrangement of the BCRs (**Figure 4D**). Following the plot for the single size assumption (**Figure 4D**, panel x), the best agreement is obtained for small BCR oligomers such as BCR dimers and trimers. This suggests that small BCR oligomers contribute significantly to the overall observed gold cluster distribution. Evaluation of related model hypotheses, $1 + x$, $2 + x$, and $1 + 2 + x$ shows that monomers plus an additional BCR oligomer size is not sufficient to explain the observed size distribution. However, accordance can be achieved for BCR dimers plus a large BCR oligomer around a size of 18 (lower, left panel). Additional BCR monomers do not further reduce the discrepancy between model and data (lower, right panel). This is also expressed in **Figure 4F**. BCR dimers dominate the small observed gold particle oligomers up to a size of 3, where BCR dimers are occasionally observed as trimers due to the pre-clustering of the gold-reagent. Underlying BCR oligomers of size 18 take over beginning from an observed gold particle size of 4. The contribution by BCR monomers is negligible. When testing a model with several BCR oligomer sizes, e.g., $1 + 2 + 18$, the maximization of the log-likelihood gives an estimate for the ratio between the abundance of the single BCR oligomer sizes. This ratio is then expressed in the percentage of receptors being contained in either of the oligomers. The number of receptors in oligomers of each size, computed from the model, indicates that 60% of all receptors are contained in BCR oligomers of size 18, 40% are contained in BCR dimers and BCR monomers are negligible (**Figures 4E,F**). In conclusion, we suggest that IgD-BCRs are arranged in pre-formed BCR oligomers on the surface of J558Lδm/mb-1flN B cells and that BCR dimers as well as large BCR oligomers of a laminar geometry co-exist.

3.6. DETERMINATION OF THE SIZE DISTRIBUTION OF A MUTANT IgD-BCR THAT MOSTLY FORMS DIMERS

To validate our combined experimental and theoretical approach, we took advantage of a transmembrane mutant IgD-BCR (IgD-hSbap BCR), which resulted in impeded BCR oligomerization as detected by Blue Native gel electrophoresis and pre-dominant detection of BCR dimers (16). Immuno-gold-labeling of the mutant BCR and sampling were performed as above. The quantification of gold clusters by TEM revealed mainly gold monomers (83%) and dimers (13%), and a smaller fraction of gold oligomers of three or more gold particles (4%) (**Figures 5A,B**). In contrast to the wt IgD-BCR, the staining efficiency was not determined as mutant IgD-BCR expression was heterogeneous (**Figure 3B**). When evaluating the log-likelihood for BCR staining efficiencies up to 40% and dominant BCR oligomer sizes up to10, the overall best log-likelihood value was achieved for BCR dimers at a

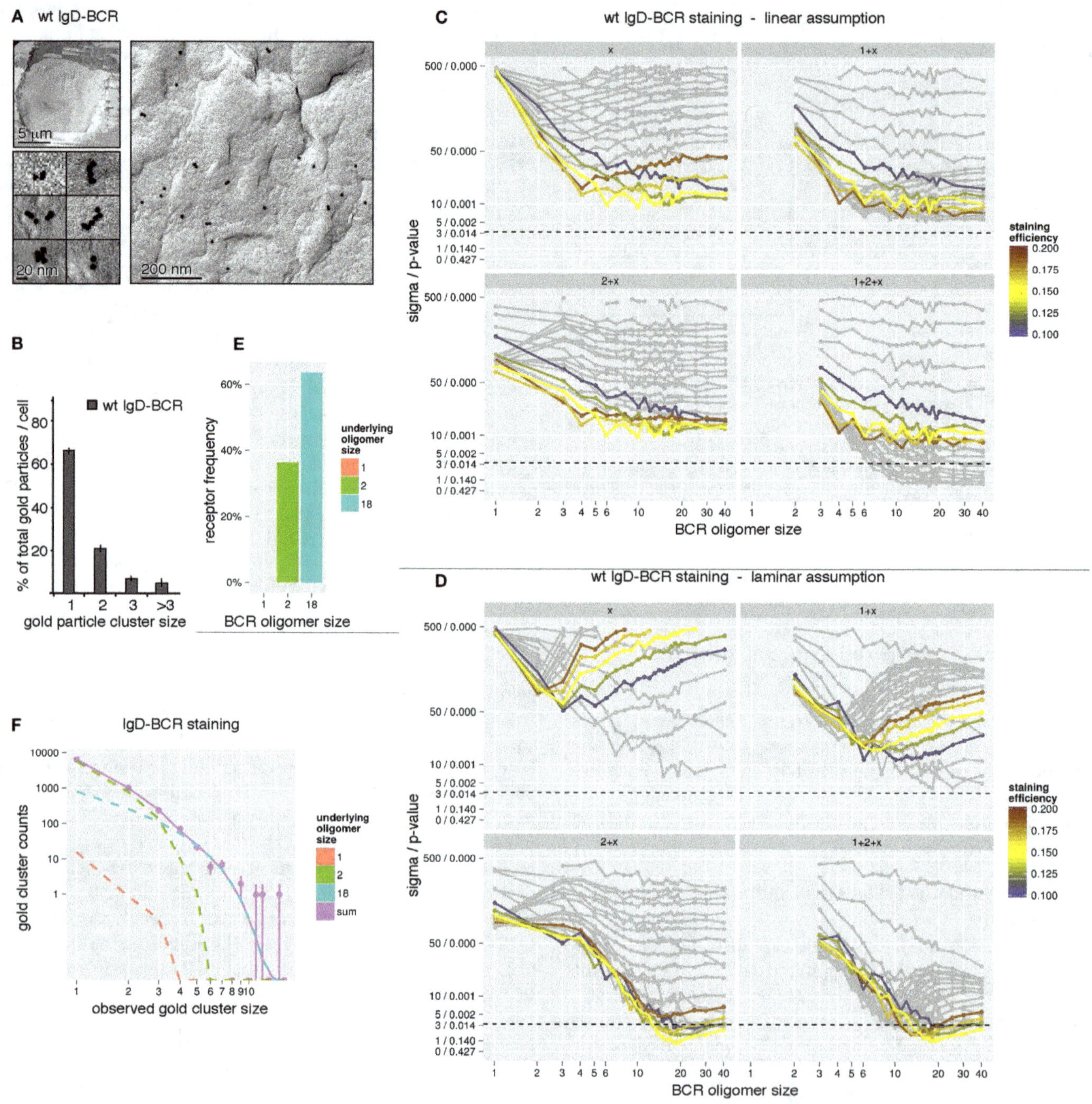

FIGURE 4 | The IgD-BCR forms differently sized oligomers on the surface of B cells. **(A)** IgD-BCR-expressing J558Lm/mb-1flN cells were immuno-gold stained using the mouse anti-BCR antibody Ac146 and anti-mouse IgG antibodies coupled to gold particles of 10 nm. The cell overview is given at low magnification (upper left panel), gold-labeling of the cell surface is shown in an overview picture (right panel) and individual gold clusters are shown at high magnification (lower left panel). **(B)** 66% of the gold particles were present as monomers, 21% formed dimers, 7.5% trimers, and 5.5% were present in clusters of sizes larger than 3. **(C)** The observed gold particle cluster size distribution was simulated with the assumption of an underlying linear BCR oligomer geometry. Simulations were performed for staining efficiencies of 15 ± 5% indicated by colored lines. The BCR oligomer sizes tested are indicated on the *x*-axis, and the sigma/*p*-values for the statistical analysis of each simulation set is given on the *y*-axis. Different hypothetical BCR oligomer size distributions are tested, namely "one BCR oligomer size only" (*x*, upper left panel), "BCR monomers + another single BCR oligomer size" (1 + *x*, upper right panel), "BCR dimers + another single BCR oligomer size" (2 + *x*, lower left panel), and "BCR monomers, dimers + another single BCR oligomer size" (1 + 2 + *x*, lower right panel). Models are rejected above the dashed line corresponding to a *p*-value of 0.01. **(D)** The observed gold particle cluster size distribution was simulated as in (C) with the assumption of an underlying laminar BCR oligomer geometry. **(E)** Our simulations predict that 60% of all receptors are part of oligomers of size 18 in a laminar geometry and 40% are BCR dimers. **(F)** Gold cluster counts (dots with error bars) compared to the prediction of best fitting model (continuous line). The number of counts originating from the different underlying BCR oligomer sizes are shown as dashed lines, indicating that observed clusters up to a size of 3 are primarily caused by BCR dimers, while gold clusters larger than 3 can be explained by BCR clusters of size 18. The impact of BCR monomers is negligible.

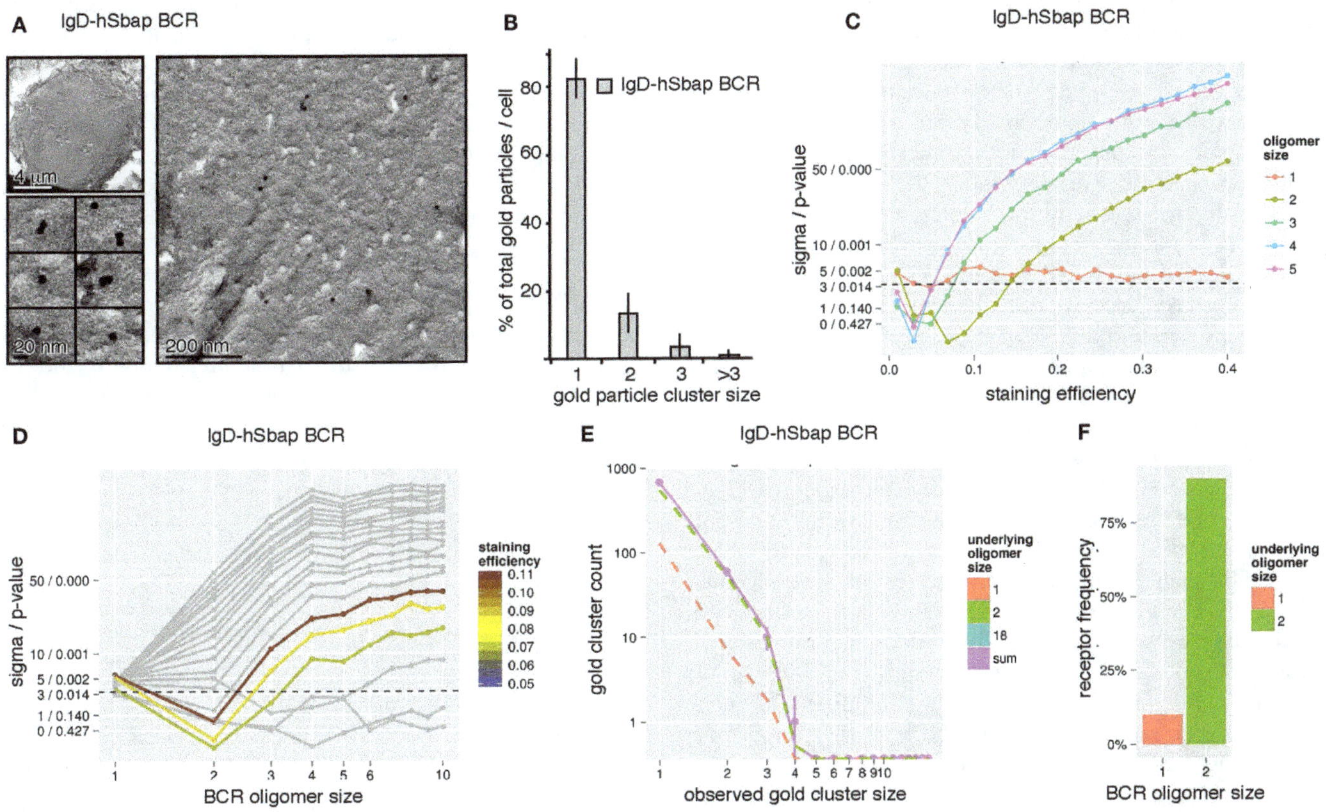

FIGURE 5 | The IgD-hSbap BCR mutant forms mainly BCR dimers on the surface of B cells. **(A)** IgD-hSbap BCR mutant-expressing J558L cells were immuno-gold stained and analyzed as in **Figure 4A**. **(B)** 83% of the gold particles were monomeric, 13% formed dimers, and 4% were present in clusters of sizes larger than 2. **(C)** The observed gold particle cluster size distribution was simulated for different BCR staining efficiencies (*x*-axis) and different underlying BCR oligomer sizes (color scale). The sigma/*p*-values for the statistical analysis of each simulation set are given on the *y*-axis. BCR dimers with a staining efficiency of 8% are identified as the most likely explanation for the observed gold cluster distribution. **(D)** Simulations were performed as in **(C)**. Assuming a staining efficiency of approximately 8% (color coding), sigma/*p*-values (*y*-axis) are plotted for the different BCR oligomer sizes (*x*-axis). **(E)** Gold cluster counts (dots with error bars) compared to prediction of best fitting model (continuous line). The number of counts originating from monomers and dimers are shown as dashed lines, indicating that the observed distribution is dominated by BCR dimers. **(F)** A model with BCR monomers and dimers was fitted to the data, predicting that 90% of all receptors are part of dimers, 10% are monomers.

staining efficiency of 8.8% (**Figure 5C**). The efficiency value is not too far from the wt IgD-BCR staining efficiency, which has been measured to be 15%. Our Monte-Carlo simulation indicated that IgD-hSbap BCR oligomers larger than two can be rejected at high confidence level unless the staining efficiency would be lower than 5% (**Figure 5D**). Also BCR monomers without larger BCR oligomers cannot explain the data, thus, confirming that the mutant BCR dimerizes. In addition to the single size model, a model with monomers and one further BCR oligomer size was tested. The observed gold cluster distribution after immuno-gold-labeling of the mutant IgD-BCR together with the model prediction of the best fitting model, i.e., monomers plus dimers, is shown in **Figure 5E**. Analogously to the wt IgD-BCR experiment, the percentage of IgD-hSbap BCR present as BCR monomers and BCR dimers was computed, demonstrating that 90% of the mutant BCRs are present as dimers and 10% as monomers (**Figure 5F**). These findings validate our approach and reflect the Blue Native gel electrophoresis data for IgD-hSbap BCR (16).

4. CONCLUSION

Here, we used a combined immuno-gold TEM and modeling approach to suggest that the IgD-BCR is expressed as BCR dimers and larger oligomers. To measure the distribution of cell surface molecules super resolution light microscopy techniques, such as high-speed photoactivated localization microscopy (5) or dSTORM (21), have been employed. Unlike these light microscopy techniques, our technique permits nano-scale resolution of cell surface molecules on the membranes that are not in contact with any support, thereby avoiding visualization of potential clustering artifacts induced by cell adherence (26). This advantage is not given in other EM methods, such as nano-probe labeling and transmission microscopy of cytoplasmic face-up sheets of cell membrane ripped off from cells to generate cytoplasmic face-up membrane sheets (27), which subsequently can be fixed and immuno-gold labeled (5,28,29). Our method can measure the distribution of any cell surface molecule, without the need to genetically modify this protein with a fluorophore, provided that antibodies against the protein are available. It is, however, not compatible with dynamic observations and, given the relatively low labeling efficiency, does not allow absolute quantifications by direct gold counting; here we present an approach to overcome the latter limitation. We assumed that the presence of one gold particle is indicative of one BCR (with the restraint that some gold particles are aggregated, which we have taken into account). There is the unlikely possibility that our staining approach with a primary anti-BCR and a secondary gold-coupled antibody could allow for double labelings of the BCRs, if the secondary antibody binds twice to the primary antibody (once to each of the two heavy chains). However, double labeling most likely did not take place: we used the IgD-hSbap BCR that only formed monomers and dimers when analyzed by Blue Native gels (16). And indeed, in our analysis this mutant BCR was exclusively detected as monomers (10% of the BCRs) and dimers (90% of the BCRs). These relative abundancies fit well to the biochemical Blue Native gel data (16). Thus, we conclude that a potential double gold-labeling of a BCR does not take place in our experiments and does not prevent drawing our conclusions from the immuno-gold TEM data. Here, we estimate that 60% of all wild type IgD-BCRs expressed on J558Lδm/mb-1flN cells are part of BCR oligomers of a size of around 18 and 40% form BCR dimers. This notion is based on the most simple BCR size distribution (i.e., assuming the lowest number of different BCR sizes) to explain the observed gold distribution. Still, the co-existence of larger number of different BCR oligomer sizes cannot be ruled out. Previously, the oligomer size of the IgM-BCR has been theoretically approached by Iber and Gruhn (30). Assuming oligomer formation and decay rates based on the literature, they calculated that IgM-BCR pentamers might exist. However, the modeling approach was not based on experimental data on BCR oligomer sizes and thus the presence of BCR pentamers is rather hypothetical. BCR pre-clustering might increase the antigen-receptor avidity, since functional antigens are mostly multimeric structures (31, 32). This increase in avidity could enhance the sensitivity of B cell activation, as suggested for TCR pre-clusters (8–10). BCR oligomers could also enhance the sensitivity of B cells by cooperativity between BCRs in one oligomer. Thus, antigen-binding to one or two BCRs could also lead to the activation of non-engaged BCRs, propagating the signal within one oligomer. In line with this, we had suggested earlier that the kinase Syk bound to one BCR can phosphorylate the neighboring BCR amplifying BCR signaling by a positive feedback loop (33). In T cells it was shown experimentally that individual TCRs cooperate in this manner within one TCR pre-cluster (34). On the other hand, enhanced sensitivity of the B cells might also bear an increased risk of reacting against abundant self-antigens and lead to autoimmunity. The presence of pre-formed BCR oligomers has important implications for the mechanism of how the BCR transmits the signal of antigen-binding into the interior of the cells. Initially, it was assumed that the BCRs are individually distributed on the B cell surface and only brought into close proximity by their multivalent antigens, leading to reciprocal phosphorylation of the cytoplasmic tyrosines in Igα and Igβ and thereby signal initiation. The idea of cross-linking as the first step in BCR activation was based on the finding that monovalent antigens do not induce BCR activation (31, 32). Now, the cross-linking model is questioned by the finding that BCR oligomers exist (16, 17, 19, 21, 35). In our analysis we hardly detected any BCR monomers, which is in line with the finding that only oligomerized are stably expressed on the cell surface (19). Our study clearly points out that BCR oligomers of different sizes co-exist on the surface of resting B cells. Activation therefore might occur according to conformational changes within the BCR oligomer, as e.g., the proposed in the dissociation activation model (20). Knowledge on the pre-clustering of a given receptor not only aids to explain the biology of the receptor, but also might open new strategies for interfering with its function for vaccination or therapeutic purposes.

ACKNOWLEDGMENTS

We thank Balbino Alarcón, Hisse M. van Santen, and Maite T. Rejas from Madrid for their help in the preparation of the electron microscopy samples. This work was funded by the Excellence Initiative of the German Research Foundation (EXC294, BIOSS Centre for Biological Signalling Studies, and GSC-4, Spemann Graduate School of Biology and Medicine). The article processing charge was funded by the open access publication fund of the Albert Ludwigs University Freiburg.

REFERENCES

1. Singer SJ, Nicolson GL. The fluid mosaic model of the structure of cell membranes. *Science* (1972) **175**:720–31. doi:10.1126/science.175.4023.720
2. Simons K, Ikonen E. Functional rafts in cell membranes. *Nature* (1997) **387**:569–72. doi:10.1038/42408
3. Lingwood D, Simons K. Lipid rafts as a membrane-organizing principle. *Science* (2010) **327**:46–50. doi:10.1126/science.1174621
4. Alarcon B, Swamy M, van Santen HM, Schamel WWA. T-cell antigen-receptor stoichiometry: pre-clustering for sensitivity. *EMBO Rep* (2006) **7**:490–5. doi:10.1038/sj.embor.7400682
5. Lillemeier BF, Mortelmaier MA, Forstner MB, Huppa JB, Groves JT, Davis MM. TCR and Lat are expressed on separate protein islands on T cell membranes and concatenate during activation. *Nat Immunol* (2010) **11**:90–6. doi:10.1038/ni.1832
6. Schamel WW, Arechaga I, Risueno RM, van Santen HM, Cabezas P, Risco C, et al. Coexistence of multivalent and monovalent TCRs explains high sensitivity and wide range of response. *J Exp Med* (2005) **202**:493–503. doi:10.1084/jem.20042155
7. Sherman E, Barr V, Manley S, Patterson G, Balagopalan L, Akpan I, et al. Functional nanoscale organization of signaling molecules downstream of the T cell antigen receptor. *Immunity* (2011) **35**:705–20. doi:10.1016/j.immuni.2011.10.004
8. Kumar R, Ferez M, Swamy M, Arechaga I, Rejas MT, Valpuesta JM, et al. Increased sensitivity of antigen-experienced T cells through the enrichment of oligomeric T cell receptor complexes. *Immunity* (2011) **35**:375–87. doi:10.1016/j.immuni.2011.08.010
9. Molnar E, Deswal S, Schamel WW. Pre-clustered TCR complexes. *FEBS Lett* (2010) **584**:4832–7. doi:10.1016/j.febslet.2010.09.004
10. Molnar E, Swamy M, Holzer M, Beck-Garcia K, Worch R, Thiele C, et al. Cholesterol and sphingomyelin drive ligand-independent T-cell antigen receptor nanoclustering. *J Biol Chem* (2012) **287**:42664–74. doi:10.1074/jbc.M112.386045
11. Hombach J, Tsubata T, Leclercq L, Stappert H, Reth M. Molecular-components of the B-cell antigen receptor complex of the IgM class. *Nature* (1990) **343**:760–2. doi:10.1038/343760a0
12. Havran WL, DiGiusto DL, Cambier JC. mIgM:mIgD ratios on B cells: mean mIgD expression exceeds mIgM by 10-fold on most splenic B cells. *J Immunol* (1984) **132**:1712–6.
13. Scher I, Titus JA, Finkelman FD. The ontogeny and distribution of B cells in normal and mutant immune-defective CBA/N mice: two-parameter analysis of surface IgM and IgD. *J Immunol* (1983) **130**:619–25.
14. Reth M. Antigen receptor tail clue. *Nature* (1989) **338**:383–4. doi:10.1038/338383b0
15. Reth M, Wienands J, Schamel WW. An unsolved problem of the clonal selection theory and the model of an oligomeric B-cell antigen receptor. *Immunol Rev* (2000) **176**:10–8. doi:10.1034/j.1600-065X.2000.00610.x

16. Schamel WW, Reth M. Monomeric and oligomeric complexes of the B cell antigen receptor. *Immunity* (2000) **13**:5–14. doi:10.1016/S1074-7613(00)00003-0
17. Reth M. Oligomeric antigen receptors: a new view on signaling for the selection of lymphocytes. *Trends Immunol* (2001) **22**:356–60. doi:10.1016/S1471-4906(01)01964-0
18. Tolar P, Sohn HW, Pierce SK. The initiation of antigen-induced B cell antigen receptor signaling viewed in living cells by fluorescence resonance energy transfer. *Nat Immunol* (2005) **6**:1168–76. doi:10.1038/ni1262
19. Yang J, Reth M. Oligomeric organization of the B-cell antigen receptor on resting cells. *Nature* (2010) **467**:465–9. doi:10.1038/nature09357
20. Yang J, Reth M. The dissociation activation model of B cell antigen receptor triggering. *FEBS Lett* (2010) **584**:4872–7. doi:10.1016/j.febslet.2010.09.045
21. Mattila PK, Feest C, Depoil D, Treanor B, Montaner B, Otipoby KL, et al. The actin and tetraspanin networks organize receptor nanoclusters to regulate B cell receptor-mediated signaling. *Immunity* (2013) **38**:461–74. doi:10.1016/j.immuni.2012.11.019
22. Reth M, Hammerling GJ, Rajewsky K. Analysis of the repertoire of anti-NP antibodies in C57BL/6 mice by cell fusion. I. Characterization of antibody families in the primary and hyperimmune response. *Eur J Immunol* (1978) **8**:393–400. doi:10.1002/eji.1830080605
23. Fiala GJ, Rejas MT, Schamel WW, van Santen HM. Visualization of TCR nanoclusters via immunogold labeling, freeze-etching and surface replication. *Methods Cell Biol* (2013) **117**:391–410. doi:10.1016/B978-0-12-408143-7.00021-9
24. Murphy RM, Slayter H, Schurtenberger P, Chamberlin RA, Colton CK, Yarmush ML. Size and structure of antigen-antibody complexes. *Biophys J* (1988) **54**:45–56. doi:10.1016/S0006-3495(88)82929-1
25. Morath V, Keuper M, Rodriguez-Franco M, Deswal S, Fiala G, Blumenthal B, et al. Semi-automatic determination of cell surface areas used in systems biology. *Front Biosci (Elite Ed)* (2013) **5**:533–45. doi:10.2741/E635
26. James JR, McColl J, Oliveira MI, Dunne PD, Huang E, Jansson A, et al. The T cell receptor triggering apparatus is composed of monovalent or monomeric proteins. *J Biol Chem* (2011) **286**:31993–2001. doi:10.1074/jbc.M111.219212
27. Sanan DA, Anderson RG. Simultaneous visualization of LDL receptor distribution and clathrin lattices on membranes torn from the upper surface of cultured cells. *J Histochem Cytochem* (1991) **39**:1017–24. doi:10.1177/39.8.1906908
28. Wilson BS, Pfeiffer JR, Oliver JM. Observing FcepsilonRI signaling from the inside of the mast cell membrane. *J Cell Biol* (2000) **149**:1131–42. doi:10.1083/jcb.149.5.1131
29. Zhang J, Leiderman K, Pfeiffer JR, Wilson BS, Oliver JM, Steinberg SL. Characterizing the topography of membrane receptors and signaling molecules from spatial patterns obtained using nanometer-scale electron-dense probes and electron microscopy. *Micron* (2006) **37**:14–34. doi:10.1016/j.micron.2005.03.014
30. Iber D, Gruhn T. Organisation of B-cell receptors on the cell membrane. *Syst Biol (Stevenage)* (2006) **153**:401–4. doi:10.1049/ip-syb:20060015
31. Dintzis HM, Dintzis RZ, Vogelstein B. Molecular determinants of immunogenicity: the immunon model of immune response. *Proc Natl Acad Sci U S A* (1976) **73**:3671–5. doi:10.1073/pnas.73.10.3671
32. Minguet S, Dopfer EP, Schamel WW. Low-valency, but not monovalent, antigens trigger the B-cell antigen receptor (BCR). *Int Immunol* (2010) **22**:205–12. doi:10.1093/intimm/dxp129
33. Rolli V, Gallwitz M, Wossning T, Flemming A, Schamel WW, Zrn C, et al. Amplification of B cell antigen receptor signaling by a Syk/ITAM positive feedback loop. *Mol Cell* (2002) **10**:1057–69. doi:10.1016/S1097-2765(02)00739-6
34. Martinez-Martin N, Risueno RM, Morreale A, Zaldivar I, Fernandez-Arenas E, Herranz F, et al. Cooperativity between T cell receptor complexes revealed by conformational mutants of CD3epsilon. *Sci Signal* (2009) **2**:ra43. doi:10.1126/scisignal.2000402
35. Treanor B, Depoil D, Gonzalez-Granja A, Barral P, Weber M, Dushek O, et al. The membrane skeleton controls diffusion dynamics and signaling through the B cell receptor. *Immunity* (2010) **32**:187–99. doi:10.1016/j.immuni.2009.12.005

6

Aspects of innate immunity and Parkinson's disease

Yue Huang[1,2] and Glenda M. Halliday[1,2]*

[1] Neuroscience Research Australia, Sydney, NSW, Australia
[2] University of New South Wales, Sydney, NSW, Australia

Edited by:
Roger A. Barker, University of Cambridge and Addenbrooke's Hospital, UK

Reviewed by:
Jason B. Wu, Cedars-Sinai Medical Center, USA
Andreas Hartmann, Assistance Publique des Hopitaux de Paris, Hopital de la Pitie-Salpetriere, France
Tamas Revesz, Institute of Neurology, University College London, UK

***Correspondence:**
Glenda M. Halliday, Neuroscience Research Australia, Barker Street, Randwick, NSW 2031, Australia.
e-mail: g.halliday@neura.edu.au

Genetic studies on PARK genes have identified dysfunction in proteasomal, lysosomal, and mitochondrial enzymes as pathogenic for Parkinson's disease (PD). We review the role of these and similar enzymes in mediating innate immune signaling. In particular, we have identified that a number of PARK gene products as well as other enzymes have roles in innate immune signaling as well as DNA repair and regulation, ubiquitination, mitochondrial functioning, and synaptic trafficking. PD enzymatic dysfunction is likely to contribute to inadequate innate immune responses to a variety of extra- and intra-cellular stimuli, with a number of the innate immunity related enzymes found in the characteristic Lewy body pathology of PD. The decrease in innate immunity in PD is associated with an increase in markers of adaptive immunity, and recent GWAS studies have identified variants in human leukocyte antigen region as associated with late-onset sporadic PD (Hamza et al., 2010; Hill-Burns et al., 2011). Intriguing new data also suggest that peripheral immune responses may be involved, giving some potential to alleviate such peripheral dysfunction more directly in patients with PD. It is now important to identify the cell type specific immune responses contributing to the initial changes that occur in PD, as well as to the propagating immune responses important for the progression of PD pathology between cells and within the brain. Overall, a complex interplay between different types of immunity appear to be involved in the underlying pathology of PD.

Keywords: immunity, mitochondrial dysfunction, Parkinson's disease, synapse dysfunction, ubiquitination

INTRODUCTION

Although Parkinson's disease (PD) is the most common progressive movement disorder in the elderly, there is still considerable uncertainty about its etiology. Recent advances in genetics have identified a number of PARK genes in families with PD, which have pointed to common underlying intrinsically driven intracellular pathways (Corti et al., 2011). These include dysfunction of the proteosome (McNaught et al., 2001), lysosome (Shin et al., 2005), and mitochondria (Muqit et al., 2006). In particular, leucine repeat rich kinase 2 (LRRK2, PARK8) and PTEN-induced kinase 1 (PINK1, PARK6) are linked to familial dominant and recessive PD respectively. PINK1 deletion causes aberrant expression of genes that regulate innate immune responses (Akundi et al., 2011). LRRK2 expression is enriched in human immune cells and is a target gene of IFN-γ (Gardet et al., 2010). Increased LRRK2 expression occurs when an immune response is required (see below). As mutations in these proteins cause PD, this suggests that innate immunity may play a more fundamental role in PD. How these systems interact to cause the fundamental pathology of PD (intracellular Lewy body inclusions made from fibrilized α-synuclein protein) to occur within affected neurons needs to be addressed.

Despite considerable organelle dysfunction, neuronal death occurs slowly, initially, and selectively targeting certain brainstem regions with a predisposition for the substantia nigra (Fearnley and Lees, 1991). Neuronal death does not occur in isolation, but is accompanied by considerable neuroinflammation (Orr et al., 2002; Wilms et al., 2003) and intrinsically driven glial cell changes (Halliday and Stevens, 2011). These changes include the accumulation of α-synuclein in glia, with many of the PARK gene proteins also concentrating in glia in the human brain (LRRK2, PINK1, DJ-1, parkin; Gandhi et al., 2006; Huang et al., 2008; Halliday and Stevens, 2011; Song et al., 2011). As glia interact most closely with the immune system, we will review how innate immunity is involved in these processes.

The innate immune system is an immediate, non-specific, first line of defense against pathogen invasion, contrasting with the delayed and targeted adaptive immune response (Stone et al., 2009). The specific molecular structure of pathogens (pathogen-associated molecular patterns or PAMPs), like lipopolysaccharides (LPS) or the bacterial DNA motif polycytosine guanine (CpG), are directly recognized by phagocytes, granulocytes, and natural killer cells of the immune system (West et al., 2006). These PAMPs

---

Abbreviations: CARD, caspase recruitment domain; CpG, polycytosine guanine; ER, endoplasmic reticulum; HDAC, histone deacetylase; IKK, IκB kinase; IRAK, interleukin-1 receptor-associated kinase; JNK, c-Jun N-terminal kinase; LPS, lipopolysaccharides; LRRK2, leucine-rich repeat kinase 2; MAPK, mitogen-activated protein kinase; MAPKK, MAPK kinase; MAVS, mitochondrial antiviral signaling; Mda5, melanoma differentiation-associated gene 5; MPTP, 1-methyl-4-phenyl-1,2,3,6-tetrahydropyridine; PAMPs, pathogen-associated molecular pattern; PARP, poly (ADP-ribose) polymerase; PD, Parkinson's disease; PINK1, PTEN-induced putative kinase 1; PKR, Protein kinase RNA-activated; RIG-I, RNA helicases protein retinoic acid-inducible gene I protein; TAK1, Transforming growth factor-beta-activated kinase 1; TBK-1, TANK-binding kinase 1; TLR, Toll-like receptor; TRAF6, tumor necrosis factor receptor-associated factor 6.

bind to Toll-like receptors (TLR) on cells, triggering a cascade of signaling that results in pro-inflammatory cytokine release and complement activation to clear the pathogen or the infected/dead cell through macroautophagy (West et al., 2006).

Pathogens activate cells by binding to specific TLRs through characteristic extracellular multiple leucine-rich repeats domains of TLR (Nguyen et al., 2002). The ultimate induction of interferons and inflammatory cytokines by different pathogens is led by several phosphorylation and subsequent ubiquitination events, with activation of TBK-1 and IKKε, JNK and p38 kinase, IKK, MAPK and MAPKK, IRAK, and TAK1 [detailed in previous reviews (Kawai and Akira, 2006; Seth et al., 2006)]. A major pathway is NF-κB activation by its release from IκB allowing its nuclear translocation and the subsequent activation of target genes to occur. IκB release occurs following IκB phosphorylation and consequent degradation through the lysine 48 linked ubiquitin–proteasome system (Silverman and Maniatis, 2001; Wu et al., 2006).

INNATE IMMUNITY AND PD

Classic PD is not considered an immune disease like multiple sclerosis, and can not be associated with common infectious agents. However, Parkinsonian symptoms can occur after Epstein–Barr virus (EBV) encephalitic infection in patients, with EBV DNA detected in the brain (Espay and Henderson, 2011). This shows that an immune activation in the brain can produce PD-like symptoms, and a number of genetic studies suggest the immune system is commonly involved. Genome-wide association studies (GWAS) show that common variants in human leukocyte antigen (HLA) region are associated with late-onset sporadic PD (Hamza et al., 2010; Hill-Burns et al., 2011). The brains of individuals with PD show upregulation of HLA-DR antigens and the presence of HLA-DR-immunopositive and highly reactive microglia (McGeer et al., 1988). Microglia are the only cells in the substantia nigra that express the initial recognition component of the complement cascade, C1q (Carlsson et al., 2011). Finally, non-steroidal anti-inflammatory drugs reduce PD risk (Wahner et al., 2007; Steurer, 2011), further supporting some involvement of the immune system in PD.

From a PARK gene perspective, it is of interest that both parkin (PARK2) and LRRK2 (PARK8) are genes associated with leprosy (Cardoso et al., 2011), which is a chronic infectious disease of peripheral nerves. LRRK2 is also a risk gene for inflammatory bowel disease (Van Limbergen et al., 2009; Torkvist et al., 2010; Umeno et al., 2011), and there is much discussion about PD being initiated from peripheral neurons within the gut (enteric nervous system; Braak et al., 2003). In an animal model of ulcerative colitis, there is an alteration of the blood–brain-barrier (BBB) permeability that leads to more substantive cell loss to pathogen-induced cell loss of the substantia nigra (Villaran et al., 2010). Interestingly, treatment of the ulcerative colitis ameliorated cell loss in the brain in this model (Villaran et al., 2010). This could suggest a more direct link between immune defense mechanisms in peripheral neurons and the later onset of PD. Deletions within PINK1 (PARK6) or DJ-1 (PARK7) genes cause aberrant expression of genes involved in the p38 MAP kinase/NF-κB signaling pathway causing changes in the regulation of the innate immune response (Cornejo Castro et al., 2010; Akundi et al., 2011). This suggests that many PARK genes also have significant influence on the immune system which may be important for the onset and/or progression of PD.

A number of animal models of the neuronal loss in PD use direct initiation of the innate immune system to model this aspect of PD. Administration of LPS induces dramatic cell loss in primary neuronal cultures and direct injection of LPS into the substantia nigra produces progressive nigrostriatal degeneration and movement abnormalities in animal models of PD (Liu, 2006; Dutta et al., 2008). These LPS PD models trigger TLR4 mediated signaling pathways (Carvey et al., 2003; Visintin et al., 2003). Even intraperitoneal and *in utero* injections of LPS cause degeneration of the nigrostriatal system (Ling et al., 2002; Perry, 2004), consistent with peripheral effects causing PD-like neurodegeneration. These innate immunity models of PD cause neurodegeneration and microglial activation in a time and LPS dose dependent manner (Liu, 2006; Dutta et al., 2008). Similar direct injections of TLR3 into the substantia nigra produce nigrostriatal degeneration (Deleidi et al., 2010). These studies show that strong stimulators of the innate immune system and increased numbers of innate immune receptors can produce significant site-specific neurodegeneration, perhaps suggesting that the nigrostriatal system is particularly vulnerable to immune activation.

Innate immune signaling also plays a role in the abnormal deposition of α-synuclein. In α-synuclein overexpressing models, ablation of TLR4 augments the deposition of α-synculein due to disruption of the ability of microglia to adequately phagocytose α-synuclein (Stefanova et al., 2011). This suggests that certain aspects of innate immunity are required for initial protection from excessive extracellular α-synuclein. Whether these mechanisms play a role in patients is more difficult to determine. Overall, these studies suggest that the innate immune system can play both neuroprotective and neurotoxic roles depending on the circumstances.

ADAPTIVE IMMUNITY AND PD

In contrast to the "non-specific" innate immune system, the adaptive immune response is cell mediated and highly specialized to remove a specific antigen. It is mainly composed of two parts: humoral immunity, which is mediated by B-lymphocytes, and cell mediated immunity, which is mediated by T-lymphocytes. The CNS was traditionally considered as an "immune privileged" site due to its protection by the BBB, which prevents toxins and infections from reaching the CNS. However, in PD the BBB is disrupted due to activated microglia and monocytes in PD brain (Stone et al., 2009). IgG, but not IgM, has been shown bound to dopamine neurons in the substantia nigra of idiopathic and familial PD patients, but not in age-matched controls (Orr et al., 2005). In addition, LRRK2, a causative gene for PD (see above), regulates B2-lymphocyte function (Kubo et al., 2010). This suggests that adaptive immunity may also be involved in the progression of PD (**Figure 1**).

Apart from B-lymphocyte involvement in PD, both $CD4^+$ and $CD8^+$ T-lymphocytes have been found in the SN of PD patients, and $CD4^+$ T-lymphocytes are responsible for the T-cell-mediated immunopathology (Brochard et al., 2009). The expression of CD95 ligand (Fas) has been shown to be important for the capacity

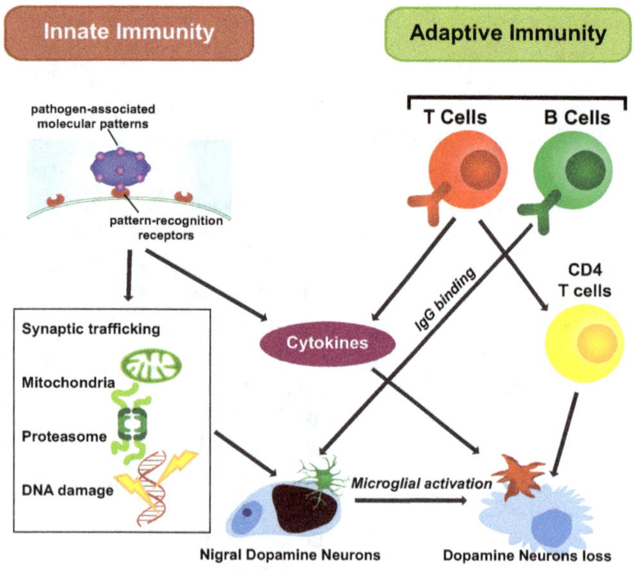

FIGURE 1 | Innate and adaptive immunity in PD. Innate and adaptive immunity are both thought to affect the cellular response to PD. Both produce cytokines facilitating microglial activation. Innate immune signaling is initiated by PAMP binding. Innate immunity influences cell functions through different organelles, such as the nucleus to affect DNA, the mitochondria and proteasome, and through impacting on synaptic trafficking. Adaptive immunity is a subsequent response. Antigen specific adaptive immune processes occur as immune cells survey the brain. In response to stimuli, B cells secrete IgG and CD4 T cells are activated impacting on selective neuronal degeneration.

of T-lymphocytes to induce neuronal death (Brochard et al., 2009). T-lymphocyte cells and T cell receptor (TCR) associated CD3, a polypeptide complex comprised of four distinct chains (CD3γ, CD3δ, CD3ε, and CD3ζ), are found in the PD characteristic Lewy body lesions (Castellani et al., 2011), providing another direct link between cell mediated immunity and PD pathology (**Figure 1**).

Through activation of both the adaptive and innate immune systems, cytokines are induced and secreted. Circulating IL-12 and IL-10 are significantly elevated in PD patients compared with controls (Rentzos et al., 2009) and our data show that the protein levels of IL-10 and GM-CSF are elevated in the cortex of patients with PD (unpublished data). Intercellular adhesion molecule-1 (ICAM-1)-positive glia are increased in the substantia nigra of PD brains (Miklossy et al., 2006). Further analysis of these immune responses in the brains of patients with PD may provide more specific cytokine targets for modifying detrimental immune responses in PD.

INNATE IMMUNITY AND DNA REPAIR AND REGULATION IN PD

The presence of genomic DNA single and double-strand breaks is very common in PD affected brain regions (Hegde et al., 2006). At early stages of DNA damage, DNA sensing molecules (such as PARP and ATM) activate and cause a signaling cascade for repair (Herceg and Wang, 2001). Histone deacetylases (HDAC) are important suppressors of gene transcription, but also deacetylates the p62 subunit of NF-κB increasing its binding to IκB and suppressing innate immunity and interferon-stimulated transcription (Babic et al., 2004; Into et al., 2010). HDACs have been localized to Lewy bodies in patients with PD (Takahashi-Fujigasaki and Fujigasaki, 2006), indicating that they are involved in PD pathogenesis. Inhibiting HDAC alleviates dopamine depletion in models of PD (Outeiro et al., 2007) and is protective by enhancing α-synuclein expression in neurons (Nusinzon and Horvath, 2003; Leng and Chuang, 2006), possibly in concert with an increased innate immune response.

Poly (ADP-ribose) polymerase catalyzes the attachment of ADP ribose units from NAD to nuclear proteins after DNA damage, resulting in three major outcomes, DNA repair, activation of transcription factors (notably NF-κB), and/or cell death due to NAD depletion and release of apoptosis releasing factor from mitochondria (Kauppinen and Swanson, 2007). PARP negatively regulates α-synuclein expression by binding to the α-synuclein promoter Rep1 region (Chiba-Falek et al., 2005) and α-synuclein protein suppresses PARP activity (Adamczyk and Kazmierczak, 2009). Inhibition of PARP activation protects mice from MPTP-induced parkinsonism (Mandir et al., 1999; Leng and Chuang, 2006). PARP may protect against PD through increasing innate immune signaling.

ATM is a kinase that is recruited to phosphorylate histones for DNA repair, signaling molecules for cell cycle arrest or apoptosis, and nuclear IKKγ (NF-κB essential modulator; Habraken and Piette, 2006; Hinz et al., 2010; Hadian and Krappmann, 2011). Phosphorylation of IKKγ leads to its ubiquitination and cytoplasmic translocation where it associates with the rest of the IKK complex, resulting in IKK activation followed by subsequent NF-κB activation and inflammatory cytokines production (Chen, 2005). ATM has also recently been shown to regulate proteasome-mediated protein turnover through suppression of the ISG15 pathway (Wood et al., 2011). ISG15 is an interferon-stimulated gene activated by viral infection and important in antiviral defense and innate immunity (Skaug and Chen, 2010). It is a ubiquitin-like protein that can be attached to both host and viral proteins (Skaug and Chen, 2010). ATM-deficient mice exhibit a selective loss of dopamine nigrostriatal neurons (Eilam et al., 1998), implicating dysfunction of ubiquitination as a factor in PD neurodegeneration, and specifically of ubiquitination in the innate immune system.

INNATE IMMUNITY AND UBIQUITINATION IN PD

The expression of ISG15 is increased in Crohn's disease (Labbe et al., 2011), an inflammatory bowel disorder sharing common genetic and environmental risk factors with PD (Bihari and Lees, 1987; Bialecka et al., 2007). Both ISG15 and LRRK2 (PARK8) are targets of interferon regulation (**Figure 2**). Interferon also regulates proteasome processing of ubiquitinated protein degradation into small peptides (Rivett et al., 2001; Piccinini et al., 2003; **Figure 2**). Ubiquitin is a small molecule and through lysine 48 and lysine 63 forms polyubiquitin chains for protein degradation and cellular localization (Ikeda and Dikic, 2008).

Among PARK genes, parkin has a variety of functions. It not only promotes lysine 48 linked ubiquitination for substrate degradation via the proteasome, but also functions in lysine 63 ubiquitin chain assembly to regulate diverse cellular processes, such as ribosome control, protein sorting and trafficking, and endocytosis of

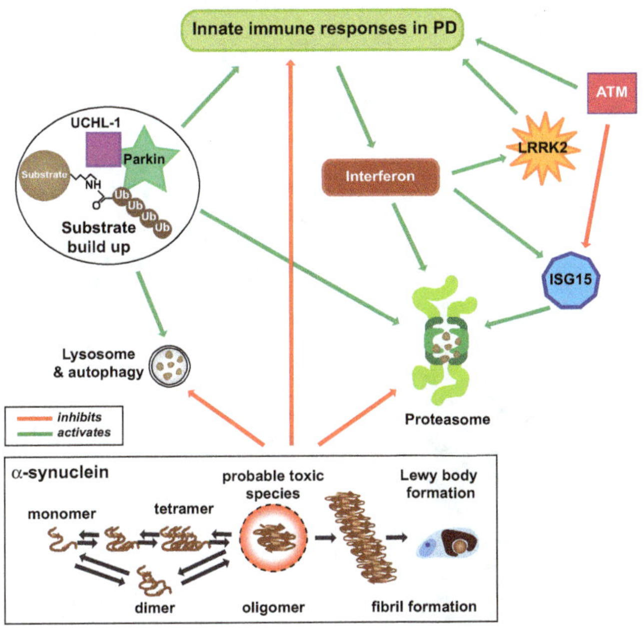

FIGURE 2 | Innate immunity and the ubiquitin–proteasome system in PD. Innate immunity is used by the cell to increase proteasome degradation of unwanted proteins by direct and indirect stimulation of the protesome through interferon-γ and ISG15, a ubiquitin-like protein that can be attached to both host and viral proteins. ATM (and appropriately functioning LRRK2) usually stimulates innate immune signaling when necessary. However, ATM also regulates proteasome-mediated protein turnover through suppression of the ISG15 pathway, and together with dysfunctional LRRK2 could decrease proteasome activity necessary for an adequate immune response and the degradation of normal cellular protein substrates, like dimer or tetramer forms of α-synuclein. As these forms are normally degraded through the ubiquitin/proteasome and lysosome/autophagy pathways, along with other cellular substrates, dysfunction in these pathways would increase α-synuclein to form toxic oligomeric species that also inhibit the proteasome and autophagy pathways, as well as innate immunity. This scenario would lead to the increase in toxic oligomers of α-synuclein that aggregate into fibrils to form Lewy bodies over time.

membrane proteins (Doss-Pepe et al., 2005). Lysine 63 linked ubiquitin chains promote the degradation of membrane proteins by the lysosome (Doss-Pepe et al., 2005). It is notable that α-synuclein is degraded via both the proteasome and lysosome pathways (Shin et al., 2005), suggestive that lysine 48 and lysine 63 linked ubiquitin chains are both important in the pathogenesis of PD (**Figure 2**). UCH-L1 has two opposing enzymatic activities, deubiquitination and ubiquityl ligase. The UCH-L1 ligase activity forms lysine 63 linked polyubiquitin chains (Liu et al., 2002). Lysine 63 multiubiquitin chains are also stimulated by α-synuclein (Doss-Pepe et al., 2005), and α-synuclein filaments and oligomers or its mutants inhibit proteasome function (Tanaka et al., 2001; Lindersson et al., 2004). These three genetically linked PD proteins all contribute to lysine 63 multiubiquitin chain formation. Dysfunction of this system is likely to decrease innate immune responses in PD.

Both lysine 48 and lysine 63 linked ubiquitin chains are known to be involved in anti-pathogen signaling cascades. In particular, lysine 63 linked ubiquitination is essential for NF-κB activation (detailed in review of Wu et al., 2006). Phosphorylation of IκB that releases NF-κB only occurs when the kinase IKKβ is released from its complex following IKKγ phosphorylation and lysine 63 linked degradation. Some other key immune response signaling molecules, such as TRAF6, also function as the lysine 63 linked ubiquitin E3 ligase to activate kinase activity (Kawai and Akira, 2006), and TRAF5 has been identified as a downstream target of VISA (see below) that mediates both IRF-3 and NF-κB activation (Tang and Wang, 2010).

INNATE IMMUNITY AND MITOCHONDRIAL FUNCTION IN PD

The proper functioning of mitochondria is crucial for adequate innate immune defense (Qi et al., 2007; Tang and Wang, 2010; West et al., 2011). Intracellular double-stranded RNA originating from viruses or virus replication is recognized by RIG-I and Mda5, which contain a caspase recruitment domain (CARD; **Figure 3**). Activated RIG-I/Mda5 passes the signal to mitochondrial antiviral signaling (MAVS/VISA) proteins via a CARD–CARD domain interaction (**Figure 3**). The C-terminal of MAVS/VISA bind to mitochondria to activate NF-κB and start interferon α and β production (Qi et al., 2007; **Figure 3**). Upon viral infection, MAVS/VISA immigrate from the outer membrane into the mitochondrial detergent-resistant membrane fraction, suggesting that mitochondria react and contribute to antiviral signaling (Qi et al., 2007; **Figure 3**). In addition to regulating antiviral signaling, there is mounting evidence that mitochondria facilitate antibacterial immunity by generating reactive oxygen species and contributing to innate immune activation following cellular damage and stress (Nakahira et al., 2011).

Most nuclear encoded PARK gene products are located within mitochondria (**Table 1**), such as PINK1, DJ-1, Omi/HtrA2, and LRRK2, suggesting mitochondrial dysfunction is common in PD. The mitochondrial complex I has been shown to be selectively reduced in PD vulnerable regions, such as the substantia nigra (Schapira et al., 1989). The mitochondrial complex I inhibitor rotenone and mitochondrial toxin MPTP (1-methyl 4-phenyl 1,2,3,6-tetrahydropyridine) induce selective dopamine neuron loss and a parkinsonian syndrome and have been used as a major model for studying the tissue aspects of PD (Langston and Ballard, 1984; Betarbet et al., 2000). These changes may decrease the cellular responses of the innate immune system in PD.

INNATE IMMUNITY AND SYNAPTIC TRAFFICKING IN PD

Most enveloped animal RNA and DNA viruses enter host cells via receptor-medicated endocytosis or viral membrane fusion with the plasma membrane in order to replicate. Endocytosis impinges on viral infection at a number of different cellular levels, from the plasma membrane to endosome to lysosome or alternatively to Golgi, and to ER (**Figure 4**; Hacker et al., 1998; Leadbetter et al., 2002; Diebold et al., 2004). Viral proteins accumulate in the ER during viral replication and elicit ER stress. Viral replication induced ER stress disturbs vesicle trafficking within the intracellular membranous web (Goodridge et al., 2011).

Many PARK genes are associated with endocytosis and synaptic vesicle trafficking. α-Synuclein, parkin and UCH-L1 concentrate in the presynapse and associate with synaptic vesicles, anchoring and regulating the undocked pool of presynaptic vesicles (Di Rosa et al., 2003; Ferrer, 2009). α-Synuclein acts as a molecular

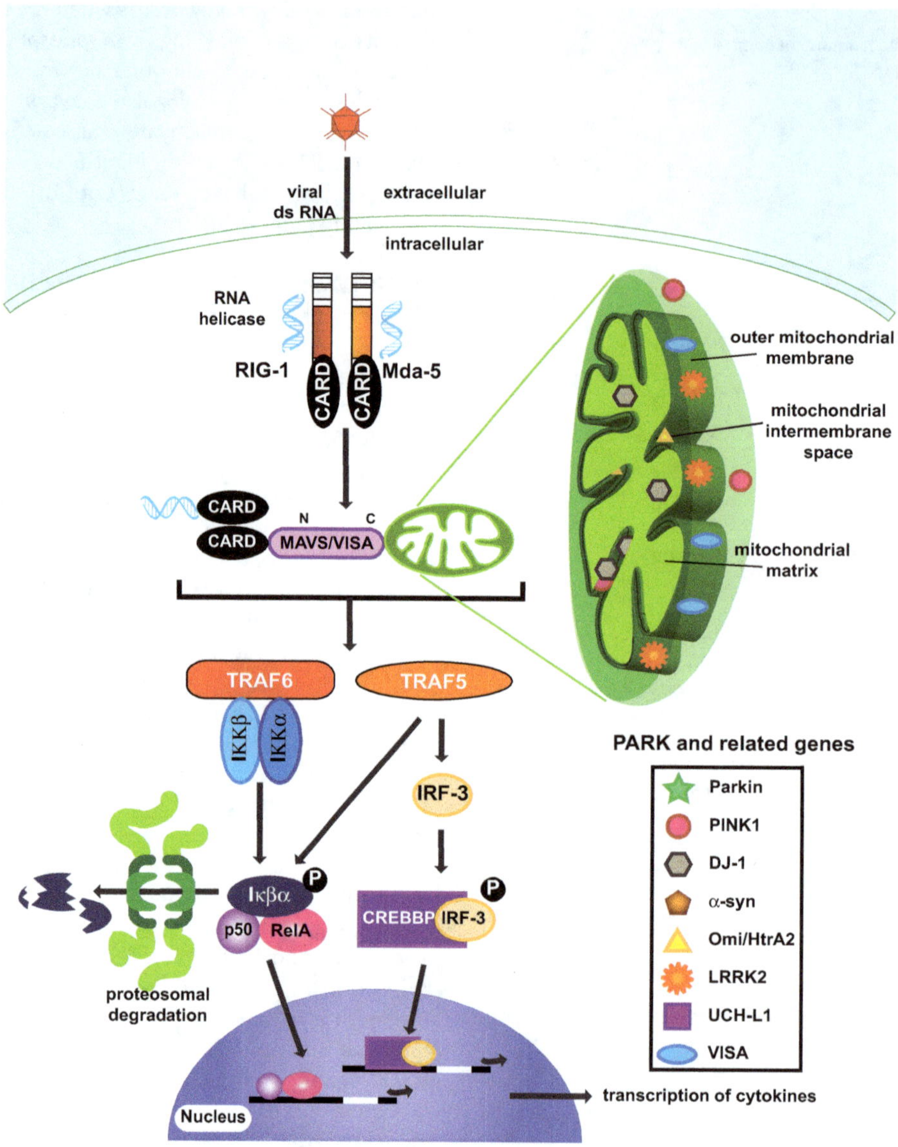

FIGURE 3 | Innate immunity and mitochondria in PD. Many PARK related gene products are located in mitochondria, implicating mitochondrial dysfunction in PD. Interestingly, MAVS/VISA that are attached to the outer membrane of mitochondria are involved in viral infection signaling by activating TRAF6 and TRAF5. Phosphorylation of Iκβα and IRF-3 leads to nuclear translocation of transcription factors and the production of cytokines.

Table 1 | Cellular localization and functions PARK and related genes

	Cellular location indicative functions in mitochondria and synaptic trafficking	**Ubiquitination**	**Reference**
Parkin	Outer mitochondrial membrane Synaptic vesicles and the synaptic membrane	Lysine 48-, 63-linked ubiquitin E3 ligase	Kubo et al. (2001); Darios et al. (2003)
DJ-1	Mitochondrial matrix and inter-membrane space	NA	Zhang et al., 2005)
PINK1	Mitochondria	Upstream of parkin	Valente et al. (2004)
Omi/HtrA2	Mitochondrial inter-membrane space	NA	Strauss et al. (2005)
LRRK2	Outer mitochondrial membrane	NA	West et al. (2005)
α-synuclein	Presynaptic terminal	Promote 63 linked ubiquitin assemble	Iwai et al. (1995)
UCH-L1	Synaptic vesicle	Lysine 63 linked ubiquitin E3 ligase	Liu et al. (2002)
VISA	Outer mitochondrial membrane	NA	Seth et al. (2005)

NA, not available.

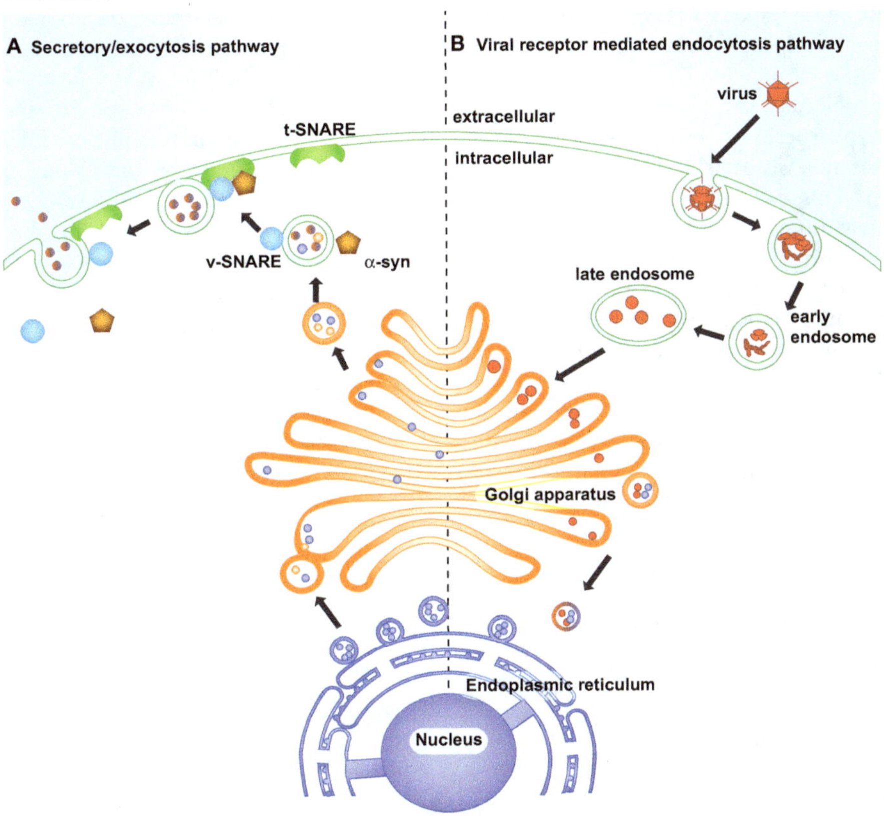

FIGURE 4 | Synaptic trafficking failure and viral intake leading to synaptic dysfunction in PD. Left: The endoplasmic reticulum is composed of a membranous network of tubes and cisternae enclosed in a membrane. It is continuous with the membrane surrounding the nuclear membrane and connects with the Golgi network via the vesicles carrying newly synthesized proteins. Certain vesicle-trafficking steps are required for the translocation of a vesicle from the Golgi apparatus to the plasma membrane. A transport vesicle is tethered and docked at the target membrane to form a tight SNARE complex, thus to merge the vesicle membrane with the target membrane and evacuate neurotransmitters into the extracellular space. The vesicle releasing process is under the assistance of α-synuclein, CDCrel-1, and synaptotagmin. Right: Viruses enter host cells through endosomes. Late endosomes fuse with or convert to lysosomes to degrade its contents, or alternatively it forms budding vesicles that pass to the trans-Golgi region and translocate to the Golgi and endoplasmic reticulum. The endoplasmic reticulum is coated with ribosomes, which assemble the viral amino acids into viral proteins.

chaperone, assisting in the folding and refolding of synaptic proteins called SNAREs, which are crucial for the release of neurotransmitters at the neuronal synapse, vesicle recycling, and synaptic integrity (Chandra et al., 2005). Upon the arrival of action potentials at the synaptic terminal, SNARE complexes, assembly of vesicle membrane (v-SNARE) and the presynaptic plasma membrane (t-SNARE), fuse the vesicle at the plasma membrane to release neurotransmitter into the synaptic cleft (Chandra et al., 2005; Fortin et al., 2005). Parkin ubiquitinates and regulates the turnover of the synaptic vesicle-associated protein, CDCrel-1, a synaptic vesicle-enriched septin GTPase implicated in the inhibition of exocytosis through its interactions with the SNARE complex component, syntaxin (Zhang et al., 2000). Another substrate of parkin is synaptotagmin XI, a member of the synaptotagmin family that is well characterized in vesicle formation and docking by interaction with SNAREs (Huynh et al., 2003). Loss of function of α-synuclein, parkin, or DJ-1 reduces neurotransmission and synaptic vesicle trafficking (Abeliovich et al., 2000; Goldberg et al., 2005). UCH-L1 deficient mice also show altered vesicle transport gene expression (Bonin et al., 2004). Reduced innate immunity allowing for pathogen replication would significantly exacerbate any loss of synaptic function caused by PARK gene products (**Figure 4**) precipitating frank degeneration.

CONCLUSION

A number of intrinsically driven cellular pathways shown to be dysfunctional in PD are important in mediating innate immune signaling. These important intracellular pathways have been identified through genetic studies in patients with PD. More recent genetic studies have also implicated immune pathways in the pathogenesis of PD. In particular, we have identified a number of PARK gene products as well as other enzymes that have dual roles in innate immune signaling as well as proteasome, lysosome, and mitochondrial functioning. The additional enzymes identified are important for DNA repair and regulation, ubiquitination, mitochondrial function, and synaptic trafficking. These pathways appear to lose their ability to mount an adequate innate immune response to PD and experimental manipulation of many of these intracellular molecules has been associated with characteristic PD pathologies in animal models. Intriguing new data also suggest that peripheral immune responses may be involved, with the potential to alleviate such peripheral dysfunction more directly in patients with PD.

Most important, the molecular pathways involved are likely to function in a cell type specific manner (Ledesma et al., 2002), a concept that has not yet been evaluated substantially in patients with PD. The cross-talk between neurons and glia is crucial for an adequate immune response, with astrocytes considered particularly important (Halliday and Stevens, 2011; Schmidt et al., 2011). Astrocytic endfeet form part of the BBB and may serve as ideal sentinel cells able to sense the appearance of toxins and viral pathogens (Scumpia et al., 2005), similar to their cousins found in the gut (Savidge et al., 2007; Daneman and Rescigno, 2009). Astroglia in both the brain and gut regulate barrier function and membrane permeability (Savidge et al., 2007; Daneman and Rescigno, 2009), functions which may be important for the cell to cell transfer of α-synuclein pathology as well as more traditional infectious agents. The increased expression of PARK gene proteins in astrocytes (see above) and their lack of activation to PD pathology in patients (Mirza et al., 2000; Halliday and Stevens, 2011) lends weight to a loss of innate immunity and BBB function in PD that potentially increases membrane and cellular permeability leading to increased toxin and pathogen infiltration in the brain. In addition to the direct cellular damage to vulnerable neurons this would initiate, pathogen exposure may also activate the alternate adaptive immune responses that are thought to participate in propagating the pathology of PD.

ACKNOWLEDGMENTS

We wish to thank Heidi Cartwight for the figurework. Yue Huang is funded by a University of New South Wales Goldstar award. Glenda M. Halliday is funded as a Senior Principal Research Fellow of the National Health and Medical Research Council of Australia.

REFERENCES

1. Abeliovich, A., Schmitz, Y., Farinas, I., Choi-Lundberg, D., Ho, W. H., Castillo, P. E., Shinsky, N., Ver- dugo, J. M., Armanini, M., Ryan, A., Hynes, M., Phillips, H., Sulzer, D., and Rosenthal, A. (2000). Mice lack- ing alpha-synuclein display func- tional deficits in the nigrostri- atal dopamine system. *Neuron* 25, 239–252.
2. Adamczyk, A., and Kazmierczak, A. (2009). Alpha-synuclein inhibits poly (ADP-ribose) polymerase-1 (PARP-1) activity via NO-dependent pathway. *Folia Neuropathol.* 47, 247–251.
3. Akundi, R. S., Huang, Z., Eason, J., Pandya, J. D., Zhi, L., Cass, W. A., Sullivan, P. G., and Bueler, H. (2011). Increased mitochondr- ial calcium sensitivity and abnormal expression of innate immunity genes precede dopaminergic defects in Pink1-deficient mice. *PLoS ONE* 6, e16038. doi:10.1371/journal.pone. 0016038
4. Babic, I., Jakymiw, A., and Fujita, J. (2004). The RNA binding protein Sam68 is acetylated in tumor cell lines, and its acety- lation correlates with enhanced RNA binding activity. *Oncogene* 23, 3781–3789.
5. Betarbet, R., Sherer, T. B., Mackenzie, G., Garcia-Osuna, M., Panov, A. V., and Greenamyre, J. T. (2000). Chronic systemic pesticide exposure reproduces features of Parkinson's disease. *Nat. Neurosci.* 3, 1301–1306.
6. Bialecka, M., Kurzawski, M., Klodowska-Duda, G., Opala, G., Juzwiak, S., Kurzawski, G., Tan, K., and Drozdzik, M. (2007). CARD15 variants in patients with sporadic Parkinson's disease. *Neurosci. Res.* 57, 473–476.
7. Bihari, K., and Lees, A. J. (1987). Cig- arette smoking, Parkinson's disease and ulcerative colitis. *J. Neurol. Neu- rosurg. Psychiatr.* 50, 635.
8. Bonin, M., Poths, S., Osaka, H., Wang, Y. L., Wada, K., and Riess, O. (2004). Microarray expression analysis of gad mice implicates involvement of Parkinson's disease associated UCH- L1 in multiple metabolic pathways. *Brain Res. Mol. Brain Res.* 126, 88–97.
9. Braak, H., Rub, U., Gai, W. P., and Del Tredici, K. (2003). Idiopathic Parkinson's disease: possible routes by which vulnerable neuronal types may be subject to neuroinvasion by an unknown pathogen. *J. Neural Transm.* 110, 517–536.
10. Brochard, V., Combadiere, B., Prigent, A., Laouar, Y., Perrin, A., Beray- Berthat, V., Bonduelle, O., Alvarez- Fischer, D., Callebert, J., Launay, J. M., Duyckaerts, C., Flavell, R. A., Hirsch, E. C., and Hunot, S. (2009). Infiltration of CD4+ lymphocytes into the brain contributes to neu- rodegeneration in a mouse model of Parkinson disease. *J. Clin. Invest.* 119, 182–192.
11. Cardoso, C. C., Pereira, A. C., De Sales Marques, C., and Moraes, M. O. (2011). Leprosy susceptibility: genetic variations regulate innate and adaptive immunity, and dis- ease outcome. *Future Microbiol.* 6, 533–549.
12. Carlsson, T., Schindler, F. R., Hollerhage, M., Depboylu, C., Arias-Carrion, O., Schnurrbusch, S., Rosler, T. W., Wozny, W., Schwall, G. P., Groebe, K., Oertel, W. H., Brundin, P., Schrattenholz, A., and Hoglinger, U. (2011). Systemic administra- tion of neuregulin-1beta1 protects dopaminergic neurons in a mouse model of Parkinson's disease. *J. Neu- rochem.* 117, 1066–1074.
13. Carvey, P. M., Chang, Q., Lipton, J. W., and Ling, Z. (2003). Prenatal exposure to the bacteriotoxin lipopolysaccharide leads to long- term losses of dopamine neurons in offspring: a potential, new model of Parkinson's disease. *Front. Biosci.* 8, s826–s837.
14. Castellani, R. J., Nugent, S. L., Mor- rison, A. L., Zhu, X., Lee, H. G., Harris, P. L., Bajic, V., Sharma, S., Chen, S. G., Oettgen, P., Perry, G., and Smith, M. A. (2011). CD3 in Lewy pathology: does the abnormal recall of neurodevelop- mental processes underlie Parkin- son's disease. *J. Neural Transm.* 118, 23–26.
15. Chandra, S., Gallardo, G., Fernandez- Chacon, R., Schluter, O. M., and Sudhof, T. C. (2005). Alpha- synuclein cooperates with CSPal- pha in preventing neurodegenera- tion. *Cell* 123, 383–396.
16. Chen, Z. J. (2005). Ubiquitin signaling in the NF-kappaB pathway. *Nat. Cell Biol.* 7, 758–765.
17. Chiba-Falek, O., Kowalak, J. A., Smul- son, M. E., and Nussbaum, R. L. (2005). Regulation of alpha- synuclein expression by poly (ADP ribose) polymerase-1 (PARP-1) binding to the NACP-Rep1 poly- morphic site upstream of the SNCA gene. *Am. J. Hum. Genet.* 76, 478–492.
18. Cornejo Castro, E. M., Waak, J., Weber, S. S., Fiesel, F. C., Ober- hettinger, P., Schutz, M., Autenri- eth, I. B., Springer, W., and Kahle, P. J. (2010). Parkinson's disease- associated DJ-1 modulates innate immunity signaling in Caenorhab- ditis elegans. *J. Neural Transm.* 117, 599–604.
19. Corti, O., Lesage, S., and Brice, A. (2011). What genetics tells us about the causes and mechanisms of Parkinson's disease. *Physiol. Rev.* 91, 1161–1218.
20. Daneman, R., and Rescigno, M. (2009). The gut immune barrier and the blood-brain barrier: are they so different? *Immunity* 31, 722–735.
21. Darios, F., Corti, O., Lucking, C. B., Hampe, C., Muriel, M. P., Abbas, N., Gu, W. J., Hirsch, E. C., Rooney, T., Ruberg, M., and Brice, A. (2003). Parkin prevents mito- chondrial swelling and cytochrome c release in mitochondria-dependent cell death. *Hum. Mol. Genet.* 12, 517–526.
22. Deleidi, M., Hallett, P. J., Koprich, J. B., Chung, C. Y., and Isacson, O. (2010). The Toll-like receptor- 3 agonist polyinosinic:polycytidylic acid triggers nigrostriatal dopamin- ergic degeneration. *J. Neurosci.* 30, 16091–16101.
23. Di Rosa, G., Puzzo, D., Sant'Angelo, A., Trinchese, F., and Arancio, O. (2003). Alpha-synuclein: between synaptic function and dysfunction. *Histol. Histopathol.* 18, 1257–1266.
24. Diebold, S. S., Kaisho, T., Hemmi, H., Akira, S., and Reis E Sousa, C. (2004). Innate antiviral responses by means of TLR7-mediated recognition of single-stranded RNA. *Science* 303, 1529–1531.
25. Doss-Pepe, E. W., Chen, L., and Madura, K. (2005). Alpha-synuclein and parkin contribute to the assembly of ubiquitin lysine 63-linked multi- ubiquitin chains. *J. Biol. Chem.* 280, 16619–16624.
26. Dutta, G., Zhang, P., and Liu, B. (2008). The lipopolysaccharide Parkinson's disease animal model: mechanis- tic studies and drug discovery. *Fundam. Clin. Pharmacol.* 22, 453–464.
27. Eilam, R., Peter, Y., Elson, A., Rot- man, G., Shiloh, Y., Groner, Y., and Segal, M. (1998). Selective loss of dopaminergic nigro-striatal neurons in brains of Atm-deficient mice. *Proc. Natl. Acad. Sci. U.S.A.* 95, 12653–12656.
28. Espay, A. J., and Henderson, K. K. (2011). Postencephalitic parkinson- ism and basal ganglia necrosis due to Epstein-Barr virus infection. *Neurol- ogy* 76, 1529–1530.
29. Fearnley, J. M., and Lees, A. J. (1991). Ageing and Parkinson's disease: substantia nigra regional selectivity. *Brain* 114 (Pt 5), 2283–2301.

30. Ferrer, I. (2009). Early involvement of the cerebral cortex in Parkin- son's disease: convergence of multi- ple metabolic defects. *Prog. Neuro- biol.* 88, 89–103.
31. Fortin, D. L., Nemani, V. M., Voglmaier, S. M., Anthony, M. D., Ryan, T. A., and Edwards, R. H. (2005). Neural activity controls the synaptic accu- mulation of alpha-synuclein. *J. Neu- rosci.* 25, 10913–10921.
32. Gandhi, S., Muqit, M. M., Stanyer, L., Healy, D. G., Abou-Sleiman, P. M., Hargreaves, I., Heales, S., Ganguly, M., Parsons, L., Lees, A. J., Latch- man, D. S., Holton, J. L., Wood, N. W., and Revesz, T. (2006). PINK1 protein in normal human brain and Parkinson's disease. *Brain* 129, 1720–1731.
33. Gardet, A., Benita, Y., Li, C., Sands, B. E., Ballester, I., Stevens, C., Korzenik, R., Rioux, J. D., Daly, M. J., Xavier, R. J., and Podolsky, D. (2010). LRRK2 is involved in the IFN-gamma response and host response to pathogens. *J. Immunol.* 185, 5577–5585.
34. Goldberg, M. S., Pisani, A., Habur- cak, M., Vortherms, T. A., Kitada, T., Costa, C., Tong, Y., Martella, G., Tscherter, A., Martins, A., Bernardi, G., Roth, B. L., Pothos, E. N., Calabresi, P., and Shen, J. (2005). Nigrostriatal dopaminergic deficits and hypokinesia caused by inactiva- tion of the familial Parkinsonism- linked gene DJ-1. *Neuron* 45, 489–496.
35. Goodridge, H. S., Reyes, C. N., Becker, C. A., Katsumoto, T. R., Ma, J., Wolf, A. J., Bose, N., Chan, A. S., Magee, A. S., Danielson, M. E., Weiss, A., Vasilakos, J. P., and Underhill, D. M. (2011). Activation of the innate immune receptor Dectin-1 upon formation of a 'phagocytic synapse'. *Nature* 472, 471–475.
36. Habraken, Y., and Piette, J. (2006). NF-kappaB activation by double- strand breaks. *Biochem. Pharmacol.* 72, 1132–1141.
37. Hacker, H., Mischak, H., Miethke, T., Liptay, S., Schmid, R., Sparwasser, T., Heeg, K., Lipford, G. B., and Wagner, H. (1998). CpG-DNA-specific activation of antigen-presenting cells requires stress kinase activity and is preceded by non-specific endo- cytosis and endosomal maturation. *EMBO J.* 17, 6230–6240.
38. Hadian, K., and Krappmann, D. (2011). Signals from the nucleus: activation of NF-kappaB by cytosolic ATM in the DNA damage response. *Sci. Signal.* 4, pe2.
39. Halliday, G. M., and Stevens, C. H. (2011). Glia: initiators and progres- sors of pathology in Parkinson's dis- ease. *Mov. Disord.* 26, 6–17.
40. Hamza, T. H., Zabetian, C. P., Tenesa, A., Laederach, A., Montimurro, J., Yearout, D., Kay, D. M., Doheny, K. F., Paschall, J., Pugh, E., Kusel, V. I., Collura, R., Roberts, J., Griffith, A., Samii, A., Scott, W. K., Nutt, J., Factor, S. A., and Payami, H. (2010). Common genetic variation in the HLA region is associated with late-onset sporadic Parkinson's disease. *Nat. Genet.* 42, 781–785.
41. Hegde, M. L., Gupta, V. B., Anitha, M., Harikrishna, T., Shankar, S. K., Muthane, U., Subba Rao, K., and Jagannatha Rao, K. S. (2006). Studies on genomic DNA topology and sta- bility in brain regions of Parkinson's disease. *Arch. Biochem. Biophys.* 449, 143–156.
42. Herceg, Z., and Wang, Z. Q. (2001). Functions of poly (ADP-ribose) polymerase (PARP) in DNA repair, genomic integrity and cell death. *Mutat. Res.* 477, 97–110.
43. Hill-Burns, E. M., Factor, S. A., Zabetian, C. P., Thomson, G., and Payami, H. (2011). Evidence for more than one Parkinson's disease-associated variant within the HLA region. *PLoS ONE* 6, e27109. doi:10.1371/jour- nal.pone.0027109
44. Hinz, M., Stilmann, M., Arslan, S. C., Khanna, K. K., Dittmar, G., and Scheidereit, C. (2010). A cyto- plasmic ATM-TRAF6-cIAP1 mod- ule links nuclear DNA damage sig- naling to ubiquitin-mediated NF- kappaB activation. *Mol. Cell* 40, 63–74.
45. Huang, Y., Song, Y. J., Murphy, K., Holton, J. L., Lashley, T., Revesz, T., Gai, W. P., and Halliday, G. M. (2008). LRRK2 and parkin immunoreactivity in multiple sys- tem atrophy inclusions. *Acta Neu- ropathol.* 116, 639–646.
46. Huynh, D. P., Scoles, D. R., Nguyen, D., and Pulst, S. M. (2003). The autosomal recessive juvenile Parkinson disease gene product, parkin, inter- acts with and ubiquitinates synap- totagmin XI. *Hum. Mol. Genet.* 12, 2587–2597.
47. Ikeda, F., and Dikic, I. (2008). Atypi- cal ubiquitin chains: new molecu- lar signals. "Protein Modifications: Beyond the Usual Suspects" review series. *EMBO Rep.* 9, 536–542.
48. Into, T., Inomata, M., Niida, S., Murakami, Y., and Shibata, K. (2010). Regulation of MyD88 aggre- gation and the MyD88-dependent signaling pathway by sequestosome 1 and histone deacetylase 6. *J. Biol. Chem.* 285, 35759–35769.
49. Iwai, A., Masliah, E., Yoshimoto, M., Ge, N., Flanagan, L., De Silva, H. A., Kit- tel, A., and Saitoh, T. (1995). The pre- cursor protein of non-A beta com- ponent of Alzheimer's disease amy- loid is a presynaptic protein of the central nervous system. *Neuron* 14, 467–475.
50. Kauppinen, T. M., and Swanson, R. A. (2007). The role of poly (ADP- ribose) polymerase-1 in CNS dis- ease. *Neuroscience* 145, 1267–1272.
51. Kawai, T., and Akira, S. (2006). Innate immune recognition of viral infection. *Nat. Immunol.* 7, 131–137.
52. Kubo, M., Kamiya, Y., Nagashima, R., Maekawa, T., Eshima, K., Azuma, S., Ohta, E., and Obata, F. (2010). LRRK2 is expressed in B-2 but not in B-1 B cells, and downregulated by cellular activation. *J. Neuroimmunol.* 229, 123–128.
53. Kubo, S. I., Kitami, T., Noda, S., Shimura, H., Uchiyama, Y., Asakawa, S., Minoshima, S., Shimizu, N., Mizuno, Y., and Hattori, N. (2001). Parkin is associated with cellular vesicles. *J. Neurochem.* 78, 42–54.
54. Labbe, C., Boucher, G., Foisy, S., Alikashani, A., Nkwimi, H., David, G., Beaudoin, M., Goyette, P., Char- ron, G., Xavier, R. J., and Rioux, J. D. (2011). Genome-wide expres- sion profiling implicates a MAST3- regulated gene set in colonic mucosal inflammation of ulcerative colitis patients. *Inflamm. Bowel Dis.* doi: 10.1002/ibd.21887. [Epub ahead of print].
55. Langston, J. W., and Ballard, P. (1984). Parkinsonism induced by 1-methyl-4-phenyl-1,2,3,6- tetrahydropyridine (MPTP): implications for treatment and the pathogenesis of Parkinson's disease. *Can. J. Neurol. Sci.* 11, 160–165.
56. Leadbetter, E. A., Rifkin, I. R., Hohlbaum, A. M., Beaudette, B. C., Shlomchik, M. J., and Marshak-Rothstein, A. (2002). Chromatin-IgG complexes activate B cells by dual engagement of IgM and Toll-like receptors. *Nature* 416, 603–607.
57. Ledesma, M. D., Galvan, C., Hellias, B., Dotti, C., and Jensen, P. H. (2002). Astrocytic but not neuronal increased expression and redistri- bution of parkin during unfolded protein stress. *J. Neurochem.* 83, 1431–1440.
58. Leng, Y., and Chuang, D. M. (2006). Endogenous alpha-synuclein is induced by valproic acid through histone deacetylase inhibition and participates in neuroprotec- tion against glutamate-induced excitotoxicity. *J. Neurosci.* 26, 7502–7512.
59. Lindersson, E., Beedholm, R., Hojrup, P., Moos, T., Gai, W., Hendil, K. B., and Jensen, P. H. (2004). Protea- somal inhibition by alpha-synuclein filaments and oligomers. *J. Biol. Chem.* 279, 12924–12934.
60. Ling, Z., Gayle, D. A., Ma, S. Y., Lipton, J. W., Tong, C. W., Hong, J. S., and Carvey, P. M. (2002). In utero bacter- ial endotoxin exposure causes loss of tyrosine hydroxylase neurons in the postnatal rat midbrain. *Mov. Disord.* 17, 116–124.
61. Liu, B. (2006). Modulation of microglial pro-inflammatory and neurotoxic activity for the treatment of Parkinson's disease. *AAPS J.* 8, E606–E621.
62. Liu, Y., Fallon, L., Lashuel, H. A., Liu, Z., and Lansbury, P. T. Jr. (2002). The UCH-L1 gene encodes two opposing enzymatic activities that affect alpha-synuclein degradation and Parkinson's disease susceptibil- ity. *Cell* 111, 209–218.
63. Mandir, A. S., Przedborski, S., Jackson-Lewis, V., Wang, Z. Q., Simbulan-Rosenthal, C. M., Smulson, M. E., Hoffman, B. E., Guastella, D. B., Dawson, V. L., and Dawson, T. M. (1999). Poly (ADP-ribose) polymerase activation mediates 1-methyl-4-phenyl-1, 2,3,6-tetrahydropyridine (MPTP)- induced parkinsonism. *Proc. Natl. Acad. Sci. U.S.A.* 96, 5774–5779.
64. McGeer, P. L., Itagaki, S., Boyes, B. E., and McGeer, E. G. (1988). Reactive microglia are positive for HLA-DR in the substantia nigra of Parkin- son's and Alzheimer's disease brains. *Neurology* 38, 1285–1291.
65. McNaught, K. S., Olanow, C. W., Hal- liwell, B., Isacson, O., and Jenner,
66. P. (2001). Failure of the ubiquitin- proteasome system in Parkinson's disease. *Nat. Rev. Neurosci.* 2, 589–594.
67. Miklossy, J., Doudet, D. D., Schwab, C., Yu, S., Mcgeer, E. G., and Mcgeer, P. L. (2006). Role of ICAM-1 in persisting inflammation in Parkinson disease and MPTP monkeys. *Exp. Neurol.* 197, 275–283.
68. Mirza, B., Hadberg, H., Thomsen, P., and Moos, T. (2000). The absence of reactive astrocytosis is indicative of a unique inflammatory process in Parkinson's disease. *Neuroscience* 95, 425–432.
69. Muqit, M. M., Gandhi, S., and Wood, N. W. (2006). Mitochondria in Parkinson disease: back in fashion with a little help from genetics. *Arch. Neurol.* 63, 649–654.
70. Nakahira, K., Haspel, J. A., Rathinam, V. A., Lee, S. J., Dolinay, T., Lam, H. C., Englert, J. A., Rabinovitch, M., Cernadas, M., Kim, H. P., Fitzger- ald, K. A., Ryter, S. W., and Choi, A. M. (2011). Autophagy proteins reg- ulate innate immune responses by inhibiting the release of mitochon- drial DNA mediated by the NALP3 inflammasome. *Nat. Immunol.* 12, 222–230.
71. Nguyen, M. D., Julien, J. P., and Rivest, S. (2002). Innate immunity: the missing link in neuroprotection and neurodegeneration? *Nat. Rev. Neu- rosci.* 3, 216–227.

72. Nusinzon, I., and Horvath, C. M. (2003). Interferon-stimulated tran- scription and innate antiviral immu- nity require deacetylase activity and histone deacetylase 1. *Proc. Natl. Acad. Sci. U.S.A.* 100, 14742–14747.
73. Orr, C. F., Rowe, D. B., and Halli- day, G. M. (2002). An inflammatory review of Parkinson's disease. *Prog. Neurobiol.* 68, 325–340.
74. Orr, C. F., Rowe, D. B., Mizuno, Y., Mori, H., and Halliday, G. M. (2005). A possible role for humoral immunity in the pathogenesis of Parkinson's disease. *Brain* 128, 2665–2674.
75. Outeiro, T. F., Kontopoulos, E., Alt- mann, S. M., Kufareva, I., Strat- hearn, K. E., Amore, A. M., Volk, C. B., Maxwell, M. M., Rochet, J. C., Mclean, P. J., Young, A. B., Abagyan, R., Feany, M. B., Hyman, B. T., and Kazantsev, A. G. (2007). Sirtuin 2 inhibitors rescue alpha- synuclein-mediated toxicity in mod- els of Parkinson's disease. *Science* 317, 516–519.
76. Perry, V. H. (2004). The influence of systemic inflammation on inflam- mation in the brain: implications for chronic neurodegenerative disease. *Brain Behav. Immun.* 18, 407–413.
77. Piccinini, M., Mostert, M., Croce, S., Baldovino, S., Papotti, M., and Rinaudo, M. T. (2003). Interferon- gamma-inducible subunits are incorporated in human brain 20S proteasome. *J. Neuroimmunol.* 135, 135–140.
78. Qi, B., Huang, Y., Rowe, D., and Halliday, G. (2007). VISA – a pass to innate immunity. *Int. J. Biochem. Cell Biol.* 39, 287–291.
79. Rentzos, M., Nikolaou, C., Andreadou, E., Paraskevas, G. P., Rombos, A., Zoga, M., Tsoutsou, A., Boufidou, F., Kapaki, E., and Vassilopoulos, D. (2009). Circulating interleukin- 10 and interleukin-12 in Parkin- son's disease. *Acta Neurol. Scand.* 119, 332–337.
80. Rivett, A. J., Bose, S., Brooks, P., and Broadfoot, K. I. (2001). Regulation of proteasome com- plexes by gamma-interferon and phosphorylation. *Biochimie* 83, 363–366.
81. Savidge, T. C., Sofroniew, M. V., and Neunlist, M. (2007). Starring roles for astroglia in barrier pathologies of gut and brain. *Lab. Invest.* 87, 731–736.
82. Schapira, A. H., Cooper, J. M., Dex- ter, D., Jenner, P., Clark, J. B., and Marsden, C. D. (1989). Mitochon- drial complex I deficiency in Parkin- son's disease. *Lancet* 1, 1269.
83. Schmidt, S., Linnartz, B., Mendritzki, S., Sczepan, T., Lubbert, M., Stichel, C. C., and Lubbert, H. (2011). Genetic mouse models for Parkinson's dis- ease display severe pathology in glial cell mitochondria. *Hum. Mol. Genet.* 20, 1197–1211.
84. Scumpia, P. O., Kelly, K. M., Reeves, W. H., and Stevens, B. R. (2005). Double-stranded RNA signals antiviral and inflammatory pro- grams and dysfunctional glutamate transport in TLR3-expressing astrocytes. *Glia* 52, 153–162.
85. Seth, R. B., Sun, L., and Chen, Z. J. (2006). Antiviral innate immunity pathways. *Cell Res.* 16, 141–147.
86. Seth, R. B., Sun, L., Ea, C. K., and Chen, Z. J. (2005). Identification and characterization of MAVS, a mitochon- drial antiviral signaling protein that activates NF-kappaB and IRF 3. *Cell* 122, 669–682.
87. Shin, Y., Klucken, J., Patterson, C., Hyman, B. T., and Mclean, P. J. (2005). The co-chaperone carboxyl terminus of Hsp70-interacting protein (CHIP) mediates alpha- synuclein degradation decisions between proteasomal and lysoso- mal pathways. *J. Biol. Chem.* 280, 23727–23734.
88. Silverman, N., and Maniatis, T. (2001). NF-kappaB signaling path- ways in mammalian and insect innate immunity. *Genes Dev.* 15, 2321–2342.
89. Skaug, B., and Chen, Z. J. (2010). Emerging role of ISG15 in antiviral immunity. *Cell* 143, 187–190.
90. Song, Y. J., Huang, Y., and Halliday, G. M. (2011). Clinical correlates of similar pathologies in parkinsonian syn- dromes. *Mov. Disord.* 26, 499–506.
91. Stefanova, N., Fellner, L., Reindl, M., Masliah, E., Poewe, W., and Wen- ning, G. K. (2011). Toll-like receptor 4 promotes alpha-synuclein clear- ance and survival of nigral dopamin- ergic neurons. *Am. J. Pathol.* 179, 954–963.
92. Steurer, J. (2011). [Nonsteroidal anal- gesics have a protective effect against Parkinson disease]. *Praxis (Bern* 1994) 100, 617–618.
93. Stone, D. K., Reynolds, A. D., Mosley, R. L., and Gendelman, H. E. (2009). Innate and adaptive immunity for the pathobiology of Parkinson's dis- ease. *Antioxid. Redox Signal.* 11, 2151–2166.
94. Strauss, K. M., Martins, L. M., Plun- Favreau, H., Marx, F. P., Kautzmann, S., Berg, D., Gasser, T., Wszolek, Z., Muller, T., Bornemann, A., Wolburg, H., Downward, J., Riess, O., Schulz, J. B., and Kruger, R. (2005). Loss of function mutations in the gene encoding Omi/HtrA2 in Parkin- son's disease. *Hum. Mol. Genet.* 14, 2099–2111.
95. Takahashi-Fujigasaki, J., and Fuji- gasaki, H. (2006). Histone deacety- lase (HDAC) 4 involvement in both Lewy and Marinesco bodies. *Neuropathol. Appl. Neurobiol.* 32, 562–566.
96. Tanaka, Y., Engelender, S., Igarashi, S., Rao, R. K., Wanner, T., Tanzi, R. E., Sawa, A., V, L. D., Daw- son, T. M., and Ross, C. A. (2001). Inducible expression of mutant alpha-synuclein decreases protea- some activity and increases sen- sitivity to mitochondria-dependent apoptosis. *Hum. Mol. Genet.* 10, 919–926.
97. Tang, E. D., and Wang, C. Y. (2010). TRAF5 is a downstream target of MAVS in antiviral innate immune signaling. *PLoS ONE* 5, e9172. doi:10.1371/journal.pone.0009172
98. Torkvist, L., Halfvarson, J., Ong, R. T., Lordal, M., Sjoqvist, U., Bresso, F., Bjork, J., Befrits, R., Lofberg, R., Blom, J., Carlson, M., Padyukov, L., D'Amato, M., Seielstad, M., and Pettersson, S. (2010). Analysis of 39 Crohn's disease risk loci in Swedish inflammatory bowel disease patients. *Inflamm. Bowel Dis.* 16, 907–909.
99. Umeno, J., Asano, K., Matsushita, T., Matsumoto, T., Kiyohara, Y., Iida, M., Nakamura, Y., Kamatani, N., and Kubo, M. (2011). Meta-analysis of published studies identified eight additional common susceptibility loci for Crohn's disease and ulcera- tive colitis. *Inflamm. Bowel. Dis.* 17, 2407–2415.
100. Valente, E. M., Abou-Sleiman, P. M., Caputo, V., Muqit, M. M., Har- vey, K., Gispert, S., Ali, Z., Del Turco, D., Bentivoglio, A. R., Healy, D. G., Albanese, A., Nussbaum, R., Gonzalez-Maldonado, R., Deller, T., Salvi, S., Cortelli, P., Gilks, W. P., Latchman, D. S., Harvey, R. J., Dallapiccola, B., Auburger, G., and Wood, N. W. (2004). Heredi- tary early-onset Parkinson's disease caused by mutations in PINK1. *Sci- ence* 304, 1158–1160.
101. Van Limbergen, J., Wilson, D. C., and Satsangi, J. (2009). The genet- ics of Crohn's disease. *Annu. Rev. Genomics Hum. Genet.* 10, 89–116.
102. Villaran, R. F., Espinosa-Oliva, A. M., Sarmiento, M., De Pablos, R. M., Arguelles, S., Delgado-Cortes, M. J., Sobrino, V., Van Rooijen, N., Ven- ero, J. L., Herrera, A. J., Cano, J., and Machado, A. (2010). Ulcerative col- itis exacerbates lipopolysaccharide- induced damage to the nigral dopaminergic system: potential risk factor in Parkinson's disease. *J. Neu- rochem.* 114, 1687–1700.
103. Visintin, A., Latz, E., Monks, B. G., Espevik, T., and Golenbock, D. T. (2003). Lysines 128 and 132 enable lipopolysaccharide binding to MD- 2, leading to Toll-like receptor-4 aggregation and signal transduction. *J. Biol. Chem.* 278, 48313–48320.
104. Wahner, A. D., Bronstein, J. M., Borde- lon, Y. M., and Ritz, B. (2007). Nonsteroidal anti-inflammatory drugs may protect against Parkinson dis- ease. *Neurology* 69, 1836–1842.
105. West, A. B., Moore, D. J., Biskup, S., Bugayenko, A., Smith, W. W., Ross, C. A., Dawson, V. L., and Dawson, T. M. (2005). Parkinson's disease- associated mutations in leucine-rich repeat kinase 2 augment kinase activity. *Proc. Natl. Acad. Sci. USA* 102, 16842–16847.
106. West, A. P., Koblansky, A. A., and Ghosh, S. (2006). Recognition and signaling by Toll-like receptors. *Annu. Rev. Cell Dev. Biol.* 22, 409–437.
107. West, A. P., Shadel, G. S., and Ghosh, S. (2011). Mitochondria in innate immune responses. *Nat. Rev. Immunol.* 11, 389–402.
108. Wilms, H., Rosenstiel, P., Sievers, J., Deuschl, G., Zecca, L., and Lucius, R. (2003). Activation of microglia by human neuromelanin is NF- kappaB dependent and involves p38 mitogen-activated protein kinase: implications for Parkinson's disease. *FASEB J.* 17, 500–502.
109. Wood, L. M., Sankar, S., Reed, R. E., Haas, A. L., Liu, L. F., Mckin- non, P., and Desai, S. D. (2011). A novel role for ATM in reg- ulating proteasome-mediated pro- tein degradation through suppres- sion of the ISG15 conjugation pathway. *PLoS ONE* 6, e16422. doi:10.1371/journal.pone.0016422
110. Wu, C. J., Conze, D. B., Li, T., Sriniva- sula, S. M., and Ashwell, J. D. (2006). NEMO is a sensor of Lys 63-linked polyubiquitination and functions in NF-kappaB activation. *Nat. Cell Biol.* 8, 398–406.
111. Zhang, Y., Gao, J., Chung, K. K., Huang, H., Dawson, V. L., and Dawson, T. M. (2000). Parkin functions as an E2- dependent ubiquitin- protein ligase and promotes the degradation of the synaptic vesicle-associated pro- tein, CDCrel-1. *Proc. Natl. Acad. Sci. U.S.A.* 97, 13354–13359.
112. Zhang, L., Shimoji, M., Thomas, B., Moore, D. J., Yu, S. W., Marupudi, N. I., Torp, R., Torgner, I. A., Ottersen, O. P., Dawson, T. M., and Dawson, V. L. (2005). Mito- chondrial localization of the Parkinson's disease related protein DJ-1: implications for patho- genesis. *Hum. Mol. Genet.* 14, 2063–2073.

7

Preparing unbiased T-cell receptor and antibody cDNA libraries for the deep next generation sequencing profiling

Ilgar Z. Mamedov[1,2†], Olga V. Britanova[1†], Ivan V. Zvyagin[1,2], Maria A. Turchaninova[1], Dmitriy A. Bolotin[1], Ekaterina V. Putintseva[1], Yuriy B. Lebedev[1] and Dmitriy M. Chudakov[1,2*]

[1] *Shemyakin-Ovchinnikov Institute of Bioorganic Chemistry, Russian Academy of Science, Moscow, Russia*
[2] *CEITEC, Masaryk University, Brno, Czech Republic*

Edited by:
Carmen Molina-Paris, University of Leeds, UK

Reviewed by:
Magadan Mompo Susana, Institut National de la Recherche Agronomique, France
Kathrin Kalies, Institute of Anatomy, Germany

****Correspondence:***
Dmitriy M. Chudakov, Shemyakin-Ovchinnikov Institute of Bioorganic Chemistry, Russian Academy of Science, Miklukho-Maklaya 16/10, 117997 Moscow, Russia
e-mail: chudakovdm@mail.ru

† Ilgar Z. Mamedov and Olga V. Britanova have contributed equally to this work.

High-throughput sequencing has the power to reveal the nature of adaptive immunity as represented by the full complexity of T-cell receptor (TCR) and antibody (IG) repertoires, but is at present severely compromised by the quantitative bias, bottlenecks, and accumulated errors that inevitably occur in the course of library preparation and sequencing. Here we report an optimized protocol for the unbiased preparation of TCR and IG cDNA libraries for high-throughput sequencing, starting from thousands or millions of live cells in an investigated sample. Critical points to control are revealed, along with tips that allow researchers to minimize quantitative bias, accumulated errors, and cross-sample contamination at each stage, and to enhance the subsequent bioinformatic analysis. The protocol is simple, reliable, and can be performed in 1–2 days.

Keywords: TCR repertoires, BCR repertoires, NGS applications, cDNA libraries, MiTCR, IG repertoires, T-cell receptor, T-cell receptor repertoire

INTRODUCTION

Next generation sequencing (NGS) technologies opened a breathtaking opportunity to perform deep analysis and comparative studies of the T-cell receptor (TCR) and antibody (IG) repertoires of the human donors and model animals, as well as of the various sorted, separated, or cultured lymphocyte subsets of interest (1–13). Still, rational NGS-analysis of such immune repertoires is critically dependent on the library preparation protocols, starting from a lymphocytes/PBMC sample and ending with the amplification of individual TCR/IG segment encoding molecules on the solid phase of a sequencing machine. Multiple sampling bottlenecks, PCR biases, and cross-contamination at different stages lie in wait to trick a researcher on his way to get the deep, clear, and congruent data.

While studying autoimmunity and hematopoietic stem cell transplantation therapy (10, 14–17), we have optimized cDNA-based protocol that allows unbiased pre-sequencing amplification of the human and murine, alpha- and beta-TCR, as well as IG heavy chain gene libraries. The protocol employs a specific oligonucleotide to prime cDNA synthesis, and template switching effect to form a universal 5′-adapter and to introduce sample barcode at the very first stage of library preparation. Subsequent two-step PCR amplification is performed with universal pairs of primers for the whole library using step-out plus PCR-suppression effect (18) on the 5′-end and nested PCR (19) on the 3′-end of the library (16).

This approach allows efficient and unbiased amplification of millions of the TCR/IG mRNA molecules in only 27–30 (21–24 considering dilution factor, see below) PCR cycles, thus providing sufficient starting material for the deep NGS-analysis of complex lymphocyte samples. Current protocol is optimal for the sequencing on Illumina MiSeq/HiSeq platforms and Roche 454 platforms.

Here we report the upgraded and tested protocol in a ready-to-use format with the technical details required for the method to be easily and uniformly reproduced in any laboratory.

ADVANTAGES OF cDNA LIBRARIES AND 5′-TEMPLATE SWITCH

Starting with cDNA synthesis using 5′-template switching (16, 20, 21) has at least two decisive advantages in comparison with the genomic DNA-based approaches (2, 12).

First, the whole diversity of variable chains (up to approximately 100 different V gene segment variants[1], can be amplified using just a pair (for TCRs) or a simple multiplex set (for IGs) of oligonucleotides, specific to the template switch adapter on the 5′-end and to the constant gene segments on the 3′-end of the library (**Figure 1**).

In contrast, the approaches starting with the genomic DNA require multiplex primer sets to be used both at the 5′ V gene segments' end, and at the 3′ introns/J-segments end of the library (2). Moreover, a subsequent nested PCR amplification, which requires

[1] http://www.imgt.org/

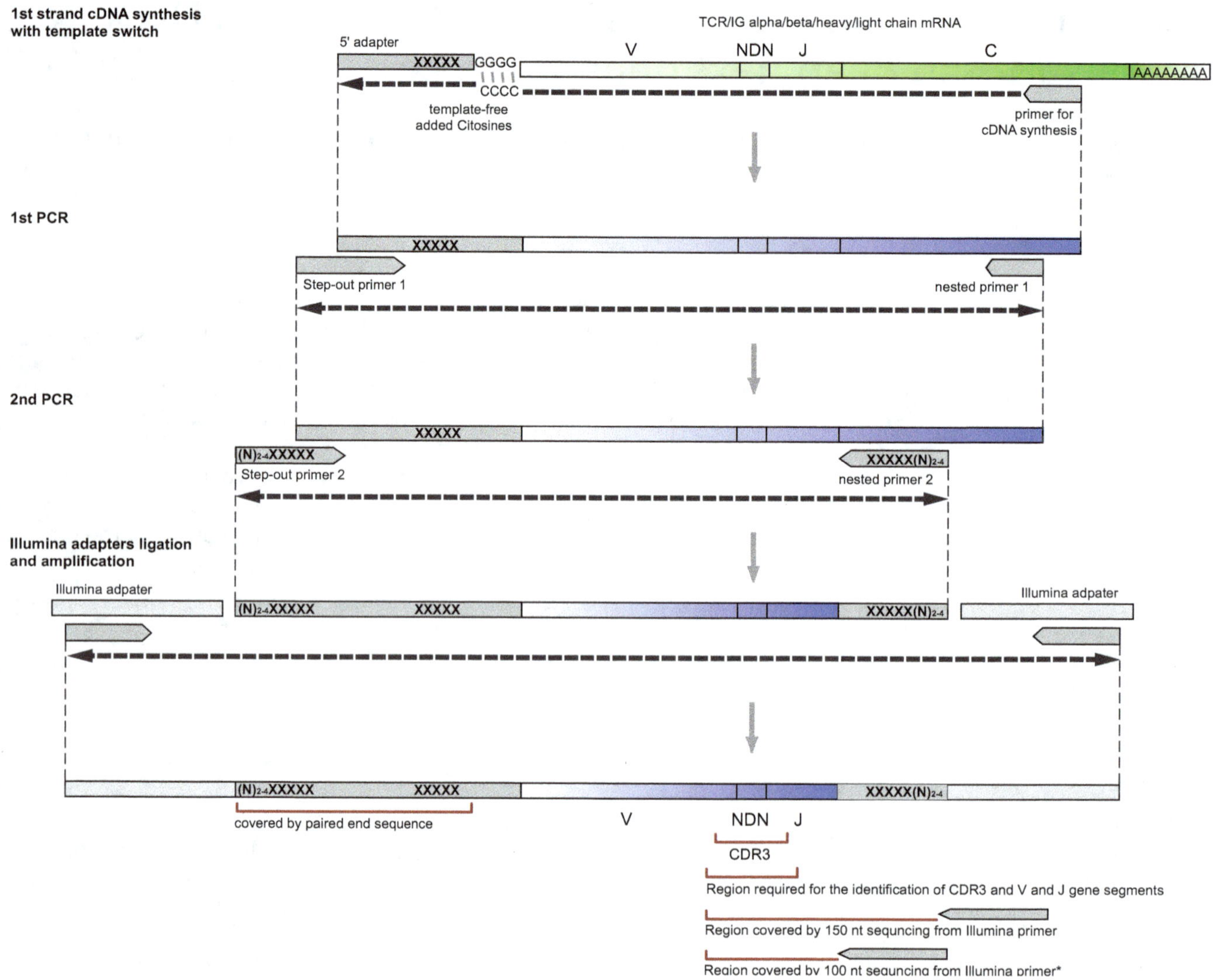

FIGURE 1 | Flow-chart of the library preparation protocol from RNA and to NGS-ready PCR product. XXXXX: optional sample barcodes (see Sample Barcoding in Appendix for details and Supplementary Material for barcodes). *For TCR alpha/beta profiling with 100 nt sequencing length, multiplexed J-segment-specific primers should be used as a reverse primer in the second PCR amplification step as described in section "Next Generation Sequencing Options."

another set of multiplex primers, can be necessary to obtain pure TCR or IG library from genomic DNA. Multiplexing inevitably leads to dramatic bias in relative efficiency of amplification of different variable segments and thus to the loss of quantitative information, and complete loss of some of the rare clonotypes (10, 16, 22, 23).

Second, abundant copies of mRNAs encoding TCR or IG chains comprise an essential portion of the total lymphocyte RNA. This practically results in an efficient amplification of a deep library starting from 10^6 mRNA molecules from a 3 μg of total RNA sample purified from three million PBMC cells (10). cDNA synthesis reaction can be performed in a volume of 10–15 μl in a single PCR tube (see Protocol), allowing multiple parallel experiments to be carried out.

In contrast, amplification of the TCR/IG library starting from 15 μg of genomic DNA of the same three million PBMC sample requires PCR to be carried out in larger volumes (since no more than 0.5 μg of genomic DNA can be taken for a 50 μl PCR reaction), and still does not provide comparable PCR efficiency, i.e., essential portion of the original sample diversity is lost due to the stochastic character of PCR, inevitably missing rare molecules.

LIMITATIONS OF THE USE OF cDNA LIBRARIES AND 5′-TEMPLATE SWITCH

We have recently demonstrated that cDNA-based template switching protocol is highly quantitative at the ensemble level – the level of relative TRBV gene segments' frequencies (10). Indeed, PCR bias is minimized and the whole approach is quite quantitative in respect of relative abundance of mRNA molecules at start and sequencing reads at the end of analysis pipeline. However, it should be noted that individual T-cell or B-cell clones can potentially be characterized by higher or lower expression levels of TCR or IG mRNA (24, 25). This limitation should be kept in mind when using NGS data for the estimation of particular lymphocyte clones' relative abundance.

It is generally important that the cells being analyzed "feel fine" and contain a sufficient amount of TCR/IG mRNA. Therefore, it is preferable to purify total RNA from a freshly isolated cell sample for the native analysis. For the frozen samples, overnight incubation of thawed cells in presence of IL2 (Roche, 15 U/ml) leads to at least twofold increase of TCR genes RNA expression levels (our unpublished observations).

Differences in the efficiency of reverse transcription and template switching may lead to a different number of cDNA molecules read per T- or B-cell. Therefore, it is important to use the same reverse transcriptase and 5′-template switch adapter and carry out all the procedures in identical experimental conditions to obtain results that can be further accurately compared at the deep level (e.g., in an analysis of relative diversity of naïve T cells or a PBMC sample, etc.).

EXPERIMENTAL DESIGN: CELLS, NUMBERS, AND BOTTLENECKS

The desirable depth of TCR or IG repertoire analysis depends on the particular experimental questions raised. For example, application of the current protocol for the deep analysis of a PBMC sample containing 10^6 T cells will provide quantitative data on those TCR clonotypes that constitute at least 0.01–0.1% of all T cells in a sample (100–1000 T cells) (10). The majority (>95%) of TCR clonotypes constituting at least 0.001% (at least 10 T cells) will be sequenced, while approximately 20–40% of TCR clonotypes represented by a single T cell in a sample may be lost (estimated according to our quantitative experiments, depends on the reverse transcriptase used). Preferably, all the synthesized cDNA should be used for the first PCR amplification step. Second PCR should result in sufficient amount of target PCR product in a reasonable number of amplification cycles (see Protocol). The desirable number of output CDR3-containing high quality sequencing reads is at least 2×10^6 per sample (see Protocol and Expected Results).

Much smaller bottleneck limits should be quite sufficient for the majority of the experimental tasks concerning more specific subpopulations of lymphocytes characterized by lower diversity [such as sorted antigen-specific T cells (26) or B cells (27)]. For example, 10,000 lymphocytes, 10 ng high quality total RNA, no more than 21 first PCR cycles, no more than 20 s PCR cycles (see Protocol and Expected Results), and at least 30,000 CDR3-containing sequencing reads (ideally 100,000 reads to achieve over-sequencing) per sample may be sufficient to identify most TCR/IG clonotypes in a low-complexity sample. It is preferable to use reverse transcriptase with high 5′-template switching efficiency (e.g., SMARTScribe, Clontech) when small cell samples/RNA amounts are analyzed.

EXPERIMENTAL DESIGN: SAMPLE BARCODES, MULTIPLEXED SEQUENCING, CROSS-CONTAMINATION

Since as few as 30,000 sequencing reads per sample may be sufficient for many experimental tasks in immune repertoire's profiling, and, for example, paired end 150 bp Illumina MiSeq run can produce more than five million good quality TCR/IG CDR3 reads, a researcher may be often interested in sequencing multiple samples in a single run. At the same time, ligating Illumina sample barcodes to 10 or more samples is rather expensive and laborious. Our design suggests that sample barcodes can be introduced within the 5′-template switch adapter during cDNA synthesis and/or second PCR amplification steps (see **Figure 1**). Samples with the barcodes inside can be then combined in equal (or unequal, if it is desirable to get more reads for some samples) proportions, and Illumina adapters can be ligated to the resulting pooled PCR library of approximately 500–600 bp length (see Protocol and Sample Barcoding in Appendix).

Sample barcodes on both ends of the library allow to eliminate most cross-contaminations between the samples sequenced in the same run/lane that may occur during the amplification of the combined sample after adapters' ligation, and potentially in course of bridge amplification on the solid phase of the sequencing machine.

To avoid contamination on the earlier stages of pre-sequencing library preparation, all procedures, including: RNA purification, cDNA synthesis, first and second PCR preparation – should be performed in separate clean PCR boxes.

PROTOCOL

PREPARING STARTING MATERIAL – TOTAL RNA

1. Use standard Trizol (Invitrogen) or QIAzol (QIAGEN), or other analogous protocol for RNA isolation. Alternatively, use RNeasy kit (QIAGEN), or other column-based RNA isolation method. Depending on the starting material, consider the following RNA purification procedures:
   A. For small amount of whole blood (less than 100 μl) use 1 ml of Trizol or specific RNA isolation kits (for example, QIAamp RNA Blood Kit, QIAGEN).
   B. For large amount of whole blood, preferably perform preliminary PBMC separation using standard procedures (Ficoll density gradient separation) and proceed to C.
   C. For large amount of white blood cells, use 1 ml of Trizol (per up to 10^7 cells). If using column-based RNA isolation method for the large amount of cells, DNase treatment is necessary (according to a manufacturer protocol) since large amounts of genomic DNA significantly affect cDNA synthesis.
   D. For small amount of cells (below 100,000 live cells, for example, sorted or bead-separated T or B cells), preferably perform isolation of total RNA shortly after cell acquisition, in order to minimize loss of live cells and mRNA. When using Trizol protocol, add a co-precipitant (e.g., Pellet Paint, Millipore) to the aqueous phase before adding isopropyl alcohol. It is highly desirable that the precipitant forms a single well-defined spot. This provides confidence that some portion of the material will not be washed off by EtOH. Do not discard EtOH used to wash the sample until you are convinced that library preparation has been performed successfully, since some portion of RNA can remain in EtOH.

All the cell/RNA isolation, cDNA synthesis and first PCR preparation steps should be carried out in a clean DNA/RNAase free room or a PCR box with no contact with any TCR-containing PCR products to prevent contamination. Standard RNA samples handling precautions should be used (gloves, labcoats, filtered tips, and certified RNAase free reagents) to avoid RNA degradation.

Time: 1–2 h.
Pause: RNA can be stored in 70% ethanol at −70°C for at least a year.

cDNA SYNTHESIS AND TEMPLATE SWITCH

2. Mix the following in a final volume of 4 μl in a sterile thin-walled reaction tube (mix1).

Component	Amount, μl	Final concentration*
RNA	1–3	Maximum 2 μg
cDNA synthesis primer(s) (20 μM)**	0.5–1.5 (0.5 each)	1 μM for each primer
mQ	0–2.5	

**Final concentration/amount in 10 μl after adding mix2 (see Step 5).*
***See **Table 1** for primers used. Simultaneous synthesis of TCR alpha and beta cDNA is possible (tested for both human and mouse) in case if limited starting material is available. Simultaneous synthesis of IgA, IgM, and IgG heavy chains cDNA is also possible (tested for human).*

Put no more than 1.5–2 μg of total RNA per 10 μl of final reaction volume. For the extra-deep profiling use proportional volume to obtain cDNA from desired amount of starting RNA.

3. Place the reaction tube(s) into a thermal cycler and incubate for 4 min at 70°C and then for 2 min at 42°C to anneal synthesis primer(s).
4. While incubating, mix the following in a separate tube in a final volume of 6 μl (mix2).

Component	Amount, μl	Final concentration*
First strand buffer (5×, Evrogen or Clontech)	2	1×
DTT (20 μM)	1	2 μM
5′-template switch adapter (10 μM)	1	1 μM
dNTP solution (10 mM each)	1	1 mM each
Mint reverse transcriptase (10×, Evrogen) or SMARTScribe reverse transcriptase (10×, Clontech)	1	1×

**Final concentration in 10 μl after adding mix 2.*

5. Add mix2 to mix1 and mix by pipetting, incubate 40–60 min at 42°C.
   Reverse transcriptases are heat sensitive. Allow the mixture to chill to 42°C after first step denaturation at least for 2 min as described.
   Reverse transcriptases are not equal in their 5′-template switching activity. We have extensive experience with Mint and SMARTScribe reverse transcriptases that provide reliable 5′-template switching.
6. (Optional, for Mint Reverse transcriptase only, to enhance template switching activity) Add 5 μl of IP solution (Evrogen) and incubate at 42°C for additional 1 h.
7. (Optional, see Unique Molecular Identifiers in Appendix) Add 1 μl of Uracyl DNA glycosylase (5 U/μl, New England Biolabs) and incubate 1 h at 37°C.

Time: 2–3 h.
Pause: although cDNA is generally stable, we prefer not to store cDNA longer than several hours at +4°C for the deep profiling experiments. Freezing small amounts of cDNA is undesirable.

FIRST PCR AMPLIFICATION

8. In a sterile thin-walled tube(s) mix the following in a final volume of 25 μl.

Component	Amount, μl	Final concentration
First strand cDNA	1	
Tersus buffer (10×, Evrogen)	2, 5	1×
dNTP (2.5 mM each)	1, 5	0.15 mM each
Primer smart20 (10 μM)	1	0.4 μM
Reverse primer(s) (10 μM)*	1–3 (1 each)	0.4 μM (each)
Tersus polymerase mix (50×, Evrogen)	0.5	1×
mQ	17.5–15.5	

See **Table 1 for primers used. Simultaneous amplification of TCR alpha and beta cDNA is possible (tested for both human and mouse) in case if limited starting material is available. Simultaneous amplification of IgA, IgM, and IgG heavy chains cDNA is also possible (tested for human).*

Put no more than 1 μl of cDNA from the synthesis reaction per 25 μl PCR reaction volume. For the deep profiling, use proportional number of tubes to amplify all the cDNA obtained.
Polymerase with high fidelity and processivity should be used for amplification.

9. Carry out 18 (when starting from large amount of cells) or 21 (when starting from small amount of cells) cycles of amplification using the following program: 95°C for 20 s, 65°C for 20 s, 72°C for 50 s.
10. Combine all the first step PCR products and purify a portion using the QIAquick PCR purification Kit (or other column-based purification system).

Time: 2–3 h.
Pause: purified first PCR product can be stored at −20°C for a month as a source for the re-amplification of material in the second PCR.

SECOND PCR AMPLIFICATION

11. Mix the following in a sterile thin-walled tube in a final volume of 25 μl.

Component	Amount, μl	Final concentration
Purified first PCR product	1	
10× polymerase buffer (e.g., Tersus buffer, Evrogen)	2.5	1×
dNTP (2.5 mM each)	1.5	0.15 mM each
Primer Step1 (10 μM)	1	0.4 μM
Reverse primer (10 μM)*	1	0.4 μM
50× polymerase (e.g., Tersus polymerase, Evrogen)	0.5	1×
mQ	17.5	

See **Table 1 for primers used. For primer design options see Sample Barcoding, Unique Molecular Identifiers, and Introducing Diversity at the Ends of the Library in Appendix. In case of simultaneous cDNA synthesis and first PCR amplification of TCR alpha and beta chain libraries, second PCR for TCR alpha and beta chain libraries preparation should be performed in separate reactions. Use an aliquot of purified first PCR product to generate TCR beta library (with beta specific primer) and TCR alpha library (with alpha specific primer).*

Polymerase with high fidelity and processivity should be used for amplification.

12. Carry out amplification using the following program: 95°C for 20 s, 65°C for 20 s, 72°C for 50 s, 9–12 cycles (up to 18–20 cycles if starting from minimal amounts of RNA); final elongation at 72°C for 5 min).
    Purify the PCR products using QIAquick PCR purification Kit (or other column-based purification system) at the same day. This step is important since it removes the residual enzyme activities that can damage the obtained PCR library.

    Time: 2 h.
    Pause: libraries can be stored at −20°C for weeks before adapter ligation.

MIXING THE BARCODED SAMPLES FOR MULTIPLEX SEQUENCING

In order to combine several PCR libraries with pre-introduced sample barcodes (see **Figure 1** and Sample Barcoding in Appendix for possible options), perform the following:

13. Determine the concentration of each library using the QuBit Fluorometer.
14. Combine samples in a sterile microcentrifuge tube proportionally to the desirable amount of sequencing reads per sample. A total amount of PCR products should be approximately 0.5–1 μg (specify the required amount of the PCR product in a sequencing center).

Alternatively, each sample can be ligated to sequencing adapters with different sample barcodes separately. Samples are mixed in desirable proportions before sequencing.

NEXT GENERATION SEQUENCING OPTIONS

Design of the current protocol is optimized for the Illumina paired end 2 × 150 nt (or 2 × 300 nt for IGs) sequencing as the most reliable way to obtain unbiased TCR/IG repertoire. The paired end sequencing is obligatory when double sample barcodes (see and Sample Barcoding in Appendix) and/or unique molecular identifiers (see Unique Molecular Identifiers in Appendix) are used. If no unique molecular identifiers are used, and sample barcoding is used on the 3′-end of the library only (**Figure 1**), then single end sequencing is possible. However, only half of obtained sequencing reads will contain the CDR3 region.

Protocol also suits well the Roche 454 sequencing technology. Frequent length-errors in reading homogenous oligonucleotide stretches on this platform should be kept in mind, and proper error-correction algorithms utilized (10).

In order to use Illumina paired end 2 × 100 nt sequencing for TCRs, the only required modification is that multiplexed J-segment-specific primers should be used instead of the reverse primer in the second PCR amplification step. This minor multiplexing within limited number of PCR cycles does not lead to essential quantitative bias and allows sequence to start closer to the CDR3 region of interest, as described (10, 16). For IG's heavy chain, the universal J-segment-specific primer (**Table 1**) is close to CDR3 already and no modifications are necessary.

Alternative strategy is that sequences for Illumina flow cell and custom sequencing primers can be introduced in the course of amplification (not shown on **Figure 1**). Although potentially beneficial, it requires thorough design in cooperation with sequencing centers.

This protocol is not adopted for Ion Torrent as these sequencing machines have limitations in the maximal length of analyzed sequencing library. Multiplex PCR mix for the V-segment is required for Ion Torrent library preparation, albeit leads to significant quantitative bias during amplification (10).

To provide better cluster differentiation, ask sequencing facility to spike the library with 10–30% of PhiX and/or design primers as described in Introducing Diversity at the Ends of the Library in Appendix.

Size selection on agarose gel after ligation of adapters is strongly recommended since even minor amounts of short non-specific PCR products can significantly reduce target sequences output.

SOFTWARE ANALYSIS OF NGS DATA

Output NGS data on TCR/IG profiling contain numerous errors accumulated during reverse transcription, PCR amplification, and sequencing. For the latter, higher Phred quality score only means lower frequency of sequencing errors. Thus, high sequence quality does not guarantee absence of sequencing errors. Generally, the more we sequence, the more erroneous TCR/IG variants we generate. Without appropriate error-correction, NGS data can generate artificial TCR/IG diversity exceeding the native diversity of complex input library up to several-fold (10).

Several approaches were proposed to correct the PCR and high quality sequencing errors in TCR datasets, suggesting to filter off low frequency TCR variants (8), to filter off the low abundance variants with single mismatch comparing to the major clonotypes (7), or to correct single mismatch errors in germline segments by

Table 1 | Oligonucleotides.

Primer	Application	Sequence*,**
FIRST STRAND cDNA SYNTHESIS		
Switch_oligo	5′ adapter: template switch adapter, universal for all libraries	AAGCAGTGGTATCAACGCAGAGTAC(XXXXX)TCTT(rG)$_5$
SmartNNN	Alternative template switch adapter with unique molecular identifier (see Unique Molecular Identifiers in Appendix), universal for all libraries	AAGCAGUGGTAUCAACGCAGAGUNNNNUNNNNUNNNNUCTT(rG)$_5$
AC1R	Primer for cDNA synthesis, human TCR alpha mRNA	ACACATCAGAATCCTTACTTTG
BC1R	Primer for cDNA synthesis, human TCR beta mRNA	CAGTATCTGGAGTCATTGA
Mus_alfa_synt1	Primer for cDNA synthesis, mouse TCR alpha mRNA	TTTCGGCACATTGATTTG
BC_mus_syn1	Primer for cDNA synthesis, mouse TCR beta mRNA	CAATCTCTGCTTTTGATG
HCA-rt	Primer for cDNA synthesis, human IgA heavy chain mRNA	GTCCGCTTTCGCTCCAGG
HCM-rt	Primer for cDNA synthesis, human IgM heavy chain mRNA	GATGTCAGAGTTGTTCTTG
HCG-rt	Primer for cDNA synthesis, human IgG heavy chain mRNA	GTGTTGCTGGGCTTGTG
FIRST PCR AMPLIFICATION		
Smart20	Step-out primer 1. Anneals on the switch_oligo, universal for all libraries	CACTCTATCCGACAAGCAGTGGTATCAACGCAG
AC2R	Nested primer 1, human TCR alpha library	TACACGGCAGGGTCAGGGT
BC2R	Nested primer 1, human TCR beta library	TGCTTCTGATGGCTCAAACAC
Mus AV2 rev	Nested primer 1, mouse TCR alpha library	GGTGCTGTCCTGAGACCGAG
BC4_mus_Rev	Nested primer 1, mouse TCR beta library	GATGGCTCAAACAAGGAGACC
HCA-n1	Nested primer 1, human IgA heavy chain library	GCGATGACCACGTTCCCATCT
HCM-n1	Nested primer 1, human IgM heavy chain library	GTGATGGAGTCGGGAAGGAAG
HCG-n1	Nested primer 1, human IgG heavy chain library	GAAGTAGTCCTTGACCAGGCA
SECOND PCR AMPLIFICATION		
Step_1	Step-out primer 2, from the Smart20, universal for all libraries	$(N)_{2-4}$(XXXXX)CACTCTATCCGACAAGCAGT
Hum bcj	Nested primer 2, human TCR beta	$(N)_{2-4}$(XXXXX)ACACSTTKTTCAGGTCCTC
Hum acj	Nested primer 2, human TCR alpha	$(N)_{2-4}$(XXXXX)GGGTCAGGGTTCTGGATAT
Mus bcj	Nested primer 2, mouse TCR beta	$(N)_{2-4}$(XXXXX)GGAGTCACATTTCTCAGATCCT
Mus acj	Nested primer 2, mouse TCR alpha	$(N)_{2-4}$(XXXXX)CAGGTTCTGGGTTCTGGATGT
IGHJ-r1	Nested primer 2, human IG heavy chain (universal for IgA, IgG, and IgM)	$(N)_{2-4}$(XXXXX)GAGGAGACGGTGACCRKGGT

XXXXX: optional sample barcode (see **Figure 1, and Sample Barcoding in Appendix for details and Supplementary Material for barcodes). U = dU (deoxyuridine).*
***$(N)_{2-4}$ – optional. Random nucleotides ("N") are introduced at the 5′ end of final library in order to generate diversity for better cluster identification on Illumina sequencer (see Introducing Diversity at the Ends of the Library in Appendix for details).*

mapping to the major clonotypes (10). Low quality sequences can be either filtered off (7, 8) or mapped to the high quality ones in order to rescue quantitative information (10).

There are currently three available software packages for NGS TCR data analysis: IMGT/HighV-QUEST web service[2], Decombinator (28), and our new software, named MiTCR[3] (29). Note that IMGT/HighV-QUEST is limited to only 50,000–150,000 sequences per batch and thus it is hardly suitable for the analysis of deep NGS profiling data. MiTCR is the only software package that considers sequence quality, performs correction of PCR and sequencing errors, and rescues low quality sequencing data. Two basic error-correction modes are currently implemented, aiming either to eliminate maximal number of accumulated errors, or to preserve maximal original TCR diversity, albeit with less efficient error-correction. Moreover, analysis parameters can be tuned by user in a wide range to obtain optimal result for the particular experimental task. Output format is a tab-delimited file or a special *.cls file for the MiTCR-Viewer software (**Figure 2**).

[2]http://www.imgt.org/IMGTindex/IMGTHighV-QUEST.html
[3]http://mitcr.milaboratory.com/

EXPECTED RESULTS

RNA

The quality and quantity of obtained RNA is critical for the library generation. Quality of total RNA is evaluated by two visible bands on electrophoresis (or two highest peaks on Agilent Bioanalyzer) corresponding to 18S and 28S rRNA. The relative amount of two bands should be between 1:2 and 1:1. The expected yield is 1–3 μg of total RNA from one million of PBMC when using Trizol protocol. If starting material is limited (10,000 cells or less) RNA should be completely used in one cDNA synthesis reaction without analyzing by electrophoresis.

NUMBER OF PCR CYCLES

In order to preserve natural TCR/IG diversity of the sample it is important to minimize the number of PCR cycles used for library

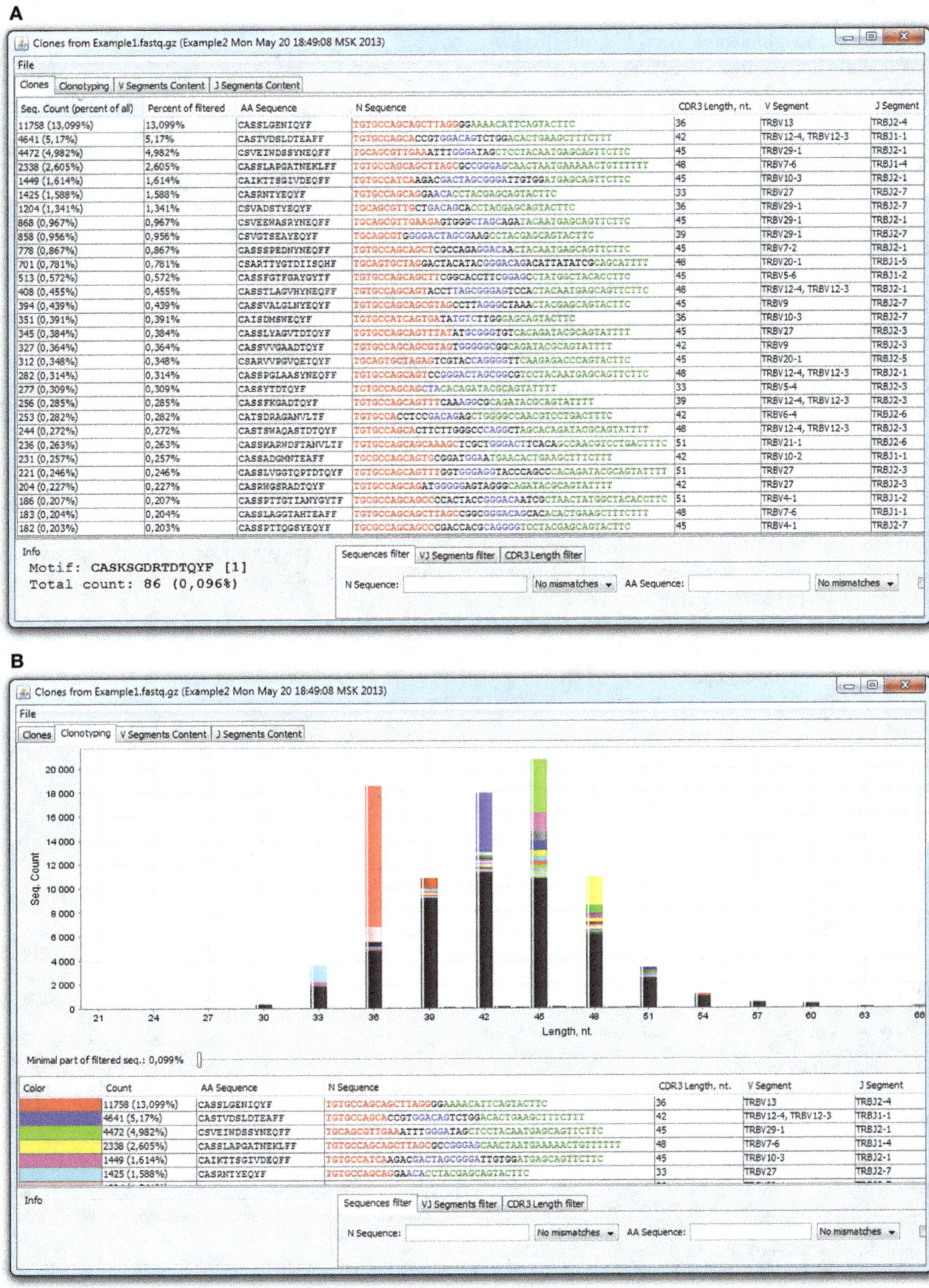

FIGURE 2 | MiTCR-viewer outputs for the analyzed TCR beta dataset. (A) Table with clonotypes. **(B)** *In silico* spectratyping.

preparation. In our system, maximal number of PCR cycles should be 18 for the first and 12 for the second amplification step if starting from 2 μg of total RNA. A well visible band is observed on electrophoresis after 12 cycles of second PCR amplification (that is at least 50 ng of PCR product per 25 μl reaction). For a minimum amount of starting material (below 10,000 cells) the maximum number of PCR cycles should be 21 for the first and 18–20 for the second amplification step. If the number of cycles needed to obtain a visible band is higher, this may indicate that low number of molecules has successfully entered amplification, thus leading to uncertain detection of CDR3 clonotypes of the input sample.

SEQUENCING OUTPUT AND ANALYSIS

With the use of the proposed protocol, at least three million of high quality CDR3-containing sequencing reads from a paired end MiSeq run and at least 100 million CDR3-containing sequencing reads from one lane of paired end HiSeq 2,000/2,500 run are expected. The number of different clonotypes depends on the nature and amount of starting material. For example, profiling of 5–10 million human PBMC cells using 1/10 of HiSeq 2000 Illumina lane (at least 10 million CDR3-containg reads) can yield from 0.5 to 2.5 million TCR beta CDR3 clonotypes after appropriate error-correction.

ACKNOWLEDGMENTS

This work was supported by the Molecular and Cell Biology Program RAS, Russian Foundation for Basic Research Grants 12-04-33139, 12-04-00229 (to Dmitriy M. Chudakov), 13-04-00998 (to Olga V. Britanova), 13-04-01124 (to Ilgar Z. Mamedov), Council of the President of the Russian Federation for young scientists CП-2039.2012.4 (to Ivan V. Zvyagin), and European Regional Development Fund CZ.1.05/1.1.00/02.0068.

REFERENCES

1. Freeman JD, Warren RL, Webb JR, Nelson BH, Holt RA. Profiling the T-cell receptor beta-chain repertoire by massively parallel sequencing. *Genome Res* (2009) **19**:1817–24. doi:10.1101/gr.092924.109
2. Robins HS, Campregher PV, Srivastava SK, Wacher A, Turtle CJ, Kahsai O, et al. Comprehensive assessment of T-cell receptor beta-chain diversity in alphabeta T cells. *Blood* (2009) **114**:4099–107. doi:10.1182/blood-2009-04-217604
3. Ravn U, Gueneau F, Baerlocher L, Osteras M, Desmurs M, Malinge P, et al. By-passing in vitro screening – next generation sequencing technologies applied to antibody display and in silico candidate selection. *Nucleic Acids Res* (2010) **38**:e193. doi:10.1093/nar/gkq789
4. Reddy ST, Ge X, Miklos AE, Hughes RA, Kang SH, Hoi KH, et al. Monoclonal antibodies isolated without screening by analyzing the variable-gene repertoire of plasma cells. *Nat Biotechnol* (2010) **28**:965–9. doi:10.1038/nbt.1673
5. Robins HS, Srivastava SK, Campregher PV, Turtle CJ, Andriesen J, Riddell SR, et al. Overlap and effective size of the human CD8+ T cell receptor repertoire. *Sci Transl Med* (2010) **2**:47ra64. doi:10.1126/scitranslmed.3001442
6. Wang C, Sanders CM, Yang Q, Schroeder HW Jr, Wang E, Babrzadeh F, et al. High throughput sequencing reveals a complex pattern of dynamic interrelationships among human T cell subsets. *Proc Natl Acad Sci U S A* (2010) **107**:1518–23. doi:10.1073/pnas.0913939107
7. Nguyen P, Ma J, Pei D, Obert C, Cheng C, Geiger TL. Identification of errors introduced during high throughput sequencing of the T cell receptor repertoire. *BMC Genomics* (2011) **12**:106. doi:10.1186/1471-2164-12-106
8. Warren RL, Freeman JD, Zeng T, Choe G, Munro S, Moore R, et al. Exhaustive T-cell repertoire sequencing of human peripheral blood samples reveals signatures of antigen selection and a directly measured repertoire size of at least 1 million clonotypes. *Genome Res* (2011) **21**:790–7. doi:10.1101/gr.115428.110
9. Baum PD, Venturi V, Price DA. Wrestling with the repertoire: the promise and perils of next generation sequencing for antigen receptors. *Eur J Immunol* (2012) **42**:2834–9. doi:10.1002/eji.201242999
10. Bolotin DA, Mamedov IZ, Britanova OV, Zvyagin IV, Shagin D, Ustyugova SV, et al. Next generation sequencing for TCR repertoire profiling: platform-specific features and correction algorithms. *Eur J Immunol* (2012) **42**:3073–83. doi:10.1002/eji.201242517
11. Klarenbeek PL, Remmerswaal EB, Ten Berge IJ, Doorenspleet ME, Van Schaik BD, Esveldt RE, et al. Deep sequencing of antiviral T-cell responses to HCMV and EBV in humans reveals a stable repertoire that is maintained for many years. *PLoS Pathog* (2012) **8**:e1002889. doi:10.1371/journal.ppat.1002889
12. Linnemann C, Heemskerk B, Kvistborg P, Kluin RJ, Bolotin DA, Chen X, et al. High-throughput identification of antigen-specific TCRs by TCR gene capture. *Nat Med* (2013) **19**:1534–41. doi:10.1038/nm.3359
13. Turchaninova MA, Britanova OV, Bolotin DA, Shugay M, Putintseva EV, Staroverov DB, et al. Pairing of T-cell receptor chains via emulsion PCR. *Eur J Immunol* (2013) **43**:2507–15. doi:10.1002/eji.201343453
14. Mamedov IZ, Britanova OV, Chkalina AV, Staroverov DB, Amosova AL, Mishin AS, et al. Individual characterization of stably expanded T cell clones in ankylosing spondylitis patients. *Autoimmunity* (2009) **42**:525–36. doi:10.1080/08916930902960362
15. Britanova OV, Staroverov DB, Chkalina AV, Kotlobay AA, Zvezdova ES, Bochkova AG, et al. Single high-dose treatment with glucosaminyl-muramyl dipeptide is ineffective in treating ankylosing spondylitis. *Rheumatol Int* (2011) **31**:1101–3. doi:10.1007/s00296-010-1663-3
16. Mamedov IZ, Britanova OV, Bolotin DA, Chkalina AV, Staroverov DB, Zvyagin IV, et al. Quantitative tracking of T cell clones after haematopoietic stem cell transplantation. *EMBO Mol Med* (2011) **3**:201–7. doi:10.1002/emmm.201100129
17. Britanova OV, Bochkova AG, Staroverov DB, Fedorenko DA, Bolotin DA, Mamedov IZ, et al. First autologous hematopoietic SCT for ankylosing spondylitis: a case report and clues to understanding the therapy. *Bone Marrow Transplant* (2012) **47**:1479–81. doi:10.1038/bmt.2012.44
18. Luk'ianov SA, Gurskaia NG, Luk'ianov KA, Tarabykin VS, Sverdlov ED. Highly-effective subtractive hybridization of cDNA. *Bioorg Khim* (1994) **20**:701–4.
19. Porter-Jordan K, Rosenberg EI, Keiser JF, Gross JD, Ross AM, Nasim S, et al. Nested polymerase chain reaction assay for the detection of *Cytomegalovirus* overcomes false positives caused by contamination with fragmented DNA. *J Med Virol* (1990) **30**:85–91. doi:10.1002/jmv.1890300202
20. Matz M, Shagin D, Bogdanova E, Britanova O, Lukyanov S, Diatchenko L, et al. Amplification of cDNA ends based on template-switching effect and step-out PCR. *Nucleic Acids Res* (1999) **27**:1558–60. doi:10.1093/nar/27.6.1558
21. Douek DC, Betts MR, Brenchley JM, Hill BJ, Ambrozak DR, Ngai KL, et al. A novel approach to the analysis of specificity, clonality, and frequency of HIV-specific T cell responses reveals a potential mechanism for control of viral escape. *J Immunol* (2002) **168**:3099–104.
22. Elnifro EM, Ashshi AM, Cooper RJ, Klapper PE. Multiplex PCR: optimization and application in diagnostic virology. *Clin Microbiol Rev* (2000) **13**:559–70. doi:10.1128/CMR.13.4.559-570.2000
23. Markoulatos P, Siafakas N, Moncany M. Multiplex polymerase chain reaction: a practical approach. *J Clin Lab Anal* (2002) **16**:47–51. doi:10.1002/jcla.2058
24. Paillard F, Sterkers G, Vaquero C. Transcriptional and post-transcriptional regulation of TcR, CD4 and CD8 gene expression during activation of normal human T lymphocytes. *EMBO J* (1990) **9**:1867–72.
25. Doskow JR, Wilkinson MF. CD3-gamma, -delta, -epsilon, -zeta, T-cell receptor-alpha and -beta transcripts are independently regulated during thymocyte ontogeny and T-cell activation. *Immunology* (1992) **77**:465–8.
26. Andersen RS, Kvistborg P, Frosig TM, Pedersen NW, Lyngaa R, Bakker AH, et al. Parallel detection of antigen-specific T cell responses by combinatorial encoding of MHC multimers. *Nat Protoc* (2012) **7**:891–902. doi:10.1038/nprot.2012.037
27. Franz B, May KF Jr, Dranoff G, Wucherpfennig K. Ex vivo characterization and isolation of rare memory B cells with antigen tetramers. *Blood* (2011) **118**:348–57. doi:10.1182/blood-2011-03-341917
28. Thomas N, Heather J, Ndifon W, Shawe-Taylor J, Chain B. Decombinator: a tool for fast, efficient gene assignment in T-cell receptor sequences using a finite state machine. *Bioinformatics* (2013) **29**:542–50. doi:10.1093/bioinformatics/btt004
29. Bolotin DA, Shugay M, Mamedov IZ, Putintseva EV, Turchaninova MA, Zvyagin IV, et al. MiTCR: software for T-cell receptor sequencing data analysis. *Nat Methods* (2013) **10**:813–4. doi:10.1038/nmeth.2555
30. Kivioja T, Vaharautio A, Karlsson K, Bonke M, Enge M, Linnarsson S, et al. Counting absolute numbers of molecules using unique molecular identifiers. *Nat Methods* (2012) **9**:72–4. doi:10.1038/nmeth.1778

8

The structural basis of antibody-antigen recognition

Inbal Sela-Culang*[†]*, Vered Kunik*[†] *and Yanay Ofran*

The Goodman Faculty of Life Sciences, Bar Ilan University, Ramat Gan, Israel

Edited by:
Michal Or-Guil, Humboldt University Berlin, Germany

Reviewed by:
Gur Yaari, Yale University, USA
Chaim Putterman, Albert Einstein College of Medicine, USA

****Correspondence:***
Yanay Ofran, The Goodman Faculty of Life Sciences, Bar Ilan University, Ramat-Gan 52900, Israel
e-mail: yanay@ofranlab.org

[†]Inbal Sela-Culang and Vered Kunik have contributed equally to this work.

The function of antibodies (Abs) involves specific binding to antigens (Ags) and activation of other components of the immune system to fight pathogens. The six hypervariable loops within the variable domains of Abs, commonly termed complementarity determining regions (CDRs), are widely assumed to be responsible for Ag recognition, while the constant domains are believed to mediate effector activation. Recent studies and analyses of the growing number of available Ab structures, indicate that this clear functional separation between the two regions may be an oversimplification. Some positions within the CDRs have been shown to never participate in Ag binding and some off-CDRs residues often contribute critically to the interaction with the Ag. Moreover, there is now growing evidence for non-local and even allosteric effects in Ab-Ag interaction in which Ag binding affects the constant region and vice versa. This review summarizes and discusses the structural basis of Ag recognition, elaborating on the contribution of different structural determinants of the Ab to Ag binding and recognition. We discuss the CDRs, the different approaches for their identification and their relationship to the Ag interface. We also review what is currently known about the contribution of non-CDRs regions to Ag recognition, namely the framework regions (FRs) and the constant domains. The suggested mechanisms by which these regions contribute to Ag binding are discussed. On the Ag side of the interaction, we discuss attempts to predict B-cell epitopes and the suggested idea to incorporate Ab information into B-cell epitope prediction schemes. Beyond improving the understanding of immunity, characterization of the functional role of different parts of the Ab molecule may help in Ab engineering, design of CDR-derived peptides, and epitope prediction.

Keywords: antibody, CDRs, antigen, paratope, epitope, framework, constant domain

INTRODUCTION

Antibodies (Abs) have two distinct functions: one is to bind specifically to their target antigens (Ags); the other is to elicit an immune response against the bound Ag by recruiting other cells and molecules. The association between an Ab and an Ag involves myriad of non-covalent interactions between the epitope – the binding site on the Ag, and the paratopes – the binding site on the Ab. The ability of Abs to bind virtually any non-self surface with exquisite specificity and high affinity is not only the key to immunity but has also made Abs an enormously valuable tool in experimental biology, biomedical research, diagnostics and therapy. The diversity of their binding capabilities is particularly striking given the high structural similarity between all Abs. The availability of increasing amounts of structural data in recent years now allows for a much better understanding of the structural basis of Ab function in general, and of Ag recognition in particular. This review surveys the recent developments and the current gaps and challenges in this field. We focus specifically on the current understanding of the determinants within the Ab structure that contribute to Ag binding. We first discuss the motivations for, and applications of, the study of the structural basis of Ag recognition. Then we describe and discuss the Ab-Ag interface, with specific focus on the paratopes and the complementarity determining regions (CDRs), and their role in Ag binding. The last part focuses on the contribution of the non-CDRs parts of the Ab [i.e., framework regions (FRs) and the constant domains] to Ag binding and on the recent suggestions regarding non-local and allosteric effects in Ab function. Over the last few years numerous reviews have addressed issues that are related or tangential to the topics we review here. This includes reviews of the engineering of Abs (1), their stability (2), affinity maturation (3), and isotype selection (4). While these important topics are relevant to the findings and ideas we review here, they are beyond the scope of this review.

THE MOTIVATIONS FOR, AND APPLICATIONS OF, THE STUDY OF Ab-Ag RECOGNITION

UNDERSTANDING IMMUNITY AND AUTOIMMUNITY

The adaptive immune response involves two types of lymphocytes: T cells, which recognizes Ags that have been processed and their fragments are presented by MHC molecules, and B cells which produce soluble Abs that can identify also the intact Ag in its native form. While the way in which T cells recognize their epitopes has been extensively studied to a level that enables the successful prediction of T-cell epitopes (5, 6), the rules that govern Ab-Ag recognition, including which parts of the Ab structure underlie Ag recognition and how and why certain determinants on the Ag are selected as epitopes, are not as well characterized. Understanding the mechanisms that underlie Ab-Ag recognition, therefore, is crucial for understanding immunity.

The immune system enables Abs to distinguish between foreign and self molecules (7). Autoimmune diseases are characterized by the inappropriate response to self-Ags. It is not always clear what role is played by Abs and what role is played by other components of the immune system in autoimmunity. A variety of molecular mechanisms have been proposed, including sequestered Ags, molecular mimicry, and polyclonal B-cell activation (8). Better understanding of the underpinnings of Ab-Ag recognition may also shed light on these questions.

A MODEL FOR STUDYING BIO-MOLECULAR RECOGNITION

A fundamental characteristic of the immune system is its ability to continuously generate novel protein recognition sites. Ab-Ag interfaces, therefore, are often considered a model system for elucidating the principles governing biomolecular recognition (9–13). For example, Keskin (14) and McCoy et al. (15) used X-ray crystallographic structures of Ab-Ag complexes to elucidate principles of the molecular architecture of protein–protein interfaces. Other studies, however, view Ab-Ag interfaces as a specific case that may not allow for generalization to all types of protein–protein interfaces (16). Thus, large scale studies of protein–protein interactions often exclude Ab-Ag complexes from the dataset analyzed (16–19). It is, therefore, important to determine to what extent Ab-Ag complexes could serve as a general model for protein–protein interactions.

ANTIBODY ENGINEERING

The specificity of the Ab molecule to its cognate Ag has been exploited for the development of a variety of immunoassays, vaccinations, and therapeutics. Ab engineering may offer to expand the application of Abs by permitting improvements of affinity (20, 21) and specificity (22, 23). Understanding of the role each structural element in the Ab plays in Ag recognition is essential for successful engineering of better binders. The engineering of Abs is also important for the clinical use of Abs from non-human sources. Early studies on the use of rodent Abs in humans determined that they can be immunogenic (24). Humanization by grafting of the CDRs from a mouse Ab to a human FR is a commonly used engineering strategy for reducing immunogenicity (25, 26). In most cases, the successful design of high-affinity, CDR-grafted, Abs requires that key residues in the human acceptor FRs that are crucial for preserving the functional conformation of the CDRs will be back-mutated to the amino acids of the original murine Ab (26, 27). Several groups (28–30) used the experimentally determined 3-D structures of Ab-Ag complexes in the Protein Data Bank (PDB) (31) to determine which residues participate in Ag recognition and binding. Such knowledge can be exploited to identify residues that are important for the function of the Ab in general and for Ag recognition in particular and may guide Ab engineering (32, 33). Residues that help maintain the functional conformation of the CDRs, for example, can be used to improve Ab humanization efforts by CDR-grafting.

Ab EPITOPE PREDICTION

Antibody epitopes (sometimes referred to as B-cell epitopes) are the molecular structures within an Ag that make specific contacts with the Ab paratope. B-cell epitopes are used in the development of vaccines and in immunodiagnostics. Correct identification of B-cell epitopes within an antigenic protein, may open the door for the design of molecules (biologic or synthetic) that mimic potentially protective epitopes and could be used to raise specific Abs or be used as a prophylactic or therapeutic vaccines. Identification of B-cell epitopes could promote protective immunity in the context of emerging and re-emerging infectious diseases and potential bioterrorist threats. This may be achieved by choosing from among the putative epitopes those that may provide immunity (e.g., by eliciting Abs that hamper the molecular function of pathogenic Ags). The choice of such epitopes is believed to be relevant for understanding and controlling protective immunity. In the case of the vaccinia virus, for example, which was used as smallpox vaccine and is the only vaccine that has led to the complete eradication of an infectious disease from the human population, individuals possessing a high frequency of memory B-cells specific for major neutralizing Ags of the vaccinia virus are better protected from smallpox than individuals with a memory B-cell pool dominated by specificities for non-protective Ags (34). Thus, understanding the way in which an Ab recognizes its cognate epitope is of particular interest for vaccine design and disease prevention (35). Existing tools for identification of Ab epitopes (such as X-ray crystallography, pepscan, phage display, expressed fragments, partial proteolysis, mass spectrometry, and mutagenesis analysis) are not only expensive, laborious, and time consuming but also fail to identify many epitopes (36). When talking about protein Ags, most of these methods typically identify linear stretches as epitopes, while, arguably, most of the epitopes on protein Ags are conformational and even discontinuous. As for computational approaches, despite more than 30 years of efforts (37), existing B-cell epitope prediction methods are not accurate enough (38, 39) and are, therefore, not widely used. This is exemplified in **Figure 1**, in which the structure of hen egg lysozyme (HEL) Ag and three Abs that bind it are shown (**Figures 1A,B**), as well as the epitopes predicted by three different methods (**Figure 1C**).

In general, current methods are trying to identify epitopic residues based on the presence of features associated with residues that bind the Ab (40–50). One possible explanation for the failure of these methods is that the differences between epitopes and other residues are not substantial. Indeed, several analyses (51–53) have shown that the amino-acid composition of epitopes is essentially indistinguishable from that of other surface-exposed non-epitopic residues.

This lack of intrinsic properties that clearly differentiate between epitopic and non-epitopic residues and the fact (demonstrated in **Figure 1**) that most of the Ag surface may become a part of an epitope under some circumstances (54–57) suggest that epitopes depend, to a great extent, on the Abs that recognize them. This is exemplified in **Figure 1**: most of the HEL surface residues are part of an epitope of at least one Ab (**Figures 1A,B**), even though this figure shows only three Abs (out of dozens known to bind HEL). Almost all the residues predicted to be epitopic may be considered as correct predictions as they bind some Ab (**Figure 1C**) but also as false predictions as they don't bind the others. Similarly, predicting that a residue is not in an epitope may be either a true negative or a false negative, depending on the Ab considered. It has recently been suggested by us (Sela-Culang et al., submitted)

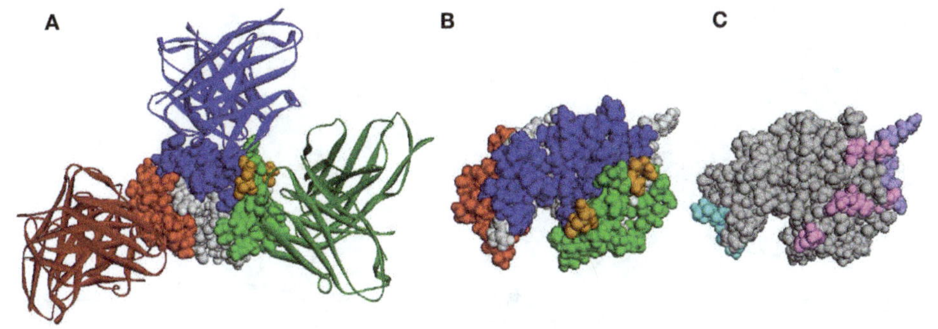

FIGURE 1 | Predicted epitopes vs. the actual epitopes of HEL. (A) The 3-D structure of HEL (CPK representation) together with three Abs (ribbon representation). PDB IDs 1JHL, 3D9A, and 1MLC were superimposed according to HEL structure. Epitope residues are colored blue, green, and red according to the corresponding Ab. Residues that are common to two epitopes are colored orange. **(B)** The structure of HEL colored according to the same three epitopes as in **(A)**, presented in a different orientation. **(C)** The structure of HEL colored according to the epitopes predicted by Discotope (light blue), ellipro (purple), and seppa (pink). Note, not all predicted residues of Discotope and ellipro are observable in the presented orientation.

and by others (58–60) that predicting epitopes should be done for a certain Ab. A similar concept was successfully applied in the case of T-cell epitope prediction methods: these methods do not examine the Ag for general features. Rather, different predictions are made, dependent on the specific MHC molecule binding and presenting the epitope to T cells.

THE ROLE OF CDRs AND THEIR DEFINITION

As shown in **Figure 2**, Abs are all-beta proteins consisting of four polypeptide chains: two identical heavy (H) chains and two identical light (L) chains (61). The light and heavy chains are linked by disulfide bonds to form the arms of a Y-shaped structure, each arm is known as a Fab (61). The Fab is composed of two variable domains (VH in the heavy chain and VL in the light chain) and two constant domains (CH1 and CL) (62). In the pairing of light and heavy chains, the two variable domains dimerize to form the Fv fragment which contains the Ag binding site. Within each variable domain lie six hypervariable loops (63), three in the light chain (L1, L2, and L3) and three in the heavy chain (H1, H2, and H3), supported by a conserved FR of β-sheets. The light and heavy variable domains fold in a manner that brings the hypervariable loops together to create the Ag binding site or paratope. Two additional domains of the heavy chain, CH2, and CH3, compose the Fc region which is responsible for mediating the biological activity of the Ab molecule.

CDRs IDENTIFICATION

As indicated by their names, CDRs are believed to account for the recognition of the Ag. Therefore, a major focus in analyzing the structural basis for Ag recognition has been in identifying the exact boundaries of the CDRs in a given Ab. It is a common practice to identify paratopes through the identification of CDRs. Kabat and co-authors (63, 64) were the first to introduce a systematic approach to identify CDRs in newly sequenced Abs. It was based on the assumption that CDRs are the most variable regions between Abs. Therefore, they aligned the (fairly limited) set of Ab sequences available at that time and identified the most variable positions. Based on the alignment, they introduced a numbering scheme for the residues in the hypervariable regions and determined which positions mark the beginning and the end of each CDR. As structural data became available, Chothia and Lesk (65, 66) manually analyzed a small number of experimentally solved 3-D structures and determined the structural location of the loop regions. The boundaries of the FRs and CDRs were determined and the latter have been shown to adopt a restricted set of conformations, based on the presence of certain residues at key positions in the CDRs and the flanking FRs. Their finding that Kabat's definitions of L1 and H1 are structurally incorrect led to the introduction of the Chothia numbering scheme. With the increase of available structural data, they ran their analysis anew and introduced a new definition of L1 (66) in 1989. In 1997 (67), however, they concluded that this correction was erroneous, and reverted to their original 1987 numbering scheme. While the Kabat and Chothia schemes treated separately the different families of immunoglobulin domains, Lefranc and colleagues (68, 69) proposed a unified numbering scheme (referred to as IMGT numbering scheme) for immunoglobulin variable domain genomic sequences, including Ab light and heavy variable domains, as well as T-cell receptor variable domains. To correlate between the sequence, structure, and domain folding behavior of all immunoglobulin variable domains, the Aho numbering scheme spatially aligned known 3-D structures of immunoglobulins and unified their numbering (70).

A drawback of the Kabat, Chothia, and IMGT numbering schemes is that CDRs length variability takes into account only the most common loop lengths; While both Kabat and Chothia schemes accommodate insertions with insertion letters (e.g., 27A), the IMGT scheme avoids the use of insertion codes for all but the least common very long loops, and the Aho numbering scheme places insertions and deletions symmetrically around a key position. However, Abs with unusually long insertions may be hard to annotate using these methods and, as a result, their CDRs may not be identified correctly. For instance, the recently determined 3-D crystal structure of two bovine Abs (71) reveal exceptionally long H3 CDRs (>60 residues), with long insertions which these methods cannot accommodate and thus cannot identify the CDRs of these Abs.

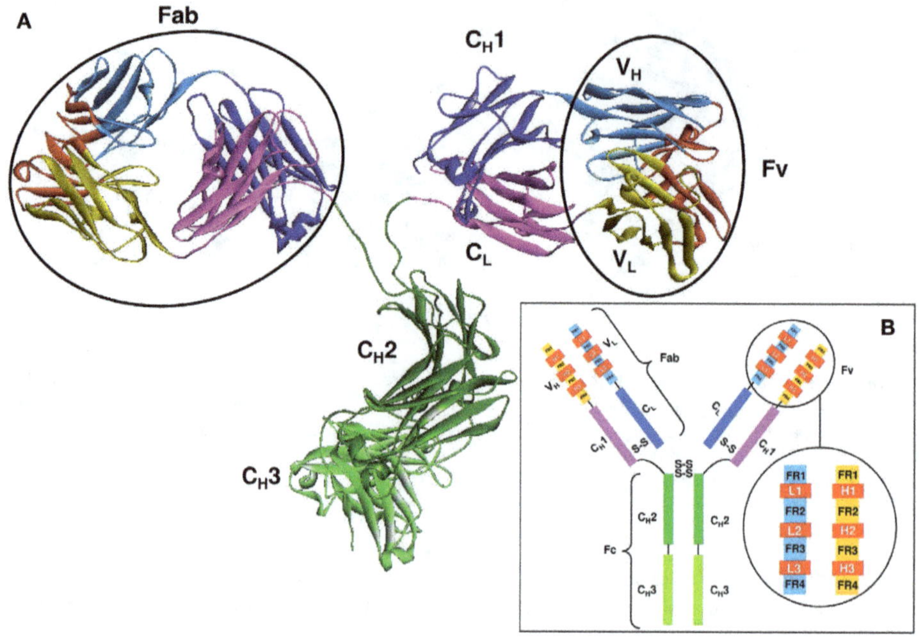

FIGURE 2 | The structure of an Ab molecule. **(A)** The 3-D structure of an Ab molecule (PDB ID: 1IGT). **(B)** A schematic representation of the Ab scaffold.

ARE CDRs GOOD PROXIES FOR THE PARATOPE?

While identification of paratopes is often done through identification of CDRs, not all the residues within the CDRs bind the Ag. In fact, an early analysis of the 3-D structures of Abs suggested that only 20–33% of the residues within the CDRs participate in Ag binding (72). In 1996, MacCallum and colleagues (73) performed a detailed residue-level analysis of Ag contacts. They suggested that contacting residues are more common at CDRs residues which are located at the center of the Ag combining site, and that non-contacting residues within the CDRs correspond with residues that are important for maintaining the structural conformations of the hypervariable loops and not necessarily for recognition of the Ag. Thus, they introduced a mapping of Ag-contacting propensities for each Ab position and proposed a new definition for CDRs based on these propensities. Padlan and co-workers (28) utilized Abs sequence and structure data to perform a by-position summary of Ag contacts. They found that the residues that are directly involved in the interaction with the Ag are also, in general, the most variable ones. They suggested that the residues that interact with the Ag should be called Specificity Determining Residues (SDRs).

The number of publicly available structures of Ab-Ag complexes increased in recent years to a level that enabled large-scale analyses. In a recent analysis (29) we utilized all available protein-Ab complexes in the PDB to identify the structural regions in which Ag binding actually occurs. This approach was implemented into a method dubbed Paratome (30, 74) that is based on a multiple structure alignment (MSTA) of all available Ab-Ag complexes in the PDB. The MSTA revealed regions of structural consensus where the pattern of structural positions that bind the Ag is highly similar among all Abs. These regions of structural binding consensus were termed antigen binding regions (ABRs). While CDRs, as identified by methods such as Kabat (63), Chothia (65), and IMGT (69), may miss ~20% of the Ag binding residues, ABRs cover ~96% of the residues that actually bind the Ag (30). To avoid confusions and cumbersome nomenclature, herein we generically refer to CDRs, SDRs, and ABRs as "CDRs" unless otherwise specified. **Figure 3** shows an example of CDRs as identified by Kabat, Chothia, IMGT, and Paratome for one Ab (anti-IL-15, PDB ID: 2XQB), compared to the actual Ag binding residues. It can be seen that in this example, some of the CDRs (e.g., L3, H3) identified by the four methods are almost identical, while in other CDRs (e.g., L2, H1, and H2) there are substantial differences between the methods. The MSTA of Abs with known 3-D structure also confirmed previous observations that there are structural positions within the CDRs in which none, or only a small percentage of the Abs contact the Ag. This is shown in **Figure 4** where an example of such a position is marked by a green arrow.

INTEGRALITY VS. MODULARITY

Designed systems are often characterized as either modular or integral. In a modular system different components, or modules, function independent of the function of other modules. The generation of Abs in the immune system is based on combining different elements, in a way that may be considered modular where each component is capable of binding the Ag regardless of the others. However, some analyses suggest that Ag binding warrants a more integrative view of the relationships between the different components of the Ab.

The binding-sites of interacting proteins are usually composed of surface patches that have good shape and electrostatic complementary (15, 75, 76). It has been shown that CDRs

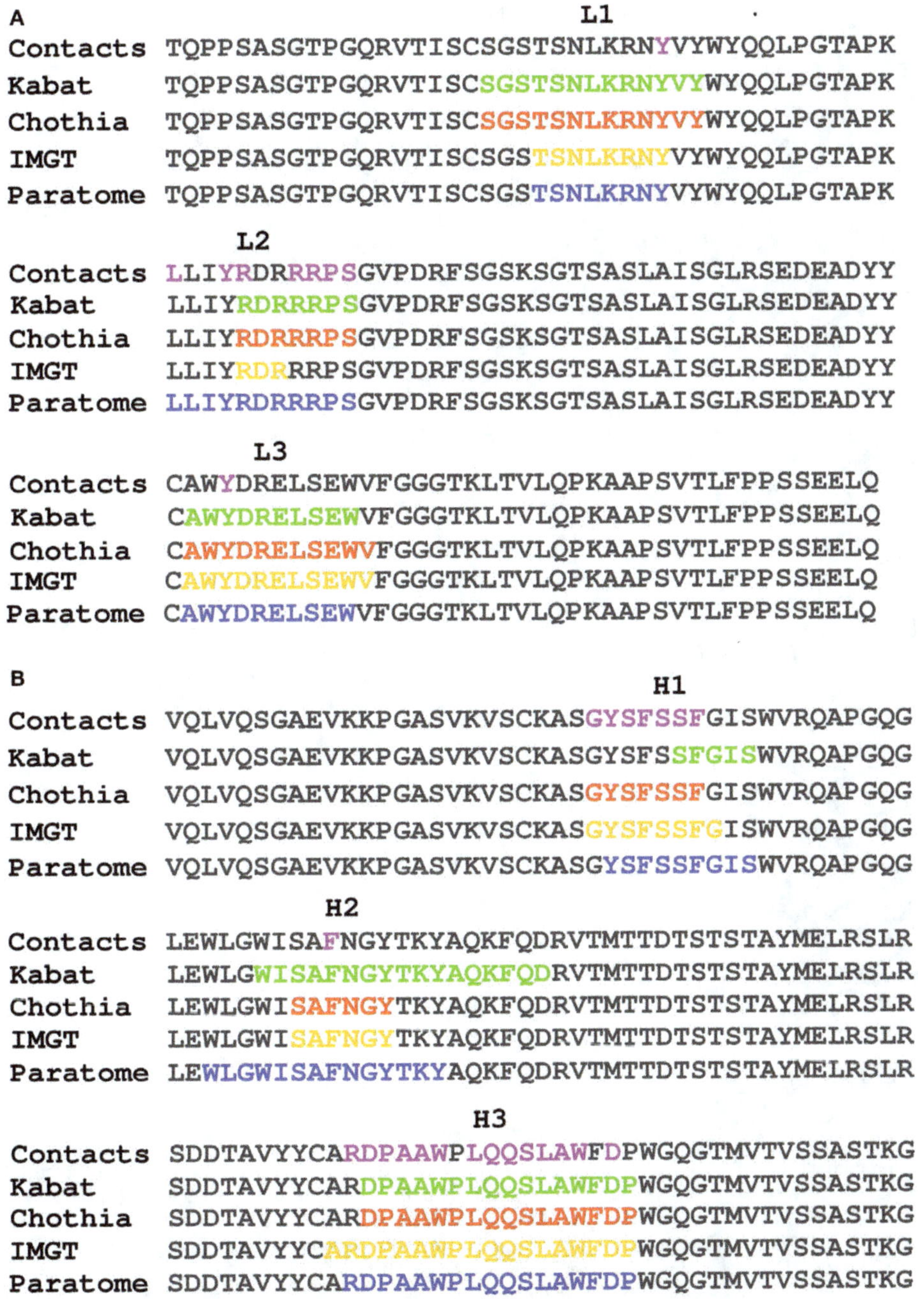

FIGURE 3 | Comparison of different CDR identification methods. The light **(A)** and heavy **(B)** chains of PDB ID 2XQB were numbered according to Kabat (colored green) and Chothia (colored red) using the Abnum tool (www.bioinf.org.uk/abs/abnum) and CDRs were extracted according to the CDR definitions table (www.bioinf.org.uk/abs/#cdrs). CDRs according to IMGT (colored orange) were identified using the IMGT-gap tool (www.imgt.org/3Dstructure-DB/cgi/DomainGapAlign.cgi). ABRs according to Paratome (colored blue) were identified using the Paratome server (www.ofranlab.org/paratome). Contacts (colored purple) between the Ab and IL-15 were defined using a 6-Å cutoff value.

are characterized by an amino-acid composition that is different from that of other protein loops (77) and also from other types of protein–protein interfaces (58). Thus, one would expect that epitopes, just like paratopes, should have a distinct amino-acid composition. However, several recent analyses (51, 53) have shown that this is not the case: while epitopes differ from other types of interfaces (10, 29, 60), their amino-acid composition is virtually the same as that of non-epitopic surface residues.

Several studies have shown that each CDR has its own unique amino-acid composition, different from the composition of the other CDRs (52, 58, 78). Additionally, we have shown that each CDR has a unique set of contact preferences, therefore, favoring

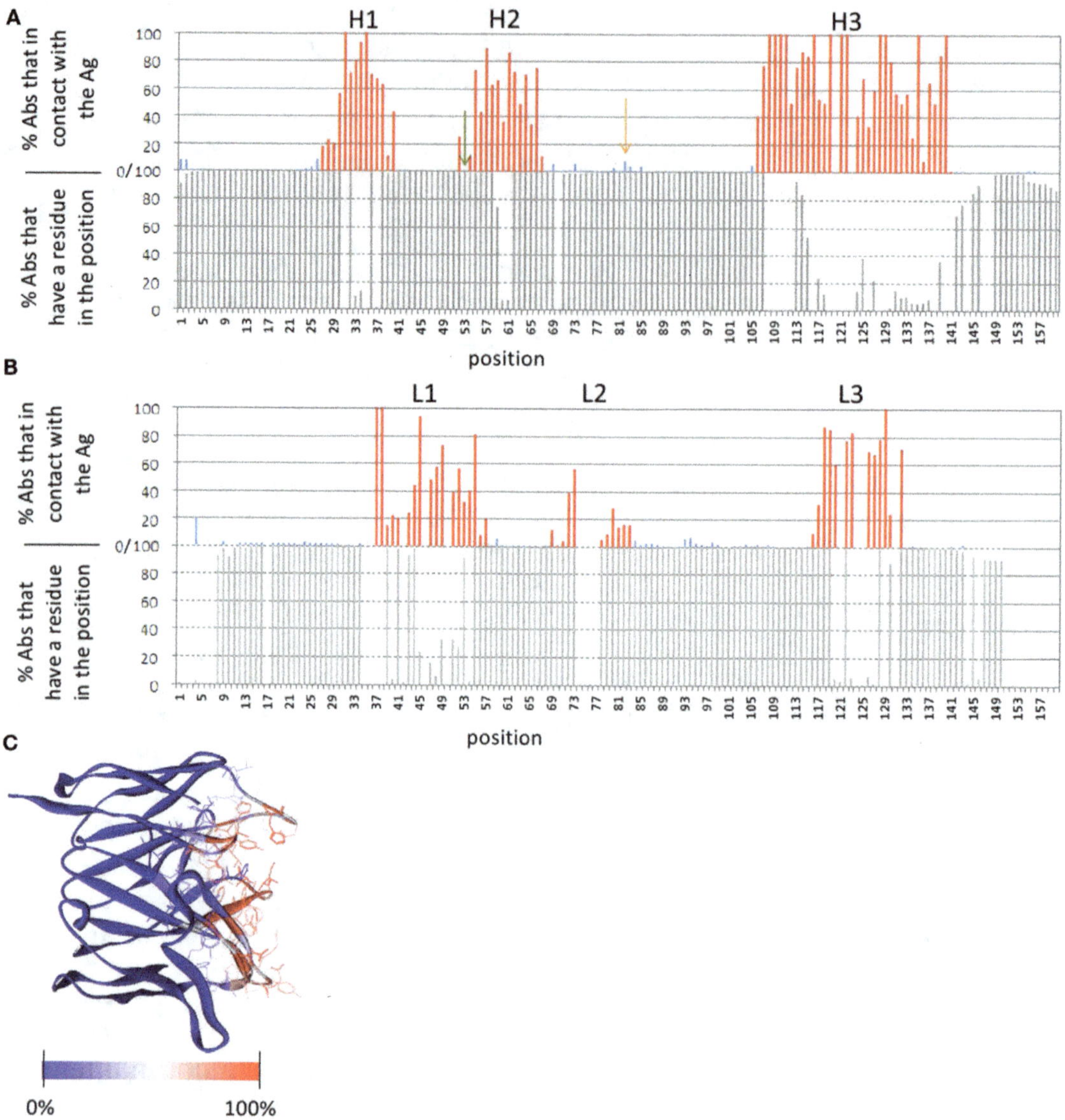

FIGURE 4 | Ab positions that contact the Ag. (A,B) The lower graphs show the percentage of Abs with known 3-D structure that have a residue in a given position (i.e., in other Abs there is a gap in the MSTA in that position). The upper graphs show the percentage of Abs that contact the Ag out of those Abs that have a residue in that position. **(A)** Depicts the heavy chain and **(B)** depicts the light chain. In the upper graphs, the ABRs are colored red and the FRs are colored blue. An example of a position within an ABR that is not in contact with the Ag in any of the Abs, is marked by a green arrow. An example of a position in the FRs that is in contact with the Ag in many (8%) of the Abs is marked by an orange arrow. **(C)** The Ab Fv domain (PDB ID: 1QFU) is colored according to the percentage of all Abs with known 3-D structure in which the residue in that position is in contact with the Ag: from red (100% of the Abs) to blue (0%). ABR residues are presented as lines. The definition of the ABRs is according to the Paratome server. A 6-Å cutoff value was used to define residues in contact. Percentages of contacts were calculated based on an MSTA of all protein Ab-Ag complexes in the PDB (30).

certain amino-acids over others (52). Dividing epitope residues into six subsets according to the CDR they bind, we found that each of the subsets has a distinct amino-acid composition, distinguishable from non-epitope surface (52). In other words, when the six subsets of epitope residues are considered together the unique composition of each subset disappears so that the overall amino-acid composition of the entire epitope is indistinguishable from the rest of the surface. Pathogenic epitopes may have evolved to resemble Ag surface to escape recognition. On the other hand, the integration of the six CDRs together, each with its own unique amino-acid composition and contact preferences, could be the evolutionary response of the immune system that enables Abs to recognize virtually any surface patch on the Ag.

Despite this integrated effect of the CDRs, Abs can be also considered as a modular system, composed of different elements (such as the Fab, VH and VL, or the six CDRs), which may bind the Ag on their own. Such smaller Ab fragments that retain Ag binding affinity and specificity, hold a great potential for drug design (79–81) as they have improved pharmacokinetics, tissue and tumor penetration, and can be produced more economically (80, 81).

They may also be combined with other fragments to yield better binders. Although such smaller fragments cannot induce effector function such as complement activation (due to the lack of the constant domains), they may neutralize the targeted Ag. Fab and single-chain variable (scFv) fragments usually maintain specific binding to the Ag (82). VH and VL fragments usually show sticky behavior, low solubility, and reduced Ag binding affinity (83–85), although, they sometime retain specificity to the Ag (83, 85–87).

The CDRs may provide additional level of modularity. According to the commonly accepted hotspot hypothesis, the binding energy of two proteins is largely determined by a very small number of critical interface residues (12, 88–90). Thus, one may wonder whether an individual CDR could bind the Ag on its own provided that it harbors hotspots. Several linear peptides containing one or more of the CDRs that retained Ag specificity have been reported (91–98). Although their affinity was usually in the micromolar range, it could be significantly improved by introducing relatively minor modifications (91, 99). However, many attempts to isolate and design such CDR derived peptides failed (100, 101). One possible reason is that a CDR, on its own, may not fold to the same conformation as in the context of the entire Fab, which may be crucial for binding. Cyclizing the CDR by adding Cys residues at its edges was suggested as a solution for this problem (96, 102–104). Another reason might lie in the fact that many attempts for the design of CDR-derived peptides are made based on CDR-H3, as it is considered to be the most important CDR for Ag binding (67, 105–107). However, the median length of ABR-H2 is substantially longer than that of H3, and both typically form the same number of interactions with the Ag (52). In addition, while ABR-H3 was shown to have the highest contribution to Ag binding energy on average (52), there are individual cases in which other CDRs are the dominant ones (52, 102). It is also possible that in some cases the binding depends on specific contacts from residues in different CDRs, which may preclude the design of CDR-derived peptides that maintain specificity. We have shown (102) that CDRs that are able to bind the Ag on their own have unique characteristics and, thus, can be computationally identified given the Ab-Ag complex structure. This may enhance the design of CDR-derived peptides that are not necessarily based on CDR-H3.

NON-CDR DETERMINANTS THAT HAVE A ROLE IN Ag BINDING

FR RESIDUES

Within the variable domain, the CDRs are believed to be responsible for Ag recognition, while the FR residues are considered a scaffold for the CDRs. However, it is now well established that some of the FR residues may play an important role in Ag binding (32, 108). As mentioned above, many such FR residues were identified during the process of Ab humanization by CDR grafting. While grafting only the CDRs usually results in a significant drop or a complete loss of binding, the binding affinity can be retained by back mutating some of the FR residues to the original murine sequence, emphasizing their role in Ag binding (26, 109–115).

Framework region residues that affect Ag binding can be divided into two categories. The first are FR residues that contact the Ag, thus are part of the binding-site (108, 109, 111, 116–123). Some of these residues are close in sequence to the CDRs (in fact they may be within the boundaries of CDRs according to some CDR identification methods, but not according to others, as shown in **Figure 3**). Other residues are those that are far from the CDRs in sequence, but are in close proximity to it in the 3-D structure. In particular, a loop in the heavy chain FR-3, sometimes referred to as CDR-H4, accounts for 1.3% of human Ab-Ag contacts (78, 124). This CDR-H4 is also enriched (in human Abs) in somatic hypermutations (Burkovitz et al., submitted). **Figure 4** shows positions that are not in the CDRs but are in contact with the Ag in many Abs [e.g., the one marked by an orange arrow (4A), which corresponds to CDR-H4].

In the second category of FR residues that affect Ag binding, are residues that are not in contact with the Ag, but affect Ag binding indirectly (108, 109, 120, 121). These residues can be further divided to those that are in spatial proximity to the CDRs, and those that are not. The former are assumed to affect binding by providing a structural support to the CDRs, enabling them to adopt the right conformation and orientation, shaping the binding-site required for Ag binding (32). For example, it has been suggested that a certain position in heavy chain FR-3, close in structure but not in sequence to CDR-H1 and CDR-H2, affects the orientation of CDR-H2 relative to CDR-H1 in such a way that a large side-chain packs between them and separates them while a small side-chain allows them to be closer to each other (109, 120). Nevertheless, this is not always true, as was shown in the case of the anti-lysozyme D1.3 Ab: while mutating Lys in this position to either Val, Ala, or Arg resulted in affinity difference, no structural change was observed (121).

Framework region residues that are more distant from the paratope are suggested to play a role in maintaining the overall structure of the Fv domains (32). However, these FR residues may also affect the Ag binding-site itself, by directing the relative orientation of the VH vs. the VL, and thus the orientation of the CDRs relative to each other (125–128). In particular, FR-2 residues were shown to play an important role in VH-VL interaction (129). Moreover, Masuda et al. (130) pointed to a specific position in the FR-2 loop, which controls the strength of the VH-VL interaction as well as its dependence on Ag binding. We have shown that the conformation of this loop changes upon Ag binding more than other residues in the FRs, and that the binding related conformational changes in this loop are similar in their magnitude to those of the CDRs (107). The potential role of the VH-VL interface in Ag binding is further supported by the observation that residues that are in the VH-VL interface (and are not a part of the Ab-Ag interface), are more likely to be mutated during the somatic hypermutation process, than residues that are not in either of these interfaces (Burkovitz et al., submitted).

Understanding the role of FR residues in Ag binding is crucial for efficient Ab design in general and for humanization in particular. Specifically, knowing in advance which FR residues may affect Ag binding, one may consider back-mutating these residues into their murine sequence, to improve affinity during CDR grafting. To this end, attempts were made to identify positions that contribute to Ag binding in multiple cases (32, 113, 119). For example, Haidar et al. (32) used a non-redundant dataset of Ab-Ag complex structures to identify positions that frequently contact the CDRs, and combined these positions with those that were back-mutated frequently in the humanization literature. The 17 FR positions they identified were successfully used to design a combinatorial library for Ab humanization. Additional Abs, for which structures of both wild-type and a mutant(s) are available, may reveal the structural mechanisms by which each FR position affects Ag binding.

CONSTANT REGION

Until recently, Ab constant domains were considered responsible for the isotype and for effector function, such as complement activation, Fc receptor binding, avidity, and serum half-life (131). However, many studies now provide a strong evidence for a role for the constant region in Ag binding (131–147). There are many examples of Abs with identical variable domains but different isotypes that bind the same Ag with a different affinity or specificity (134–146). For instance, two Abs sharing identical variable domains but expressing different isotypes were shown to bind tubulin with significantly different affinities (135). Consistent with these studies, it has been shown that the complex of HEL and the Fv version of the HyHEL-10 Ab has an order of magnitude lower dissociation constant than the complex of HEL with the Fab version of this Ab (147). A probable explanation for this phenomenon would be an allosteric influence of the constant domains on the structure of the variable domains. Indeed, several structural studies provided some evidence for such structural effects (133, 146, 147). For example, Janda et al. (133) analyzed by Circular Dichroism (CD) spectra four different Ab isotypes of the 3E5 family that share identical variable domains, and showed that the different isotypes undergo different structural changes upon binding a common Ag. Similar results were obtained for anti-nuclear Abs as well: Xia et al. (146) compared four different isotypes of the PL9–11 anti-nuclear Ab sharing the same variable region, and found that the changes in secondary structure content (as revealed by CD analysis) as well as the wave length shifts of tryptophan fluorescence emission, upon Ag binding, are both isotype dependent. Recently, Tudor et al. (144) showed that this allosteric effect may control not only Ag binding affinity and specificity, but also the epitope recognized. They showed that two anti-HIV-1 IgG1 and IgA2 Abs with identical variable regions, recognize only partially overlapping epitopes.

Differences in affinity and specificity of Abs with the same variable region but different isotypes may play a role in autoimmunity if they occur in a self-reactive Ag. For example, different isotypes have been shown to be associated with different clinical outcomes for lupus erythematosus: a set of anti-PL9–11 Abs sharing the same variable domain but different isotypes were shown to bind DNA and chromatin, as well as the renal Ags, with different affinities that were associated with significant differences in renal pathogenicity *in vivo* and survival (148).

Several studies have suggested that allosteric effects in Abs may occur on the other direction as well: structural changes in the variable region caused by Ag binding may be transferred into the constant domains, potentially influencing effector activation and cellular response (131, 149–151). For example, Oda et al. (149) showed that the binding of staphylococcal protein A (SPA) or streptococcal protein G (SPG) to the constant region was inhibited by hapten binding in several Abs. A different example was provided by Horgan et al. (151) who observed differences in complement activation of two Abs which differ only in their VH domain.

An allosteric effect in Abs is further supported by a systematic computational analysis we have performed on all available free and Ag-bound pairs of structures (107). Many of the Ag-binding-related structural changes occur distant from the Ag binding-site, including changes in the relative orientation of the heavy and light chains in both the variable and constant domains as well as a change in the elbow angle between the variable and the constant domains. Moreover, the most consistent and substantial conformational change outside of the binding site was found in a loop in the heavy chain constant domain, which is a part of the CH1-CL interface, and is involved in complement binding (152).

What could be the mechanism for these allosteric effects? Changes in the constant domains sequence (different isotypes of the same Ab) or in its conformation (e.g., by effector binding) may lead to a rearrangement of the constant domains relative to each other and relative to the variable domains, which may result in a change to the VH-VL relative orientation (72), thus re-shaping the Ag binding-site (153–155).

The potential influence of the constant region on Ag affinity or specificity suggests that the process of class-switch may be considered, in combination with somatic hypermutations, as a mechanism for Ab diversity (131, 132). Engineering of an Ab of interest is usually associated with the optimization of its affinity to the Ag. Since the constant region may affect this affinity, the isotype selected should be carefully considered. Moreover, the constant region should be taken into account in vaccine design as well since different isotypes may bind the pathogenic Ag with different affinities, thus affecting the response to infection. For example, the anti HIV-1 IgG1 and IgA2 Abs mentioned above share the same variable region, nevertheless, they have been shown to block HIV-1 infection differently (144). While IgA2 blocked HIV-1 transcytosis and $CD4^+$ cell infection more efficiently, IgG1 and IgA2 act synergistically to block HIV-1 transfer from Langerhans cells to T cells. Thus, it has been suggested that a mucosal IgA-based vaccine response should complement an IgG-based vaccine response in blocking HIV-1 transmission.

CONCLUDING REMARKS

As Abs are one of the most versatile naturally occurring biosensors, it is of high importance to decipher the structural and molecular mechanisms by which they recognize and bind their Ags. Such knowledge is crucial for understanding immunity, may enable better prediction of Ab epitopes, and assist in Ab engineering.

While the commonly accepted view has been that CDRs hold the key for Ab-Ag recognition, recent findings indicate that not all the positions in the traditionally defined CDRs are important for binding. Furthermore, it has been shown that many positions that contribute critically to the binding energy reside outside of the transitional CDRs. Moreover, different CDR identification methods may often identify radically different stretches as "CDRs," indicating that CDRs are not well defined and thus are not necessarily a good proxy for the binding site. The hypervariable loops that accommodate the CDRs differ significantly from each other on various aspects. Understanding the way in which their binding preferences are integrated to yield the overall specificity of the Ab is an intriguing structural and biophysical challenge.

Accumulation of recent data suggests that elements that may be spatially distant from the Ag binding site also play a crucial role in Ag recognition. The unorthodox suggestion that non-local and even allosteric effects influence epitope recognition warrants additional analysis and research.

Addressing the open questions regarding the structural basis of Ag recognition requires additional structural data in the form of crystal structures of Abs bound to Ags of different types (proteins, peptides, nucleic acids, and haptens). Large-scale analysis of such structures will allow for the generation and testing of new hypotheses regarding the way in which Abs find and bind their epitopes.

ACKNOWLEDGMENTS

The authors are supported in part by NIAID contract N01-AI-90048C (http://www.niaid.nih.gov/).

REFERENCES

1. Vincent KJ, Zurini M. Current strategies in antibody engineer- ing: Fc engineering and pH- dependent antigen binding, bis- pecific antibodies and antibody drug conjugates. *Biotechnol J* (2012) 7:1444–50. doi:10.1002/biot.201200250
2. Wang W, Singh S, Zeng DL, King K, Nema S. Antibody structure, instability, and formulation. *J Pharm Sci* (2007) 96:1–26. doi:10.1002/ jps.20727
3. Sheedy C, MacKenzie CR, Hall JC. Isolation and affinity maturation of hapten-specific antibodies. *Biotechnol Adv* (2007) 25:333–52. doi:10.1016/j.biotechadv.2007.02. 003
4. Salfeld JG. Isotype selection in antibody engineering. *Nat Biotech- nol* (2007) 25:1369–72. doi:10. 1038/nbt1207-1369
5. Brusic V, Bajic VB, Petrovsky N. Computational methods for pre- diction of T-cell epitopes – a framework for modelling, test- ing, and applications. *Methods* (2004) 34:436–43. doi:10.1016/j. ymeth.2004.06.006
6. Kim Y, Sette A, Peters B. Applications for T-cell epi- tope queries and tools in the Immune Epitope Database and Analysis Resource. *J Immunol Methods* (2011) 374:62–9. doi:10.1016/j.jim.2010.10.010
7. Frank SA. Specificity and cross- reactivity (Chapter 4). In: *Immunology and Evolution of Infectious Disease*. Princeton, NJ: Princeton University Press (2002). p. 33–54.
8. Rose NR, MacKay IR, editors. T- cells and autoimmunity. In: *The Autoimmune Diseases*, 4th ed. San Diego: Elsevier Academic Press (2006). 1160 p.
9. Jones S, Thornton JM. Principles of protein-protein interactions. *Proc Natl Acad Sci U S A* (1996) 93: 13–20. doi:10.1073/pnas.93.1.13
10. Jones S, Thornton JM. Analysis of protein-protein interaction sites using surface patches. *J Mol Biol* (1997) 272:121–32. doi:10.1006/ jmbi.1997.1234
11. Lo Conte L, Chothia C, Janin J. The atomic structure of protein- protein recognition sites. *J Mol Biol* (1999) 285:2177–98. doi:10.1006/ jmbi.1998.2439
12. Bogan AA, Thorn KS. Anatomy of hot spots in protein interfaces. *J Mol Biol* (1998) 280:1–9. doi:10. 1006/jmbi.1998.1843
13. Chakrabarti P, Janin J. Dissecting protein-protein recognition sites. *Proteins* (2002) 47:334–43. doi:10. 1002/prot.10085
14. Keskin O. Binding induced confor- mational changes of proteins cor- relate with their intrinsic fluctu- ations: a case study of antibod- ies. *BMC Struct Biol* (2007) 7:31. doi:10.1186/1472-6807-7-31
15. McCoy AJ, Chandana Epa V, Colman PM. Electro- static complementarity at protein/protein interfaces. *J Mol Biol* (1997) 268:570–84. doi:10.1006/ jmbi.1997.0987
16. Neuvirth H, Raz R, Schreiber G. ProMate: a structure based predic- tion program to identify the loca- tion of protein-protein binding sites. *J Mol Biol* (2004) 338:181–99. doi:10.1016/j.jmb.2004.02.040
17. Ma B, Elkayam T, Wolfson H, Nussinov R. Protein–protein inter- actions: structurally conserved residues distinguish between bind- ing sites and exposed protein sur- faces. *Proc Natl Acad Sci U S A* (2003) 100:5772–7. doi:10.1073/ pnas.1030237100
18. Bordner AJ, Abagyan R. Statis- tical analysis and prediction of protein-protein interfaces. *Proteins* (2005) 60:353–66. doi:10.1002/ prot.20433
19. Ofran Y, Rost B. Analysing six types of protein-protein interfaces. *J Mol Biol* (2003) 325:377–87. doi: 10.1016/S0022-2836(02)01223-8
20. Marks JD, Griffiths AD, Malmqvist M, Clackson TP, Bye JM, Winter G. By-passing immunization: build- ing high affinity human antibod- ies by chain shuffling. *Biotechnol- ogy (N Y)* (1992) 10:779–83. doi: 10.1038/nbt0792-779
21. Soderlind E, Ohlin M, Carlsson R. Complementarity-determining region (CDR) implantation: a theme of recombination. *Immunotechnology* (1999) 4:279–85.
22. Hemminki A, Niemi S, Hau- toniemi L, Soderlund H, Takkinen K. Fine tuning of an anti- testosterone antibody binding site by stepwise optimisation of the CDRs. *Immunotechnology* (1998) 4:59–69. doi:10.1016/S1380-2933(98)00002-5
23. Ohlin M, Owman H, Mach M, Borrebaeck CA. Light chain shuffling of a high affinity anti- body results in a drift in epitope recognition. *Mol Immunol* (1996) 33:47–56. doi:10.1016/0161- 5890(95)00123-9
24. Mirick GR, Bradt BM, Denardo SJ, Denardo GL. A review of human anti-globulin antibody (HAGA, HAMA, HACA, HAHA) responses to monoclonal antibodies. Not four letter words. *Q J Nucl Med Mol Imaging* (2004) 48:251–7.
25. Jones PT, Dear PH, Foote J, Neu- berger MS, Winter G. Replacing the complementarity-determining regions in a human antibody with those from a mouse. *Nature* (1986) 321:522–5. doi:10.1038/321522a0
26. Queen C, Schneider WP, Selick HE, Payne PW, Landolfi NF, Duncan JF, et al. A humanized antibody that binds to the interleukin 2 recep- tor. *Proc Natl Acad Sci U S A* (1989) 86:10029–33. doi:10.1073/ pnas.86.24.10029
27. Co MS, Queen C. Humanized anti- bodies for therapy. *Nature* (1991) 351:501–2. doi:10.1038/351501a0
28. Padlan EA, Abergel C, Tipper JP. Identification of specificity- determining residues in antibod- ies. *FASEB J* (1995) 9:133–9.
29. Ofran Y, Schlessinger A, Rost B. Automated identification of com- plementarity determining regions (CDRs) reveals peculiar charac- teristics of CDRs and B cell epi- topes. *J Immunol* (2008) 181: 6230–5.
30. Kunik V, Peters B, Ofran Y. Struc- tural consensus among antibod- ies defines the antigen binding site. *PLoS Comput Biol* (2012) 8:e1002388. doi:10.1371/journal. pcbi.1002388
31. Berman HM, Westbrook J, Feng Z, Gilliland G, Bhat TN, Weissig H, et al. The Protein Data Bank. *Nucleic Acids Res* (2000) 28:235–42. doi: 10.1093/nar/28.1.235
32. Haidar JN, Yuan QA, Zeng L, Snavely M, Luna X, Zhang H, et al. A universal combinatorial design of antibody framework to graft distinct CDR sequences: a bioinformatics approach. *Proteins* (2012) 80:896–912. doi:10.1002/prot.23246
33. Hanf KJ, Arndt JW, Chen LL, Jarpe M, Boriack-Sjodin PA, Li Y, et al. Antibody humanization by redesign of complementarity- determining region residues prox- imate to the acceptor frame- work. *Methods* (2013). doi:10. 1016/j.ymeth.2013.06.024
34. Amanna IJ, Slifka MK, Crotty S. Immunity and immunolog- ical memory following small- pox vaccination. *Immunol Rev* (2006) 211:320–37. doi:10.1111/j.0105-2896.2006. 00392.x
35. Yang XD, Yu XL. An introduc- tion to epitope prediction methods and software. *Rev Med Virol* (2009) 19:77–96. doi:10.1002/rmv.602
36. Xu XL, Sun J, Liu Q, Wang XJ, Xu TL, Zhu RX, et al. Evaluation of spatial epitope computational tools based on experimentally- confirmed dataset for protein antigens. *Chin Sci Bull* (2010) 55:2169–74. doi:10.1007/s11434- 010-3199-z
37. Hopp TP, Woods KR. Prediction of protein antigenic determinants from amino acid sequences. *Proc Natl Acad Sci U S A* (1981) 78:3824–8. doi:10.1073/pnas.78.6. 3824
38. Ponomarenko JV, Bourne PE. Antibody-protein interac- tions: benchmark datasets and prediction tools evaluation. *BMC Struct Biol* (2007) 7:64. doi:10.1186/1472-6807-7-64
39. Blythe MJ, Flower DR. Bench- marking B cell epitope pre- diction: underperformance of existing methods. *Pro- tein Sci* (2005) 14:246–8. doi:10.1110/ ps.041059505
40. Ansari HR, Raghava GP. Iden- tification of conformational B- cell epitopes in an antigen from its primary sequence. *Immunome Res* (2010) 6:6. doi:10.1186/1745- 7580-6-6
41. Kulkarni-Kale U, Bhosle S, Kolaskar AS. CEP: a con- formational epitope predic- tion server. *Nucleic Acids Res* (2005) 33:W168–71. doi:10.1093/nar/gki460
42. Liang SD, Zheng DD, Zhang C, Zacharias M. Prediction of anti- genic epitopes on protein surfaces by consensus scoring. *BMC Bioin- formatics* (2009) 10:302. doi:10. 1186/1471-2105-10-302
43. Ponomarenko J, Bui HH, Li W, Fusseder N, Bourne PE, Sette A, et al. ElliPro: a new structure- based tool for the prediction of antibody epitopes. *BMC Bioinfor- matics* (2008) 9:514. doi:10.1186/ 1471-2105-9-514

44. Rubinstein ND, Mayrose I, Pupko T. A machine-learning approach for predicting B-cell epitopes. *Mol Immunol* (2009) 46:840–7. doi:10. 1016/j.molimm.2008.09.009
45. Rubinstein ND, Mayrose I, Martz E, Pupko T. Epitopia: a web-server for predict- ing B-cell epitopes. *BMC Bioinformatics* (2009) 10:287. doi:10.1186/1471-2105-10-287
46. Sun J, Wu D, Xu T, Wang X, Xu X, Tao L, et al. SEPPA: a computational server for spa- tial epitope prediction of pro- tein antigens. *Nucleic Acids Res* (2009) 37:W612–6. doi:10.1093/ nar/gkp417
47. Sweredoski MJ, Baldi P. PEPITO: improved discontinuous B-cell epitope prediction using multi- ple distance thresholds and half sphere exposure. *Bioinformatics* (2008) 24:1459–60. doi:10.1093/ bioinformatics/btn199
48. Ambroise J, Giard J, Gala JL, Macq B. Identification of rele- vant properties for epitopes detec- tion using a regression model. *IEEE/ACM Trans Comput Biol Bioinform* (2011) 8:1700–7. doi:10. 1109/TCBB.2011.77
49. Liang S, Zheng D, Standley DM, Yao B, Zacharias M, Zhang C. EPSVR and EPMeta: prediction of antigenic epitopes using sup- port vector regression and multi- ple server results. *BMC Bioinfor- matics* (2010) 11:381. doi:10.1186/ 1471-2105-11-381
50. Zhang W, Xiong Y, Zhao M, Zou H, Ye X, Liu J. Prediction of confor- mational B-cell epitopes from 3D structures by random forests with a distance-based feature. *BMC Bioinformatics* (2011) 12:10. doi: 10.1186/1471-2105-12-341
51. Janin J, Chothia C. The struc- ture of protein-protein recogni- tion sites. *J Biol Chem* (1990) 265:16027–30.
52. Kunik V, Ofran Y. The indistin- guishability of epitopes from pro- tein surface is explained by the dis- tinct binding preferences of each of the six antigen-binding loops. *Protein Eng Des Sel* (2013). doi:10. 1093/protein/gzt027
53. Kringelum JV, Nielsen M, Padkjær SB, Lund O. Structural analysis of B-cell epitopes in antibody:protein complexes. *Mol Immunol* (2013) 53:24–34. doi:10.1016/j.molimm. 2012.06.001
54. Benjamin DC, Berzofsky JA, East IJ, Gurd FR, Hannum C, Leach SJ, et al. The antigenic structure of proteins: a reappraisal. *Annu Rev Immunol* (1984) 2:67–101. doi:10.1146/annurev.iy.02.040184. 000435
55. Greenbaum JA, Andersen PH, Blythe M, Bui HH, Cachau RE, Crowe J, et al. Towards a consensus on datasets and evaluation met- rics for developing B-cell epitope prediction tools. *J Mol Recognit* (2007) 20:75–82. doi:10.1002/ jmr. 815
56. Novotný J, Handschumacher M, Haber E, Bruccoleri RE, Carlson WB, Fanning DW, et al. Antigenic determinants in proteins coincide with surface regions accessible to large probes (antibody domains). *Proc Natl Acad Sci U S A* (1986) 83:226–30. doi:10.1073/pnas.83.2. 226
57. Thornton JM, Edwards MS, Taylor WR, Barlow DJ. Location of "con- tinuous" antigenic determinants in the protruding regions of proteins. *EMBO J* (1986) 5:409–13.
58. Zhao L, Li JY. Mining for the antibody-antigen interacting asso- ciations that predict the B cell epitopes. *BMC Struct Biol* (2010) 10(Suppl 1):S6. doi:10.1186/1472- 6807-10-S1-S6
59. Zhao L, Wong L, Li JY. Antibody- specified b-cell epitope predic- tion in line with the principle of context-awareness. *IEEE/ACM Trans Comput Biol Bioinform* (2011) 8:1483–94. doi:10.1109/ TCBB.2011.49
60. Soga S, Kuroda D, Shirai H, Kobori M, Hirayama N. Use of amino acid composition to pre- dict epitope residues of individ- ual antibodies. *Protein Eng Des Sel* (2010) 23:441–8. doi:10.1093/ protein/gzq014
61. Edelman GM, Benacerraf B. On structural and functional rela- tions between antibodies and proteins of the gamma-system. *Proc Natl Acad Sci U S A* (1962) 48:1035–42. doi:10.1073/pnas.48. 6.1035
62. Putnam FW, Liu YS, Low TL. Pri- mary structure of a human IgA1 immunoglobulin. IV. Streptococ- cal IgA1 protease, digestion, Fab and Fc fragments, and the com- plete amino acid sequence of the alpha 1 heavy chain. *J Biol Chem* (1979) 254:2865–74.
63. Wu TT, Kabat EA. An analysis of the sequences of the variable regions of Bence Jones proteins and myeloma light chains and their implications for antibody com- plementarity. *J Exp Med* (1970) 132:211–50. doi:10.1084/ jem.132. 2.211
64. Kabat EA, Wu TT, Bilofsky H, Reid-Miller M, Perry H. *Sequence of Proteins of Immunological Inter- est*. Bethesda: National Institute of Health (1983).
65. Chothia C, Lesk AM. Canonical structures for the hypervariable regions of immunoglobulins. *J Mol Biol* (1987) 196:901–17. doi:10. 1016/0022-2836(87)90412-8
66. Chothia C, Lesk AM, Tra- montano A, Levitt M, Smith- Gill SJ, Air G, et al. Con- formations of immunoglob- ulin hypervariable regions. *Nature* (1989) 342:877–83. doi:10.1038/342877a0
67. Al-Lazikani B, Lesk AM, Chothia C. Standard con- formations for the canonical structures of immunoglobulins. *J Mol Biol* (1997) 273:927–48. doi:10.1006/jmbi.1997.1354
68. Giudicelli V, Chaume D, Bodmer J, Muller W, Busin C, Marsh S, et al. IMGT, the international ImMuno- GeneTics database. *Nucleic Acids Res* (1997) 25:206–11. doi:10. 1093/nar/25.1.206
69. Lefranc MP, Pommié C, Ruiz M, Giudicelli V, Foulquier E, Truong L, et al. IMGT unique numbering for immunoglobulin and T cell receptor variable domains and Ig superfamily V-like domains. *Dev Comp Immunol* (2003) 27:55–77. doi:10.1016/S0145- 305X(02)00039-3
70. Honegger A, Pluckthun A. Yet another numbering scheme for immunoglobulin variable domains: an automatic mod- eling and analysis tool. *J Mol Biol* (2001) 309:657–70. doi:10.1006/jmbi.2001.4662
71. Wang F, Ekiert DC, Ahmad I, Yu W, Zhang Y, Bazirgan O, et al. Reshaping antibody diversity. *Cell* (2013) 153:1379–93. doi:10.1016/ j.cell.2013.04.049
72. Padlan EA. Anatomy of the anti- body molecule. *Mol Immunol* (1994) 31:169–217. doi:10.1016/ 0161-5890(94)90001-9
73. MacCallum RM, Martin AC, Thornton JM. Antibody-antigen interactions: contact analysis and binding site topography. *J Mol Biol* (1996) 262:732–45. doi:10.1006/ jmbi.1996.0548
74. Kunik V, Ashkenazi S, Ofran Y. Paratome: an online tool for systematic identification of anti- gen binding regions in antibod- ies based on sequence or struc- ture. *Nucleic Acids Res* (2012) 40(Web Server issue):W521–4. doi:10.1093/nar/gks480
75. Jones S, Thornton JM. Prediction of protein-protein interaction sites using patch analysis. *J Mol Biol* (1997) 272:133–43. doi:10.1006/ jmbi.1997.1234
76. Cohen GH, Silverton EW, Padlan EA, Dyda F, Wibbenmeyer JA, Willson RC, et al. Water molecules in the antibody-antigen inter- face of the structure of the Fab HyHEL-5-lysozyme complex at 1.7 A resolution: comparison with results from isothermal titration calorimetry. *Acta Crystallogr D Biol Crystallogr* (2005) 61: 628–33. doi:10.1107/ S0907444905007870
77. Collis AV, Brouwer AP, Martin AC. Analysis of the antigen com- bining site: correlations between length and sequence composi- tion of the hypervariable loops and the nature of the antigen. *J Mol Biol* (2003) 325:337–54. doi:10.1016/S0022-2836(02) 01222-6
78. Raghunathan G, Smart J, Williams J, Almagro J. Antigen-binding site anatomy and somatic mutations in antibodies that recognize differ- ent types of antigens. *J Mol Recog- nit* (2012) 25:103–13. doi:10.1002/ jmr.2158
79. Nelson AL, Reichert JM. Devel- opment trends for therapeutic antibody fragments. *Nat Biotech- nol* (2009) 27:331–7. doi:10.1038/ nbt0409-331
80. Holliger P, Hudson PJ. Engineered antibody fragments and the rise of single domains. *Nat Biotechnol* (2005) 23:1126–36. doi:10.1038/ nbt1142
81. Hudson PJ, Souriau C. Engineered antibodies. *Nat Med* (2003) 9:129–34. doi:10.1038/nm0103-129
82. Jain M, Kamal N, Batra SK. Engineering antibodies for clin- ical applications. *Trends Biotech- nol* (2007) 25:307–16. doi:10.1016/ j.tibtech.2007.05.001
83. Ward ES, Güssow D, Griffiths AD, Jones PT, Winter G. Bind- ing activities of a repertoire of single immunoglobulin variable domains secreted from *Escherichia coli. Nature* (1989) 341:544–6. doi: 10.1038/341544a0
84. Rinfret A, Horne C, Dorrington KJ, Klein M. Noncovalent association of heavy and light chains of human immunoglobulins. IV. The roles of the CH1 and CL domains in idio- typic expression. *J Immunol* (1985) 135:2574–81.
85. Berry MJ, Davies J. Use of anti- body fragments in immunoaffinity chromatography. Comparison of FV fragments, VH fragments and paralog peptides. *J Chromatogr* (1992) 597:239–45. doi:10.1016/ 0021-9673(92)80116-C
86. Pereira B, Benedict CR, Le A, Shapiro SS, Thiagarajan P. Car- diolipin binding a light chain from lupus-prone mice. *Biochem- istry* (1998) 37:1430–7. doi:10. 1021/bi972277q
87. Dubnovitsky AP, Kravchuk ZI, Chumanevich AA, Cozzi A, Arosio P, Martsev SP. Expression, refold- ing, and ferritin-binding activ- ity of the isolated VL-domain of monoclonal antibody F11. *Biochemistry (Mosc)* (2000) 65: 1011–8.
88. Clackson T, Wells JA. A hot spot of binding energy in a hormone-receptor interface. *Sci- ence* (1995) 267:383–6. doi:10. 1126/science.7529940
89. Sheinerman FB, Norel R, Honig B. Electrostatic aspects of protein- protein interactions. *Curr Opin Struct Biol* (2000) 10:153–9. doi: 10.1016/S0959-440X(00)00065-8
90. Ofran Y. *Prediction of Protein Interaction Sites. Computational Protein-Protein Interactions R Nussinov and G Schreiber*. Boca Raton: CRC Press (2009). p. 167–84.
91. Park BW, Zhang HT, Wu C, Berezov A, Zhang X, Dua R, et al. Rationally designed anti- HER2/neu peptide mimetic disables P185HER2/neu tyrosine kinases in vitro and in vivo. *Nat Biotechnol* (2000) 18:194–8. doi:10.1038/72651

92. Polonelli L, Pontón J, Elguezabal N, Moragues MD, Casoli C, Pilotti E, et al. Antibody complementarity- determining regions (CDRs) can display differential antimi- crobial, antiviral and antitumor activities. *PLoS One* (2008) 3(6):e2371. doi:10.1371/journal. pone.0002371
93. Kang CY, Brunck TK, Kieber- Emmons T, Blalock JE, Kohler H. Inhibition of self-binding anti- bodies (autobodies) by a VH- derived peptide. *Science* (1988) 240:1034–6. doi:10.1126/science. 3368787
94. Taub R, Hsu JC, Garsky VM, Hill BL, Erlanger BF, Kohn LD. Peptide sequences from the hypervariable regions of two monoclonal anti-idiotypic anti- bodies against the thyrotropin (TSH) receptor are similar to TSH and inhibit TSH-increased cAMP production in FRTL-5 thy- roid cells. *J Biol Chem* (1992) 267:5977–84.
95. Saragovi HU, Fitzpatrick D, Rak- tabutr A, Nakanishi H, Kahn M, Greene MI. Design and synthesis of a mimetic from an antibody complementarity-determining region. *Science* (1991) 253:792–5. doi:10.1126/science.1876837
96. Levi M, Sällberg M, Rudén U, Herlyn D, Maruyama H, Wigzell H, et al. A complementarity- determining region synthetic pep- tide acts as a miniantibody and neutralizes human immunodefi- ciency virus type 1 in vitro. *Proc Natl Acad Sci U S A* (1993) 90:4374–8. doi:10.1073/ pnas.90.10.4374
97. Tsumoto K, Misawa S, Ohba Y, Ueno T, Hayashi H, Kasai N, et al. Inhibition of hepatitis C virus NS3 protease by peptides derived from complementari-ty- determining regions (CDRs) of the monoclonal antibody 8D4: tolerance of a CDR peptide to conformational changes of a tar- get. *FEBS Lett* (2002) 525:77–82. doi:10.1016/S0014-5793(02) 03090-9
98. Feng Y, Chung D, Garrard L, McEnroe G, Lim D, Scardina J, et al. Peptides derived from the complementarity-determining regions of anti-Mac-1 antibod- ies block intercellular adhesion molecule-1 interaction with Mac-1. *J Biol Chem* (1998) 273:5625–30. doi:10.1074/jbc.273. 10.5625
99. Feng J, Li Y, Zhang W, Shen B. Rational design of potent mimic peptide derived from mono- clonal antibody: antibody mimic design. *Immunol Lett* (2005) 98:311–6. doi:10.1016/j.imlet. 2004.12.006
100. Lasonder E, Bloemhoff W, Welling GW. Interaction of lysozyme with synthetic anti-lysozyme D1.3 anti- body fragments studied by affin- ity chromatography and surface plasmon resonance. *J Chromatogr A* (1994) 676:91–8. doi:10.1016/ 0021-9673(94)00125-1
101. Schellekens GA. *Molecular Aspects of Antibody-Antigen Interactions: Size Reduction of a Herpes Simplex Virus Neutralizing Antibody and its Antigen.* Groningen: University of Groningen (1996).
102. Burkovitz A, Leiderman O, Sela- Culang I, Byk G, Ofran Y. Compu- tational identification of antigen- binding antibody fragments. *J Immunol* (2013) 190:2327–34. doi: 10.4049/jimmunol.1200757
103. Bourgeois C, Bour JB, Aho LS, Pothier P. Prophylactic admin- istration of a complementarity- determining region derived from a neutralizing monoclonal anti- body is effective against respi- ratory syncytial virus infection in BALB/c mice. *J Virol* (1998) 72:807–10.
104. Williams WV, Kieber-Emmons T, VonFeldt J, Greene MI, Weiner DB. Design of bioactive pep- tides based on antibody hyper- variable region structures. Devel- opment of conformationally con- strained and dimeric peptides with enhanced affinity. *J Biol Chem* (1991) 266:5182–90.
105. Barrios Y, Jirholt P, Ohlin M. Length of the antibody heavy chain complementarity determin- ing region 3 as a specificity- determining factor. *J Mol Recognit* (2004) 17:332–8. doi:10.1002/jmr. 679
106. Kuroda D, Shirai H, Kobori M, Nakamura H. Structural classifica- tion of CDR-H3 revisited: a les- son in antibody modeling. *Pro- teins* (2008) 73:608–20. doi:10. 1002/prot.22087
107. Sela-Culang I, Alon S, Ofran Y. A systematic comparison of free and bound antibodies reveals binding- related conformational changes. *J Immunol* (2012) 189:4890–9. doi: 10.4049/jimmunol.1201493
108. Sedrak P, Hsu K, Mohan C. Mol- ecular signatures of anti-nuclear antibodies – contribution of heavy chain framework residues. *Mol Immunol* (2003) 40:491–9. doi:10. 1016/S0161-5890(03)00223-2
109. Xiang J, Sha Y, Jia Z, Prasad L, Delbaere L. Framework residue- 71 and residue-93 of the chimeric B72.3 antibody are major deter- minants of the conformation of heavy-chain hypervariable loops. *J Mol Biol* (1995) 253:385–90. doi: 10.1006/jmbi.1995.0560
110. Verhoeyen M, Milstein C, Winter G. Reshaping human antibodies: grafting an antilysozyme activity. *Science* (1988) 239:1534–6. doi:10. 1126/science.2451287
111. Kettleborough CA, Saldanha J, Heath VJ, Morrison CJ, Bendig MM. Humanization of a mouse monoclonal antibody by CDR- grafting: the importance of frame- work residues on loop con- formation. *Protein Eng* (1991) 4:773–83. doi:10.1093/protein/4.7. 773
112. Carter P, Presta L, Gorman CM, Ridgway JB, Henner D, Wong WL, et al. Humanization of an anti- p185HER2 antibody for human cancer therapy. *Proc Natl Acad Sci U S A* (1992) 89:4285–9. doi:10. 1073/pnas.89.10.4285
113. Baca M, Presta L, O'Connor S, Wells J. Antibody humanization using monovalent phage display. *J Biol Chem* (1997) 272:10678–84. doi:10.1074/ jbc.272.16.10678
114. Rodríguez-Rodríguez ER, Ledezma-Candanoza LM, Contreras-Ferrat LG, Olamendi- Portugal T, Possani LD, Becerril B, et al. A single mutation in framework 2 of the heavy variable domain improves the properties of a diabody and a related single-chain antibody. *J Mol Biol* (2012) 423:337–50. doi:10.1016/j.jmb.2012.07.007
115. Chiu WC, Lai YP, Chou MY. Humanization and characteriza- tion of an anti-human TNF-alpha murine monoclonal antibody. *PLoS One* (2011) 6:e16373. doi:10. 1371/journal.pone.0016373
116. Davies DR, Chacko S. Antibody structure. *Acc Chem Res* (1993) 26:421–7. doi:10.1021/ar00032a005
117. Schroeder H, Hillson J, Perlmut- ter R. Structure and evolution of mammalian VH families. *Int Immunol* (1990) 2:41–50. doi:10. 1093/intimm/2.1.41
118. Amit A, Mariuzza R, Phillips S, Poljak R. 3-Dimensional struc- ture of an antigen-antibody com- plex at 2.8 a resolution. *Science* (1986) 233:747–53. doi:10.1126/ science.2426778
119. Foote J, Winter G. Antibody framework residues affecting the conformation of the hypervari- able loops. *J Mol Biol* (1992) 224:487–99. doi:10.1016/0022- 2836(92)91010-M
120. Tramontano A, Chothia C, Lesk Framework residue-71 is a major determinant of the position and conformation of the 2nd hypervariable region in the VH domains of immunoglobulins. *J Mol Biol* (1990) 215:175–82. doi:10.1016/S0022-2836(05) 80102-0
121. Holmes M, Buss T, Foote J. Structural effects of framework mutations on a humanized anti- lysozyme antibody. *J Immunol* (2001) 167:296–301.
122. Potter K, Hobby P, Klijn S, Stevenson F, Sutton B. Evidence for involvement of a hydropho- bic patch in framework region 1 of human v4-34-encoded igs in recognition of the red blood cell I antigen. *J Immunol* (2002) 169:3777–82.
123. Pospisil R, Youngcooper G, Mage R. Preferential expansion and survival of B-lymphocytes based on VH framework-1 and framework-3 expression: "pos- itive" selection in appendix of normal and VH-mutant rabbits. *Proc Natl Acad Sci USA* (1995) 92:6961–5. doi:10.1073/pnas.92. 15.6961
124. Capra J, Kehoe J. Variable region sequences of 5 human immunoglobulin heavy chains of VH3 subgroup: definitive identification of four heavy chain hypervariable regions. *Proc Natl Acad Sci USA* (1974) 71:845–8. doi:10.1073/pnas.71.3.845
125. Banfield M, King D, Mountain A, Brady R. V-L:V-H domain rota- tions in engineered antibodies: crystal structures of the Fab frag- ments from two murine antitumor antibodies and their engineered human constructs. *Proteins* (1997) 29:161–71. doi:10.1002/(SICI) 1097-0134(199710)29:2<161: :AID-PROT4>3.0.CO;2-G
126. Nakanishi T, Tsumoto K, Yokota A, Kondo H, Kumagai I. Critical contribution of VH-VL interaction to reshaping of an antibody: the case of humanization of anti-lysozyme antibody, HyHEL-10. *Protein Sci* (2008) 17:261–70. doi:10.1110/ps. 073156708
127. Stanfield R, Takimotokamimura M, Rini J, Profy A, Wilson I. Major antigen-induced domain rearrangements in an antibody. *Structure* (1993) 1:83–93. doi:10. 1016/0969-2126(93)90024-B
128. Tan P, Sandmaier B, Stayton P. Contributions of a highly con- served VHNL hydrogen bonding interaction to scFv folding stability and refolding efficiency. *Biophys J* (1998) 75:1473–82. doi:10.1016/ S0006-3495(98)74066-4
129. Essen L, Skerra A. The de-novo design of an antibody combin- ing site – crystallographic analy- sis of the V-L domain confirms the structural model. *J Mol Biol* (1994) 238:226–44. doi:10.1006/ jmbi.1994.1284
130. Masuda K, Sakamoto K, Kojima M, Aburatani T, Ueda T, Ueda H. The role of interface frame- work residues in determining anti- body V-H/V-L interaction strength and antigen-binding affinity. *Febs J* (2006) 273:2184–94. doi:10.1111/ j.1742-4658.2006.05232.x
131. Torres M, Casadevall A. The immunoglobulin constant region contributes to affinity and speci- ficity. *Trends Immunol* (2008) 29: 91–7. doi:10.1016/j. it.2007.11.004
132. Casadevall A, Janda A. Immunoglobulin isotype influences affinity and speci- ficity. *Proc Natl Acad Sci U S A* (2012) 109:12272–3. doi:10.1073/ pnas.1209750109
133. Janda A, Casadevall A. Circu- lar dichroism reveals evidence of coupling between immunoglobu- lin constant and variable region secondary structure. *Mol Immunol* (2010) 47:1421–5. doi:10.1016/j. molimm.2010.02.018

134. Dam TK, Torres M, Brewer CF, Casadevall A. Isothermal titra- tion calorimetry reveals differen- tial binding thermodynamics of variable region-identical antibod- ies differing in constant region for a univalent ligand. *J Biol Chem* (2008) 283:31366–70. doi: 10.1074/jbc.M806473200
135. Pritsch O, Hudry-Clergeon G, Buckle M, Petillot Y, Bou- vet JP, Gagnon J, et al. Can immunoglobulin C(H)1 constant region domain modulate antigen binding affinity of antibodies? *J Clin Invest* (1996) 98:2235–43. doi:10.1172/JCI119033
136. Pritsch O, Magnac C, Dumas G, Bouvet JP, Alzari P, Dighiero G. Can isotype switch modulate antigen-binding affinity and influence clonal selection? *Eur J Immunol* (2000) 30(12):3387–95. doi:10.1002/1521-4141(2000012) 30:12<3387::AID-IMMU3387>3. 0.CO;2-K
137. Torres M, May R, Scharff MD, Casadevall A. Variable-region- identical antibodies differ- ing in isotype demonstrate differences in fine specificity and idiotype. *J Immunol* (2005) 174:2132–42.
138. Torres M, Fernández-Fuentes N, Fiser A, Casadevall A. The immunoglobulin heavy chain constant region affects kinetic and thermodynamic parame- ters of antibody variable region interactions with antigen. *J Biol Chem* (2007) 282:13917–27. doi:10.1074/jbc.M700661200
139. McLean GR, Torres M, Elgueza- bal N, Nakouzi A, Casadevall A. Isotype can affect the fine speci- ficity of an antibody for a polysac- charide antigen. *J Immunol* (2002) 169:1379–86.
140. Cooper LJ, Shikhman AR, Glass DD, Kangisser D, Cunningham MW, Greenspan NS. Role of heavy chain constant domains in antibody-antigen interaction. Apparent specificity differences among streptococcal IgG anti- bodies expressing identical vari- able domains. *J Immunol* (1993) 150:2231–42.
141. McCloskey N, Turner MW, Steffner P, Owens R, Goldblatt D. Human constant regions influence the antibody binding character- istics of mouse-human chimeric IgG subclasses. *Immunology* (1996) 88:169–73. doi:10.1111/j. 1365-2567.1996.tb00001.x
142. Michaelsen TE, Ihle Ø, Beckstrøm KJ, Herstad TK, Sandin RH, Kol- berg J, et al. Binding properties and anti-bacterial activities of V- region identical, human IgG and IgM antibodies, against group B *Neisseria meningitidis*. *Biochem Soc Trans* (2003) 31:1032–5. doi:10. 1042/BST0311032
143. Liu F, Bergami PL, Duval M, Kuhrt D, Posner M, Cavacini L. Expression and functional activity of isotype and subclass switched human monoclonal antibody reactive with the base of the V3 loop of HIV-1 gp120. *AIDS Res Hum Retro- viruses* (2003) 19:597–607. doi:10.1089/088922203322230969
144. Tudor D, Yu H, Maupetit J, Drillet AS, Bouceba T, Schwartz-Cornil I, et al. Isotype modulates epi- tope specificity, affinity, and antivi- ral activities of anti-HIV-1 human broadly neutralizing 2F5 anti- body. *Proc Natl Acad Sci U S A* (2012) 109:12680–5. doi:10.1073/ pnas.1200024109
145. Torosantucci A, Chiani P, Bro- muro C, De Bernardis F, Palma AS, Liu Y, et al. Protection by anti- beta-glucan antibodies is associ- ated with restricted beta-1,3 glu- can binding specificity and inhi- bition of fungal growth and adherence. *PLoS One* (2009) 4: e5392. doi:10.1371/journal.pone. 0005392
146. Xia Y, Janda A, Eryilmaz E, Casade- vall A, Putterman C. The con- stant region affects antigen bind- ing of antibodies to DNA by altering secondary structure. *Mol Immunol* (2013) 56:28–37. doi:10. 1016/j.molimm.2013.04.004
147. Adachi M, Kurihara Y, Nojima H, Takeda-Shitaka M, Kamiya K, Umeyama H. Interaction between the antigen and antibody is con- trolled by the constant domains: normal mode dynamics of the HEL-HyHEL-10 complex. *Protein Sci* (2003) 12:2125–31. doi:10. 1110/ps.03100803
148. Xia Y, Pawar RD, Nakouzi AS, Her- litz L, Broder A, Liu K, et al. The constant region contributes to the antigenic specificity and renal pathogenicity of murine anti-DNA antibodies. *J Autoim- mun* (2012) 39:398–411. doi:10. 1016/j.jaut.2012.06.005
149. Oda M, Kozono H, Morii H, Azuma T. Evidence of allosteric conformational changes in the antibody constant region upon antigen binding. *Int Immunol* (2003) 15:417–26. doi:10.1093/ intimm/dxg036
150. Piekarska B, Drozd A, Konieczny L, Król M, Jurkowski W, Roterman I, et al. The indirect generation of long-distance structural changes in antibodies upon their binding to antigen. *Chem Biol Drug Des* (2006) 68:276–83. doi:10.1111/j. 1747-0285.2006.00448.x
151. Horgan C, Brown K, Pincus SH. Effect of H-chain V-region on complement activation by immobilized immune-complexes. *J Immunol* (1992) 149:127–35.
152. Vidarte L, Pastor C, Mas S, Blazquez AB, de los Rios V, Guer- rero R, et al. Serine 132 is the C3 covalent attachment point on the CH1 domain of human IgG1. *J Biol Chem* (2001) 276(41): 38217–23.
153. Braden BC, Poljak RJ. Structural features of the reactions – between antibodies and protein antigens. *FASEB J* (1995) 9:9–16.
154. Pellequer JL, Chen SW, Roberts VA, Tainer JA, Getzoff ED. Unrav- eling the effect of changes in conformation and compactness at the antibody V-L-V-H interface upon antigen binding. *J Mol Recog* (1999) 12:267–75. doi:10.1002/ (SICI)1099-1352(199907/08)12: 4<267::AID-JMR465>3.3. CO;2-0
155. Wilson IA, Stanfield RL. Antibody- antigen interactions – new struc- tures and new conformational- changes. *Curr Opin Struct Biol* (1994) 4:857–67. doi:10.1016/ 0959-440X(94)90267-4

9

Role of heat shock protein 70 in innate alloimmunity

Walter G. Land*

German Academy of Transplantation Medicine, Munich, Germany

Edited by:
Willem Van Eden, Utrecht University, Netherlands

Reviewed by:
Cristina Bonorino, Pontificia Universidade Catolica do Rio Grande do Sul, Brazil
Ruurd Van Der Zee, Universiteit Utrecht, Netherlands

Correspondence:
Walter G. Land, Köglweg 32, 82024 Taufkirchen, Germany.
e-mail: walterland@aol.com

This article briefly describes our own experience with the proven demonstration of heat shock protein 70 (HSP70) in reperfused renal allografts from brain-dead donors and reflects about its potential role as a typical damage-associated molecular pattern (DAMP) in the setting of innate alloimmunity. In fact, our group was able to demonstrate a dramatic up-regulation of HSP70 expression after postischemic reperfusion of renal allografts. Of note, up-regulation of this stress protein expression, although to a lesser extent, was already observed after cold storage of the organ indicating that this molecule is already induced in the stressed organism of a brain-dead donor. However, whether or not the dramatic up-regulation of HSP70 expression contributes to mounting an innate alloimmune response cannot be judged in view of these clinical findings. Nevertheless, HSP70, since generated in association with postischemic reperfusion-induced allograft injury, can be called a typical DAMP – as can every molecule be termed a DAMP that is generated in association with any stressful tissue injury regardless of its final positive or negative regulatory function within the innate immune response elicited by it. In fact, as we discuss in this article, the context-dependent, even contradistinctive activities of HSP70 reflect the biological phenomenon that, throughout evolution, mammals have developed an elaborate network of positive and negative regulatory mechanisms, which provide balance between defensive and protective measures against unwarranted destruction of the host. In this sense, up-regulated expression of HSP70 in an injured allograft might reflect a pure protective response against the severe oxidative injury of a reperfused donor organ. On the other hand, up-regulated expression of this stress protein in an injured allograft might reflect a (futile) attempt of the innate immune system to restore homeostasis with the aim to eliminate the "unwanted foreign allograft invader" by contributing to development of an adaptive alloimmune response. However, this adaptive immune response against donor histocompatibility alloantigens – in its evolutionary sense aimed to restore homeostasis – is by no means protective from a recipient's view point but tragically ends up with allograft rejection. Indeed: in this sense, allograft rejection is the result of a fateful confusion by the immune system of danger and benefit!

Keywords: injury hypothesis, innate alloimmunity, DAMPs, HSP72

INTRODUCTION: ALLOGRAFT INJURY-INDUCED INNATE ALLOIMMUNITY

FIRST CLUE TO THE EXISTENCE OF INNATE ALLOIMMUNITY: THE INJURY HYPOTHESIS (1994)

Originally, the immune system was regarded as a host defense system that is primarily directed against invading pathogens with the aim to prevent/cure infection. Following the re-discovery of innate immunity in the mid/late 1990s, this concept was confirmed and extended: Infection of cells by microorganisms was seen to activate the innate immune system that elicits an inflammatory response merging into an adaptive immune response. The initial sensing of infection was recognized to be mediated by pattern recognition receptors (PRRs) in/on innate immune cells that play a pivotal role in the first line of this host defense system. PRRs were found to recognize distinct pathogen-derived motifs, the pathogen-associated molecular patterns (PAMPs) to initiate and regulate innate and adaptive immune responses (for review, see Kumar et al., 2011).

First notions that the immune system has evolved the capacity to detect *any* tissue injury in ways that stimulate the initiation and generation of adaptive immune responses to antigens were addressed and discussed by two hypotheses nearly simultaneously published early in 1994 (Land et al., 1994; Matzinger, 1994). These two hypotheses postulated that the adaptive immune system evolved to respond not only to pathogen-mediated "infectious" tissue injury *per se* but also to non-physiological cell death, tissue injury, or stress, as, for example, mediated by postischemic reperfusion injury (IRI). As a matter of fact, it was Matzinger (1994) who proposed her famous "Danger Hypothesis." Her model – proposed on theoretical grounds – suggested that the primary driving force of the immune system is the need to detect and protect against danger. Danger, however, equals tissue destruction, that is, tissue injury. Our "Injury Hypothesis" – proposed on statistically significant data from a prospective clinical trial in kidney transplant patients (the "Munich SOD Trial") – discussed the possibility that it is the primary injury to an allograft that – via activation of antigen-presenting cells – induces pathways leading to an adaptive alloimmune response (Land et al., 1994). In fact, this hypothesis was based on our pivotal clinical observation that (antioxidative) treatment of a non-specific tissue injury [here: the reactive oxygen species (ROS)-mediated IRI to allografts] leads to a significant reduction in subsequent specific, adaptive immunity-mediated processes (here: reduction of alloimmune-mediated allograft rejection).

Under the line, the two hypotheses postulated the same scenario: The initial tissue injury, that is, the injurious inflammatory tissue environment, alerts the immune system, and is a mandatory prerequisite to mount an efficient adaptive immune response against foreign antigens.

ROLE OF DAMAGE-ASSOCIATED MOLECULAR PATTERNS AND PATTERN RECOGNITION RECEPTORS IN OXIDATIVE INJURY – INDUCED ALLOGRAFT ("STERILE") INFLAMMATION

Over the past decade, increasing evidence has been published in support of the notion that PRRs recognize non-infectious but injurious agents that can cause tissue damage (for reviews, see: Beutler, 2007; Manfredi et al., 2009; Chen and Nuñez, 2010; Bauernfeind et al., 2011; Jaeschke, 2011; Yanai et al., 2011). In this scenario, PRRs sense injury-induced, host-derived endogenous molecules in terms of damage-associated molecular patterns, that is, DAMPs, an acronym that was coined by us in analogy to PAMPs 8 years ago (Land, 2003a). These DAMPs are released following tissue injury or cell death and have similar functions as PAMPs in terms of their ability to activate pro-inflammatory pathways in innate immune cells.

Of note, ROS-mediated IRI to allografts can be regarded as a model of a non-pathogen-induced oxidative tissue injury that activates the innate immune system. In fact, an emerging role of innate immune events in adaptive alloimmunity-mediated allograft rejection (= innate alloimmunity) has been noted (for reviews, see Land, 2011a,b). However, the situation in the allograft setting is more complex as two individually different categories of DCs are involved: (1) donor-derived PRR-bearing innate immune cells such as DCs, vascular, and epithelial cells already residing in the transplant and (2) recipient-derived PRR-bearing innate immune cells such as DCs and neutrophils invading the allograft during reperfusion in the recipient. Moreover, various DAMPs such as high mobility group box 1 (HMGB1) and heat shock protein 70 (HSP70) are generated already in the brain-dead organ donor (Arbogast et al., 2002; Krüger et al., 2009; Kaminska et al., 2011), however, their up-regulated expression culminate during allograft reperfusion in the recipient (Arbogast et al., 2002; Kaczorowski et al., 2009; Klune and Tsung, 2010). Indeed, according to new insights into mechanisms of innate immunity, a brain-dead organism, characterized by the demonstration of DAMPs, PRRs, and circulating cytokines, may be defined as an acute systemic innate immunity-mediated autoinflammatory syndrome (Land, 2011b). To add yet another level of complexity in the allograft setting, it can be assumed that further DAMPs are released from necrotic cells caused by allograft reperfusion injury which may include nucleic acids, oxidation-specific DAMPs such as thioredoxin (TRX)-interacting protein (TXNIP) and purine metabolites such as ATP (Schröder et al., 2010; Bours et al., 2011; Kis-Toth et al., 2011). In addition to those DAMPs derived from an intracellular source, IRI leads to release of extracellular located DAMPs such as extracellular matrix fragments including hyaluronan and heparan sulfate. The prototypical PRRs recognizing all those various DAMPs include Toll-like receptors (TLRs) such as TLR2 and TLR4 and the receptor for advanced glycation end-products (RAGE) as well as PRRs able to recognize nucleic acids such as RIG-I-like receptors (RLRs) and AIM2-like receptors (for review, see Land, 2011e).

There is a special role for the cytosolic nucleotide-binding domain leucine-rich repeats (NLR) receptors because one of its members represents the core structure of the NOD, LRR, and pyrin domain-containing 3 (NLRP3) inflammasome, the most widely studied inflammasome now known to be activated by various DAMPs (for review, see Bauernfeind et al., 2011). In fact, the well-known creation of "sterile" inflammation in reperfused organs (and solid allografts have to be included here) is now believed to be induced by inflammasomes. Most important in regard to the topic of IRI are recent studies in both *Nlrp3*- and *ASC*-deficient mice clearly demonstrating that the NLRP3 inflammasome contributes to the IRI-mediated acute inflammatory response (Iyer et al., 2009). These studies revealed that non-lethal renal IRI results in a significant up-regulation of *Nlrp3* gene expression, which is accompanied by pronounced acute tubular necrosis that is similar between wild-type (WT) and *Nlrp3*-deficient animals. Importantly, the studies showed that *Nlrp3*-deficiency protected animals from lethal renal IRI. Similarly, *ASC*-deficiency protected animals from lethal renal IRI, although the difference, compared to WT mice, was less pronounced than in *Nlrp3*-deficient mice.

Activation of the NLRP3 inflammasome is currently thought to consist of two steps: a first priming step that consists of stimulation of PRRs which leads to the up-regulation of NLRP3 expression and also induces pro-IL-1β expression. Stimuli priming NLRP3 appear to include all ligands for TLRs, RLRs, and NLRs, that lead to enhanced NLRP3 expression (Bauernfeind et al., 2011). Thus, theoretically, HSP70, as a ligand of TLR4 and TLR2, can be counted to those priming DAMPs (The LPS-contamination debate in regard to TLR2 and TLR4 is not dealt with here but discussed elsewhere; Land, 2011e). The second step consists of the activation of NLRP3 itself which is distinct from this initial priming step. Three presumably distinct pathways have been postulated that can lead to the activation of NLRP3 (activation step): (1) extracellular ATP that is often seen to be largely increased during cell death, can bind to purinergic receptor P2X7 and leads to NLRP3 activation via ion flux effects (including intracellular K^+ depletion) mediated by the P2X7-receptor-associated hemi-channel pannexin-1; (2) endocytosis of sterile particulates, such as cholesterol crystals, resulting in lysosomal disintegration which leads to the leakage of lysosomal enzymes into the cytosol (activation of the protease cathepsin B); and (3) generation of ROS during cellular stress or death leading to the activation of NLRP3 through the release of TXNIP from thioredoxin and then binds to NLRP3 (for review, see Bauernfeind et al., 2011). Although the role of ROS in NLRP3 activation is still not quite clear, this potential activation mechanism is of considerable attraction in regard to ROS-mediated reperfusion injury to allografts.

ALLOGRAFT INJURY-INDUCED, DAMPs-MEDIATED GENERATION OF DONOR- AND RECIPIENT-DERIVED IMMUNOSTIMULATORY DCs

In fact, growing evidence suggests that allograft injury induces innate immune events which precede adaptive alloimmunity. Within an innate immune-mediated intragraft inflammatory milieu, donor- and recipient-derived DCs get activated, migrate to the secondary lymphoid tissue of the recipient to translate innate immunity to an adaptive alloimmune response. The generation of these immunostimulatory DCs is the result of innate immune pathways initiated and induced by various DAMPs which, as reviewed (Land, 2011b), may be divided into four different classes of DAMPs: (1) class I DAMPs such as HMGB1 and HSP70 that, when recognized by PRRs of immature DCs (iDCs), trigger their activation to immunostimulatory DCs; (2) class II DAMPs such as MHC class I chain-related molecules A and B that, when recognized by special activating receptors (NKG2D) on innate lymphocytes may contribute to generation of immunostimulatory DCs in terms of a cross-talk; (3) class III DAMPs such as TXNIP and extracellular ATP that are recognized by PRRs involved in the activation of the NLRP3 inflammasome, and (4) class IV DAMPs in terms of neoantigens that are recognized by pre-existing natural immunoglobulin M antibodies, which – via complement activation – are able to aggravate the oxidative tissue injury and, thereby, may indirectly promote metamorphosis of iDCs into immunostimulatory DCs.

In fact, there seems to be a complex collaboration between various membrane-bound and cytosolic PRRs on one side and their different cognate DAMPs on the other side which results in those well-known vigorous innate alloimmune responses. Most likely, this complex orchestration of intragraft DAMP–PRR interactions may finely regulate the maturation process of donor- and recipient-derived iDCs into immunostimulatory DCs, that, via processes of direct and indirect allorecognition, may stimulate naïve T cells of the recipient, thereby mounting, and fine-tuning adaptive alloimmune responses of various intensities.

ROLE OF HEAT SHOCK PROTEIN 70 IN INNATE ALLOIMMUNITY

DONOR BRAIN DEATH-MEDIATED AND REPERFUSION INJURY-INDUCED UP-REGULATION OF HSP70 EXPRESSION IN HUMAN ALLOGRAFTS

The first DAMP shown to be involved in the setting of clinical organ transplantation was the inducible HSP70 that was up-regulated following renal allograft reperfusion injury, that is, a condition in which contamination with pathogen-derived exogenous ligands of PRRs can be totally ruled out (Arbogast et al., 2002). In fact, our group was able to demonstrate a dramatic up-regulation of HSP70 expression after postischemic reperfusion of renal allografts from deceased (brain-dead) donors (**Figure 1**). Interestingly, up-regulation of HSP70 expression, although to a lesser extent, was already observed after cold storage of the organ indicating that this stress protein is already induced in the stressed organism of a brain-dead donor (**Figure 1**). These findings prompted us to discuss a role of HSP70 in innate alloimmunity by proposing that HSPs (1) in their function as endogenous ligands of TLRs may lead to DC maturation and (2) in their function as chaperokines may facilitate cross-presentation of HSP-chaperoned allopeptides on MHC class I molecules of recipient-derived DCs (Land, 2002, 2003b). Whether or not dramatic up-regulation of HSP70 expression in an allograft contributes to mounting an innate alloimmune response cannot be judged in view of these clinical findings alone, but a brief look at the more recent literature may help in interpreting our earlier findings.

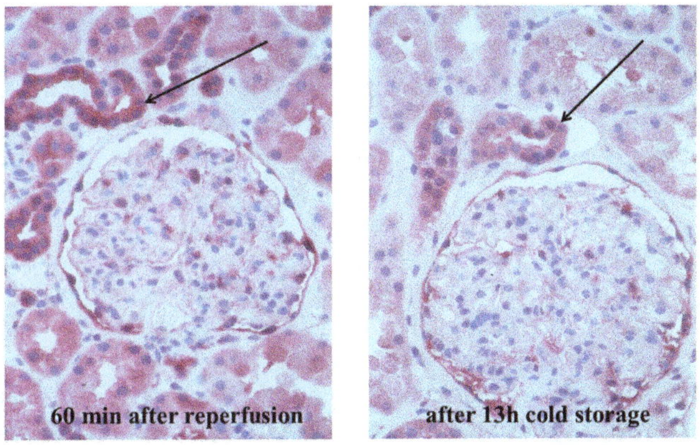

FIGURE 1 | Immunohistochemical demonstration of expression of the inducible heat shock protein 70. The renal biopsy specimen shows a human kidney removed from a brain-dead donor, perfused with the University Wisconsin preservation solution, and cold-stored over 13 h. The biopsy was taken before (right) and 60 min after reperfusion (left) following implantation into the recipient. Demonstration was performed using the monoclonal antibody HSP 6B3 (GSF, non-commercially available), specific for inducible heat shock component HSP 70 (formerly HSP72c) in a dilution of 1:150, at room temperature, for 1 h. A detection system APAAP (alkaline phosphatase–antialkaline phosphatase) from the rat (Fa Dako) is used, by incubation with linking antibody and staining with fast red. Sources: Further properties (e.g., specificity) of the monoclonal antibodies are described in: Milani et al. (2002) and Arbogast et al. (2002). Permission: Reproduced with permission of: Land WG. *Innate Alloimmunity, Part 2. Innate Immunity and Allograft Rejection*, and Başkent University, Pabst Science Publishers, 2011.

ROLE OF HSP70 FAMILY MEMBERS IN ENHANCING ADAPTIVE IMMUNE RESPONSES

In general, extracellular HSPs released from damaged cells are immunogenic and have been shown to enhance TH1 adaptive immune responses and, therefore, have been used for improved vaccination procedures against infectious diseases and cancer (for review, see Binder, 2006). For example, a novel HSP70 family member, termed Hsp70-like protein 1 (Hsp70L1) was recently identified as a potent TH1 polarizing adjuvant that contributes to antitumor immune responses (Fang et al., 2011). In another line of experiments on a fusion cell model (DC and tumor cell fusion), efficient cytotoxic T lymphocyte productivity of modified fusion cells was demonstrated and supposed to be due to an up-regulation of HSP70 (Koide et al., 2009).

Such enhancement of adaptive immune responses by HSP70 is thought to be preferentially mediated by its capacity to promote maturation of immunostimulatory DCs as well as to enhance cross-presentation of peptide antigens, that is, a crucial pathway of exogenous antigen presentation on the HLA class I molecules by DCs, enabling adaptive antiviral or antitumor responses.

In fact, in earlier studies, it was already shown that human HSP70 preparations are able to induce DC maturation (Kuppner et al., 2001; Bethke et al., 2002). In a more recent study on an *in vitro*-induced ischemia model, bone marrow–derived DCs were shown to augment allogeneic T-cell proliferation as well as the interferon-gamma response (Jurewicz et al., 2010). In this study, TLR4 ligation was also shown to occur in ischemic DCs, most likely – as concluded by the authors – in response to HSP70, which was found to be elevated in DCs after ischemic injury.

In addition to contributing to the generation of immunostimulatory DCs in terms of a ligand of TLR2/4, extracellular HSP70 has been shown in models of antitumor T-cell responses to promote the cross-presentation of peptide antigens to MHC class I molecules in DCs, leading to efficient induction of antigen-specific cytotoxic T-lymphocytes (Castelli et al., 2001; Srivastava, 2002; Ueda et al., 2004). Of particular importance for the discussion of a role of cross-presentation in innate alloimmunity are recent studies demonstrating that HSP70 binds HLA class I and class II epitope precursors, which further strengthens the role of HSP70 in the HLA class I and class II antigen presentation process (Stocki et al., 2010). In fact, these studies lent support to a more general characteristic of the HSP70-chaperoned peptides and suggest involvement of HSP70 as a more general phenomenon in the antigen presentation process.

HEAT SHOCK PROTEINS AND ALLOGRAFT SURVIVAL

Most interesting for our early assumption in 2002/2003 that HSP70 may be involved in innate alloimmunity would be the provision of data from experimental studies on allograft models. However, there are only a few such data published so far and, unfortunately, they are even controversial. Thus, it could be shown that targeted gene disruption of the *hsp72* gene in donor tissue is associated with significantly but modestly prolonged rejection-free survival in a murine skin allograft model, the difference between *hsp72*-deficient mice and controls being 3 days only (Oh et al., 2004). Nonetheless, these experimental data suggest that HSP70 in terms of a pro-inflammatory acting DAMP contributes to an innate alloimmune response although only in a moderate way.

On the other hand, data from another experimental allograft model indicate that HSP70 in terms of an anti-inflammatory acting DAMP may even exert a beneficial effect on allograft survival, although again quite modestly (Borges et al., 2010). In this study, *Mycobacterium tuberculosis* HSP70 (TBHSP70) was shown to inhibit allograft rejection in a skin allograft model in which the donor skin was immersed in a PBS solution containing TBHSP70 before transplantation. Interestingly, however, TBHSP70-induced prolongation of skin allograft survival was associated with the demonstration of T regulatory cells (Tregs), a finding supposed by the authors to mediate the graft-prolonging effect. Interestingly, the authors discuss (although not conclusive from their observations) whether or not the Tregs observed in their studies are specific for TBHSP70, by referring to growing evidence in support of the notion that HSPs possess inherent immunoregulatory properties (van Eden et al., 2005).

SYNOPSIS

In my opinion, HSPs, since generated in *association* with any stressful tissue injury, can be called typical damage-*associated* molecular patterns, that is, DAMPs. Their evolutionarily determined, inherent protective role in concert with a large panoply of other molecules in commission of the innate immune system lies in defense against any cell/tissue injury (including elimination of the injurious agent concerned, e.g., viruses, tumor cells).

In regard to innate alloimmunity, it can be concluded from our own experience that the expression of HSP70 is moderately increased in kidneys from brain-dead donors but dramatically up-regulated after IRI to human renal allografts, thus, fulfilling the criteria of a DAMP. No more, no less. However, the exact biological activity of HSP70 in innate alloimmunity remains elusive. Without addressing the "contamination debate" here, one may discuss that, in the excessively inflammatory milieu of a postischemically reperfused allograft, this DAMP – in concert and collaboration with a variety of other DAMPs such as HMGB1 and nucleic acids released from necrotic graft cells – may operate as an immunity-initiating, -promoting, and -facilitating stress protein to allograft rejection [the originally protective role of HSPs here is being converted to a harmful response from a recipient's point of view, caused by a fateful confusion of "invading" foreign antigens (alloantigens) within an injured organ and foreign antigens derived from invading dangerous pathogens]. Potential pro-inflammatory properties of HSP70 may lie in its capacities (1) to act as a "priming" DAMP of the NLRP3 inflammasome contributing to the typical inflammatory environment of a reperfused allograft, (2) to contribute to maturation of donor- and recipient-derived DCs by engagement with TLR4/2, and (3) to intensify re-presentation of allopeptides within donor MHC class II molecules on donor- and recipient-derived DCs as well as promote cross-presentation of allopeptides within donor MHC class I molecules on recipient-derived DCs.

In contrast, in a non-injurious or weakly injurious tissue microenvironment, for example, when HSP70 is added to skin grafts immersed in culture prior to transplantation (Borges et al., 2010), this DAMP may elicit negative regulation mechanisms in graft-containing antigen-presenting cells on the level of TLR signaling. As known, in order to prevent catastrophic host immune overreactions, such negative feedback regulations exist that control the intensity and duration of TLR-triggered innate immune responses – best known as the classic negative regulation in response to LPS, the "LPS or endotoxin tolerance." In fact, molecular feedback inhibitors operating at different levels of TLR-signaling pathways can be divided into three major groups: extracellular regulators such as soluble decoy TLRs, transmembrane protein regulators such as the *suppressor of tumorigenicity 2*, and intracellular negative regulators such *as IL-1 receptor-associated kinase-M* (IRAK-M) and members of the *suppressors of cytokine signaling* (SOCS) family (for review, see Land, 2011d).

For example, the well-known anti-inflammatory effect of preconditioning procedures including heat preconditioning associated with the expression of HSP70 (Jo et al., 2006) has been thought to be due to elicitation of regulatory feedback inhibitors of TLR signaling (for review, see also Karikó et al., 2004). In fact, in earlier studies, it was demonstrated that prior exposure to HSP70, here the *Toxoplasma gondii*-derived HSP70, induces a hyporesponse in macrophages to subsequent stimulation with this HSP70 by expression of SOCS1 via TLR4 (Mun et al., 2005). Of note, as shown in more recent studies on a model of hepatic IRI, preconditioning using the TLR4 agonist LPS elicited the up-regulation of specific negative regulators including SOCS1 and IRAK-M in the TLR4-signaling pathway (Sano et al., 2011). Impressively, molecules operating in those regulatory feedback loops have been shown to also prevent DC maturation, that is, to promote generation of tolerogenic DCs known to induce Tregs (for reviews, see Maldonado and von Andrian, 2010; Land, 2011c). Thus, data from an experimental model of SOCS1-gene overexpression in bone marrow-derived DCs showed that SOCS1 inhibits DC maturation and induces generation of regulatory DCs, which – via generation of $CD4^+CD25^+$Tregs – resulted in prolongation of allograft survival (Fu et al., 2009). First evidence of a similar feedback inhibiting effect of SOCS2 on TLR-induced activation in human monocyte-derived DCs has also been recently reported (Posselt et al., 2011).

Altogether, the context-dependent, even contradistinctive activities of HSP70 reflect the biological phenomenon that, throughout evolution, mammals have developed an elaborate network of positive and negative regulatory mechanisms, which provide balance between defensive measures against dangerous bacterial and viral pathogens and protective measures against unwarranted destruction of the host by the activated immune system. Fine-tuning of TLR signaling in amplitude, space, time, and character is a key aspect of inflammatory reactions in health, homeostasis, and pathology. What is becoming more and more apparent is that positive and negative regulators within immune responses do not work as a single entity, but rather, similar to an orchestral score, each component is reliant on its other tools such as HSP70 to produce a harmonious melody instead of a crashing cacophony.

REFERENCES

Arbogast, H., Arbogast, S., Fertmann, J., and Land, W. (2002). Expression of heat shock proteins in cadav- eric human renal allografts – a role in activation of innate immunity? *Transplantation* 74(Suppl.),266.

Bauernfeind, F., Ablasser, A., Bartok, E., Kim, S., Schmid-Burgk, J., Cavlar, T., and Hornung, V. (2011). Inflamma- somes: current understanding and open questions. *Cell. Mol. Life Sci.* 68, 765–783.

Bethke, K., Staib, F., Distler, M., Schmitt, U., Jonuleit, H., Enk, A. H., Galle, P. R., and Heike, M. (2002). Differ- ent efficiency of heat shock proteins (HSP) to activate human monocytes and dendritic cells: superiority of HSP60. *J. Immunol.* 169, 6141–6148. Beutler, B. (2007). Neo-ligands for innate immune receptors and the etiology of sterile inflammatory disease. *Immunol. Rev.* 220, 113–128.

Binder, R. J. (2006). Heat shock protein vaccines: from bench to bedside. *Int. Rev. Immunol.* 25,353–375.

Borges, T. J., Porto, B. N., Teixeira, C. A., Rodrigues, M., Machado, F. D., Ornaghi, A. P., de Souza, A. P., Maito, F., Pavanelli, W. R., Silva, J. S., and Bonorino, C. (2010). Prolonged survival of allografts induced by mycobacterial HSP70 is dependent on CD4CD25 regula- tory T cells. *PLoS ONE* 5, e14264. doi:10.1371/journal.pone.0014264

Bours, M. J., Dagnelie, P. C., Giuliani, A. L., Wesselius, A., and Di Virgilio, F. (2011). P2 receptors and extracellu- lar ATP: a novel homeostatic path- way in inflammation. *Front. Biosci. (Schol. Ed).* 3, 1443–1456.

Castelli, C., Ciupitu, A. M., Rini, F., Rivoltini, L., Mazzocchi, A., Kiessling, R., and Parmiani, G. (2001). Human heat shock protein 70 peptide complexes specifically activate antimelanoma T cells. *Can- cer Res.* 61, 222–227.

Chen, G. Y., and Nuñez, G. (2010). Ster- ile inflammation: sensing and react- ing to damage. *Nat. Rev. Immunol.* 10, 826–837.

Fang, H., Wu, Y., Huang, X., Wang,., Ang, B., Cao, X., and Wan, T. (2011). Toll-like receptor 4 (TLR4) is essential for Hsp70-like protein 1 (HSP70L1) to activate dendritic cells and induce Th1 response. *J. Biol. Chem.* 286, 30393–30400.

Fu, H., Song, S., Liu, F., Ni, Z., Tang, Y., Shen, X., Xiao, L., Ding, G., and Wang, Q. (2009). Dendritic cells transduced with SOCS1 gene exhibit regulatory DC properties and pro- long allograft survival. *Cell. Mol. Immunol.* 6,87–95.

Iyer, S., Pulskensc, W., Sadler, J., Butter, L. M., Teske, G. J., Ulland, T. K., Eisenbarth, S. C., Florquin, S., Flavell, R. A., Leemans, J. C., and Sutterwala, F. S. (2009). Necrotic cells trigger a sterile inflammatory response through the Nlrp3 inflammasome. *Proc. Nat. Acad. Sci. U.S.A.* 106, 20388–20393.

Jaeschke, H. (2011). Reactive oxygen and mechanisms of inflammatory liver injury: present concepts. *J. Gastroenterol. Hepatol.* 26(Suppl. 1), 173–179.

Jo, S. K., Ko, G. J., Boo, C. S., Cho, W. Y., and Kim, H. K. (2006). Heat pre- conditioning attenuates renal injury in ischemic ARF in rats: role of heat- shock protein 70 on NF-kappaB- mediated inflammation and on tubular cell injury. *J. Am. Soc. Nephrol.* 17, 3082–3092.

Jurewicz, M., Takakura, A., Augello, A., Naini, S. M., Ichimura, T., Zandi- Nejad, K., and Abdi, R. (2010). Ischemic injury enhances dendritic cell immunogenicity via TLR4 and NF-kappa B activation. *J. Immunol.* 184, 2939–2948.

Kaczorowski, D. J., Nakao, A., Val- labhaneni, R., Mollen, K. P., Sug- imoto, R., Kohmoto, J., Zucker- braun, B. S., McCurry, K. R., and Billiar, T. R. (2009). Mechanisms of Toll-like receptor 4 (TLR4) mediated inflammation after cold ischemia/reperfusion in the heart. *Transplantation* 87, 1455–1463.

Kaminska, D., Koscielska-Kasprzak, K., Drulis-Fajdasz, D., Halon, A., Polak, W., Chudoba, P., Janczak, D., Mazanowska, O., Patrzalek, D., and Klinger, M. (2011). Kidney ischemic injury genes expressed after donor brain death are predictive for the outcome of kidney transplantation. *Transplant. Proc.* 43, 2891–2894.

Karikó, K., Weissman, D., and Welsh, F. A. (2004). Inhibition of Toll-like receptor and cytokine signaling – a unifying theme in ischemic toler- ance. *J. Cereb. Blood Flow Metab.* 24, 1288–1304.

Kis-Toth, K., Szanto, A., Thai, T. H., and Tsokos, G. C. (2011). Cytoso- lic DNA-activated human den- dritic cells are potent activators of the adaptive immune response. *J. Immunol.* 187, 1222–1234.

Klune, J. R., and Tsung, A. (2010). Molecular biology of liver ischemia/reperfusion injury: established mechanisms and recent advancements. *Surg. Clin. North Am.* 90, 665–677.

Koide, T., Iinuma, H., and Fukushima, (2009). Efficient CTL produc- tivity of modified fusion cells by increase of heat shock protein 70. *Oncol. Rep.* 21, 737–746.

Krüger, B., Krick, S., Dhillon, N., Lerner, M., Ames, S., Bromberg, J. S., Lin, M., Walsh, L., Vella, J., Fischereder, M., Krämer, B. K., Colvin, R. B., Heeger, P. S., Murphy, B. T., and Schröppel, B. (2009). Donor Toll-like receptor 4 contributes to ischemia and reperfusion injury fol- lowing human kidney transplanta- tion. *Proc. Natl. Acad. Sci. U.S.A.* 106, 3390–3395.

Kumar, H., Kawai, T., and Akira, S. (2011). Pathogen recognition by the innate immune system. *Int. Rev. Immunol.* 30,16–34.

Kuppner, M. C., Gastpar, R., Gelwer, S., Nössner, E., Ochmann, O., Scharner, A., and Issels, R. D. (2001). The role of heat shock protein (hsp70) in den- dritic cell maturation: hsp70 induces the maturation of immature den- dritic cells but reduces DC differen- tiation from monocyte precursors. *Eur. J. Immunol.* 31, 1602–1609.

Land, W. (2002). Postischemic reperfusion injury to allografts – a case for "innate immunity"? *Eur. Surg. Res.* 34, 160–169.

Land, W. (2003a). Allograft injury mediated by reactive oxygen species: from conserved proteins of *Drosophila* to acute and chronic rejection of human transplants. Part III: interaction of (oxidative) stress-induced heat shock proteins with Toll-like receptor-bearing cells of innate immunity and its consequences for the development of acute and chronic allograft rejection. *Transplant. Rev.* 17, 67–86.

Land, W. (2003b). Allograft injury mediated by reactive oxygen species: from conserved proteins of *Drosophila* to acute and chronic rejection of human transplants. Part II: role of reactive oxygen species in the induction of the heat shock response as a regulator of innate immunity. *Transplant. Rev.* 17, 31–44.

Land, W., Schneeberger, H., Schleib- ner, S., Illner, W. D., Abendroth, D., Rutili, G., Arfors, K. E., and Messmer, K. (1994). The benefi- cial effect of human recombinant superoxide dismutase on acute and chronic rejection events in recipients of cadaveric renal transplants. *Transplantation* 57, 211–217.

Land, W. G. (2011a). Emerging role of innate immunity in organ transplan- tation. Part I: evolution of innate immunity and oxidative allograft injury. *Transplant. Rev. (Orlando).* doi: 10.1016/j.trre.2011.05.001. [Epub ahead of print].

Land, W. G. (2011b). Emerging role of innate immunity in organ transplantation.

Part II: Potential of DAMPs to generate immunostimulatory dendritic cells. *Transplant. Rev. (Orlando).* doi: 10.1016/jtrre.2011.02.003. [Epubahead of print].

Land, W. G. (2011c). Emerging role of innate immunity in organ transplantation. Part III: the quest for transplant tolerance via prevention of oxidative allo- graft injury and its consequences. *Transplant. Rev. (Orlando).* doi: 10.1016/j. trre.2011.07.001. [Epubahead of print].

Land, W. G. (2011d). "Negative regula- tion of TLR-signaling pathways," in *Innate Alloimmunity, Part I: Innate Immunity and Host Defence*, ed. W. G. Land (Lengerich: Başkent Uni- versity, Pabst Science Publishers), 267–285.

Land, W. G. (2011e). "Oxidative injury-induced, damage-associated molecular pattern molecules and their pattern recognition receptors," in *Innate Alloimmunity, Part II: InnateImmunityandAllograftRejec- tion*, ed. W. G. Land (Lengerich: Başkent University, Pabst Science Publishers),229–337.

Maldonado, R. A., and von Andrian, U. H. (2010). How tolerogenic den- dritic cells induce regulatory T cells. *Adv. Immunol.* 108, 111–165.

Manfredi, A. A., Capobianco, A., Bianchi, M. E., and Rovere-Querini, P. (2009). Regulation of dendritic- and T-cell fate by injury-associated endogenous signals. *Crit. Rev. Immunol.* 29,69–86.

Matzinger, P. (1994). Tolerance, danger, and the extended family. *Annu. Rev. Immunol.* 12, 991–1045.

Milani, V., Noessner, E., Ghose, S., Kup- pner, M., Ahrens, B., Scharner, A., Gastpar, R., and Issels, R. D. (2002). Heat shock protein 70 role in antigen presentation and immune stimula- tion. *Int. J. Hyperthermia* 18,563.

Mun, H. S., Aosai, F., Norose, K., Piao, L.., Fang, H., Akira, S., and Yano, A. (2005). Toll-like receptor 4 mediates tolerance in macrophages stimulated with *Toxoplasma gondii*-derivedheat shock protein 70. *Infect. Immun.* 73, 4634–4642.

Oh, K. H., Kim, J. Y., Kim, D., Lee, E.M., Oh, H. Y., Seo, J. S., Han, J. S., Kim, S., Lee, J. S., and Ahn, C. (2004). Targeted gene disruption of the heat shock protein 72 gene (hsp70.1) in the donor tissue is associated with a prolonged rejection-free survival in the murine skin allograft model. *Transpl. Immunol.* 13, 273–281.

Posselt, G., Schwarz, H., Duschl, A., and Horejs-Hoeck, J. (2011). Suppressor of cytokine signaling 2 is a feed- back inhibitor of TLR-induced acti- vation in human monocyte-derived dendritic cells. *J. Immunol.* 187, 2875–2884.

Sano, T., Izuishi, K., Hossain, M. A., Inoue, T., Kakinoki, K., Hagiike, M., Okano, K., Masaki, T., and Suzuki, Y. (2011). Hepatic preconditioning using lipopolysaccharide: associa- tion with specific negative regula- tors of the Toll-like receptor 4 sig- naling pathway. *Transplantation* 91, 1082–1089.

Schröder, K., Zhou, R., and Tschopp, J. (2010). The NLRP3 inflamma- some: a sensor for metabolic danger? *Science* 327, 296–300.

Srivastava, P. (2002). Interaction of heat shock proteins with peptides and antigen presenting cells: chap- eroning of the innate and adap- tive immune responses. *Annu. Rev. Immunol.* 20, 395–425.

Stocki, P., Morris, N. J., Preisinger, C., Wang, X. N., Kolch, W., Multhoff, G., and Dickinson, A. M. (2010). Identi- fication of potential HLA class I and class II epitope precursors associated with heat shock protein 70 (HSPA). *Cell Stress Chaperones* 15, 729–741.

Ueda, G., Tamura, Y., Hirai, I., Kamiguchi, K., Ichimiya, S., Torigoe, T., Hiratsuka, H., Sunakawa, H., and Sato, N. (2004). Tumor-derived heat shock protein 70-pulsed dendritic cells elicit tumor-specific cytotoxic T lymphocytes (CTLs) and tumor immunity. *Cancer Sci.* 95, 248–253.

van Eden, W., van der Zee, R., and Prakken, B. (2005). Heat-shock pro- teins induce T cell regulation of chronic inflammation. *Nat. Rev. Immunol.* 5,318–330.

Yanai, H., Ban, T., and Taniguchi, T. (2011). Essential role of high- mobility group box proteins in nucleic acid-mediated innate immune responses. *J. Intern. Med.* 270, 301–308.

10

Beneficial autoimmunity at body surfaces – immune surveillance and rapid type 2 immunity regulate tissue homeostasis and cancer

***Tim Dalessandri* and *Jessica Strid* ***

Division of Immunology and Inflammation, Department of Medicine, Imperial College London, London, UK

Edited by:
Fang-Ping Huang, Imperial College London, UK

Reviewed by:
Masaaki Murakami, Hokkaido University, Japan
Yasmina Laouar, University of Michigan, USA

***Correspondence:**
Jessica Strid, Division of Immunology and Inflammation, Department of Medicine, Imperial College London, London W12 0NN, UK
e-mail: j.strid@imperial.ac.uk

Epithelial cells (ECs) line body surface tissues and provide a physicochemical barrier to the external environment. Frequent microbial and non-microbial challenges such as those imposed by mechanical disruption, injury or exposure to noxious environmental substances including chemicals, carcinogens, ultraviolet-irradiation, or toxins cause activation of ECs with release of cytokines and chemokines as well as alterations in the expression of cell-surface ligands. Such display of epithelial stress is rapidly sensed by tissue-resident immunocytes, which can directly interact with self-moieties on ECs and initiate both local and systemic immune responses. ECs are thus key drivers of immune surveillance at body surface tissues. However, ECs have a propensity to drive type 2 immunity (rather than type 1) upon non-invasive challenge or stress – a type of immunity whose regulation and function still remain enigmatic. Here, we review the induction and possible role of type 2 immunity in epithelial tissues and propose that rapid immune surveillance and type 2 immunity are key regulators of tissue homeostasis and carcinogenesis.

Keywords: immune surveillance, Type 2 immunity, epithelial cells, tissue homeostasis, carcinogenesis, IgE, intraepithelial lymphocytes, sterile stress

Epithelial cells (ECs) are the main constituent of tissues lining body surfaces like the skin, intestine, lungs, and genitourinary tract. They regulate crucial life processes such as micronutrient absorption, gaseous exchange, and thermo- and hydro-control whilst also providing a physiochemical barrier to the external environment against microbes and a plethora of non-microbial stressors. ECs are extremely dynamic and versatile cells and it is becoming increasingly clear that they are also intimately involved in the induction and regulation of local tissue- and systemic immune responses. Disruption of epithelial surfaces may therefore result in dysregulated body processes and penetrance to deeper tissues by microbes or noxious moieties. In addition, the direct response of ECs to tissue disruption strongly affects resident immunocytes and their subsequent regulation of both local and systemic innate and adaptive immunity. A growing body of evidence both from mouse models and human genetics suggest that EC dysregulation can be a primary cause of pathology in different tissues. Given the multifaceted biological actions of ECs and the multitude of challenges imposed on epithelial tissues, it is reasonable to think that ECs in conjunction with tissue-resident immunocytes possess mechanisms, both immunological and non-immunological, to maintain healthy barrier homeostasis and to minimize inflammation and cellular dysregulation. Indeed, ECs are now known to be highly immunomodulatory by virtue of the cytokines, chemokines, damage-associated molecular pattern (DAMP) molecules, and major histocompatibility (MHC) gene products they express; a repertoire that has collectively been termed the "epimmunome" (1). ECs express pattern-recognition receptors (PRRs) including toll-like receptors (TLRs), NOD-like receptors (NLRs), RIG-I-like receptors (RLRs), and a variety of "NK" receptor ligands, enabling them to respond to a wide variety of microbial and non-microbial (including self) moieties and disseminate the response to immunocytes. The NLR–inflammasome complex allows ECs to respond to non-microbial sterile stress elicited by toxins, irritants, and (for skin keratinocytes) ultraviolet (UV) light (2); the most pervasive environmental DNA-damaging agent (3). Thus, ECs express a suite of sensors for detecting differing insults and challenges at the body surfaces, and an armory of soluble and cell-surface molecules to direct an appropriate, restorative response. These epithelial-driven responses in health sculpt and modulate tissue homeostasis and local tissue immunity, in a manner that aids morphological tissue homeostasis, restoration of the epithelial barrier following injury, and elimination or expulsion of microbial and non-microbial insults. Here, we review how ECs drive immunity at body surfaces and how this is involved in regulating immune surveillance, tissue immune homeostasis, and cancer.

EPITHELIAL CELLS AND THEIR RESPONSE TO CHALLENGE

The vast majority of environmental challenges occur at epithelial surfaces. The repertoire of responses available to ECs to combat these daily challenges is immense. For example, EC-derived cytokines include IL-1, IL-6, IL-10, IL-18, IL-25, IL-33, TNFα, and thymic stromal lymphopoietin (TSLP). Pro-IL-1α and pro-IL-1β are constitutively produced by ECs, particularly skin keratinocytes, and are secreted following exposure to noxious stimuli or tissue damage. Corneocytes (non-nucleated skin ECs) release IL-1α in the skin in response to disruption of the outermost surface, the stratum corneum (4), while UV-irradiation induces IL-1β. In addition to agonistic effects on tissue macrophages, IL-1α induces growth-factor expression from tissue fibroblasts, prompting a replicative burst in neighboring ECs to repair damage (5). The pro-inflammatory cytokines IL-6 and TNFα are produced in large quantities by damaged ECs; the former of which can also be used as a STAT-3-dependant autocrine growth factor, in healthy and cancerous epithelium (6). The most robustly expressed cytokines upon any EC insult however are IL-25, IL-33, and TSLP. In common, these three cytokines can drive type 2 immune responses, which thus impart a particular propensity of epithelial tissues to induce type 2 immunity. Such predisposition of stressed ECs may underlie the high frequency of allergic and atopic disease at the skin and mucosal surfaces. However, despite the intense interest in this area, the cellular and molecular linkage of type 2 immunity to barrier- and EC disruption is not clearly understood – nor is the functional role of this type of immunity to EC homeostasis or immune surveillance yet fully elucidated.

IL-25, also know as IL-17E, is a member of the IL-17 cytokine family. Despite bearing some amino acid sequence homology to the best-characterized IL-17 cytokines, IL-17A and IL-17F, IL-25 has divergent biological functions and promotes Th2 rather than Th17 responses *in vivo*. IL-25 directly amplifies expression of the Th-2 mediators IL-4, IL-5, and IL-13, and supports production of Th2 serum immunoglobulins (7). IL-25 was first reported with high steady-state mRNA expression in the kidney, and moderate to low expression in other organs and the peripheral tissue (8). Subsequently, it was found by multiple groups to be important in type 2-mediated immunity to enteric parasites, such as *Trichuris muris* (9), and is upregulated in the gut upon EC-sensing of commensal bacteria (10). The mouse gut parasite *Heligmosomoides polygyrus bakeri* elicits the EC-derived cytokine, IL-1β, which suppresses IL-25 and IL-33 and promotes pathogen chronicity by attenuating expulsive type 2 responses (11), suggesting that IL-25 is particularly important in maintaining immunity to gut pathogens. Similarly, mice and humans subjected to parenteral nutrition have impaired mucosal immunity, due to reduced gut luminal levels of antimicrobial effectors, but administration of exogenous IL-25 to parenteral nutrition-fed mice was found to be protective against enteric bacterial invasion (12). In allergic models, IL-25 expression is upregulated upon exposure to allergens both in murine or human lung EC lines and in primary murine lung ECs (13). Elevated protein levels have also been found in tissues of patients with allergic disease in the lung and skin (14). IL-25 has been found to drive tissue (airway) remodeling, and expression of the other major EC cytokines IL-33 and TSLP in a house dust mite model of allergy (15), and drive pulmonary fibrosis by inducing IL-13 expression from lung innate lymphoid cells (ILCs) in mice challenged with lung *Schistosoma mansoni* eggs (16). In addition to production by ECs, dermal dendritic cells (DCs) have been reported to be a major source of IL-25 in atopic dermatitis (AD) patients (17), while IL-25 and IL-33-activated ILC2s in mouse skin promote AD-like inflammation (18). These reports and others highlight an interesting crosstalk and autocrine regulation of EC-derived effectors, as well as a role for IL-25 in augmenting epithelial barrier immunity, or conversely promoting pathological Th2 tissue inflammation, in differing settings.

IL-33 is a multi-functional protein. The full length protein is localized in the nucleus but following cleavage the c-terminal fragment acts as a cytokine which binds the receptor ST2. IL-33 was recently discovered as an IL-1 family member with type 2-promoting functions similar to IL-25. It is expressed by ECs, macrophages, DCs, and mast cells *in vivo* and its cytokine function drives IL-4, IL-5, and IL-13 expression and differentiation of Th2 $CD4^+$ T cells (19). IL-33-induced IL-4 production appears to be mainly from innate cells and together these two cytokines will induce proliferation of B cells and amplify IgE synthesis (20). Similar to IL-25, IL-33 acts in an autocrine fashion to promote TSLP expression by ECs, particularly in response to gut nematodes, where IL-33 mRNA can be detected rapidly following colonization (21). Interestingly, the efficacy of IL-33 in this infection model (and others) seems to be highly time-dependent, with administration of exogenous IL-33 at late time points post-infection being ineffective in promoting type 2 responses that would otherwise resolve infection. IL-33 is highly expressed by intestinal ECs and inflammatory infiltrates in ulcerative colitis, with IL-33 cleavage products being detected in the serum (22). IL-33 is also rapidly released and detectable in bronchoalveolar lavage fluid following lung allergen exposure in humans, suggesting it is a rapid type 2 mediator in sites additional to the gut (23). Protective as well as immunopathological roles of EC-derived IL-33 have been described in the skin. Transgenic over-expression of IL-33 in mouse skin, driven by a keratinocyte-specific promoter, induces a spontaneous dermatitis-like disease and activates ILC2s in the dermis (24). It has also been shown in a phorbol 12-myristate 13-acetate model of skin inflammation that mice deficient for the IL-33 receptor, ST2, do not exhibit IL-33-dependant skin inflammation (25). Similarly in human inflammatory conditions, IL-33 has been reported to be upregulated in clinical psoriatic lesions and the serum of skin sclerosis patients (26). Conversely, mice treated with exogenous IL-33, following full-thickness skin wounding, demonstrate dramatically improved wound-healing, collagen deposition, and expression of extracellular matrix proteins indicative of tissue repair (27). These reports suggest a particularly rapid and acute role for IL-33 in cutaneous homeostasis and gut integrity whereas constitutive, late, or dysregulated expression may be involved in a variety of chronic inflammatory conditions. This temporally coordinated aspect fits well with current thinking of IL-33 as an "alarmin," whereby its immediate release from intranuclear stores by damaged, apoptotic, or necrotic cells rather than a classic Golgi-mediated secretion pathway (19) facilitates a rapid and restorative response to tissue damage.

TSLP is produced almost exclusively by ECs of the lung, tonsils, intestine, and skin (13), and is upregulated in response to tissue damage (28), various TLR ligands and infection, or exposure to type 2 cytokines such as IL-4, IL-13, IL25, and IL-33 (29). A protective role of TSLP in intestinal immunity to *T. muris* has been well described; mice which are knockouts for IKKβ fail to produce TSLP in response to infection, and subsequently develop chronic intestinal inflammation (30). Mechanistically, EC-derived TSLP suppresses p40 and upregulates OX40L expression in DCs, a costimulatory molecule with a propensity to license Th2 responses in $CD4^+$ T cells (31). TSLP also augments Th2 cytokine production by direct effects on $CD4^+$ T cells and has indirect, agonist effects on a variety of granulocyte populations including mast cells and basophils. Similar to IL-25 and IL-33, inappropriate expression or dysregulation of TSLP is implicated in a number of inflammatory diseases including the triad of atopic diseases; asthma, allergic rhinitis, and AD (31). TSLP is required for allergic lung inflammation in mice exposed to inhaled antigen, and TSLP receptor knockout animals do not develop lung inflammation in this model. Interestingly, these animals do develop strong Th1 responses with high IFNγ, IL-12, and IgG2a (32), highlighting how a single epithelial-derived molecule can skew adaptive immune responses in response to tissue-challenge. In humans, AD sufferers show high TSLP expression in lesional skin (33), and mice with induced expression of TSLP in the epidermis develop spontaneous AD-like pathology (34). Production of TSLP is however critically important for resistance to skin carcinogenesis in mouse models (35, 36).

Further to cytokines and chemokines, ECs can release other proteins upon cellular stress. Of note, they can produce hedgehog morphogens, which are a family of secreted proteins that regulate a wide variety of physiological processes including tissue development during embryogenesis and tissue homeostasis as well as being implicated in carcinogenesis (37). Sonic Hedgehog h (Hh) expression was recently found to be upregulated in lung ECs in models of allergic disease, and lung resident T cells were shown to respond locally to EC-derived Hh by upregulating IL-4 (38). This demonstrates that ECs also produce non-classical immune modulators, such as tissue morphogens, which appear to contribute to the robust induction of type 2 immunity in epithelial tissues.

In addition to the secreted and soluble molecules produced by ECs, they also express a variety of cell-surface molecules enabling them to directly interact with resident and infiltrating immunocytes. For example, ECs express E-cadherin that engage CD103, which is constitutively expressed on intraepithelial lymphocytes (IELs) and tissue DCs such as the epidermal Langerhans cells (LCs). ECs also express T cell costimulatory ligands, although it remains unclear as to what extent ECs express the classical B7.1 and 2 molecules, they clearly express PD-L1 and PD-L2 (39). Some members of a novel family of B7-related molecules, the butyrophilins, appear to be preferentially expressed on ECs and have been implicated in EC-immune regulation (40) as have *Skint* family members which are exclusively expressed on ECs and have profound impact on IEL development and function (41, 42). Thus via appropriate receptor–ligand interactions ECs are capable of initiating and sculpting both local tissue immunity and further downstream systemic immunity. Under conditions of physiochemical tissue disruption or barrier perturbation (1), infection (43), genotoxic stress (44), sterile inflammation, or heavy proliferation (45), ECs respond by upregulating additional self-encoded and cell-surface markers, which are often termed as "'stress antigens" as they are indicative of a dysregulated state of the epithelium. The EC stress antigens have an important role in initiating and directing tissue immune responses during perturbations and as such these will be discussed in more detail in the Section "Immune Surveillance" below.

EPITHELIAL CELLS AND THEIR NEIGHBORS

In close association with ECs, the epithelial tissues are home to several specialized subsets of immunocytes. IELs are found in all epithelial tissues, but have most notably been studied in the intestine and skin. IELs are adaptive T cells carrying RAG-dependent rearranged T cell receptors (TCRs), nevertheless they are often MHC non-restricted cells and express many innate receptors allowing them to react to stress antigen with "innate-like" response kinetics. The IELs are a mixture of αβ and γδ T cells, which are either $CD4^-CD8^-$ or coexpress a CD8αα coreceptor. The ratio of αβ to γδ T cells depends on the anatomical site as well as the species. IEL compartments are often much less diverse than systemic T cells (for example in the mouse skin and uterus they are essentially monoclonal), implying that these cells recognize predictable antigens encountered in specific tissues – these antigens could be either pathogen encoded or self-encoded molecules that reflect a dysregulated state of the tissue they inhabit. Not many IEL TCR-specificities have yet been defined, but it seems clear that both their recognition capabilities and mode of activation are distinct from systemic T cells (46). Particularly, it has been proposed that IELs are primarily autoreactive T cells that have been agonist-selected, recognize tissue stress antigens, and have regulatory properties (47). The murine skin for example contains a specialized subset of $\gamma\delta\ (TCR)^+$ IELs called dendritic epidermal T cells (DETC) that exclusively carry a Vγ5Vδ1 TCR – a TCR arrangement only found on epidermal IELs (and on the progenitor fetal thymic population). The skin epithelia also contain a specialized subset of DCs, the epidermal LCs. Both LC and DETC infiltrate the epithelium very early during stratification of the skin ECs, and are long-lived and likely self-renewing immune compartments, which clearly integrate and physically interact with the ECs.

In addition to the "unconventional" T cells in the epithelium, more conventional $CD8\alpha\beta^+$ αβ T cells have been shown to rapidly accumulate in tissues upon infection, where they can become resident memory T cells and provide protective antigen-specific responses. This was elegantly shown in the skin following local infection with herpes simplex virus (48) or vaccinia virus (49), which induced a rapid influx of antigen-specific $CD8^+$ αβ T cells both into the epithelial epidermal layer and the underlying dermis. Interestingly, these infiltrating $CD8^+$ αβ T cells were shown to populate the entire skin and provide long-lasting protection against re-infection as a continuing tissue-resident memory T cell population. In steady state, the subepithelial layer of most tissues contains a diverse set of immunocytes that can all contribute to epithelial-immune surveillance. These include tissue-specific resident populations of myeloid cells, such as DC, macrophages and mast cells, lymphoid cells, such as $CD4^+$ or $CD8^+$ αβ T cells, γδ T cells, and ILCs, as well as stromal fibroblasts. In fact, it is becoming increasingly apparent that different tissues constitutively harbor a variety of specialized immunocytes in the subepithelial space. For example, in human skin a population of IL-22 and growth factor producing T cells (Th22) can rapidly enter the epithelium upon challenge and be involved in epidermal remodeling (50). Similarly, the gut contains a resident IL-22 producing population of NK-like cells (51). In recent years, an array of different ILCs has been discovered that are resident in the subepithelial tissue layer. Different subsets of ILCs dominate in particular tissues and their specialized functions are starting to be elucidated; many of them contribute to both homeostatic and pathophysiological conditions in the tissue they inhabit (52). The subepithelial immunocytes can respond to epithelial cues and be recruited into the epithelium upon damage – in addition systemic immune cells can be recruited both to the subepithelial and epithelial layer. In sum, the epithelium and body surface tissues are home to an intricate array of immunocytes, which can interact and integrate activities in numerous complex ways that likely differ substantially depending on the anatomical site and the challenge encountered. Additional research is required to understand the interaction between different resident immunocytes in the tissues and how their responses may be integrated to regulate local and systemic immunity.

TYPE 2 IMMUNITY AND ITS TRIGGERS

Epithelial cells and EC-associated leukocytes such as IELs can clearly drive local and systemic type 2 immunity (53). More conventionally, however, type 2 immunity is thought to be mediated primarily by Th2 cells, IgE and IgG1 antibodies, as well as a host of innate immune cells such as mast cells, basophils, eosinophils, alternatively activated macrophages, and ILCs. The type 2 immune response *in vivo* is accordingly extremely heterogeneous and it is surprisingly poorly understood how type 2 immunity is induced, regulated – and indeed what its primary physiological function is. Type 2 immune responses are classically induced by macroparasites and conventional thinking holds that type 2 immunity has evolved to protect against infection by parasites such as helminthes and ticks. However, this is probably a too simple explanation, as it is not true that all parasites are fought by IgE and type 2 immunity. Although IgE levels are raised in people as well as mice with helminth infections, IgE is dispensable for immunity to many helminthes and much of the IgE raised is not specific to the parasite (54). Type 2 immunity is also notoriously activated in response to a broad range of different environmental challenges and antigens. Such non-infectious stimuli that trigger type 2 immunity are collectively termed allergens and form the basis of a host of allergic disorders like asthma, allergic rhinitis, food allergies, and AD. Type 2 immune responses have been explored largely in the context of helminth infections and allergic diseases. They have been thought to provide a host-beneficial role only as defense against macroparasites, whereas allergic reactions are most commonly explained as a detrimental consequence of a misdirected response mimicking parasite immunity. This paradigm is now changing and with more triggers of type 2 immunity being elucidated (**Figure 1**) it seems plausible that type 2 immunity can provide host-benefits in settings other than against parasites. In 1991, Profet published an inspired hypothesis suggesting that the physiological role of allergic responses was an immunological defense against toxins (55). This idea is resonating with recent data (56, 57) and the hypothesis has been recharged and expanded into a broader model of intentional allergic host defense not only against helminthes but also

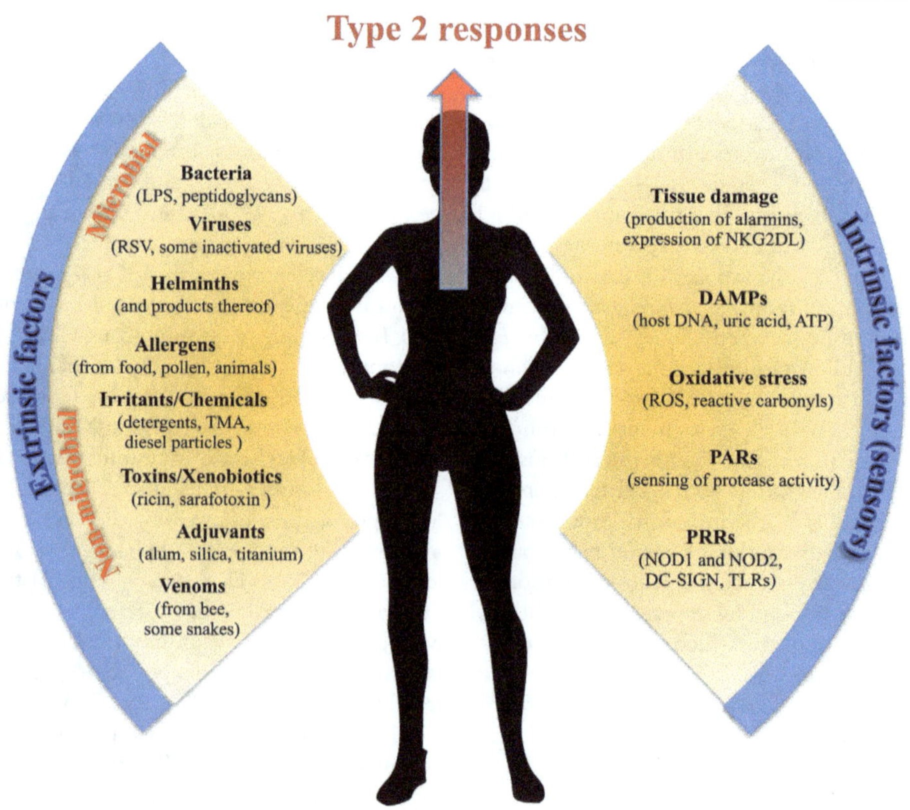

FIGURE 1 | Extrinsic and intrinsic factors promoting type 2 immunity. Type 2 immunity can be triggered by an array of diverse extrinsic stimuli from both infectious and non-infectious sources and is most potently induced at the body surface tissues. Equally, the intrinsic cellular mechanisms inducing and/or sensing type 2-triggering extrinsic stimuli are many and diverse. In common, most of the extrinsic factors promoting type 2 immunity, as well as the intrinsic factors sensing them, are founded on a breach of the protective barrier of the body and thus on tissue and cellular damage.

non-infectious environmental factors such as venoms, chemical irritants, and xenobiotics (58). Accordingly, there may be multiple pathways that lead to type 2 immunity and IgE – some more classically "adaptive" and some more "innate" (59). The route to type 2 immunity and whether protection or allergic sensitization is the outcome may depend on tissue context, allergen, dose, genetics, and species. Common for all type 2 immune responses is that their effector functions converge at the epithelial surfaces (skin and mucosa), vasculature, and smooth muscles where they promote barrier defenses and expulsion. Conspicuously, allergic disorders, unlike other immune pathologies, exclusively affect epithelial tissues that interface with the environment.

Type 2 immunity can be triggered by a bewildering array of molecules from both infectious and non-infectious sources (**Figure 1**). Much work has been done to try and identify a unifying framework for what makes a substance "an allergen" (60), but common allergens such as peanut, shellfish, pollen, nickel, bee venom, latex, house dust mite, and penicillin appear to have little in common in terms of their chemical structure or origin. In addition, type 2 immunity can be triggered by certain vaccine adjuvants [alum most notably (61)], noxious toxins (56, 58), environmental irritants and chemicals (62, 63), as well as certain infections or bacterial products (64). One commonality between both infectious and non-infectious triggers of type 2 immunity that may have been less well appreciated is that many are insults inducing some level of physical trauma that breaches the protective barrier of the body. Tissue damage, at least in the absence of strong type 1-promoting pathogen-associated molecular pattern (PAMP) signaling, appears to be a potent mechanism driving type 2 immunity. Tissue damage induces rapid release of several epithelium-derived cytokine alarmins, such as IL-33, TSLP, and IL-25 (reviewed above) – all of which can drive downstream type 2 immunity. In a macroparasite infection, the large size of the parasite and the consequent tissue damage it causes during invasion may be the most important factor in inducing type 2 immunity (65), although some parasite-derived products with direct type 2 polarizing capacity may also exist (66). The tissue-damage caused by macroparasites may be modeled by ingestion of large inert particle structures. Interestingly, it has been shown that inert silica and titanium particles induce innate type 2 immunity and can be used as adjuvants promoting Th2 responses by pathways independent of TLR4 and MyD88 (67, 68). These particles may induce cellular damage and consequently activate endogenous danger- or stress-signals. That "injury" or cellular stress alone can support induction of type 2 immunity is strongly supported by results showing that transgenic up-regulation of the NKG2D stress-ligand Rae-1 on ECs promote potent type 2 immunity and IgE to innocuous antigens (53). This rapid innate-like IgE response is also independent of MyD88 (53). Cellular damage may also explain the type 2-inducing effect of the adjuvant alum as injection of alum causes the release of DAMPs, like uric acid and host cell DNA (61, 69). Uric acid has been shown to drive type 2 immunity and again this is via pathways independent of both MyD88 and the inflammasome (69). Host DNA signaling intriguingly appears to differentially regulate IgG1 and IgE production following alum-adjuvanted immunization, where host DNA induces primary B cell responses with IgG1 through interferon response factor 3 (Irf3)-independent mechanism but more canonical Th2 responses and IgE through an Irf3-dependent mechanism (70). Furthermore, extracellular ATP, presumably released from damaged cells, binds to P2 purinergic receptors and triggers IL-33 release and innate type 2 immune responses in the lung (71). Oxidative stress, which is widespread and entwined with pathological processes, has also been shown to be involved in orchestrating type 2 immunity. For example, induction of reactive oxygen species (ROS) in ECs induces oxidation of lipids that in turn triggers TSLP release by ECs (72) and oxidative stress has been shown to induce reactive carbonyl adduction, which is reported to be a potent driver of type 2 immunity (73). DAMPs thus appear to be part of both the initiation and amplification of type 2 immunity and may as such also play an important role in allergic diseases.

Another feature that contributes to the induction of type 2 immunity by some allergens is their serine or cysteine protease activity. Allergens such as Der P1 (from house dust mite) and papain (from papaya fruit) appear to rely on their protolytic function as inactive forms of these proteins do not induce type 2 immunity (60). A cysteine protease from the parasite *Leishmania Mexicana* has also been shown to induce type 2 immunity and this could be blocked by protease inhibitors (66). The importance of controlling enzymatic activity at epithelial surfaces is dramatically demonstrated in patients with Netherton syndrome. Netherton syndrome, which is caused by hereditary mutations in the serine protease inhibitor, LEKTI, presents with severe disruption in barrier function and persistent atopy, allergic disease, and AD (74, 75). The mutation in LEKTI results in persistent activation of protease-activated receptor (PAR)-2 and induction of TSLP and type 2 immunity (76).

Other endogenous stress-signals, for example the NLR receptors, NOD-1, and NOD-2, can polarize antigen-specific immune responses toward Th2 and thus contribute to the onset of adaptive immunity (77, 78). Interestingly, NOD-1 and NOD-2 expression within the stromal compartment is necessary to prime effector $CD4^+$ Th2 responses and full Th2 induction is dependent on stromal TSLP (79). The type 2-inducing innate immune sensing is in these cases recognition of bacterial-derived products (peptidoglycans) and not self- or environmental antigens. Although the role of PAMPs and PRRs such as TLRs are usually associated with type 1 immunity, there are other examples in which TLR stimuli can induce type 2 responses. For example, low doses of lipopolysaccharides (LPS) have been proposed to promote Th2 cell responses (whereas high doses promote Th1) (80) for which stromal expression of TLR4 is critical (81). Certain microbial stimuli that signal via DC-SIGN induce Th2 biased responses and many TLR2 agonists have also been shown to suppress Th1 and promote Th2 responses (82). Furthermore, in the case of allergens, there is evidence that some can be directly sensed by PRRs; house dust mite allergens (83) as well as nickel (84) can signal via TLR4 for instance.

Given the vast array of molecules that can trigger type 2 immunity and the many innate and adaptive immune cells involved in orchestrating the response it seems reasonable that there are several routes to inducing type 2 responses and that these may yield a qualitatively different kind of type 2 immunity. The conventional mode of inducing type 2 immunity and high affinity antigen-specific IgG1 and IgE antibody has since long been described and substantiated. Activated $CD4^+$ αβ Th cells upregulate CD40L and secrete IL-4 and IL-13, whereby they promote germ-line transcription of the γ1 and ε heavy chain to initialize class switching. This requires cognate interactions between B cell MHC II molecules and the TCR–CD3 complex. However, perhaps especially with regards to IgE, there appears to be additional non-conventional modes of inducing class switching and the requirement for T cell help may differ. In contrast to orthodox belief, mice that are deficient in αβ T cells have highly elevated levels of IgE antibodies and class switch particularly efficient to IgG1 and IgE (85, 86). Mice lacking the linker for activation of T cells (LAT) adapter protein (87) or the Tec kinase ltk also have elevated levels of IgE (88, 89), which may be regulated non-conventionally by γδ T cells. Evidence for a non-conventional route to IgE has also been demonstrated during the γδ T cell dependent "lymphoid stress-surveillance response" in the context of stressed skin epithelium (53). It has been established that the IgE produced in immunodeficient mice differ from conventional adaptive IgE not only by being MHC II-mediated T cell cognate independent but also by lacking dependence on germinal centers and thus producing IgE without significant somatic hypermutations (90). Moreover, this "natural" IgE also appears to be mainly self-reactive (85, 90). It may be that in a given circumstance a mixture of conventional adaptive routes and less-adaptive non-conventional routes to IgE are operating simultaneously. For example, infection with a helminth produces not only high affinity antigen-specific IgE but also a lot of "non-specific" IgE and similarly NKG2D-dependent induction of IgE from stressed skin produces not only antigen-specific IgE to an antigen encountered simultaneously but also "non-specific" IgE (53). Analysis of IgE repertoires and the particular requirements for development of IgE-secreting B cells is needed to further elucidate conventional (via Th2) and non-conventional routes to IgE. This may also provide invaluable information as to what actually constitutes a host-protective response (against tissue stress, toxins, parasites) versus allergic Th2 immunity.

IMMUNE SURVEILLANCE

To address the role of EC-driven type 2 immunity in tissue immune surveillance it is useful to first define "immune surveillance." Immune surveillance refers to the capacity of the immune system to sense cellular dysregulation and respond by activating a stress response to restore homeostasis. This continued "quality control" mechanism has most commonly been applied to and studied in relation to cancer. The cancer immuosurveillance hypothesis was first proposed by Ehrlich in 1909 when he predicted that the immune system could repress or destroy the outgrowth of tumors that arise spontaneously on a continued basis (91). This proposal initiated a century of debate over the immune systems role in controlling neoplasia. The idea of a natural immune response against neoplasms or pre-malignant and dysregulated cells was revisited and expanded by Burnet and Thomas in the 1950s (92, 93). They proposed that lymphocytes form the basis of a "cancer immunosurveillance" process that protects immunocompetent hosts against primary tumor development. Although the hypothesis grew in recognition with the expansion of knowledge about the immune system and tumor-antigen recognition, the architects themselves pointed to "the problem with the idea of immunosurveillance is that it cannot be shown to exist in experimental animals" (94) – and it is of course rarely appreciated in a clinical setting. By the early 1990s, little attention was paid to the idea that natural immunity could control tumor establishment *de novo*. However, by the mid-1990s and onward several observations were made that rekindled the interest in this early aspect of tumor immunity [reviewed in Ref. (95)]. In short, the physiological importance of immune surveillance was well revealed by the pathological consequences of its failure: the neutralization of IFNγ with antibodies (96) and later the use of mice lacking IFNγ responsiveness was shown to enhance tumor growth (97). Lymphocytes were unequivocally proven to play an essential role in immune surveillance by seminal observations in $rag2^{-/-}$ mice (98) and subsets of lymphocytes such as NK, NKT cells (99), and γδT cells (100) were shown to play prominent roles in the control of malignancy. These new data prompted a refinement of the cancer immunosurveillance concept (95) and an ongoing quest to understand the triggers and mechanistic action of this early and continuous immune response against altered self.

ELICITORS AND EFFECTORS OF IMMUNE SURVEILLANCE

Epithelial-derived cancers, called carcinomas, make up about 85% of all cancers. The epithelial barriers of our body surfaces are also where the majority of exogenous stresses and challenges occur. Both sterile and microbial insults are encountered daily at epithelial surfaces and prompt EC and immune activation. Cancer development is, however, a multifactorial and multistep process. Most solid cancers only emerge following a sequential accumulation of somatic mutations over many years, which eventually may overwhelm the barriers that normally restrain their growth and thus clonal expansion of transformed cells can occur. Cumulative mutational load, telomere dysfunction, and altered stromal milieu are all required before a solid tumor presents (101). Fortunately, numerous intrinsic and extrinsic tumor-supressor mechanisms exist to prevent the development and outgrowth of malignant cells and all cells continuously undergo these rigorous "health checks." The normal health control mechanisms can be triggered both by endogenous and exogenous stress and are executed by a cell-autonomous intrinsic surveillance system (such as delay in cell-cycle progression, repair of DNA-damage/genetic mutations, and induction of senescence or apoptosis) – and backed up by extrinsic immune surveillance mechanisms triggered by manifestations of EC dysregulation. The cell intrinsic responses to stress and the cell-extrinsic responses of the immune system are therefore intimately linked.

Damage-associated molecular patterns are mainly intracellular components of cells that are released or exposed upon physical or metabolic stress or cell death (102). For example ATP released from dying cells can act as a chemoattractant on macrophages drawing them to the stressed tissue (103). Extracellular ATP can bind to P2 purinergic receptors, which dependent on the cell engaged, can induce inflammatory (104) or anti-inflammatory (71) immune responses. Release of ROS or DNA from damaged cells can also powerfully initiate immune surveillance responses (105). Upon stress, ECs also rapidly and potently increase their synthesis of complement C3 (106), which due to its action on a multitude of innate and adaptive immune cells is likely to play a role in early immune surveillance, although its role in cancer as well as tissue homeostasis is as yet relatively unexplored.

In addition to the release of DAMPs, complement and cytokines/chemokines ECs can in response to numerous forms of cell-dysregulation dynamically alter cell-surface antigens to engage with receptors on innate and adaptive immune cells. Ligand–receptor interactions between ECs and tissue-resident immunocytes are thus important not only for homestatic interactions but are key regulators and elicitors of immune surveillance. One of the most important and best-characterized families of stress-induced EC ligands includes Rae-1, H60, and MULT1 (mouse), MICA, MICB and ULBPs (human). These are members of the larger family of MHC class Ib molecules and are reported upregulated on ECs by stresses such as heat-shock, UV-irradiation, DNA-damage, viral and bacterial infection, and autoimmunity. These unconventional MHC molecules engage the activating lectin-type receptor NKG2D, which is constitutively expressed by tissue-resident T cells and NK, NKT cells but is also expressed on $CD8^+$ T cells and in some circumstances subsets of $CD4^+$ T cells. The NKG2D-pathway has proven important in numerous settings of cell-dysregulation, such as cancer (107), infection (108), autoimmunity (109), and transplantation [reviewed in Ref. (110)], and its key role in immune surveillance is supported by the plethora of strategies tumors and viruses have adopted to evade it (111, 112). In relation to cancer, NKG2D-ligands are expressed by most epithelial tumors and the NKG2D-pathway is strongly associated with anti-tumor responses in both humans and mice (113). NKG2D-ligands are often upregulated early upon cellular dysregulation or transformation, it has however been controversial whether immune cells could be activated by such self-moieties alone. By generating transgenic mice where an autologous NKG2D-ligand, Rae-1, could be upregulated on keratinocytes by administration of doxycycline it was shown that even in the absence of any overt microbial stress (or overt tissue/cellular dysregulation as in a tumor setting) engagement of NKG2D on the epidermal IELs (DETCs) activated these cells and caused profound changes in the local immune compartment (114). This demonstrates that resident immunocytes can recognize and act solely on alterations in autologous stress antigens and thus survey the "health-status" of a given EC, pre-malignancy. The data support the cancer immune surveillance theory as it was also shown that the tissue-resident IELs have a key role in host-protection against skin carcinogenesis (114). Afferent sensing is normally attributed to innate myeloid cells, perhaps particularly to DCs that are often viewed as the primary orchestrator of adaptive immunity. To highlight the capacity of tissue-resident T cells (as demonstrated by the epidermal γδT cells discussed above) to perform an equivalent function as sensors of dysregulation, this mode of afferent sensing has been termed "lymphoid stress-surveillance" (115, 116). Lymphoid stress-surveillance may particularly be engaged in recognition of "stressed-self" and as such confer "beneficial autoimmune" responses in our body surface tissues. It is intriguing that NKG2D is expressed primarily, perhaps exclusively, by lymphoid cells (γδT, NKT, $CD8^+$ αβT, and NK cells), suggesting that engagement of NKG2D could elicit an acute lymphocyte stress response to EC damage perhaps engaging different cells in different tissues.

In addition to the NKG2D-pathway, many other ligand–receptor pathways modulating epithelial-immune cell interactions and contributing to immune surveillance and tissue homeostasis are emerging. One such emerging family of regulators is the nectin and nectin-like (necl) proteins. Nectins are immunoglobulin-like cell–cell adhesion molecules involved in the formation of adherens junctions in ECs and fibroblast. Both nectin and the necl molecules play important roles not only in adhesion but also in migration, proliferation, and wound healing (117, 118). The group of receptors that engage these nectin molecules are therefore now being intensely studied in relation to cancer and immune surveillance (119). The major receptors that bind nectin and necl family members are DNAM-1 (CD226, PTA-1, TLiSA1), class I-restricted T cell-associated molecule (CRTAM), CD96, and TIGIT (WUCAM, VSIG9, Vstm3). All of these receptors are expressed on NK cells, γδT cells and $CD8^+$ αβT cells and can mediate effector functions in these cells upon engagement. DNAM-1 ligands are frequently upregulated on tumor cells and have been reported to be regulated through the DNA-damage response pathway (120). Activation of DNAM-1 can evoke potent cytotoxicity in both T cells and NK cells (121) and control tumor growth (122). CRTAM binds necl2, which have been shown to regulate wound healing in the skin (118) and be involved in metastasis of human tumors (123). Expression and activation of CRTAM on immunocytes is likely highly important in early control of tissue homeostasis and cancer immune surveillance. *In vitro* studies have shown CRTAM to induce IFNγ from T cells and *in vivo* ncl2 expressing tumors have been shown to be controlled by NK and $CD8^+$ T cells. Less is currently known about CD96 and TIGIT, but interestingly TIGIT appears to have an inhibitory function on NK and T cells (119).

Another example of an immune surveillance stimulator displayed by stressed ECs is the Coxsackie and adenovirus receptor (CAR). CAR is also a junctional adhesion molecule, it is upregulated on damaged ECs and potentially revealed when integrity of the tight junction is compromised. It binds junction adhesion molecule-like (JAML), which is expressed on neutrophils, tissue-resident γδT cells, and to a lesser extent on monocytes and some activated $CD8^+$ αβT cells. Resident skin and intestinal γδT cells upregulate their expression of JAML upon tissue injury and binding of JAML to CAR lead to proliferation, cytokine, and growth factor production (124). Inhibiting costimulation of resident γδT cells by blocking JAML significantly delayed wound healing, akin to the total absence of these resident T cells, suggesting that CAR-JAML interactions are important for initiation of immune surveillance and tissue homeostasis. Interestingly, it has been shown that interaction of JAML with CAR recruits the central cell signal transducer PI3K, as is known for the αβT cell costimulator CD28, further emphasizing JAMLs role as a costimulator for tissue-resident T cells with implications for immune surveillance of dysregulated ECs (125).

Similar to the role of CAR-JAML interactions between ECs and resident T cells, it has recently been shown that plexin-B2-CD100 interactions are important for regulating the activity of IELs in both the skin and intestine (126, 127). CD100 (also know as Sema4D) is a member of the large family of semaphorin proteins. These proteins interact with plexins, which were first shown to play a fundamental role in the nervous system directing axon guidance. Intriguingly though, semaphorin–plexin interactions are also extensively involved in regulating immune responses and analysis of CD100-deficient animals have revealed a crucial role for this semaphorin in both humoral and cellular immunity (128). In relation to EC-immunocyte interactions, plexin-B2 is expressed on ECs in the epidermis and in the colon and interaction with CD100 on resident γδ IELs promotes wound repair in the skin (126) and protects against dextran sulfate sodium (DSS)-induced colitis in the intestine (127). In both tissues, CD100$^{-/-}$ mice failed to mount a proliferative EC response to tissue damage, which was attributable to the lack of activation and growth factor production by the γδ IELs required to heal the epithelium.

Tissue-resident immunocytes are in a unique position to carry out a continued maintenance function such as tissue stress-surveillance. Innate immune cells have the capacity to recognize antigens that are displayed in tissues following a variety of stressors and can respond rapidly in large numbers without requiring clonal expansion. The early stages of an immune response – the afferent phase – are therefore conventionally ascribed to myeloid cells or NK cells. However, as highlighted above tissue-resident T cells can also be afferent sensors of cellular dysregulation. The importance of a tissue-specific resident population in cancer immune surveillance has nevertheless been difficult to verify. This was addressed experimentally by taking advantage of the unique tissue location of specific γδTCR-expressing IELs in the mouse, where the epidermal population of Vγ5Vδ1^{+} IELs can be specifically knocked out (leaving all other T cell populations intact). These *vg5vd1*$^{-/-}$ mice are significantly more susceptible to cutaneous carcinogenesis than wild-type mice, demonstrating a key role for resident tissue-specific IELs in cancer immune surveillance. Consistent with the cancer immune surveillance hypothesis the γδ IEL act early and significantly suppress the development of papillomas but cannot suppress the progression from papilloma to carcinoma (114). Thus, myeloid cells, NK cells, and IELs all act as afferent sensors of dysregulation and initiators of immune surveillance in epithelial tissues. These cells can then also contribute to the downstream effector and regulatory phases of immunity. Clearly, both CD4^{+} and CD8^{+} αβT cells as well as B cells play important roles in cancer immune surveillance in the effector phase.

FUNCTIONS AND MECHANISMS OF IMMUNE SURVEILLANCE

The afferent phase of immune surveillance – the sensing of dysregulated self – applies to many other stresses than purely oncogenic stress. Thus the concept of immune surveillance not only pertains to cancer; accumulating evidence suggests that it can be more broadly applied to other non-malignant pathologies. For example, liver fibrosis, as a result of liver damage, is exacerbated when NK or NKT cells are depleted or the gene for perforin (required for cytotoxicity) is deleted as the stressed hepatic stellar cells cannot be controlled (129, 130). Stressed hepatic stellar cells express NKG2D-ligands upon damage, as described for ECs, facilitating their recognition by immune surveillance cells. Interestingly, natural activation of hepatic iNKT cells inhibits fibrosis whereas non-natural "over-stimulation" of iNKT cells appears to have the opposite effect and accelerate liver injury (129). Equally in the liver, tissue-resident macrophages have been shown to protect against ischemia reperfusion injury and be critical for tissue homeostasis (131).

Mice lacking normal resident IEL repertoires, such as *Tcrd*$^{-/-}$ mice, develop spontaneous chronic dermatitis, which can only be downregulated when *Tcrd*$^{-/-}$ mice are reconstituted with the tissue-specific resident IEL (the Vγ5Vδ1 TCR-expressing epidermal DETC) (132). Interestingly, these *Tcrd*$^{-/-}$ mice also show a defect in the integrity of the epidermal barrier, as measured by hydration status and transepidermal water loss (TEWL). However, the epidermal barrier defect is obvious only upon environmental challenge, consistent with the notion that the IELs survey the health-status of the ECs and promote tissue homeostasis (133). Skin IELs were also the first T cells to be implicated in promoting EC growth. Closure of full-thickness skin wounds is significantly delayed in *Tcrd*$^{-/-}$ mice, and this is attributed to the skin IELs capacity to rapidly produce EC growth factors such as insulin-like growth factor-1 (IGF-1) and keratinocyte growth factors (KGF) (134, 135). Intriguingly, it has also been shown in humans that T cells isolated from healthy or acutely wounded skin actively produce EC growth factors and participate in wound repair, whereas T cells from patients with chronic wound-healing problems are anergic and unable to produce EC growth factors (136). Similarly, *Tcrd*$^{-/-}$ mice lacking the γδ IEL population, which represents a major intestinal T cell population, are more susceptible to DSS-induced mucosal injury of the gut and demonstrate delayed tissue repair due to the lack of localized delivery of EC growth factors from the missing γδ IEL compartment (137).

The examples above clearly demonstrate that immune surveillance is not only a mechanism to control the development and outgrowth of tumors but is also a key regulator of tissue homeostasis more generally [reviewed in Ref. (138)]. The implication of immune surveillance mechanisms in the maintenance and re-establishment of tissue homeostasis thus broadens its scope and it is likely that similar cell-extrinsic immune surveillance mechanisms are important at disease-initiating (pre-disease) stages in many pathophysiological settings other than cancer.

Immune surveillance can function by many (non-exclusive) mechanisms (**Figure 2**): (1) recognize and remove damaged, stressed, senescent, and (pre)-malignant cells, (2) remove damaging substances, waste, and dead cells, (3) facilitate re-establishment of homeostasis by repair mechanisms, (4) neutralize potential harmful environmental substances, or (5) dampen detrimental inflammatory reactions.

In relation to cancer immune surveillance, the main focus has been on type 1 immunity and cytotoxic mechanisms, both of which have overwhelming experimental support for playing a role in extrinsic tumor suppression. In both genetic and carcinogen-induced tumor models, cytotoxic molecules such as perforin and TRAIL, as well as NKG2D engagement, have repeatedly been shown to be important in tumor control. Likewise mice lacking type 1 molecules such as IFNγ, IFNGR, IL-12, or type I IFN receptors are significantly more susceptible to carcinogenesis in several models. Mice lacking IFNγ, perforin, TRAIL, functioning FasL or IL-12 responsiveness can also develop spontaneous tumors of variable origin [extensively reviewed in Ref. (139)].

However, the repair functions of immune surveillance are clearly also very important in the early phases of immune

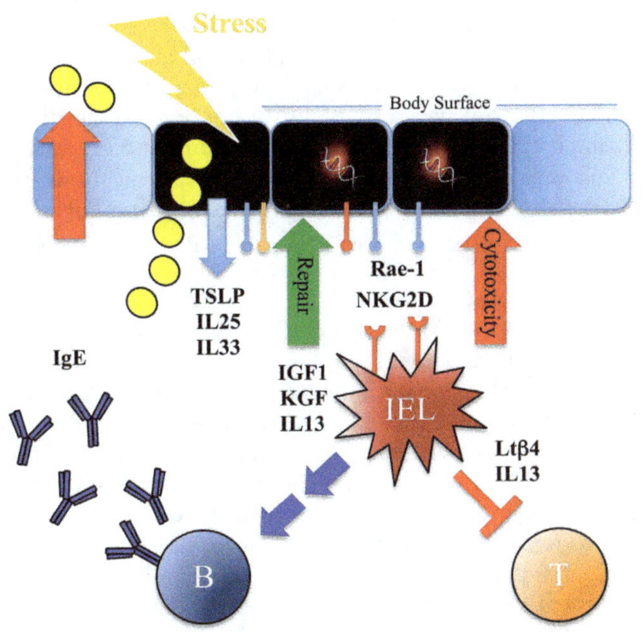

FIGURE 2 | Immune surveillance with type 2 immunity promotes tissue homeostasis and protects against carcinogenesis using numerous layers of control. Scheme illustrating possible mechanisms whereby tissue-resident IELs can provide rapid host-protective immune surveillance and re-establish tissue homeostasis at body surfaces. Tissue stress as imposed by mechanical disruption, injury, or exposure to noxious environmental substances such as chemicals, carcinogens, UV-irradiation or toxins prompts ECs to release IL-25, IL-33, and TSLP cytokines, and upregulate expression of stress-ligands such as Rae-1, CAR, and plexins. This activates the resident IELs and their responses include cytolytic effects, release of growth factors (for example IGF-1, KGF), dampening of αβ T cell-mediated inflammation [for example by release of thymosin-β4 lymphoid splice variant (LTβ4)], rapid and potent production of IL-13, as well as promoting humoral IgE responses. Stress surveillance by IELs can thus recognize and remove damaged and possibly (pre-)malignant cells, promote tissue repair, and induce type 2 immunity, which in turn controls inflammation, expels or inactivates noxious substances, and promotes morphological tissue homeostasis.

surveillance. This is illustrated by the link between wounding and tumor development. It has been observed that tumors can develop at the site of chronic skin wounds or untreated mouth ulcers (140) and there are several case reports of lung metastasis at sites of accidental trauma (141). A clear illustration of the link between a defective wound-healing response and the development of cancer comes from patients with epidermolysis bullosa. These patients have mutations in genes encoding skin extracellular matrix components and suffer from chronic skin blistering and sores – and as a result of the chronic tissue damage are at increased risk of developing squamous cell carcinoma (142, 143). A diminished capacity to repair a damaged barrier can thus predispose to the development of cancer. Such associations between chronic damage/wounds and cancer as well as the histological similarities of wounds and tumors led to the often-cited phrase that "tumors are wounds that do not heal" (144).

The association between chronic wounds and development of cancer may of course not only pertain to the lack of repair *per se* but also to the onset of a detrimental chronic inflammation as a consequence. There is a close association between chronic inflammation and cancer, and once a malignant cell has escaped the early phase of immune surveillance, inflammation can exert prominent pro-carcinogenic effects (145). The tumor-promoting effects of inflammation are being intensively studied and are starting to have implications for the treatment of cancers (145, 146). An important feature of early tumor immune surveillance could thus be the release of anti-inflammatory products in the tissue. Stressed ECs promptly release many anti-inflammatory products such as IL-33, TSLP, and IL-25 – all with the propensity to drive anti-inflammatory type 2 immune responses. The role of such anti-inflammatory DAMPs and type 2 immunity in early cancer immune surveillance remains to be clarified but intriguingly when tumor-protective skin-resident IELs are activated by stressed ECs they promptly release high levels of IL-13 (53) (and Strid-J unpublished data). Interestingly, this IL-13 and a following production of IgE is dependent on engagement of NKG2D on the IELs (53), perhaps suggesting that the tumor-suppressive effect of NKG2D and skin-resident IELs may not solely be via cytotoxic/type 1-mediated immune surveillance mechanisms. The surprising association between NKG2D and anti-inflammatory type 2 immune responses (and IgE) was recently corroborated in a model of allergic pulmonary inflammation, where mice lacking NKG2D were resistant to the induction of allergic inflammation and showed reduced Th2 and IgE responses (147). The association between a stress-sensor such as NKG2D, which has been intimately linked to anti-tumor responses, and induction of type 2 immunity demands a closer look at the role of early type 2 immunity in cancer immune surveillance. The possible role of such early type 2 responses in tissue homeostasis and immune surveillance of cancer as well as its possible pro- and anti-tumor growth functions are discussed in more detail below.

ROLE OF TYPE 2 IMMUNITY IN TISSUE HOMEOSTASIS AND IMMUNE SURVEILLANCE

What is known so far of the physiological role of type 2 responses is that their host-protection properties converge in different forms of barrier defenses (58). This seems logical as epithelial surfaces have a propensity to drive type 2 immunity (rather than type 1) upon non-invasive/non-penetrating challenge or stress and type 2 immune mediators are thus well poised to play a role in early immune surveillance as well as homeostatic tissue regulation. IL-13 is the best-characterized inducer of mucus production and goblet cell hyperplasia in the respiratory and intestinal mucosa. In the skin, transgenic over-expression of IL-13 induces skin remodeling, which is primarily driven by TSLP (148). In both circumstances, hyperplasia results in improved resistance to damage and damaging substances at the body barrier either via production of mucus at the mucosal surfaces or thickening of the skin. IL-13 may also be involved in homeostatic EC differentiation/proliferation in the skin. Epidermal IELs, which are non-redundant for normal tissue homeostasis and wound-healing, are rapid and potent producers of IL-13 following skin challenge (UV-radiation, tape-stripping, NKG2D-ligand expression, and exposure to carcinogen) and mice deficient in IL-13 have delayed barrier repair following epidermal tape-stripping as measured by TEWL (Strid-J unpublished).

Removal or expulsion is another host defense strategy induced by type 2 immunity, which can directly protect against noxious toxins or parasites, as well as limiting their systemic dissemination. The removal/expulsive actions of allergic and type 2 immunity through sneezing/coughing/itching/vomiting/diarrhea are partly induced by EC-derived mediators including TSLP, which acts directly on sensory neurons in the skin triggering itching (149), and by the effect of mast cell-derived histamine on smooth muscles. Type 2 immune mediators can also confer host-protection by inactivation, neutralization, and destruction of noxious substances. This is most notably shown by the requirement for mast cells in the detoxification of snake and bee venom (150) and the evidence that mast cell proteases can specifically attack snake venom at the structures required for toxicity and thereby neutralizing it (151). Recent data strongly suggest that IgE mediates or at least contributes to protection against venoms as for example the protective responses against re-challenge with high doses of bee venom is abrogated in mice lacking B cells, FcεRI, or IgE (56, 57). It is likely that this protection is partly via the very rapid IgE-mediated degranulation of mast cells. Encapsulation and restriction is another layer of barrier defense regulated by type 2 mediators, which can help prevent the spread of noxious substances if elimination or expulsion has been insufficient. Endothelial leakage and exudate formation can be induced by mast cell-derived products and such local tissue edema may impede parasite invasion. For example it has been shown that the edema caused by IgE-mediated mast cell degranulation is important in the defense against macroparasites such as ticks (152). Another restriction mechanism, which may restrict the spread of noxious substance as well as macroparasites, involves sequestration through granuloma formation. Type 2 immune responses protect the host during infection with schistosomiasis by inducing granulomas that sequester the tissue-damaging toxins from the parasite eggs (153).

Perhaps most importantly, much of type 2 immunity seems dedicated to tissue repair and promoting tolerance to damage. Indeed, it has been hypothesized that type 2 immunity has evolved to direct innate wound repair mechanisms (154). The rationale for the induction of tissue repair as a part of type 2 immune defense is obvious. It may also explain the extreme urgency of some type 2 responses (which is not easily explained if directed only toward a slow replicating macroparasite), as damage control may well be more important than pathogen control. In evolutionary terms, it makes sense to be able to quickly expel or neutralize noxious substances as well as rapidly repair the life-essential body barrier. EC-derived cytokine alarmins and cell-ligands can activate and direct the resident tissue cells to promote repair responses; IELs rapidly sense stress and can produce growth factors locally in the absence of further inflammation and tissue-resident ILCs can amplify the type 2 response and produce amphiregulin. Indeed, depletion of ILC2 compromises lung epithelial barrier integrity (155) just as depletion of γδ IEL compromises skin and gut epithelial integrity during homeostasis as well as delaying wound healing (127, 133, 134). Almost all of the cells associated with type 2 immunity are also associated with the wound-healing response. Alternatively activated macrophages produce vascular endothelial growth factor (VEGF), arginase 1, and IGF-1; Eosinophils store preformed growth factors, matrix metalloproteinases, and lipid mediators, all of which can mediate wound healing (156). Amphiregulin is produced by mast cells following FcεRI signaling, potentially also linking IgE responses to wound repair (157). In sum, the effects of type 2 immunity at our body surface tissues play important roles in eliminating, restricting, and neutralizing noxious environmental substances as well as repairing the damage caused and minimizing inflammation – as such this type of immunity is critical for tissue homeostasis and responses to challenges that have breached the epithelial barrier.

In terms of early cancer immune surveillance, the role of type 2 immunity has been little explored. However, the effects of rapid type 2 immune responses as outlined above could indeed play a prominent role in cancer immune surveillance. It has been demonstrated that the same tissue-resident IELs act as key components of tumor resistance and potent inducers of type 2 immunity and IgE antibodies (53, 114). The humoral component of this lymphoid stress-surveillance response may limit tissue damage by targeting noxious foreign substances, such as toxins that may be the root cause of the tissue dysregulation. The IgE effector response may promote toxin expulsion and limit their systemic dissemination. Simultaneously, the cellular response can direct cytotoxicity toward dysregulated cells as well as promoting repair of the damaged tissue and dampening inflammation (**Figures 2** and **3**). To limit the likelihood of cancer, it is clearly important to repair a wound or breached barrier quickly and efficiently as is demonstrated by the close association between chronic tissue damage and cancer. Less efficient wound repair may lead to inefficient immune surveillance against (pre-)malignant cells with damaged cells being allowed to stay longer in the tissue before being replaced. Additionally, slow repair of tissue damage may lead to inflammation, which as discussed can have potent pro-carcinogenic effects.

Although one can imagine a role for type 2 immunity and its regenerative capacity in early cancer immune surveillance this may indeed be a double-edged sword in further development of cancer (**Figure 3**). Failure of the type 2 response to adequately contain or eliminate the initiating substance may lead to a chronic wound-healing response and exacerbation of inflammation. Such continued tissue damage, repair, and regeneration may ultimately result in fibrosis. Fibrotic tissue is a highly permissive environment for tumor formation and it is also well established that continuous wound-healing responses and tumorigenesis are two processes that rely on similar molecular mechanisms (158). As such it is perhaps not surprising that the literature on type 2/IgE responses and cancer is somewhat bewildering.

ROLE OF TYPE 2 IMMUNITY AND IgE IN CANCER

Both positive and negative effects of type 2 immunity on tumor growth and carcinogenesis have been reported in the literature (**Table 1**). Contrasting results are clearly in part due to the differing experimental approaches and models but most likely also reflects the divergent roles that type 2 immunity may play at different stages of carcinogenesis and in different tissues. $CD4^+$ T cell-derived IL-4 has been reported to induce granulocyte infiltration, thereby promoting tumor clearance (an action enhanced by IL-13), and conversely increase tumor cells' resistance to apoptosis by up-regulation of anti-apoptotic proteins (159). Many

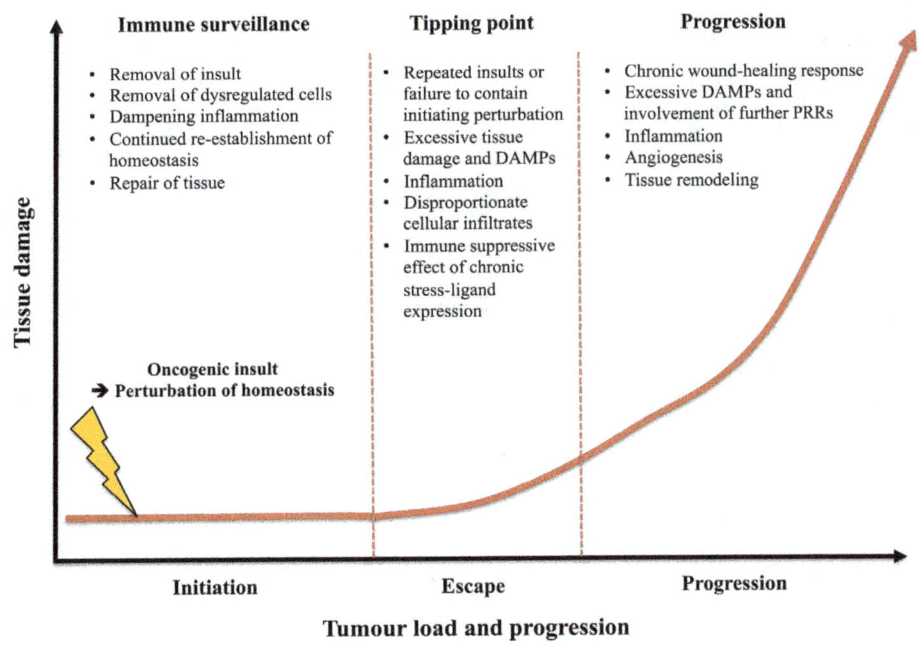

FIGURE 3 | Contrasting role of type 2 immunity in immune surveillance of early tissue dysregulation versus tumor progression. The type 2 component of immune surveillance may aid in host-protection against carcinogenesis at epithelial surfaces by removing the oncogenic insult, eliminating the dysregulated cells, dampening excessive inflammation, repairing tissue, re-establishing homeostasis, as well as improving resistance to future damage. However, following continuous perturbations, failure to eliminate the initial insult or dysregulated immune surveillance a tipping point may be reached where excessive tissue damage and DAMPs lead to inflammation, disproportionate cellular infiltrates, and escape from immune surveillance and tissue homeostasis. Once a certain level of tissue damage is reached, a perpetual type 2 response may be detrimental to the host by transitioning to aid carcinogenesis by promoting a chronic wound-healing response and fibrosis as well as supporting neo-angiogenesis.

studies carried out in the 1990s and early 2000s demonstrated that tumors or tumor cell lines engineered to produce IL-4 would exhibit increased rejection and retarded growth *in vivo*; curiously a phenotype often dependent on $CD8^+$ cytotoxic T cells (160–163). IL-10 has been reported to be both "pro-tumorigenic" by inhibiting tumor cell lysis by cytotoxic T cells and "anti-tumorigenic" by promoting NK-cell-mediated tumor clearance and inhibiting angiogenesis (164). The EC-derived cytokines IL-33 and TSLP have been shown to enhance tumorigenesis by promoting epithelial-mesenchycmal transition (EMT) in organotypic culture of *ex vivo* carcinoma-associated fibroblasts (CAFs) and squamous cell carcinoma cells (165) and by enhancing Th2 inflammation (166). On the contrary TSLP has convincingly been shown in mouse *in vivo* models to be critically important for resistance to skin carcinogenesis (35, 36) establishing TSLP as a tumor suppressor in the skin. Many epithelial cancers express receptors for type 2 mediators such as IL-4 and IL-13, allowing for a direct effect on tumor growth, death, and proliferation that is independent of their effect on immunocytes (167). This perhaps also explains the likely divergent effects of type 2 immunity in early cancer immune surveillance versus in established tumors. Human breast and renal cancer cell lines treated with exogenous IL-13 *in vitro* demonstrate reduced proliferation (168–170) – although an ovarian cancer line demonstrated enhanced invasive and enzyme (protease) activity (171) suggesting IL-13 aids primary tumor invasion and metastasis in this model. No doubt the heterogeneity of cancer cell lines and *ex vivo* tumors derived from patients and experimental animals clouds a consistent description of how potent type 2 cytokines may affect growth and immune surveillance of tumors *in vivo*. Cellular type 2 players, such as eosinophils, have an extensive description in the cancer literature, and have been shown to play a protective role against chemically induced tumors *in vivo* – and directly kill chemically induced fibrosarcomas *in vitro* (172), suggesting efficacious tissue immune surveillance. Mast cells frequently infiltrate the tumor microenvironment and are usually correlated with a poor prognosis in human cancers (173), although both tumor rejection and promotion has been attributed to them in the mouse. Interestingly, the ancient and highly conserved (174) immunoglobulin isotype IgE has been shown to play a significant role in immune surveillance of tumors. Since the 1990s IgE mAbs have been considered for cancer immunotherapy; particularly given IgE's extreme biological potency and presence of high and low affinity receptors on various effector cell types (175). Indeed, animals deficient in IgE show drastically altered susceptibility to cutaneous chemical carcinogenesis, and an altered tumor cytokine microenvironment (Dalessandri-T and Strid-J; unpublished). IgE-coated irradiated tumor cells has also been shown to generate protective, eosinophil, and T cell immunity to subsequently administered non-irradiated tumors (176). In addition, the type 2 immunoglobulin IgG1 has been reported to be potently tumoricidal when not "blocked" by competing IgG4 antibodies (177).

Table 1 | Examples of type 2 cytokines and immunoglobulins influencing tumor pathology.

Type 2 mediator	Experimental approach	Model	Tumor growth
IL-4	Tumors engineered to produce IL-4, IL-4 ↑	Primary murine renal cancer	↓ Enhanced $CD8^+$ T cell-dependent rejection (160)
		Injection of syngeneic tumor cell lines	↓ Enhanced $CD8^+$ T cell-dependent rejection (161) ↑ Delayed primary tumor clearance, increased secondary tumor development (178) ↑ Reduced $CD8^+$ T cell-mediated clearance (178)
		Primary murine adenocarcinoma	↓ Enhanced $CD8^+$ T cell-dependent and eosinophil-mediated rejection (162)
		Vaccination with irradiated tumor cells	↓ Enhanced $CD8^+$ T cell-dependent clearance of lung metastases (163)
	Exogenous rIL-4 treatment, IL-4 ↑	Prostate, breast and bladder cancer cell lines	↑ Enhanced resistance to apoptosis and chemotherapeutic agents (159)
IL-13	Tumors engineered to produce IL-13, IL-13 ↑	Injection of P815 mastocytoma cell line	↓ Improved rejection and development of systemic anti-tumor immunity (179)
	Exogenous IL-13 treatment, IL-13 ↑	*Ex vivo* leukemic B blasts	↓ Reduced proliferation and cell-cycle progression assessed by DNA content (168)
		Human breast cancer cell line	↓ Inhibition of estrogen-induced cell proliferation, unchanged basal proliferation (169)
		Human renal carcinoma cell line	↓ Reduced proliferation and colony formation (170)
		Ovarian cancer cell line	↑ Increased MMP and AP-1-dependant invasion and protease activity in matrigel invasion assay (171)
	Antibody-mediated IL-13 neutralization, IL-13 ↓	Hodgkin lymphoma cell line	↓ Decreased proliferation and STAT6 phosphorylation (180)
IL-33	IL-33 receptor knockout ($ST2^{-/-}$), IL-33-signaling ↓	$ST2^{-/-}$ mammary carcinoma-bearing mice	↓ Attenuated tumor growth and metastasis, increased number and cytotoxic activity of NK cells (181)
	Exogenous IL-33 treatment, IL-33 ↑	4T1 cell line tumor-bearing mice	↑ Reduced intra-tumoral tumoricidal NK cells, increased splenic MDSCs and M2 macrophages (182)
	IL-33 co-admin, with HPV DNA vaccine, IL-33 ↑	TC-1 cell line (HPV-16 E7-positive) tumor-bearing mice	↓ Improved HPV antigen-specific CD4 and CD8 T cells, increased TC-1 regression (183)
	Organotypic culture, IL-33 ↑	*Ex vivo* human carcinoma-associated fibroblasts (CAFs)	↑ CAFs promote carcinoma invasion via IL-33 signaling and EMT induction (165)
TSLP	Antibody-mediated TSLP neutralization, TSLP ↓	Murine breast tumor xenograft	↓ Inhibition of tumor development (166)
	K14-$TSLP^{Tg}$ or calcipotriol induced TSLP, TSLP ↑	DMBA/TPA chemical skin carcinogenesis	↓ Delayed tumor onset and significantly reduced tumor number and growth (35)
	TSLP receptor knockout or TSLP neutralization, TSLP-signaling ↓	Notchl/Notch2 receptor knockout	↑ Loss of TSLP-signaling in Notch-deficient epidermis leads to tumor formation (36)
IgE	IgE-loaded tumor cell vaccine, IgE ↑	Post-vaccination challenge with RMA lymphoma or MC38 adenocarcinoma	↓ Improved protective eosinophil, $CD4^+$ and $CD8^+$ T cell responses to tumor challenge (176, 184)
IgGI	Engineered tumor-antigen-specific IgG4, IgGI ↓	Human melanoma xenograft model	↑ IgG4 blocked potent IgGI-mediated anti-tumor effector functions (177)

EPIDEMIOLOGICAL AND CLINICAL ASSOCIATIONS BETWEEN TYPE 2 IMMUNITY, IgE AND CANCER

Associations between allergy history and cancer risk have been investigated in numerous epidemiological studies and their association is being defined in the nascent field of "AllergoOncology" (**Table 2**). Recent overviews of the epidemiological literature demonstrate that both potent inverse and positive associations exist, which point to complex underlying interactions as well as reflecting the heterogeneity of these diseases. Accordingly, although the relationship between cancer and allergy has intrigued researchers for decades, the biological nature of this association remains unclear.

Table 2 | Proposed hypotheses explaining associations between type 2 immunity/allergy and cancer.

Hypothesis	Predicted allergy–cancer relationship	Predicted affected tissue site	Proposed mechanisms
Antigenic stimulation or chronic inflammation (185)	Positive, causal	All sites	• Allergic inflammation and oxidative damage promote pro-tumorigenic gene mutations • Type 2-induced tissue remodeling and angiogenesis promotes tumor growth and invasion
Inappropriate Th2 skewing (186)	Positive, causal	All sites	• Diversion away from protective cytolytic type 1 responses • Non-protective IgE clonality, or poorly tumoricidal IgG4 class switching with immunosuppressive IL-10
Immune surveillance (93)	Inverse, causal	All sites	• Potent effector cells, including γδT cells, mast cells and eosinophils eradicate tumors • Tumor-specific IgE potently cytolytic via ADCC • Type 2 immunity repairs tissue damage and dampens inflammation hereby restricting tumor formation
Prophylaxis (55)	Inverse, causal	Mucosal and external surfaces	• Tissue type 2 immunity removes or neutralizes noxious and potentially carcinogenic environmental moieties before they cause genotoxicity • Type 2 immunity restricts systemic dissemination of noxious substances and enhances natural barrier defenses

Two hypotheses put forward to explain positive allergy–cancer associations are the "antigenic stimulation"/"chronic inflammation" hypothesis and the "inappropriate Th2 skewing" hypothesis (**Table 2**). The "antigenic stimulation" hypothesis was first proposed in the late 1980s (185) and has been reiterated numerous times, also termed the "chronic inflammation" hypothesis (186). This hypothesis proposes that inflammation associated with allergic disease establishes a tissue environment conducive to tumor growth. Indeed, more than 100 years ago a link between inflammation and cancer was first proposed by Virchow (146), who noted the presence of leukocytes in neoplastic tissues and suggested cancer originated at sites of chronic inflammation. Tissue damage with the release of DAMPs, chronic infection, and inflammation are all believed to contribute to the development of malignant disease. Mechanistically, cellular Th2-mediators such as macrophages promote oxidative damage through production of iNOS and hydrogen peroxide via the respiratory burst, increasing the likelihood of damage and mutation of tumor-suppressor genes or cell-cycle regulator genes. Tissue remodeling and pro-angiogenesis factors such as vasoactive mediators from tissue-resident mast cells and eosinophils, as well as VEGF, arginase and matrix metalloproteases released by macrophages, may promote local invasion of outgrowing tumors, and eventual metastasis with establishment of distal secondary loci worsening clinical outcome. Thus, the "antigenic stimulation/chronic inflammation" hypothesis predicts a positive relationship between allergic disease and cancer in any tissue site and this relationship is directly causal, i.e., inflammation secondary to or as a result of allergic disease directly promotes oncogenesis. The "inappropriate Th2 skewing" hypothesis (186) suggests that type 2 mediators – such as IL-4, IL-10, IL-13 – may redirect tissue immunity away from a potently anti-tumor and cytolytic Th1 response, toward an ineffective Th2 response, where IgE is produced and directed toward allergens and not tumor-specific or tumor-associated antigens. Additionally, with production of immunomodulatory IL-10, Th2-immunogloublin IgG4 class-switch recombination is favored over IgE, the former being far less potently tumoricidal, further attenuating anti-tumor responses. This hypothesis therefore also predicts a positive relationship between allergic disease and cancer, in any tissue site, and this relationship is directly causal – skewing to type 2 responses that are non-protective and aids oncogenesis.

Two hypotheses put forward to explain inverse allergy–cancer associations are the "immune surveillance" hypothesis, and the "prophylaxis" hypothesis (**Table 2**). Prophylaxis was first proposed by Profet (55), and suggests that the symptoms and mechanisms of allergic disease serve to repel and clear potentially mutagenic substances at the external body surfaces before mutagenesis can occur; a coopted function of type 2 immunity which also serves to expel parasites and helminths. Itch induced by type 2 mediators such as TSLP, goblet cell hypersecretion of mucus, sneezing, coughing, vomiting, and diarrhea all act as repulsive mechanisms and are particularly common allergy symptoms. In additional to physical expulsion, type 2 cellular players directly deactivate noxious xenobiotics. In mice at least, mast cells have been shown to degrade venom components through release of carboxypeptidases (150), and IgE raised to a conserved component (and allergen) of many venoms is protective against a repeat exposure (56, 57). The unpleasantness of allergy symptoms also conditions the animal to avoid potentially carcinogenic triggers. Thus, the "prophylaxis" hypothesis predicts an inverse, causal relationship between allergic disease and cancer, particularly at the exposed body barrier surfaces. This hypothesis requires that moieties encountered at the body surfaces are directly carcinogenic, or are pro-carcinogens, and predicts that individuals with allergy symptoms should present with (i) lower levels of carcinogens in their blood and (ii) restrictive or obstructive disease at mucosal surfaces – or that treatment to reduce allergic symptoms results in greater vulnerability to cancer at those sites (187). These corollaries of the "prophylaxis" hypothesis have been poorly investigated. The "immune surveillance" hypothesis, first proposed by Burnet (93), also predicts an inverse allergy–cancer relationship and inverse associations are predicted at any body site. It suggests that allergy and atopic symptoms are indicative of an immune system that is generally hyper-responsive to challenge, and has enhanced immune surveillance capability. Potently cytolytic type 2 responses raised against tumor-associated or -specific antigens can rapidly eradicate dysregulated and proto-neoplastic cells; hence allergy symptoms are a fortuitous, albeit unpleasant, result of an individual's potent immune system, which also controls dysregulated cells and results in an inverse allergy–cancer relationship. Although the inverse allergy–cancer relationship proposed by the "immune surveillance" hypothesis was originally thought to be purely correlational, as argued in this review, type 2 immunity is also likely to play an important role in early immune surveillance in a direct casual manner by virtue of its ability to remove noxious substances, repair tissue damage and dampen initial inflammation.

In spite of many speculations and associations there is little evidence for a strong association between allergy and *overall* cancer risk (188). However, given that allergic disease occurs primarily at outer epithelial surfaces it is logical to examine the incidence of cancer at specific tissue sites, particularly those at which allergic disease is prevalent; such as the skin, respiratory, and gastrointestinal tracts. A recent large meta-analysis of more than 400 studies of relationships between allergy and cancer reported a preponderance of inverse allergy–cancer associations, and interestingly this was particularly strong for cancers of tissues that interface with the external environment, such as skin, mouth, throat, colon, and cervix (187). These results support the "prophylaxis" as well as the "immune surveillance" hypotheses. Intriguingly, while most studies investigate the link between specifically Type I allergic disease and cancer, a significant inverse association between contact (Type IV) hypersensitivity and breast and non-melanoma skin cancer has been reported, and the authors suggested these data support the "immune surveillance" hypothesis (189).

The large number of published association studies nevertheless often paints a conflicting picture, some of which may be due to methodological constraints. Most retrospective studies on allergy–cancer associations have investigated self-reported or clinician-diagnosed allergy, methodologies particularly prone to recollection and reporting bias (former) and subject selection bias (latter). Researchers have attempted to alleviate these concerns at least in part by discriminating subjects on the basis of physiological indices of allergic disease, such as serum IgE titers (190, 191) and skin-prick testing. Of course, serum total or allergen-specific IgE suffers less from human biases, but these are not a definite metric of allergic status in all individuals, all of the time; in addition this methodology potentially precludes the possibility of examining significant non-Type I hypersensitivities in the analysis. Another concern is that if variation between individual's allergy symptoms is due more to differences in individual's exposure to antigens and/or carcinogens (the environment as a confounding variable), rather than individual differences in immunity ("immune surveillance" hypothesis), then positive correlations between allergic symptoms and cancer may occur – even if the "prophylaxis" or "immune surveillance" hypotheses are true. Particularly, given that exposure to carcinogenic allergens (such as cigarette smoke or vehicle exhaust) results in increased cancer and allergic disease (187). In addition, the genetic and phenotypic heterogeneity of tumors, and the complex inflammatory niche in which they reside, may also confound epidemiological association studies.

CONCLUDING REMARKS

Epithelial cancers are products of a series of events starting with dysregulated and stressed ECs. It is now clear that challenges to ECs can trigger discrete pathways promoting the release of specific cytokines, chemokines, and expression of stress antigens on the EC surface. Together this can powerfully drive immune responses, initially from cells resident in the epithelial and subepithelial compartment. The initial response to EC challenge and damage is often a very rapid type 2 immune response. This may serve to remove or neutralize noxious challenging substances, clear waste, repair the tissue, dampen inflammation, and re-establish tissue homeostasis. It may also directly contribute to the elimination of damaged cells together with cytolytic mechanisms from resident IELs and other immunocytes. Rapid type 2 immune responses at body surfaces thus prominently contribute to immune surveillance of dysregulated ECs. Since epithelial dysregulation contributes notably to a multitude of inflammatory diseases, this may not only be important in control of (pre-)malignancy but could be important at disease-initiating stages in a variety of diseases.

Immune surveillance by its nature is mainly important in the initiation phase of tissue damage and tumor control – for maintenance of tissue homeostasis. The same effector molecules and mechanisms may play a very different role during the progression phase of tissue damage and tumor growth. Failure to eliminate the original damaging substance, damaged cells, or to repair the tissue may lead to a continual stress response with excessive release of DAMPs, persistent stress-ligand expression, inflammation, and a chronic wound-healing response and this may determine the transition point between beneficial and detrimental functions of type 2 immunity in the course of disease. Similarly, continual exposure to noxious environmental substances may eventually overwhelm the immune surveillance mechanisms keeping the damage in check and result in pathology or tumor growth. Further research is needed to study whether the balance between tumor cell growth and elimination may be tipped back upon immune manipulations aimed at enhancing naturally occurring immune surveillance.

ACKNOWLEDGMENTS

We thank colleagues within our laboratory and beyond for insightful discussions and especially Dr. Olga Sobolev for critical review of the manuscript. Apologies to colleagues whose work has inadvertently been overlooked or that were a victim of space constraints. We thank the Wellcome Trust for funding and declare no competing financial interests.

REFERENCES

1. Swamy M, Jamora C, Havran W, Hayday A. Epithelial decision makers: in search of the "epimmunome." *Nat Immunol* (2010) **11**(8):656–65. doi:10.1038/ni.1905

2. Nestle FO, Di Meglio P, Qin J-Z, Nickoloff BJ. Skin immune sentinels in health and disease. *Nat Rev Immunol* (2009) **9**(10):679–91. doi:10.1038/nri2622
3. Jackson SP, Bartek J. The DNA-damage response in human biology and disease. *Nature* (2009) **461**(7267):1071–8. doi:10.1038/nature08467
4. Wood LC, Elias PM, Calhoun C, Tsai JC, Grunfeld C, Feingold KR. Barrier disruption stimulates interleukin-1 alpha expression and release from a pre-formed pool in murine epidermis. *J Invest Dermatol* (1996) **106**(3):397–403. doi:10.1111/1523-1747.ep12343392
5. Jerde TJ, Bushman W. IL-1 induces IGF-dependent epithelial proliferation in prostate development and reactive hyperplasia. *Sci Signal* (2009) **2**(86):ra49. doi:10.1126/scisignal.2000338
6. Culig Z, Puhr M. Interleukin-6: a multifunctional targetable cytokine in human prostate cancer. *Mol Cell Endocrinol* (2012) **360**(1–2):52–8. doi:10.1016/j.mce.2011.05.033
7. Fort MM, Cheung J, Yen D, Li J, Zurawski SM, Lo S, et al. IL-25 induces IL-4, IL-5, and IL-13 and Th2-associated pathologies in vivo. *Immunity* (2001) **15**(6):985–95. doi:10.1016/S1074-7613(01)00243-6
8. Lee J, Ho WH, Maruoka M, Corpuz RT, Baldwin DT, Foster JS, et al. IL-17E, a novel proinflammatory ligand for the IL-17 receptor homolog IL-17Rh1. *J Biol Chem* (2001) **276**(2):1660–4. doi:10.1074/jbc.M008289200
9. Owyang AM, Zaph C, Wilson EH, Guild KJ, McClanahan T, Miller HRP, et al. Interleukin 25 regulates type 2 cytokine-dependent immunity and limits chronic inflammation in the gastrointestinal tract. *J Exp Med* (2006) **203**(4):843–9. doi:10.1084/jem.20051496
10. Zaph C, Du Y, Saenz SA, Nair MG, Perrigoue JG, Taylor BC, et al. Commensal-dependent expression of IL-25 regulates the IL-23-IL-17 axis in the intestine. *J Exp Med* (2008) **205**(10):2191–8. doi:10.1084/jem.20080720
11. Zaiss MM, Maslowski KM, Mosconi I, Guenat N, Marsland BJ, Harris NL. IL-1β suppresses innate IL-25 and IL-33 production and maintains helminth chronicity. *PLoS Pathog* (2013) **9**(8):e1003531. doi:10.1371/journal.ppat.1003531
12. Heneghan AF, Pierre JF, Gosain A, Kudsk KA. IL-25 improves luminal innate immunity and barrier function during parenteral nutrition. *Ann Surg* (2014) **259**(2):394–400. doi:10.1097/SLA.0b013e318284f510
13. Angkasekwinai P, Park H, Wang Y-H, Wang Y-H, Chang SH, Corry DB, et al. Interleukin 25 promotes the initiation of proallergic type 2 responses. *J Exp Med* (2007) **204**(7):1509–17. doi:10.1084/jem.20061675
14. Wang Y-H, Angkasekwinai P, Lu N, Voo KS, Arima K, Hanabuchi S, et al. IL-25 augments type 2 immune responses by enhancing the expansion and functions of TSLP-DC-activated Th2 memory cells. *J Exp Med* (2007) **204**(8):1837–47. doi:10.1084/jem.20070406
15. Gregory LG, Jones CP, Walker SA, Sawant D, Gowers KHC, Campbell GA, et al. IL-25 drives remodelling in allergic airways disease induced by house dust mite. *Thorax* (2013) **68**(1):82–90. doi:10.1136/thoraxjnl-2012-202003
16. Hams E, Armstrong ME, Barlow JL, Saunders SP, Schwartz C, Cooke G, et al. IL-25 and type 2 innate lymphoid cells induce pulmonary fibrosis. *Proc Natl Acad Sci U S A* (2014) **111**(1):367–72. doi:10.1073/pnas.1315854111
17. Deleuran M, Hvid M, Kemp K, Christensen GB, Deleuran B, Vestergaard C. IL-25 induces both inflammation and skin barrier dysfunction in atopic dermatitis. *Chem Immunol Allergy* (2012) **96**:45–9. doi:10.1159/000331871
18. Salimi M, Barlow JL, Saunders SP, Xue L, Gutowska-Owsiak D, Wang X, et al. A role for IL-25 and IL-33-driven type-2 innate lymphoid cells in atopic dermatitis. *J Exp Med* (2013) **210**(13):2939–50. doi:10.1084/jem.20130351
19. Schmitz J, Owyang A, Oldham E, Song Y, Murphy E, McClanahan TK, et al. IL-33, an interleukin-1-like cytokine that signals via the IL-1 receptor-related protein ST2 and induces T helper type 2-associated cytokines. *Immunity* (2005) **23**(5):479–90. doi:10.1016/j.immuni.2005.09.015
20. Komai-Koma M, Brombacher F, Pushparaj PN, Arendse B, McSharry C, Alexander J, et al. Interleukin-33 amplifies IgE synthesis and triggers mast cell degranulation via interleukin-4 in naïve mice. *Allergy* (2012) **67**(9):1118–26. doi:10.1111/j.1398-9995.2012.02859.x
21. Humphreys NE, Xu D, Hepworth MR, Liew FY, Grencis RK. IL-33, a potent inducer of adaptive immunity to intestinal nematodes. *J Immunol* (2008) **180**(4):2443–9. doi:10.4049/jimmunol.180.4.2443
22. Pastorelli L, Garg RR, Hoang SB, Spina L, Mattioli B, Scarpa M, et al. Epithelial-derived IL-33 and its receptor ST2 are dysregulated in ulcerative colitis and in experimental Th1/Th2 driven enteritis. *Proc Natl Acad Sci U S A* (2010) **107**(17):8017–22. doi:10.1073/pnas.0912678107
23. Fux M, Pecaric-Petkovic T, Odermatt A, Hausmann OV, Lorentz A, Bischoff SC, et al. IL-33 is a mediator rather than a trigger of the acute allergic response in humans. *Allergy* (2014) **69**(2):216–22. doi:10.1111/all.12309
24. Imai Y, Yasuda K, Sakaguchi Y, Haneda T, Mizutani H, Yoshimoto T, et al. Skin-specific expression of IL-33 activates group 2 innate lymphoid cells and elicits atopic dermatitis-like inflammation in mice. *Proc Natl Acad Sci U S A* (2013) **110**(34):13921–6. doi:10.1073/pnas.1307321110
25. Hueber AJ, Alves-Filho JC, Asquith DL, Michels C, Millar NL, Reilly JH, et al. IL-33 induces skin inflammation with mast cell and neutrophil activation. *Eur J Immunol* (2011) **41**(8):2229–37. doi:10.1002/eji.201041360
26. Yanaba K, Yoshizaki A, Asano Y, Kadono T, Sato S. Serum IL-33 levels are raised in patients with systemic sclerosis: association with extent of skin sclerosis and severity of pulmonary fibrosis. *Clin Rheumatol* (2011) **30**(6):825–30. doi:10.1007/s10067-011-1686-5
27. Yin H, Li X, Hu S, Liu T, Yuan B, Gu H, et al. IL-33 accelerates cutaneous wound healing involved in upregulation of alternatively activated macrophages. *Mol Immunol* (2013) **56**(4):347–53. doi:10.1016/j.molimm.2013.05.225
28. Allakhverdi Z, Comeau MR, Jessup HK, Yoon B-RP, Brewer A, Chartier S, et al. Thymic stromal lymphopoietin is released by human epithelial cells in response to microbes, trauma, or inflammation and potently activates mast cells. *J Exp Med* (2007) **204**(2):253–8. doi:10.1084/jem.20062211
29. Saenz SA, Taylor BC, Artis D. Welcome to the neighborhood: epithelial cell-derived cytokines license innate and adaptive immune responses at mucosal sites. *Immunol Rev* (2008) **226**:172–90. doi:10.1111/j.1600-065X.2008.00713.x
30. Zaph C, Troy AE, Taylor BC, Berman-Booty LD, Guild KJ, Du Y, et al. Epithelial-cell-intrinsic IKK-beta expression regulates intestinal immune homeostasis. *Nature* (2007) **446**(7135):552–6. doi:10.1038/nature05590
31. Ziegler SF, Artis D. Sensing the outside world: TSLP regulates barrier immunity. *Nat Immunol* (2010) **11**(4):289–93. doi:10.1038/ni.1852
32. Al-Shami A, Spolski R, Kelly J, Keane-Myers A, Leonard WJ. A role for TSLP in the development of inflammation in an asthma model. *J Exp Med* (2005) **202**(6):829–39. doi:10.1084/jem.20050199
33. Indra AK. Epidermal TSLP: a trigger factor for pathogenesis of atopic dermatitis. *Expert Rev Proteomics* (2013) **10**(4):309–11. doi:10.1586/14789450.2013.814881
34. Yoo J, Omori M, Gyarmati D, Zhou B, Aye T, Brewer A, et al. Spontaneous atopic dermatitis in mice expressing an inducible thymic stromal lymphopoietin transgene specifically in the skin. *J Exp Med* (2005) **202**(4):541–9. doi:10.1084/jem.20041503
35. Demehri S, Turkoz A, Manivasagam S, Yockey LJ, Turkoz M, Kopan R. Elevated epidermal thymic stromal lymphopoietin levels establish an antitumor environment in the skin. *Cancer Cell* (2012) **22**(4):494–505. doi:10.1016/j.ccr.2012.08.017
36. Di Piazza M, Nowell CS, Koch U, Durham A-D, Radtke F. Loss of cutaneous TSLP-dependent immune responses skews the balance of inflammation from tumor protective to tumor promoting. *Cancer Cell* (2012) **22**(4):479–93. doi:10.1016/j.ccr.2012.08.016
37. Jiang J, Hui C-C. Hedgehog signaling in development and cancer. *Dev Cell* (2008) **15**(6):801–12. doi:10.1016/j.devcel.2008.11.010
38. Furmanski AL, Saldana JI, Ono M, Sahni H, Paschalidis N, D'Acquisto F, et al. Tissue-derived hedgehog proteins modulate Th differentiation and disease. *J Immunol* (2013) **190**(6):2641–9. doi:10.4049/jimmunol.1202541
39. Kim J, Myers AC, Chen L, Pardoll DM, Truong-Tran Q-A, Lane AP, et al. Constitutive and inducible expression of b7 family of ligands by human airway epithelial cells. *Am J Respir Cell Mol Biol* (2005) **33**(3):280–9. doi:10.1165/rcmb.2004-0129OC
40. Bas A, Swamy M, Abeler-Dörner L, Williams G, Pang DJ, Barbee SD, et al. Butyrophilin-like 1 encodes an enterocyte protein that selectively regulates functional interactions with T lymphocytes. *Proc Natl Acad Sci U S A* (2011) **108**(11):4376–81. doi:10.1073/pnas.1010647108
41. Boyden LM, Lewis JM, Barbee SD, Bas A, Girardi M, Hayday AC, et al. Skint1, the prototype of a newly identified immunoglobulin superfamily gene cluster, positively selects epidermal γδ T cells. *Nat Genet* (2008) **40**(5):656–62. doi:10.1038/ng.108
42. Turchinovich G, Hayday AC. Skint-1 identifies a common molecular mechanism for the development of interferon-γ-secreting versus interleukin-17-secreting γδ T cells. *Immunity* (2011) **35**(1):59–68. doi:10.1016/j.immuni.2011.04.018

43. Rölle A, Mousavi-Jazi M, Eriksson M, Odeberg J, Söderberg-Nauclér C, Cosman D, et al. Effects of human cytomegalovirus infection on ligands for the activating NKG2D receptor of NK cells: up-regulation of UL16-binding protein (ULBP)1 and ULBP2 is counteracted by the viral UL16 protein. *J Immunol* (2003) **171**(2):902–8. doi:10.4049/jimmunol.171.2.902
44. Raulet DH, Gasser S, Gowen BG, Deng W, Jung H. Regulation of ligands for the NKG2D activating receptor. *Annu Rev Immunol* (2013) **31**(1):413–41. doi:10.1146/annurev-immunol-032712-095951
45. Jung H, Hsiung B, Pestal K, Procyk E, Raulet DH. RAE-1 ligands for the NKG2D receptor are regulated by E2F transcription factors, which control cell cycle entry. *J Exp Med* (2012) **209**(13):2409–22. doi:10.1084/jem.20120565
46. Vantourout P, Hayday A. Six-of-the-best: unique contributions of γδ T cells to immunology. *Nat Rev Immunol* (2013) **13**(2):88–100. doi:10.1038/nri3384
47. Cheroutre H, Lambolez F, Mucida D. The light and dark sides of intestinal intraepithelial lymphocytes. *Nat Rev Immunol* (2011) **11**(7):445–56. doi:10.1038/nri3007
48. Gebhardt T, Wakim LM, Eidsmo L, Reading PC, Heath WR, Carbone FR. Memory T cells in nonlymphoid tissue that provide enhanced local immunity during infection with herpes simplex virus. *Nat Immunol* (2009) **10**(5):524–30. doi:10.1038/ni.1718
49. Jiang X, Clark RA, Liu L, Wagers AJ, Fuhlbrigge RC, Kupper TS. Skin infection generates non-migratory memory CD8+ T(RM) cells providing global skin immunity. *Nature* (2012) **483**(7388):227–31. doi:10.1038/nature10851
50. Eyerich S, Eyerich K, Pennino D, Carbone T, Nasorri F, Pallotta S, et al. Th22 cells represent a distinct human T cell subset involved in epidermal immunity and remodeling. *J Clin Invest* (2009) **119**(12):3573–85. doi:10.1172/JCI40202
51. Cella M, Fuchs A, Vermi W, Facchetti F, Otero K, Lennerz JKM, et al. A human natural killer cell subset provides an innate source of IL-22 for mucosal immunity. *Nature* (2008) **457**(7230):722–5. doi:10.1038/nature07537
52. Björkström NK, Kekäläinen E, Mjösberg J. Tissue-specific effector functions of innate lymphoid cells. *Immunology* (2013) **139**(4):416–27. doi:10.1111/imm.12098
53. Strid J, Sobolev O, Zafirova B, Polic B, Hayday A. The intraepithelial T cell response to NKG2D-ligands links lymphoid stress surveillance to atopy. *Science* (2011) **334**(6060):1293–7. doi:10.1126/science.1211250
54. Harris N, Gause WC. To B or not to B: B cells and the Th2-type immune response to helminths. *Trends Immunol* (2011) **32**(2):80–8. doi:10.1016/j.it.2010.11.005
55. Profet M. The function of allergy: immunological defense against toxins. *Q Rev Biol* (1991) **66**(1):23–62. doi:10.1086/417049
56. Marichal T, Starkl P, Reber LL, Kalesnikoff J, Oettgen HC, Tsai M, et al. A beneficial role for immunoglobulin in host defense against honeybee venom. *Immunity* (2013) **39**(5):963–75. doi:10.1016/j.immuni.2013.10.005
57. Palm NW, Rosenstein RK, Yu S, Schenten DD, Florsheim E, Medzhitov R. Bee venom phospholipase A2 induces a primary type 2 response that is dependent on the receptor ST2 and confers protective immunity. *Immunity* (2013) **39**(5):976–85. doi:10.1016/j.immuni.2013.10.006
58. Palm NW, Rosenstein RK, Medzhitov R. Allergic host defences. *Nature* (2012) **484**(7395):465–72. doi:10.1038/nature11047
59. Gutierrez DA, Rodewald H-R. A sting in the tale of Th2 immunity. *Immunity* (2013) **39**(5):803–5. doi:10.1016/j.immuni.2013.10.015
60. Traidl-Hoffmann C, Jakob T, Behrendt H. Determinants of allergenicity. *J Allergy Clin Immunol* (2009) **123**(3):558–66. doi:10.1016/j.jaci.2008.12.003
61. Kool M, Lambrecht BN. Alum adjuvant boosts adaptive immunity by inducing uric acid and activating inflammatory dendritic cells. *J Exp Med* (2008) **205**(4):869–82. doi:10.1084/jem.20071087
62. Fukuyama T, Tajima Y, Ueda H, Hayashi K, Shutoh Y, Saito TR, et al. Investigation of the chemical-induced selective type II (TH2) allergic response in mice: effect of the length of the sensitizing phase. *J Immunotoxicol* (2009) **6**(2):75–83. doi:10.1080/15476910902891319
63. Dearman RJ, Basketter DA, Kimber I. Selective induction of type 2 cytokines following topical exposure of mice to platinum salts. *Food Chem Toxicol* (1998) **36**(3):199–207. doi:10.1016/S0278-6915(97)00143-9
64. Jotwani R, Pulendran B, Agrawal S, Cutler CW. Human dendritic cells respond to *Porphyromonas gingivalis* LPS by promoting a Th2 effector response in vitro. *Eur J Immunol* (2003) **33**(11):2980–6. doi:10.1002/eji.200324392
65. Salgame P, Yap GS, Gause WC. Effect of helminth-induced immunity on infections with microbial pathogens. *Nat Immunol* (2013) **14**(11):1118–26. doi:10.1038/ni.2736
66. Bryson K, Besteiro S, McGachy HA, Coombs GH, Mottram JC, Alexander J. Overexpression of the natural inhibitor of cysteine peptidases in *Leishmania mexicana* leads to reduced virulence and a Th1 response. *Infect Immun* (2009) **77**(7):2971–8. doi:10.1128/IAI.00558-08
67. Kuroda E, Ishii KJ, Uematsu S, Ohata K, Coban C, Akira S, et al. Silica crystals and aluminum salts regulate the production of prostaglandin in macrophages via NALP3 inflammasome-independent mechanisms. *Immunity* (2011) **34**(4):514–26. doi:10.1016/j.immuni.2011.03.019
68. Mishra PK, Wu W, Rozo C, Hallab NJ, Benevenia J, Gause WC. Micrometer-sized titanium particles can induce potent Th2-type responses through TLR4-independent pathways. *J Immunol* (2011) **187**(12):6491–8. doi:10.4049/jimmunol.1101392
69. Kool M, Willart MAM, van Nimwegen M, Bergen I, Pouliot P, Virchow JC, et al. An unexpected role for uric acid as an inducer of T helper 2 cell immunity to inhaled antigens and inflammatory mediator of allergic asthma. *Immunity* (2011) **34**(4):527–40. doi:10.1016/j.immuni.2011.03.015
70. Marichal T, Ohata K, Bedoret D, Mesnil C, Sabatel C, Kobiyama K, et al. DNA released from dying host cells mediates aluminum adjuvant activity. *Nat Med* (2011) **17**(8):996–1002. doi:10.1038/nm.2403
71. Kouzaki H, Iijima K, Kobayashi T, O'Grady SM, Kita H. The danger signal, extracellular ATP, is a sensor for an airborne allergen and triggers IL-33 release and innate Th2-type responses. *J Immunol* (2011) **186**(7):4375–87. doi:10.4049/jimmunol.1003020
72. Tang H, Cao W, Kasturi SP, Ravindran R, Nakaya HI, Kundu K, et al. The T helper type 2 response to cysteine proteases requires dendritic cell-basophil cooperation via ROS-mediated signaling. *Nat Immunol* (2010) **11**(7):608–17. doi:10.1038/ni.1883
73. Moghaddam AE, Gartlan KH, Kong L, Sattentau QJ. Reactive carbonyls are a major Th2-inducing damage-associated molecular pattern generated by oxidative stress. *J Immunol* (2011) **187**(4):1626–33. doi:10.4049/jimmunol.1003906
74. Chavanas S, Bodemer C, Rochat A, Hamel-Teillac D, Ali M, Irvine AD, et al. Mutations in SPINK5, encoding a serine protease inhibitor, cause Netherton syndrome. *Nat Genet* (2000) **25**(2):141–2. doi:10.1038/75977
75. Walley AJ, Chavanas S, Moffatt MF, Esnouf RM, Ubhi B, Lawrence R, et al. Gene polymorphism in Netherton and common atopic disease. *Nat Genet* (2001) **29**(2):175–8. doi:10.1038/ng728
76. Briot A, Deraison C, Lacroix M, Bonnart C, Robin A, Besson C, et al. Kallikrein 5 induces atopic dermatitis-like lesions through PAR2-mediated thymic stromal lymphopoietin expression in Netherton syndrome. *J Exp Med* (2009) **206**(5):1135–47. doi:10.1084/jem.20082242
77. Fritz JH, Le Bourhis L, Sellge G, Magalhaes JG, Fsihi H, Kufer TA, et al. Nod1-mediated innate immune recognition of peptidoglycan contributes to the onset of adaptive immunity. *Immunity* (2007) **26**(4):445–59. doi:10.1016/j.immuni.2007.03.009
78. Magalhaes JG, Fritz JH, Le Bourhis L, Sellge G, Travassos LH, Selvanantham T, et al. Nod2-dependent Th2 polarization of antigen-specific immunity. *J Immunol* (2008) **181**(11):7925–35. doi:10.4049/jimmunol.181.11.7925
79. Magalhaes JG, Rubino SJ, Travassos LH, Le Bourhis L, Duan W, Sellge G, et al. Nucleotide oligomerization domain-containing proteins instruct T cell helper type 2 immunity through stromal activation. *Proc Natl Acad Sci U S A* (2011) **108**(36):14896–901. doi:10.1073/pnas.1015063108
80. Eisenbarth SC, Piggott DA, Huleatt JW, Visintin I, Herrick CA, Bottomly K. Lipopolysaccharide-enhanced, Toll-like receptor 4-dependent T helper cell type 2 responses to inhaled antigen. *J Exp Med* (2002) **196**(12):1645–51. doi:10.1084/jem.20021340
81. Tan AM, Chen HC, Pochard P, Eisenbarth SC, Herrick CA, Bottomly HK. TLR4 signaling in stromal cells is critical for the initiation of allergic Th2 responses to inhaled antigen. *J Immunol* (2010) **184**(7):3535–44. doi:10.4049/jimmunol.0900340
82. Agrawal S, Agrawal A, Doughty B, Gerwitz A, Blenis J, Van Dyke T, et al. Cutting edge: different toll-like receptor agonists instruct dendritic cells to induce distinct Th responses via differential modulation of extracellular signal-regulated kinase-mitogen-activated protein kinase and c-Fos. *J Immunol* (2003) **171**(10):4984–9. doi:10.4049/jimmunol.171.10.4984
83. Hammad H, Chieppa M, Perros F, Willart MA, Germain RN, Lambrecht BN. House dust mite allergen induces asthma via Toll-like receptor 4 triggering of airway structural cells. *Nat Med* (2009) **15**(4):410–6. doi:10.1038/nm.1946

84. Schmidt M, Raghavan B, Müller V, Vogl T, Fejer G, Tchaptchet S, et al. Crucial role for human Toll-like receptor 4 in the development of contact allergy to nickel. *Nat Immunol* (2010) **11**(9):814–9. doi:10.1038/ni.1919
85. Wen L, Roberts SJ, Viney JL, Wong FS, Mallick C, Findly RC, et al. Immunoglobulin synthesis and generalized autoimmunity in mice congenitally deficient in alpha beta(+) T cells. *Nature* (1994) **369**(6482):654–8. doi:10.1038/369654a0
86. Wen L, Pao W, Wong FS, Peng Q, Craft J, Zheng B, et al. Germinal center formation, immunoglobulin class switching, and autoantibody production driven by "non alpha/beta" T cells. *J Exp Med* (1996) **183**(5):2271–82. doi:10.1084/jem.183.5.2271
87. Aguado E, Richelme S, Nuñez-Cruz S, Miazek A, Mura A-M, Richelme M, et al. Induction of T helper type 2 immunity by a point mutation in the LAT adaptor. *Science* (2002) **296**(5575):2036–40. doi:10.1126/science.1069057
88. Qi Q, Xia M, Hu J, Hicks E, Iyer A, Xiong N, et al. Enhanced development of CD4+ gammadelta T cells in the absence of Itk results in elevated IgE production. *Blood* (2009) **114**(3):564–71. doi:10.1182/blood-2008-12-196345
89. Felices M, Yin CC, Kosaka Y, Kang J, Berg LJ. Tec kinase Itk in gamma delta T cells is pivotal for controlling IgE production in vivo. *Proc Natl Acad Sci U S A* (2009) **106**(20):8308–13. doi:10.1073/pnas.0808459106
90. McCoy KD, Harris NL, Diener P, Hatak S, Odermatt B, Hangartner L, et al. Natural IgE production in the absence of MHC class II cognate help. *Immunity* (2006) **24**(3):329–39. doi:10.1016/j.immuni.2006.01.013
91. Ehrlich P. Über den jetzigen Stand der Karzinomforschung. *Ned Tijdschr Geneeskd* (1909) **5**:273–90.
92. Burnet M. Cancer; a biological approach. I. The processes of control. *Br Med J* (1957) **1**(5022):779–86. doi:10.1136/bmj.1.5022.779
93. Burnet M. Cancer: a biological approach. III. Viruses associated with neoplastic conditions. IV. Practical applications. *Br Med J* (1957) **1**(5023):841–7. doi:10.1136/bmj.1.5023.841
94. Thomas L. On immunosurveillance in human cancer. *Yale J Biol Med* (1982) **55**(3–4):329–33.
95. Dunn GP, Old LJ, Schreiber RD. The three Es of cancer immunoediting. *Annu Rev Immunol* (2004) **22**(1):329–60. doi:10.1146/annurev.immunol.22.012703.104803
96. Dighe AS, Richards E, Old LJ, Schreiber RD. Enhanced in vivo growth and resistance to rejection of tumor cells expressing dominant negative IFN gamma receptors. *Immunity* (1994) **1**(6):447–56. doi:10.1016/1074-7613(94)90087-6
97. Kaplan DH, Shankaran V, Dighe AS, Stockert E, Aguet M, Old LJ, et al. Demonstration of an interferon gamma-dependent tumor surveillance system in immunocompetent mice. *Proc Natl Acad Sci U S A* (1998) **95**(13):7556–61. doi:10.1073/pnas.95.13.7556
98. Shankaran V, Ikeda H, Bruce AT, White JM. IFNγ and lymphocytes prevent primary tumour development and shape tumour immunogenicity. *Nature* (2001) **410**(6832):1107–11. doi:10.1038/35074122
99. Smyth MJ, Thia KY, Street SE, Cretney E, Trapani JA, Taniguchi M, et al. Differential tumor surveillance by natural killer (NK) and NKT cells. *J Exp Med* (2000) **191**(4):661–8. doi:10.1084/jem.191.4.661
100. Girardi M, Oppenheim DE, Steele CR, Lewis JM, Glusac E, Filler R, et al. Regulation of cutaneous malignancy by gamma delta T cells. *Science* (2001) **294**(5542):605–9. doi:10.1126/science.1063916
101. DePinho RA. The age of cancer. *Nature* (2000) **408**(6809):248–54. doi:10.1038/35041694
102. Matzinger P. The danger model: a renewed sense of self. *Science* (2002) **296**(5566):301–5. doi:10.1126/science.1071059
103. Chao MP, Majeti R, Weissman IL. Programmed cell removal: a new obstacle in the road to developing cancer. *Nat Rev Cancer* (2012) **12**(1):58–67. doi:10.1038/nrc3171
104. Ma Y, Galluzzi L, Zitvogel L, Kroemer G. Autophagy and cellular immune responses. *Immunity* (2013) **39**(2):211–27. doi:10.1016/j.immuni.2013.07.017
105. Zitvogel L, Kepp O, Galluzzi L, Kroemer G. Inflammasomes in carcinogenesis and anticancer immune responses. *Nat Immunol* (2012) **13**(4):343–51. doi:10.1038/ni.2224
106. Schonthaler HB, Guinea-Viniegra J, Wculek SK, Ruppen I, Ximénez-Embún P, Guío-Carrión A, et al. S100A8-S100A9 protein complex mediates psoriasis by regulating the expression of complement factor C3. *Immunity* (2013) **39**(6):1171–81. doi:10.1016/j.immuni.2013.11.011
107. Ullrich E, Koch J, Cerwenka A, Steinle A. New prospects on the NKG2D/NKG2DL system for oncology. *Oncoimmunology* (2013) **2**(10):e26097. doi:10.4161/onci.26097
108. Cerwenka A, Lanier LL. NKG2D ligands: unconventional MHC class I-like molecules exploited by viruses and cancer. *Tissue Antigens* (2003) **61**(5):335–43. doi:10.1034/j.1399-0039.2003.00070.x
109. Van Belle TL, von Herrath MG. The role of the activating receptor NKG2D in autoimmunity. *Mol Immunol* (2009) **47**(1):8–11. doi:10.1016/j.molimm.2009.02.023
110. Suárez-Alvarez B, López-Vázquez A, Baltar JM, Ortega F, López-Larrea C. Potential role of NKG2D and its ligands in organ transplantation: new target for immunointervention. *Am J Transplant* (2009) **9**(2):251–7. doi:10.1111/j.1600-6143.2008.02526.x
111. Groh V, Wu J, Yee C, Spies T. Tumour-derived soluble MIC ligands impair expression of NKG2D and T-cell activation. *Nature* (2002) **419**(6908):734–8. doi:10.1038/nature01112
112. Lodoen MB, Lanier LL. Viral modulation of NK cell immunity. *Nat Rev Microbiol* (2005) **3**(1):59–69. doi:10.1038/nrmicro1066
113. Champsaur M, Lanier LL. Effect of NKG2D ligand expression on host immune responses. *Immunol Rev* (2010) **235**(1):267–85. doi:10.1111/j.0105-2896.2010.00893.x
114. Strid J, Roberts SJ, Filler RB, Lewis JM, Kwong BY, Schpero W, et al. Acute upregulation of an NKG2D ligand promotes rapid reorganization of a local immune compartment with pleiotropic effects on carcinogenesis. *Nat Immunol* (2008) **9**(2):146–54. doi:10.1038/ni1556
115. Strid J, Tigelaar RE, Hayday AC. Skin immune surveillance by T cells – a new order? *Semin Immunol* (2009) **21**(3):110–20. doi:10.1016/j.smim.2009.03.002
116. Hayday AC. Gammadelta T cells and the lymphoid stress-surveillance response. *Immunity* (2009) **31**(2):184–96. doi:10.1016/j.immuni.2009.08.006
117. Takai Y, Irie K, Shimizu K, Sakisaka T, Ikeda W. Nectins and nectin-like molecules: roles in cell adhesion, migration, and polarization. *Cancer Sci* (2003) **94**(8):655–67. doi:10.1111/j.1349-7006.2003.tb01499.x
118. Giangreco A, Jensen KB, Takai Y, Miyoshi J, Watt FM. Necl2 regulates epidermal adhesion and wound repair. *Development* (2009) **136**(20):3505–14. doi:10.1242/dev.038232
119. Chan CJ, Andrews DM, Smyth MJ. Receptors that interact with nectin and nectin-like proteins in the immunosurveillance and immunotherapy of cancer. *Curr Opin Immunol* (2012) **24**(2):246–51. doi:10.1016/j.coi.2012.01.009
120. Soriani A, Zingoni A, Cerboni C, Iannitto ML, Ricciardi MR, Di Gialleonardo V, et al. ATM-ATR-dependent up-regulation of DNAM-1 and NKG2D ligands on multiple myeloma cells by therapeutic agents results in enhanced NK-cell susceptibility and is associated with a senescent phenotype. *Blood* (2009) **113**(15):3503–11. doi:10.1182/blood-2008-08-173914
121. Shibuya A, Campbell D, Hannum C, Yssel H, Franz-Bacon K, McClanahan T, et al. DNAM-1, a novel adhesion molecule involved in the cytolytic function of T lymphocytes. *Immunity* (1996) **4**(6):573–81. doi:10.1016/S1074-7613(00)70060-4
122. Ramsbottom KM, Hawkins ED, Shimoni R, McGrath M, Chan CJ, Russell SM, et al. Cutting edge: DNAX accessory molecule 1-deficient CD8+ T cells display immunological synapse defects that impair antitumor immunity. *J Immunol* (2014) **192**(2):553–7. doi:10.4049/jimmunol.1302197
123. Takahashi Y, Iwai M, Kawai T, Arakawa A, Ito T, Sakurai-Yageta M, et al. Aberrant expression of tumor suppressors CADM1 and 4.1B in invasive lesions of primary breast cancer. *Breast Cancer* (2012) **19**(3):242–52. doi:10.1007/s12282-011-0272-7
124. Witherden DA, Verdino P, Rieder SE, Garijo O, Mills RE, Teyton L, et al. The junctional adhesion molecule JAML is a costimulatory receptor for epithelial gamma delta T cell activation. *Science* (2010) **329**(5996):1205–10. doi:10.1126/science.1192698
125. Verdino P, Witherden DA, Havran WL, Wilson IA. The molecular interaction of CAR and JAML recruits the central cell signal transducer PI3K. *Science* (2010) **329**(5996):1210–4. doi:10.1126/science.1187996
126. Witherden DA, Watanabe M, Garijo O, Rieder SE, Sarkisyan G, Cronin SJF, et al. The CD100 receptor interacts with its plexin B2 ligand to regulate epidermal γδ T cell function. *Immunity* (2012) **37**(2):314–25. doi:10.1016/j.immuni.2012.05.026
127. Meehan TF, Witherden DA, Kim C-H, Sendaydiego K, Ye I, Garijo O, et al. Protection against colitis by CD100-dependent modulation of intraepithelial γδ T lymphocyte function. *Mucosal Immunol* (2014) **7**(1):134–42. doi:10.1038/mi.2013.32
128. Shi W, Kumanogoh A, Watanabe C, Uchida J, Wang X, Yasui T, et al. The class IV semaphorin CD100 plays nonredundant roles in the immune system:

defective B and T cell activation in CD100-deficient mice. *Immunity* (2000) **13**(5):633–42. doi:10.1016/S1074-7613(00)00063-7

129. Park O, Jeong W-I, Wang L, Wang H, Lian Z-X, Gershwin ME, et al. Diverse roles of invariant natural killer T cells in liver injury and fibrosis induced by carbon tetrachloride. *Hepatology* (2009) **49**(5):1683–94. doi:10.1002/hep.22813
130. Sagiv A, Biran A, Yon M, Simon J, Lowe SW, Krizhanovsky V. Granule exocytosis mediates immune surveillance of senescent cells. *Oncogene* (2013) **32**(15):1971–7. doi:10.1038/onc.2012.206
131. Devey L, Ferenbach D, Mohr E, Sangster K, Bellamy CO, Hughes J, et al. Tissue-resident macrophages protect the liver from ischemia reperfusion injury via a heme oxygenase-1-dependent mechanism. *Mol Ther* (2009) **17**(1):65–72. doi:10.1038/mt.2008.237
132. Girardi M, Lewis J, Glusac E, Filler RB, Geng L, Hayday AC, et al. Resident skin-specific gamma delta T cells provide local, non-redundant regulation of cutaneous inflammation. *J Exp Med* (2002) **195**(7):855–67. doi:10.1084/jem.20012000
133. Girardi M, Lewis JM, Filler RB, Hayday AC, Tigelaar RE. Environmentally responsive and reversible regulation of epidermal barrier function by γδ T cells. *J Invest Dermatol* (2006) **126**(4):808–14. doi:10.1038/sj.jid.5700120
134. Sharp LL, Jameson JM, Cauvi G, Havran WL. Dendritic epidermal T cells regulate skin homeostasis through local production of insulin-like growth factor 1. *Nat Immunol* (2005) **6**(1):73–9. doi:10.1038/ni1152
135. Jameson J, Havran WL. Skin gammadelta T-cell functions in homeostasis and wound healing. *Immunol Rev* (2007) **215**:114–22. doi:10.1111/j.1600-065X.2006.00483.x
136. Jameson J, Ugarte K, Chen N, Yachi P, Fuchs E, Boismenu R, et al. A role for skin gamma delta T cells in wound repair. *Science* (2002) **296**(5568):747–9. doi:10.1126/science.1069639
137. Chen Y, Chou K, Fuchs E, Havran WL, Boismenu R. Protection of the intestinal mucosa by intraepithelial gamma delta T cells. *Proc Natl Acad Sci U S A* (2002) **99**(22):14338–43. doi:10.1073/pnas.212290499
138. Senovilla L, Galluzzi L, Zitvogel L, Kroemer G. Immunosurveillance as a regulator of tissue homeostasis. *Trends Immunol* (2013) **34**(10):471–81. doi:10.1016/j.it.2013.06.005
139. Vesely MD, Kershaw MH, Schreiber RD, Smyth MJ. Natural innate and adaptive immunity to cancer. *Annu Rev Immunol* (2011) **29**(1):235–71. doi:10.1146/annurev-immunol-031210-101324
140. Dunham LJ. Cancer in man at site of prior benign lesion of skin or mucous membrane: a review. *Cancer Res* (1972) **32**(7):1359–74.
141. Walter ND, Rice PL, Redente EF, Kauvar EF, Lemond L, Aly T, et al. Wound healing after trauma may predispose to lung cancer metastasis: review of potential mechanisms. *Am J Respir Cell Mol Biol* (2011) **44**(5):591–6. doi:10.1165/rcmb.2010-0187RT
142. Ortiz-Urda S. Type VII collagen is required for ras-driven human epidermal tumorigenesis. *Science* (2005) **307**(5716):1773–6. doi:10.1126/science.1106209
143. South AP, O'Toole EA. Understanding the pathogenesis of recessive dystrophic epidermolysis bullosa squamous cell carcinoma. *Dermatol Clin* (2010) **28**(1):171–8. doi:10.1016/j.det.2009.10.023
144. Dvorak HF. Tumors: wounds that do not heal. Similarities between tumor stroma generation and wound healing. *N Engl J Med* (1986) **315**(26):1650–9. doi:10.1056/NEJM198612253152606
145. Coussens LM, Zitvogel L, Palucka AK. Neutralizing tumor-promoting chronic inflammation: a magic bullet? *Science* (2013) **339**(6117):286–91. doi:10.1126/science.1232227
146. Balkwill F, Mantovani A. Inflammation and cancer: back to Virchow? *Lancet* (2001) **357**(9255):539–45. doi:10.1016/S0140-6736(00)04046-0
147. Farhadi N, Lambert L, Triulzi C, Openshaw PJ, Guerra N. Natural killer cell NKG2D and granzyme B are critical for allergic pulmonary inflammation. *J Allergy Clin Immunol* (2014) **133**(3):827–35. doi:10.1016/j.jaci.2013.09.048
148. Oh M-H, Oh SY, Yu J, Myers AC, Leonard WJ, Liu YJ, et al. IL-13 induces skin fibrosis in atopic dermatitis by thymic stromal lymphopoietin. *J Immunol* (2011) **186**(12):7232–42. doi:10.4049/jimmunol.1100504
149. Wilson SR, Thé L, Batia LM, Beattie K, Katibah GE, McClain SP, et al. The epithelial cell-derived atopic dermatitis cytokine TSLP activates neurons to induce itch. *Cell* (2013) **155**(2):285–95. doi:10.1016/j.cell.2013.08.057
150. Metz M, Piliponsky AM, Chen CC, Lammel V, Abrink M, Pejler G, et al. Mast cells can enhance resistance to snake and honeybee venoms. *Science* (2006) **313**(5786):526–30. doi:10.1126/science.1128877
151. Schneider LA, Schlenner SM, Feyerabend TB, Wunderlin M, Rodewald H-R. Molecular mechanism of mast cell mediated innate defense against endothelin and snake venom sarafotoxin. *J Exp Med* (2007) **204**(11):2629–39. doi:10.1084/jem.20071262
152. Matsuda H, Watanabe N, Kiso Y, Hirota S, Ushio H, Kannan Y, et al. Necessity of IgE antibodies and mast cells for manifestation of resistance against larval *Haemaphysalis longicornis* ticks in mice. *J Immunol* (1990) **144**(1):259–62.
153. Pearce EJ, Cheever A, Leonard S, Covalesky M, Fernandez-Botran R, Kohler G, et al. *Schistosoma mansoni* in IL-4-deficient mice. *Int Immunol* (1996) **8**(4):435–44. doi:10.1093/intimm/8.4.435
154. Gause WC, Wynn TA, Allen JE. Type 2 immunity and wound healing: evolutionary refinement of adaptive immunity by helminths. *Nat Rev Immunol* (2013) **13**(8):607–14. doi:10.1038/nri3476
155. Monticelli LA, Sonnenberg GF, Abt MC, Alenghat T, Ziegler CGK, Doering TA, et al. Innate lymphoid cells promote lung-tissue homeostasis after infection with influenza virus. *Nat Immunol* (2011) **12**(11):1045–54. doi:10.1031/ni.2131
156. Rosenberg HF, Dyer KD, Foster PS. Eosinophils: changing perspectives in health and disease. *Nat Rev Immunol* (2013) **13**(1):9–22. doi:10.1038/nri3341
157. Okumura S, Sagara H, Fukuda T, Saito H, Okayama Y. FcεRI-mediated amphiregulin production by human mast cells increases mucin gene expression in epithelial cells. *J Allergy Clin Immunol* (2005) **115**(2):272–9. doi:10.1016/j.jaci.2004.12.835
158. Arwert EN, Hoste E, Watt FM. Epithelial stem cells, wound healing and cancer. *Nat Rev Cancer* (2012) **12**(3):170–80. doi:10.1038/nrc3217
159. Conticello C, Pedini F, Zeuner A, Patti M, Zerilli M, Stassi G, et al. IL-4 protects tumor cells from anti-CD95 and chemotherapeutic agents via up-regulation of antiapoptotic proteins. *J Immunol* (2004) **172**(9):5467–77. doi:10.4049/jimmunol.172.9.5467
160. Golumbek PT, Lazenby AJ, Levitsky HI, Jaffee LM, Karasuyama H, Baker M, et al. Treatment of established renal cancer by tumor cells engineered to secrete interleukin-4. *Science* (1991) **254**(5032):713–6. doi:10.1126/science.1948050
161. Hock H, Dorsch M, Kunzendorf U, Qin Z, Diamantstein T, Blankenstein T. Mechanisms of rejection induced by tumor cell-targeted gene transfer of interleukin 2, interleukin 4, interleukin 7, tumor necrosis factor, or interferon gamma. *Proc Natl Acad Sci U S A* (1993) **90**(7):2774–8. doi:10.1073/pnas.90.7.2774
162. Pericle F, Giovarelli M, Colombo MP, Ferrari G, Musiani P, Modesti A, et al. An efficient Th2-type memory follows CD8+ lymphocyte-driven and eosinophil-mediated rejection of a spontaneous mouse mammary adenocarcinoma engineered to release IL-4. *J Immunol* (1994) **153**(12):5659–73.
163. Rodolfo M, Zilocchi C, Accornero P, Cappetti B, Arioli I, Colombo MP. IL-4-transduced tumor cell vaccine induces immunoregulatory type 2 CD8 T lymphocytes that cure lung metastases upon adoptive transfer. *J Immunol* (1999) **163**(4):1923–8.
164. Ellyard JI, Simson L, Parish CR. Th2-mediated anti-tumour immunity: friend or foe? *Tissue Antigens* (2007) **70**(1):1–11. doi:10.1111/j.1399-0039.2007.00869.x
165. Chen S-F, Nieh S, Jao S-W, Wu M-Z, Liu C-L, Chang Y-C, et al. The paracrine effect of cancer-associated fibroblast-induced interleukin-33 regulates the invasiveness of head and neck squamous cell carcinoma. *J Pathol* (2013) **231**(2):180–9. doi:10.1002/path.4226
166. Pedroza-Gonzalez A, Xu K, Wu T-C, Aspord C, Tindle S, Marches F, et al. Thymic stromal lymphopoietin fosters human breast tumor growth by promoting type 2 inflammation. *J Exp Med* (2011) **208**(3):479–90. doi:10.1084/jem.20102131
167. Hallett MA, Venmar KT, Fingleton B. Cytokine stimulation of epithelial cancer cells: the similar and divergent functions of IL-4 and IL-13. *Cancer Res* (2012) **72**(24):6338–43. doi:10.1158/0008-5472.CAN-12-3544
168. Renard N, Duvert V, Banchereau J, Saeland S. Interleukin-13 inhibits the proliferation of normal and leukemic human B-cell precursors. *Blood* (1994) **84**(7):2253–60.
169. Blais Y, Gingras S, Haagensen DE, Labrie F, Simard J. Interleukin-4 and interleukin-13 inhibit estrogen-induced breast cancer cell proliferation and stimulate GCDFP-15 expression in human breast cancer cells. *Mol Cell Endocrinol* (1996) **121**(1):11–8. doi:10.1016/0303-7207(96)03843-9

170. Obiri NI, Husain SR, Debinski W, Puri RK. Interleukin 13 inhibits growth of human renal cell carcinoma cells independently of the p140 interleukin 4 receptor chain. *Clin Cancer Res* (1996) **2**(10):1743–9.

171. Fujisawa T, Joshi BH, Puri RK. IL-13 regulates cancer invasion and metastasis through IL-13Rα2 via ERK/AP-1 pathway in mouse model of human ovarian cancer. *Int J Cancer* (2012) **131**(2):344–56. doi:10.1002/ijc.26366

172. Simson L, Ellyard JI, Dent LA, Matthaei KI, Rothenberg ME, Foster PS, et al. Regulation of carcinogenesis by IL-5 and CCL11: a potential role for eosinophils in tumor immune surveillance. *J Immunol* (2007) **178**(7):4222–9. doi:10.4049/jimmunol.178.7.4222

173. Dalton DK, Noelle RJ. The roles of mast cells in anticancer immunity. *Cancer Immunol Immunother* (2012) **61**(9):1511–20. doi:10.1007/s00262-012-1246-0

174. Vernersson M, Aveskogh M, Hellman L. Cloning of IgE from the echidna (*Tachyglossus aculeatus*) and a comparative analysis of epsilon chains from all three extant mammalian lineages. *Dev Comp Immunol* (2004) **28**(1):61–75. doi:10.1016/S0145-305X(03)00084-3

175. Jensen-Jarolim E, Achatz G, Turner MC, Karagiannis S, Legrand F, Capron M, et al. AllergoOncology: the role of IgE-mediated allergy in cancer. *Allergy* (2008) **63**(10):1255–66. doi:10.1111/j.1398-9995.2008.01768.x

176. Reali E, Greiner JW, Corti A, Gould HJ, Bottazzoli F, Paganelli G, et al. IgEs targeted on tumor cells: therapeutic activity and potential in the design of tumor vaccines. *Cancer Res* (2001) **61**(14):5517–22.

177. Karagiannis P, Gilbert AE, Josephs DH, Ali N, Dodev T, Saul L, et al. IgG4 subclass antibodies impair antitumor immunity in melanoma. *J Clin Invest* (2013) **123**(4):1457–74. doi:10.1172/JCI65579

178. Olver S, Groves P, Buttigieg K, Morris ES, Janas ML, Kelso A, et al. Tumor-derived interleukin-4 reduces tumor clearance and deviates the cytokine and granzyme profile of tumor-induced CD8+ T cells. *Cancer Res* (2006) **66**(1):571–80. doi:10.1158/0008-5472.CAN-05-1362

179. Lebel-Binay S, Laguerre B, Quintin-Colonna F, Conjeaud H, Magazin M, Miloux B, et al. Experimental gene therapy of cancer using tumor cells engineered to secrete interleukin-13. *Eur J Immunol* (1995) **25**(8):2340–8. doi:10.1002/eji.1830250833

180. Skinnider BF, Elia AJ, Gascoyne RD, Patterson B, Trumper L, Kapp U, et al. Signal transducer and activator of transcription 6 is frequently activated in Hodgkin and Reed-Sternberg cells of Hodgkin lymphoma. *Blood* (2002) **99**(2):618–26. doi:10.1182/blood.V99.2.618

181. Jovanovic I, Radosavljevic G, Mitrovic M, Juranic VL, McKenzie ANJ, Arsenijevic N, et al. ST2 deletion enhances innate and acquired immunity to murine mammary carcinoma. *Eur J Immunol* (2011) **41**(7):1902–12. doi:10.1002/eji.201141417

182. Jovanovic IP, Pejnovic NN, Radosavljevic GD, Pantic JM, Milovanovic MZ, Arsenijevic NN, et al. Interleukin-33/ST2 axis promotes breast cancer growth and metastases by facilitating intratumoral accumulation of immunosuppressive and innate lymphoid cells. *Int J Cancer* (2013) **134**(7):1669–82. doi:10.1002/ijc.28481

183. Villarreal D, Wise MC, Walters JN, Reuschel E, Choi MJ, Obeng-Adjei N, et al. Alarmin IL-33 acts as an immunoadjuvant to enhance antigen-specific tumor immunity. *Cancer Res* (2014) **74**(6):1–12. doi:10.1158/0008-5472.CAN-13-2729

184. Nigro EA, Brini AT, Soprana E, Ambrosi A, Dombrowicz D, Siccardi AG, et al. Antitumor IgE adjuvanticity: key role of Fc RI. *J Immunol* (2009) **183**(7):4530–6. doi:10.4049/jimmunol.0900842

185. McWhorter WP. Allergy and risk of cancer. A prospective study using NHANESI follow up data. *Cancer* (1988) **62**(2):451–5. doi:10.1002/1097-0142(19880715)62:2<451::AID-CNCR2820620234>3.0.CO;2-D

186. Josephs DH, Spicer JF, Corrigan CJ, Gould HJ, Karagiannis SN. Epidemiological associations of allergy, IgE and cancer. *Clin Exp Allergy* (2013) **43**(10):1110–23. doi:10.1111/cea.12178

187. Sherman PW, Holland E, Sherman JS. Allergies: their role in cancer prevention. *Q Rev Biol* (2008) **83**(4):339–62. doi:10.1086/592850

188. Rittmeyer D, Lorentz A. Relationship between allergy and cancer: an overview. *Int Arch Allergy Immunol* (2012) **159**(3):216–25. doi:10.1159/000338994

189. Engkilde K, Thyssen JP, Menné T, Johansen JD. Association between cancer and contact allergy: a linkage study. *BMJ Open* (2011) **1**(1):e000084. doi:10.1136/bmjopen-2011-000084

190. Van Hemelrijck M, Garmo H, Binda E, Hayday A, Karagiannis SN, Hammar N, et al. Immunoglobulin E and cancer: a meta-analysis and a large Swedish cohort study. *Cancer Causes Control* (2010) **21**(10):1657–67. doi:10.1007/s10552-010-9594-6

191. Lindelof B, Granath F, Tengvall-Linder M, Ekbom A. Allergy and cancer. *Allergy* (2005) **60**(9):1116–20. doi:10.1111/j.1398-9995.2005.00808.x

11

Receptor pre-clustering and T cell responses: insights into molecular mechanisms

Mario Castro[1]*, Hisse M. van Santen[2]*, María Férez[2], Balbino Alarcón[2], Grant Lythe[3] and Carmen Molina-París[3]

[1] Grupo de Dinámica No-Lineal and Grupo Interdisciplinar de Sistemas Complejos (GISC), Escuela Técnica Superior de Ingeniería (ICAI), Universidad Pontificia Comillas, Madrid, Spain
[2] Departamento de Biología Celular e Inmunología, Centro de Biología Molecular Severo Ochoa, Consejo Superior de Investigaciones Científicas, Universidad Autónoma de Madrid, Madrid, Spain
[3] Department of Applied Mathematics, School of Mathematics, University of Leeds, Leeds, UK

Edited by:
Rob J. De Boer, Utrecht University, Netherlands

Reviewed by:
Daniel Coombs, University of British Columbia, Canada
Barbara Szomolay, University of Warwick, UK

***Correspondence:**
Mario Castro, Universidad Pontificia Comillas, C/ Alberto Aguilera 25, Madrid E28015, Spain
e-mail: marioc@upcomillas.es;
Hisse M. van Santen, Centro Biología Molecular Severo Ochoa, Calle Nicolás Cabrera 1, Campus de Cantoblanco, Madrid 28049, Spain
e-mail: hvansanten@cbm.csic.es

T cell activation, initiated by T cell receptor (TCR) mediated recognition of pathogen-derived peptides presented by major histocompatibility complex class I or II molecules (pMHC), shows exquisite specificity and sensitivity, even though the TCR–pMHC binding interaction is of low affinity. Recent experimental work suggests that TCR pre-clustering may be a mechanism via which T cells can achieve such high sensitivity. The unresolved stoichiometry of the TCR makes TCR–pMHC binding and TCR triggering, an open question. We formulate a mathematical model to characterize the pre-clustering of T cell receptors (TCRs) on the surface of T cells, motivated by the experimentally observed distribution of TCR clusters on the surface of naive and memory T cells. We extend a recently introduced stochastic criterion to compute the timescales of T cell responses, assuming that ligand-induced cross-linked TCR is the minimum signaling unit. We derive an approximate formula for the mean time to signal initiation. Our results show that pre-clustering reduces the mean activation time. However, additional mechanisms favoring the existence of clusters are required to explain the difference between naive and memory T cell responses. We discuss the biological implications of our results, and both the compatibility and complementarity of our approach with other existing mathematical models.

Keywords: T cell receptor, clustering, stochastic dynamics, signaling, naive T cells, memory T cells

1. INTRODUCTION

A hallmark of the adaptive immune system is the ability of T cells, making use of the T cell receptors (TCRs) on their surface, to recognize a given agonist peptide–MHC ligand complex (pMHC) with high sensitivity (1). Some aspects of TCR–pMHC molecular interactions that are of current research interest are the frequency of encounters between T cells and the agonist pMHC, how cell–cell interactions determine the activation of lymphocytes (2), how early interactions change the state of the T cell receptor (3), what are the mechanisms of modulation of receptor–ligand interactions at cell–cell interfaces (4), and how protein organization in the cell membrane (for instance, protein islands or lipid rafts) affects the recognition process (5). Some recent experiments have explored the role of dimensionality on T cell activation and have highlighted the significance of the events taking place at the receptor level [see Refs. (1) and (6) for comprehensive reviews].

These open questions have been addressed with the use of mathematical modeling. Different theories can be classified according to the level of description (7). At the individual TCR–pMHC bond level, the kinetic proof-reading model (8) assumes that the TCR needs to undergo a series of consecutive (phosphorylation) steps before being triggered. Also at the TCR level, the optimal dwell time model (9) reconciles the concurrence of different timescales, providing an *optimal* timescale between the very short times related to the off rate of TCR–pMHC binding, and the long times related to kinetic proof-reading mechanisms. The TCR occupancy model (10) considers the cell as a *counting device* in which multiple TCR–pMHC interactions are required to activate a T cell. In a similar fashion, the serial triggering model (11) proposed that the same pMHC can engage *serially* different TCRs. This model enriches the viewpoint of the TCR occupancy model, by giving greater relevance to the role of the pMHC itself. Finally, the serial encounter model (12) and the confinement time model (13) combine several of the ideas above and provide some appealing explanations by relaxing some restrictions in those models.

While antigen presenting cells (APCs), such as dendritic cells or B cells, present 10^3–10^4 times more self-pMHC than antigenic pMHC, self-pMHC ligands by themselves do not usually elicit a T cell response, even though their affinity for TCR$\alpha\beta$ is only 10 times lower than the affinity of the antigenic pMHC (14). This illustrates how a small difference in affinity results in high specificity, when there is only a few antigenic pMHC molecules in a background of self-pMHC ligands (15).

The T cell signaling process begins with (extracellular) TCR–pMHC binding, followed by phosphorylation of the intracellular ITAM domains of the TCR–CD3 complex. When a TCR binds a pMHC molecule, the TCR$\alpha\beta$ hetero-dimer binds the peptide, while the CD4 or CD8 co-receptor binds the MHC molecule. The binding of the co-receptor activates the tyrosine kinase Lck, which phosphorylates the ITAMs of the CD3 complex. ITAM phosphorylation allows recruitment of intracellular signaling components that mediate downstream signaling events (16).

It has recently been suggested that, contrary to what happens in TCR micro-clusters and the immunological synapse, clustering is not only induced by the ligand but by an *avidity maturation* mechanism (or pre-clustering) (17), allowing the aggregation of chains of TCRs as long as 20 units (around 200 nm long), and referred to as *nano-clusters* (3, 18). Specifically, multimeric TCR–CD3 complexes are activated at low agonistic pMHC concentrations and monomeric TCRs remain unaffected at low ligand concentration. The TCR nano-clusters could enhance T cell sensitivity by the mechanisms proposed in the models of T cell activation (7), as their existence would reduce the time needed for two (or more) receptors to aggregate (by diffusion). This pre-cluster formation could be explained by three different mechanisms (3):

- Multimeric complexes (or clusters) enhance the TCR *avidity* toward the ligand, which is expressed in clusters on the surface of APCs (19–21). At low ligand concentration, only multimeric TCR clusters are bound to ligand, as TCR monomers require higher ligand concentration. Monomeric TCRs might only be activated at high agonist doses.
- Multimeric complexes allow the propagation of the activation signal from ligand-bound TCR$\alpha\beta$ to neighboring receptors in the same TCR *multimer.*
- Linear arrays of multimeric TCR complexes help a single pMHC serially trigger several receptors (11).

The existence of these nano-clusters does not exclude additional mechanisms of T cell activation, as long as they involve the *cooperation* of receptors when they aggregate. Thus, while models such as kinetic proof-reading [and improvements as described in Ref. (22)] operate at the level of a single receptor, other models might be used in combination with the fact that the pre-cluster distribution of naive and memory T cells is different.

Additionally, the fact that the TCR stoichiometry has not been resolved under physiological conditions, yet, makes it even more difficult to understand, at a molecular level, the dynamics of TCR pre-clustering (23). TCR pre-clustering could be an example of a more general mechanism of membrane-bound molecular pre-clustering, as clustering prior to cell–cell interaction has also been observed on the surface of APCs (19–21). It is worth mentioning that monomeric TCRs can still be activated at increasing ligand concentrations, thus, conferring the T cell with a capacity to generate a dose-dependent response at very high pMHC doses, when multimeric TCR–CD3 complexes are already saturated (18). Such mechanisms have been previously described for chemotactic bacteria, as a cellular mechanism to control sensitivity (24).

Various mechanisms have already been suggested, at the population, cellular or molecular level, to explain the capacity of T cells to respond, faster and more strongly, to a second antigenic encounter. However, the underlying mechanisms of the observed changes in the sensitivity of the T cell for pMHC ligand-mediated TCR stimulation (25) have not yet been clearly elucidated. Interestingly, the distribution of clusters in naive and memory T cells is different: memory T cells accommodate larger linear TCR clusters than naive ones. This could explain why memory T cells elicit more rapid responses than naive T cells (17) (see **Figure 1** below).

In this paper, we explore the consequences of TCR pre-clustering in signaling and in distinguishing naive from memory T cell responses. We present some experimentally obtained distributions of TCR clusters for both types of cells (see **Figure 1**), and two complementary theoretical models: (i) a simple model of receptor oligomerization that describes cluster size distributions, and (ii) a generalization of the stochastic T cell response criterion of Ref. (26), to accommodate the hypothesis that the minimum signaling unit is composed of a TCR receptor cluster that is bound by the same cross-linked multivalent ligand. We find that this signaling unit is able to discriminate between agonist and antagonist pMHC ligands (with greater sensitivity than in the monomeric case), and to explain some of the advantages that higher cluster sizes can provide to memory T cells. The model also points at the need to invoke additional cooperativity mechanisms, to explain the experimentally observed role of clustering in T cell responses (27). Finally, this model of ligand-induced TCR cross-linking can be relevant in physiological conditions, according to the defective ribosomal products (DRiP) hypothesis (28, 29), which provides a rapid source of peptide precursors to optimize immuno-surveillance of pathogens and tumors (30).

2. MATHEMATICAL MODELING OF TCR PRE-CLUSTERING AND T CELL ACTIVATION

2.1. MODEL 1: T CELL RECEPTOR PRE-CLUSTERING

The TCR–CD3 complex consists of the pMHC binding TCR$\alpha\beta$ hetero-dimer, associated with the hetero-dimers CD3$\gamma\epsilon$ and CD3$\delta\epsilon$, and the homo-dimer CD3$\zeta\zeta$. Binding of a stimulating pMHC ligand by the extracellular domain of TCR$\alpha\beta$ results in conformational changes in the intracellular part of the CD3ϵ chain, and phosphorylation of the immuno-receptor tyrosine-based activation motifs (ITAMs) in the intracellular domains of the CD3$\gamma\epsilon$, CD3$\delta\epsilon$, and CD3$\zeta\zeta$ dimers, which in turn lead to initiation of downstream signaling cascades and T cell activation.

It has long been recognized that the TCR–CD3 complex forms clusters upon ligand binding (31–36). More recently, it has been shown that in the absence of stimulating pMHC ligand, TCR–CD3 complexes are already expressed at the cell surface as a combination of monomeric and oligomeric TCR complexes or TCR nano-clusters (18). Electron microscopy (EM) analysis of immuno-gold-labeled human and murine T cells showed that these nano-clusters consist of up to 20 TCR–CD3 complexes. The exact stoichiometry of the nano-clusters has not been resolved yet.

The integrity of TCR nano-clusters depends on cholesterol present at the cell surface membrane (18). The formation of the clusters depends, at least, on the trans-membrane region of the CD3$\zeta\zeta$ homo-dimer (17), perhaps due to the capacity of $\zeta\zeta$ dimers to form dimers of dimers (37). Other possible mechanisms of cluster formation rely on the capacity of the extracellular domain of TCRα to dimerize (38).

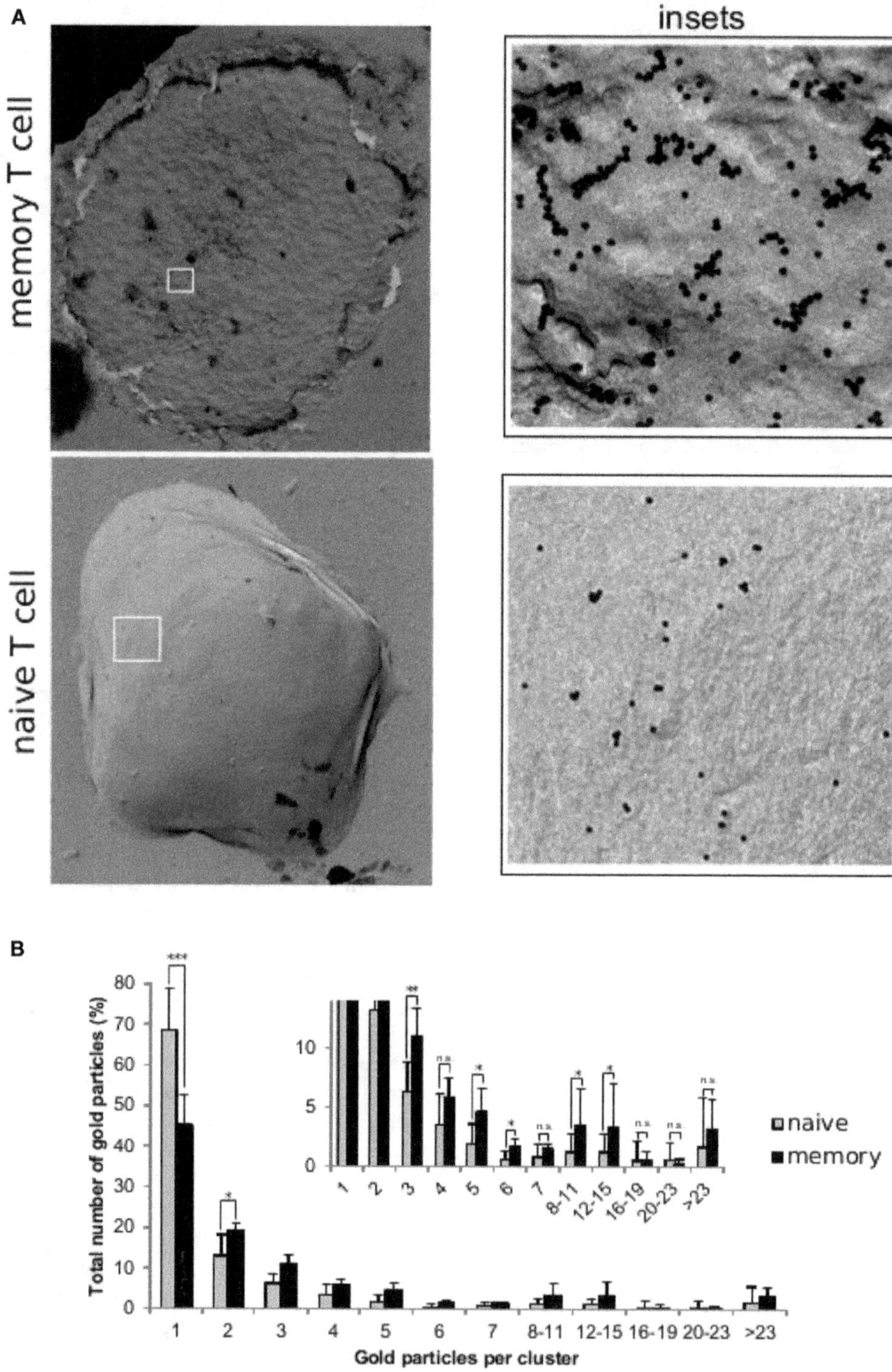

FIGURE 1 | Distribution of TCRs at the surface of naive and memory T cells. Resting naive and memory $CD8^+$ OT-1 T cells were labeled with the CD3ϵ-specific mAb 2C11 and 10 nm gold-conjugated protein-A. Cell surface replicas of the labeled T cells were analyzed by transmission electron microscopy and the number and size of the observed gold clusters were recorded. **(A)** TEM image of surface replicas of a memory and a naive OT-1 T cell. The insets to the right show an enlargement of the boxed areas. **(B)** Quantification (mean ± SD) of gold particles in clusters of the indicated sizes for resting naive T cells (gray bars, 7 cells, 9190 particles) and memory T cells (black bars, 5 cells, 3001 particles). The inset shows a detailed view of the distribution of clusters of three or more gold particles and statistical analysis (2-tailed Student's *t*-test: $^*p < 0.05$, $^{**}p < 0.01$, and $^{***}p < 0.001$). All naive and memory T cells had clusters with gold. However, whereas in naive T cells the maximum gold cluster size shared by all cells was four, this was eight for memory T cells. Also clusters bigger than twenty three particles were present in four out of five memory T cells, and only two out of seven naive T cells.

This body of experimental evidence allows us to conclude that multimeric TCR–CD3 complexes are co-expressed with TCR monomers on the surface of resting T cells.

A simple model of aggregation of TCR$\alpha\beta$ units is depicted in the left panel of **Figure 2**. Given a chain of length n (with n heterodimers linked), in a small time interval Δt, with probability $q_+ \Delta t$, the chain increases to length $n+1$, and with probability $q_- \Delta t$, the chain decreases to length $n-1$. Thus, by probability conservation, the probability to remain the same length n is $1-(q_+ + q_-)\Delta t$.

Mathematically, the dynamics of the process can be described by a continuous time Markov chain (39) (or birth and death process, as we assume that polymerization takes place in unit steps). The state space is $\{1, 2, 3, \ldots, n-1, n, n+1, \ldots\}$, where the number denotes the number of TCRs in a cluster:

$$1 \underset{q_+}{\overset{q_-}{\leftrightharpoons}} 2 \underset{q_+}{\overset{q_-}{\leftrightharpoons}} 3 \underset{q_+}{\overset{q_-}{\leftrightharpoons}} \cdots \underset{q_+}{\overset{q_-}{\leftrightharpoons}} n-1 \underset{q_+}{\overset{q_-}{\leftrightharpoons}} n \underset{q_+}{\overset{q_-}{\leftrightharpoons}} n+1 \cdots .$$

The forward Kolmogorov equations for the probability of having a cluster of size n are given by (40)

$$\frac{dp_n(t)}{dt} = q_+ p_{n-1}(t) + q_- p_{n+1}(t) - (q_+ + q_-)p_n(t)\,, \ \forall n \geq 2,$$
$$\frac{dp_1(t)}{dt} = q_- p_{2(t)} - q_+ p_1(t).$$

The stationary probability distribution is then given by

$$\lim_{t\to+\infty} p_n(t) \equiv \pi_n = \frac{b^{n-1}(1-b)}{(1-b^{N_{\max}})}\,,$$
$$b<1\,, \quad n \in \{1,2,3,\ldots,N_{\max}\}\,, \tag{1}$$

with $b = \frac{q_+}{q_-}$, and π_n the probability (in thermodynamic equilibrium) to have a cluster of size n. When $b<1$ (the number of clusters with a given size, n, decreases as n increases), and taking into account that peripheral T cells have around $N_{\max} \simeq 3 \times 10^4$ receptors, the latter expression can be further simplified to

$$\pi_n = b^{n-1}(1-b)\,, \quad b<1\,, \quad n \in \{1,2,3,\ldots\}\,. \tag{2}$$

2.2. MODEL 2: A BIVALENT MODEL FOR T CELL ACTIVATION

The TCR–pMHC binding model introduced in Ref. (26) considered monovalent pMHC ligands binding to TCR monomers on the surface of a T cell. Monovalent ligands have been reported to elicit a T cell response (41–43), but only when they are immobilized on a surface (which makes it difficult to assess whether they are truly monovalent or not). Yet, multivalent receptor–ligand interactions are required to elicit T cell responses in both CD4$^+$ and CD8$^+$ T cells. In what follows, and supported by a body of experimental work (3, 24, 44), we adopt the hypothesis that the minimum activating unit is a TCR–pMHC cross-linked dimeric complex (31, 45–47). We make use of the binding model (Model 2) with pMHC dimers (ligands) and dimeric TCRs (receptors), described in the right panel of **Figure 2**.

Gold-labeling experiments support the existence of nano-clusters with more than two TCRs, yet it can be shown (see Section 5.2) that the key parameter of the mathematical model is the fraction of monomeric to multimeric TCR clusters. Thus, without loss of generality, we will assume that all TCR clusters are dimeric.

The biochemical reactions encoded by the right panel of **Figure 2** are as follows:

- A (bivalent) ligand can bind a free receptor with monomeric binding reaction rates (k_{on} and k_{off}). Although not shown in the figure, we allow for a second ligand to bind the free receptor of the cluster. However, at low concentrations of ligands, this reaction can be safely neglected.
- Cross-linking of a singly bound ligand follows with rates k_2 (forward reaction) and k_{-2} (backward reaction).
- If the complex formed by the ligand cross-linked to the dimeric TCR cluster lasts at least a time τ, *dwell time*, we count that event. When we reach N such events, we will assume that a T cell response is initiated. The rationale behind this T cell response criterion follows the work of Palmer et al. (48), where the concepts of minimum dwell time and productive binding were introduced. This model combines aspects of the kinetic proof-reading (8) and the serial triggering models (7, 11). The

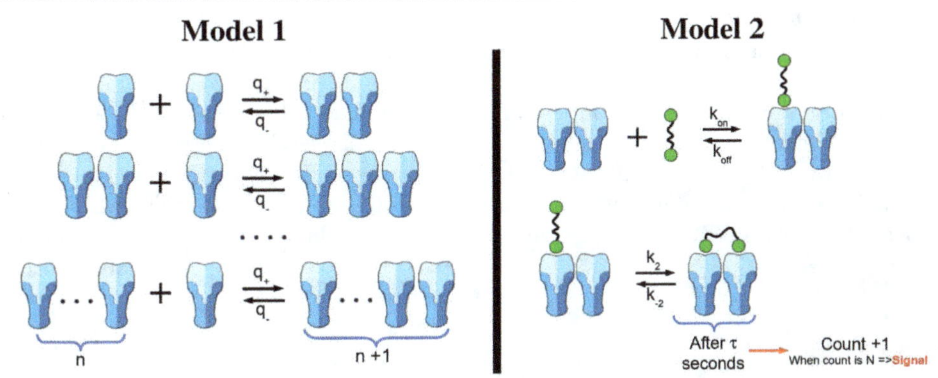

FIGURE 2 | Oligomerization and signaling models. Left panel: oligomerization model not mediated by ligand (Model 1). We assume that receptors are able to diffuse and aggregate to an existing cluster. However, we exclude the possibility of clusters with size larger than one to diffuse. Clusters grow one monomeric unit at a time. Right panel: reactions included in the stochastic activation model (Model 2). Ligands in solution are able to attach monovalently to any receptor in a cluster (top reaction). In addition, ligand-induced TCR cross-linking can occur once a ligand is bound to a TCR in a given nano-cluster (bottom reaction). Following Ref. (26), once the bivalently bound ligand has been attached for a time τ, we count that state as a signaling unit. After N of these units have been generated, the cell becomes activated.

minimum dwell time for a TCR–pMHC complex is the time the complex must remain bound in order to reach a level of ITAM phosphorylation, which will allow TCR triggering. Any binding, which persists for longer than the minimum dwell time is classified as a productive binding [see Refs. (48) and (26) for further details].

- From an immunological perspective, the relevant parameter is the *mean time to signal initiation*, or MTSI (26). Namely, the MTSI is the average time needed for a T cell response according to the criterion that at least N TCR dimers should be bivalently engaged to a bivalent ligand (pMHC) for at least a time τ.

Here we assume that N is around 10–100. That is, 10–100 TCRs are required for signaling and $N_B = b \times N_R$ is of the order of 10^4, with N_B the total number of clusters on the T cell surface. This means, under the assumptions of Model 2, that at most, there can be $N = 100$ internalization events, as this is the number of triggered TCRs. Thus, in this approximation, the loss of TCR due to internalization after triggering can be safely neglected. Nevertheless, internalization is an important step in early signaling, and a proper mechanistic model to justify the value of τ will require internalization to be considered. This analysis is out of the scope of this article.

We implement these reactions as a Markov process, and solve them numerically using the standard Gillespie algorithm (49), and with the parameters summarized in **Table 1**. We have made use of three different ligands: 4A, 4P, and 4N, which were also used in Ref. (26). For these ligands, that bind the same TCR with different affinities, a simple estimation of the number of cross-linking events required to elicit a T cell response is summarized in **Table 2**.

There is some evidence that, under physiological conditions, the chance of two specific peptides being presented by two MHC molecules in sufficient proximity and long enough to act as a dimer is very small (46). This will make ligand-induced TCR cross-linking a rare event. However, some recent experimental work on the distribution of cognate pMHC molecules on the surface of APCs shows that both for MHC class I (virus infection models), and for MHC class II (antigen uptake via the endocytic route) clusters of cognate pMHC can be detected (19–21).

We also note that ligand concentration is not the only factor that depends on physiological conditions. According to the DRiP hypothesis (28, 29), rapid viral antigen presentation is possible because antigenic peptides originate from defective ribosomal products that have short half-lives. Although this phenomenon affects the time between viral challenge and antigen presentation, we assume it is independent of the subsequent signaling dynamics of T cell activation.

Table 1 | Summary of the parameters used in the stochastic simulations.

Parameter	Value	Comment
N_A	6.023×10^{23}	Avogadro's number
N_R	30,000	Average number of TCRs per T cell (34)
V	50 μl	Volume of the experiment
N_C	10^5 cells	Number of T cells in the experiment
V_C	V/N_C	Average extracellular volume per cell
k_{-2}	k_{off}	Cross-linking off rate
k_2	$k_{off}(k_d/k_d^{dimer})$	Cross-linking rate[a]
N	10	Minimum number of bound dimer-bivalent clusters to elicit a T cell response
τ	1–4 s	Dwell time

For typical values of the dissociation rate, k_d, we find that k_2 is about 10–50 times k_{off}. We have assumed $k_{-2} = k_{off}$ following Ref. (44). When not explicitly shown, we have used the same parameters as in Ref. (26).

[a]The cross-linking rate k_2 is adapted from Ref. (44) for bivalent receptors.

Table 2 | Estimated mean number of cross-linking events, $N' \simeq Ne^{2k_{-2}\tau}$, required to elicit a T cell response (SP thymocytes).

Ligand		N'	
	τ (s)	$N = 10$	$N = 100$
4P	1	3	12
($k_{on} = 153{,}691\ M^{-1}\ s^{-1}$)	4	3	13
($k_{off} = 0.0169\ s^{-1}$)	8	3	14
4A	1	7	58
($k_{on} = 157{,}533\ M^{-1}\ s^{-1}$)	4	$\sim 10^3$	$\sim 10^4$
($k_{off} = 0.8664\ s^{-1}$)	8	$\sim 10^6$	$\sim 10^7$
4N	1	$\sim 10^7$	$\sim 10^8$
($k_{on} = 149{,}385\ M^{-1}\ s^{-1}$)	4	$\sim 10^{30}$	$\sim 10^{31}$
($k_{off = 8.6643}\ s^{-1}$)	8	$\sim 10^{60}$	$\sim 10^{61}$

3. RESULTS

3.1. DISTRIBUTION OF TCR CLUSTERS

The mathematical model described in Section 2.1, or Model 1, allows us to obtain the value of b that best fits the experimental data. We have used a weighted (by the variance) minimum-square regression to fit the experimental distributions to equation (2). This kind of fit minimizes the value of χ^2. Thus, in **Figure 3**, we show the agreement between theory and experiment, with values: $b_{\text{naive}} = 0.32$ and $b_{\text{memory}} = 0.55$. The difference between b_{naive} and b_{memory} can be explained by the existence of larger (or at least more localized) lipid rafts on the membrane of memory T cells (50, 51). Thus, the rates $q_\pm$ could be the effective combination of two mechanisms: one related to the diffusion of receptors on the membrane, and the other related to the aggregation of the receptors at the molecular level. The presence of cholesterol on the membrane changes the diffusion coefficient of the TCR receptors, as receptor diffusion within the raft is inhibited due to protein anchorage (52) and, thus, stabilizes the formation of clusters (a larger value of b means that, once two receptors are embedded in the same lipid raft, it is more difficult for them to become separated from each other).

A consequence of Model 1 is that, as the stationary probabilities need to sum up to one, the fraction of clusters of size larger than one is, precisely, b. This fraction is 72% higher for memory T cells than for naive T cells: $b_{\text{memory}}/b_{\text{naive}} = 1.72$.

3.2. MEAN TIME TO SIGNAL INITIATION

In **Figures 4A–D**, we show how the stochastic criterion is able to provide a ligand hierarchy according to their *potency*. Namely,

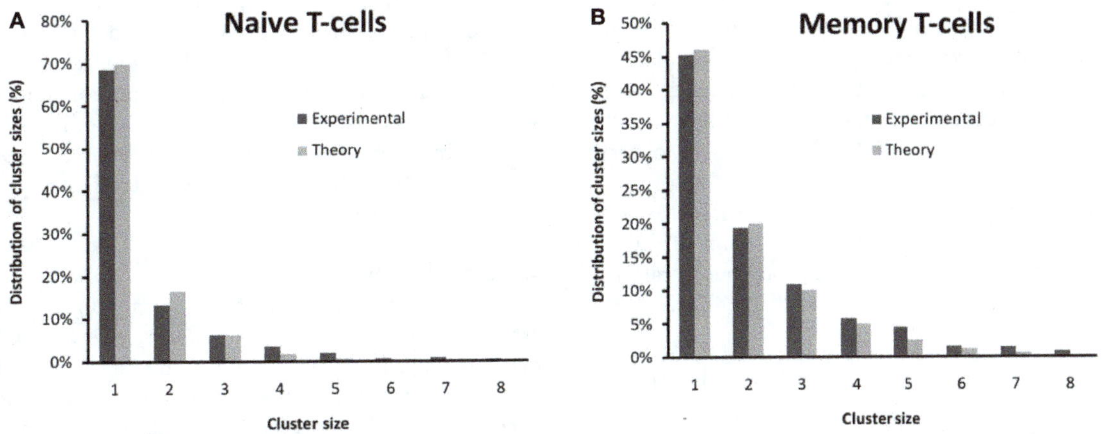

FIGURE 3 | Comparison between the experimental distribution of clusters (see also Figure 1) and those from Model 1 for (A) naive T cells and (B) memory T cells. The theoretical distribution has been fitted to equation (2) using a weighted (by the variance) minimum-square regression. The fitted values are $b_{naive} = 0.32$ and $b_{memory} = 0.55$.

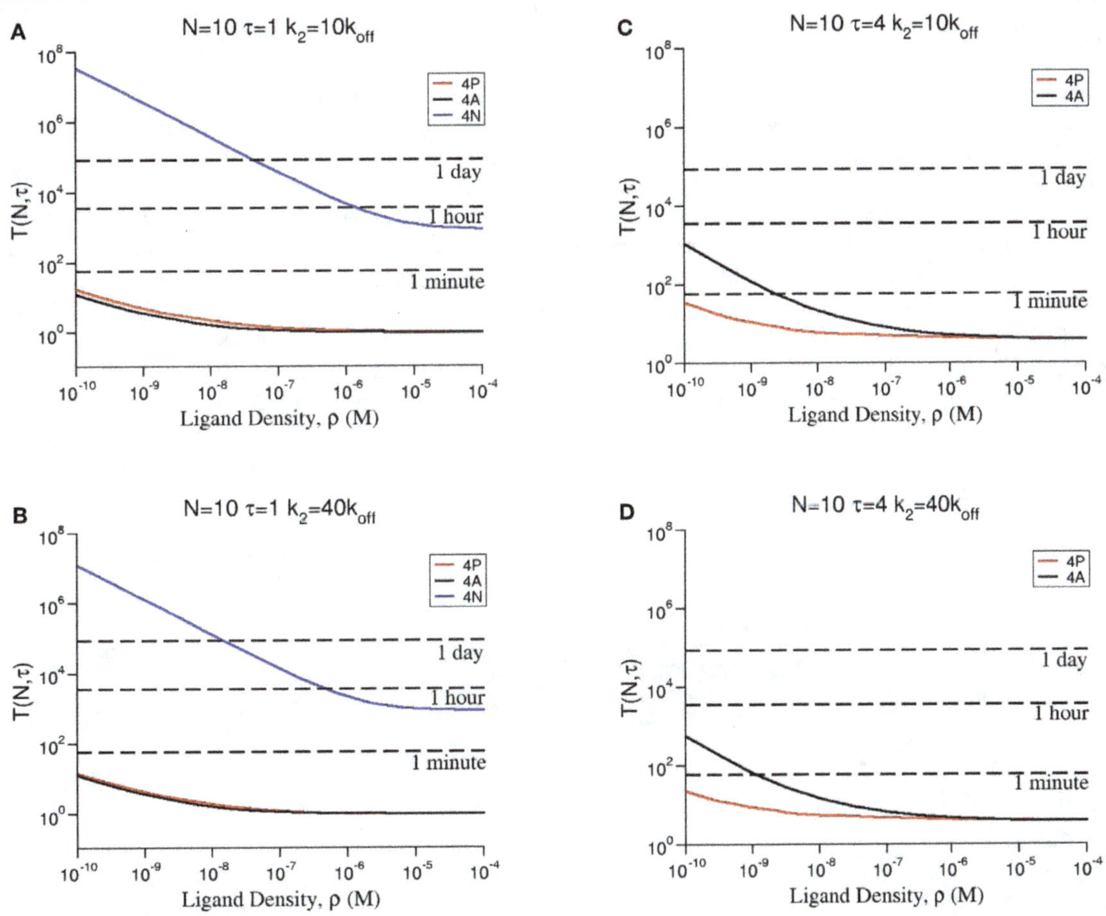

FIGURE 4 | Dependence of the mean time to signal initiation (MTSI), $T(N, \tau)$ to have N cross-linked ligand–receptor complexes bound for at least a dwell time τ for different model parameters as shown in every panel. The results have been obtained by making use of a Gillespie algorithm, after averaging over 100 realizations for each set of the parameters, summarized in **Table 2** (a python code for the stochastic integration is available upon request). Units of time are seconds. All parameters are taken from **Tables 1** and **2** except **(A)** $N = 10$, $\tau = 1$ and $k_2 = 10 \times k_{off}$; **(B)** $N = 10$, $\tau = 1$ and $k_2 = 40 \times k_{off}$; **(C)** $N = 10$, $\tau = 4$ and $k_2 = 10 \times k_{off}$; **(D)** $N = 10$, $\tau = 4$ and $k_2 = 40 \times k_{off}$.

the most agonistic ligand, 4P, elicits a T cell response in times of the order of a few seconds in all cases. On the contrary, the most antagonistic ligand, 4N, takes extremely large times to do so (in practical terms, this means it does not elicit a T cell response). Thus, TCR clustering can enhance the *potency* of ligands, when compared to the monomeric case (26), as experimentally observed and theoretically shown.

Following a similar approach to that of Ref. (26), we can derive an approximate formula for the mean time to signal initiation (MTSI), $T(N, \tau)$, for different ranges of ligand concentration, ρ. We write (see **Figure 5A** and Section 5.3 for further details):

$$T(N,\tau) \simeq \begin{cases} \tau & \text{at high concentration} \\ \tau + \left[\frac{N\exp(2k_{-2}\tau)}{2\rho N_B k_{\mathrm{on}} k_2}\right]^{1/2} & \text{at intermediate concentration} \\ \tau + \frac{N\exp(2k_{-2}\tau)}{4\rho N_B k_{\mathrm{on}}(k_2/k_{-2})} & \text{at low concentration} \end{cases} \quad (3)$$

These three regimes correspond to different immunological scenarios. In the case of high concentration of ligand, ligand is in great excess, so that the required number of *signaling units* is reached, almost as soon as the first signaling unit is formed (time of order τ). At low ligand concentration, the dynamics is limited by the first binding event, as cross-linking occurs in a slower timescale. So, the MTSI has the same functional form as that for the monomeric case (26). Finally, for intermediate ligand concentration, the competition between binding and cross-linking implies a more complicated mathematical relationship. Of greater relevance to the discussion is the nature of the ligand (with different k_{on} and k_{off} rates), and the number of TCR clusters on the membrane of the T cell (encoded in the parameter $N_B = b \times N_R$, with N_R, the average number of TCRs per T cell, see **Table 1**).

An expression for the variance of the time to signal initiation (TSI) cannot be provided in a closed form [as done in Ref. (26)]. However, the fact that the variance decreases as the ligand concentration increases, suggests that the mathematical formula for the variance in the monovalent case can provide an upper bound to the present (dimeric) case.

Using equation (3), we also can deduce the role of pre-clustering in the signaling time, or MTSI. As the number of bivalent clusters is $b \times N_R$, the larger b is, the shorter the response time becomes. The model predicts that, for physiological conditions (not too high ligand concentrations), the ratio of the MTSI for naive and memory T cells is inversely proportional to the ratio of their corresponding values of b. Namely, memory cells would respond up to 72% faster than naive ones (**Figure 5B**).

4. DISCUSSION

TCR triggering mechanisms are currently under debate [see, for example, Ref. (53) and (7) for recent reviews]. TCR clustering may be invoked as a description of the experimental results (27). The requirement for multivalent engagement of TCRs by pMHC ligands in $CD4^+$ T cells has been widely shown (45, 47, 54, 55). The same requirement was shown in $CD8^+$ T cells by Stone and Stern (56).

In this paper, we have made use of the concept of *mean time to signal initiation* (MTSI or stochastic criterion) as a method to quantify the effect of TCR clustering on the timescales of T cell responses and, thus, to compare the behavior of naive and memory T cells. This criterion has also allowed us to compare the results in Section 3 for dimeric binding with those of Ref. (26) for monomeric binding. The introduction of the cross-linked ligand–receptor complex as the minimum *signaling* unit gives the response greater sensitivity to small differences in ligand affinity.

A recent and novel feature of TCR immunology is the existence of TCR nano-clusters that are pre-formed, independently of ligand (3). This suggests that a simple stoichiometric clustering model (oligomerization of free TCRs diffusing on the T cell membrane) is enough to account for the distribution of TCR nano-clusters. In the case of naive T cells, Model 1 predicts an effective non-dimensional parameter, $b = q_+/q_-$, that allows us to explain the experimentally observed TCR cluster distributions. The presence of larger lipid rafts on the membrane of memory T cells might provide support for the different values of b for naive and memory cells, b_{naive} and b_{memory}, respectively. It has recently been shown that receptor diffusion within the raft is inhibited due to protein anchorage (52). This reduction in the TCR diffusion coefficient

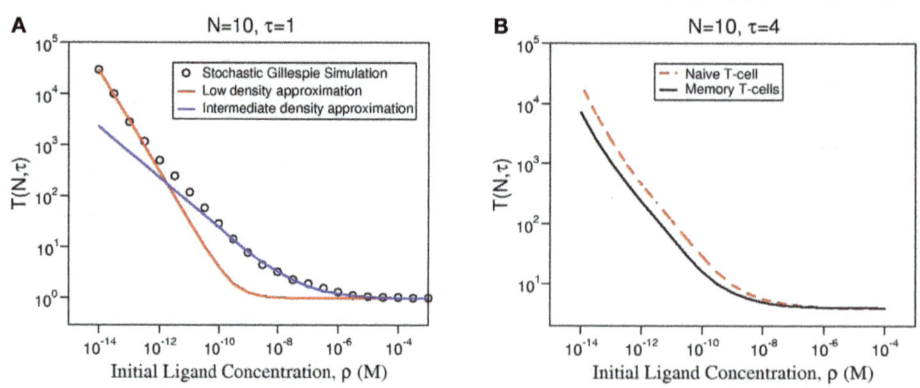

FIGURE 5 | (A) Comparison of the numerical solution of Model 2 (Gillespie algorithm with the parameters summarized in **Table 2**) and the approximate solution [equation (3)] for ligand 4P and the same parameters as in **Figure 4**. **(B)** Comparison of the mean MTSI for naive (red dashed line) and memory (solid black line) T cells.

would increase the time required for the receptor to escape from the raft [in a similar fashion as other escape problems (57)]. This escape time is inversely proportional to the diffusion coefficient itself. A smaller TCR diffusivity, as would be the case for memory T cells, will imply a larger residence time in the raft, which in turn will increase the probability of receptor aggregation in a given TCR cluster. A more detailed model of TCR diffusion and aggregation on the T cell membrane will be the subject of future work.

Equation (3) shows the explicit dependence of the MTSI, $T(N, \tau)$, on the parameter N_B, for given values of N and τ. N_B is the average number of dimeric receptor clusters per T cell, so that $N_B = b \times N_R$, with N_R, the average number of TCRs per T cell (see **Table 1**). For large ligand concentration, the predicted T cell response time for memory and naive T cells is the same, and is equal to τ. In the case of intermediate concentrations, the MTSI is proportional to $\frac{1}{\sqrt{b}}$. Finally, for low ligand concentration the MTSI is proportional to $\frac{1}{b}$. This implies that, at low ligand concentration, TCR pre-clustering alone can only account for at most 72% of the reduction in the response time between memory and naive T cells. This behavior is illustrated in **Figure 5A**. This difference is not so large as to be able to account for the observed higher responsiveness of memory T cells. Our results, thus, point to the need for additional mechanisms beyond TCR pre-clustering.

A potential candidate to explain the large differences between memory and naive T cell responses is the conformational change of the CD3 complex (58). This conformational change is essential to enable ITAM phosphorylation and, thus, the transfer of the TCR signal from the ecto-domain to the cytoplasmic tail of the TCR (58). Conformational changes in the CD3 complex occur as a result of the $\alpha\beta$ hetero-dimer binding to pMHC. These conformational changes allow the subunits of the CD3 complex (the $\gamma\epsilon$ and $\delta\epsilon$ hetero-dimers and the $\zeta\zeta$ homo-dimer) to become accessible to Lck, which can then phosphorylate their cytoplasmic domains at the ITAMs, leading to T cell signaling (59). In this way, the ligand-induced conformational change of the receptors can be propagated to all the receptors in the same cluster, so that larger clusters would benefit from this conformational change as a *cascade* [see, for example, Ref. (60) and references therein]. Thus, differences in the distribution of cluster sizes could, indeed, explain the immunological differences between memory and naive cells.

Other membrane receptors also exhibit pre-clustering and ligand-induced receptor cross-linking. For instance, in the case of the vascular endothelial growth factor receptor (VEGFR), it has been shown (61) that there are two distinct pathways to receptor dimerization: (i) dynamic pre-dimerization (as the one described in Model 1), and (ii) ligand-induced receptor dimerization. The main conclusion in Ref. (61) is that both mechanisms are almost indistinguishable at low ligand concentration. However, the first mechanism is more sensitive to changes in the binding affinity at large ligand concentration. Although the biological system studied in Ref. (61) is different from the T cell receptor considered here, their conclusions might be generalized as both receptors are tyrosine kinases.

Bachmann et al. (62, 63) considered a model of diffusion and ligand-induced TCR clustering. Their model suggests that the existence of large enough clusters greatly inhibits subsequent multimer diffusion, thus, reducing the relevance that this mechanism might have. This inhibition might be experimentally tested by exploiting the differences between naive (small and few clusters) and memory (large and many clusters). It will be interesting to make use of the models introduced in this paper to investigate the different roles of ligand binding and cellular activation (62), and TCR turnover (64).

Finally, the existence of TCR pre-clusters [and the knowledge of their membrane distribution given by π_n, equation (2)] can be considered in the kinetic-segregation model (65). In this model, diffusion out of close-contact zones would be inhibited by the existence of nano-clusters, thus, enhancing the number of triggered receptors. In a similar way, consecutive receptor phosphorylation events (66) in TCR nano-clusters would also amplify receptor signaling.

5. MATERIALS AND METHODS

5.1. EXPERIMENTS

Naive $CD8^+$ OT-1 T cells, which recognize an ovalbumin-derived peptide presented by the MHC class I molecule $H\text{-}2K^b$, were isolated from superficial and mesenteric lymph nodes of OT-1 TCR transgenic mice (67), via depletion of $CD19^+$ B cells, $CD4^+$ helper T cells and $CD11b^+$ macrophages, using antibodies and Dynal magnetic beads (Invitrogen). Memory OT-1 T cells were generated by adoptively transferring 10^6 naive OT-1 T cells into congenic C57BL/6 Ly5.1 Pep3b mice, which were simultaneously immunized with 10^7 PFU MVA-OVA (68). After 6 months, resting memory OT-1 T cells were isolated from the spleen and lymph nodes of these mice by antibody-mediated depletion of macrophages, B cells, and $CD4^+$ T cells, followed by separation of the OT-1 memory T cells from host-derived $Ly5.1^+$ $CD8^+$ T cells via fluorescence-activated cell sorting, using a Ly5.1-specific antibody. Labeling of cells with the $CD3\epsilon$-specific antibody 2C11 and 10 nm gold-conjugated protein-A, replica generation and analysis were performed as previously described (17).

5.2. MODELS OF SIGNALING WITH DIMERIC AND TRIMERIC RECEPTOR CLUSTERS

In Section 2, we introduced a model in which ligands are bivalent and receptor clusters are dimeric (that is, composed of two monomeric TCRs). This is, of course, a first approximation that neglects the distribution of cluster sizes experimentally observed. Yet, the results of our mathematical study only change in a quantitative way, but not qualitatively, when we include TCR clusters of larger sizes. In this Section, we illustrate this by considering a system in which clusters of size 1, 2, and 3 coexist and the ligands are bivalent. **Table 3** provides the notation introduced to describe the molecular species considered in the model, as well as a graphical representation.

At large initial ligand concentration, under the stochastic criterion, the MTSI tends to τ. On the other hand, at low initial ligand concentration, the number of receptors, compared to the number of ligands, is so large that we can neglect molecular species x_4, y_4, y_6, and y_7, which involve more than one bivalent ligand. This has also been confirmed experimentally. Given our stochastic T cell response criterion, in this case, the signaling units correspond to molecular species x_5, y_5, and y_7. Molecular species z_1 and z_3 do

Table 3 | Summary of variables for a model in which clusters of size 1, 2, and 3 coexist.

Variable	Description	Molecular representation
z_1	Free monomeric receptor	
z_2	Free ligand (dimer)	
z_3	Ligand-bound to a monomeric receptor	
x_1	Free dimeric cluster	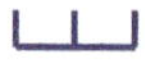
x_2	Same as z_2 (defined for convenience of notation)	
x_3	Ligand singly bound to a dimeric cluster	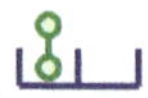
x_4	Two ligands bound to a dimeric cluster	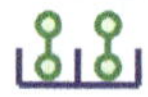
x_5	Cross-linked ligand in a dimeric cluster	
y_1	Free trimeric receptor	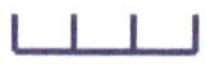
y_2	Same as z_2 (defined for convenience of notation)	
y_3	Ligand singly bound to a trimeric cluster	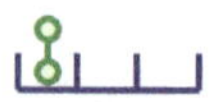
y_4	Two ligands bound to a trimeric cluster	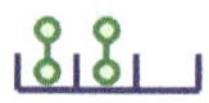
y_5	Cross-linked ligand in a trimeric cluster	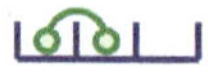
y_6	Three ligands bound to a trimeric cluster	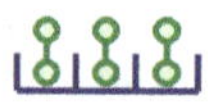
y_7	One ligand singly bound to a trimeric cluster and another cross-linked	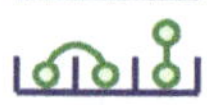

All the variables correspond to the total number of molecular species (not concentrations). Hence, all the rates in the mathematical model have units of s^{-1}.

not contribute to the T cell response and will be neglected in what follows. Thus, we only need to consider the dynamics of dimeric and trimeric T cell receptor clusters.

We introduce the total number of *signaling units*, $S_5(t) \equiv x_5(t) + y_5(t)$. The set of ordinary differential equations for the model is given by:

$$\begin{aligned}
\dot{x}_1 &= -4k_+ x_1 x_2 + k_{\text{off}} x_3, \\
\dot{x}_2 &= -4k_+ x_1 x_2 + k_{\text{off}} x_3, \\
\dot{x}_3 &= 4k_+ x_1 x_2 - k_{\text{off}} x_3 - k_2 x_3 + 2k_{-2} x_5, \\
\dot{x}_5 &= k_2 x_3 - 2k_{-2} x_5, \\
\dot{y}_1 &= -6k_+ y_1 y_2 + k_{\text{off}} y_3, \\
\dot{y}_2 &= -6k_+ y_1 y_2 + k_{\text{off}} y_3, \\
\dot{y}_3 &= 6k_+ y_1 y_2 - k_{\text{off}} y_3 - 2k_2 y_3 + 2k_{-2} y_5, \\
\dot{y}_5 &= 2k_2 y_3 - 2k_{-2} y_5,
\end{aligned}$$

where $k_+ = k_{\text{on}}/(VN_A)$, V is the volume of the experiment and N_A is Avogadro's number.

Given the symmetry of the problem, and in the limit of low initial ligand concentration, we will assume that the ratio of x_3 to y_3 is that of the initial ratio of free TCR dimers to free TCR trimers, namely,

$$\frac{y_3}{x_3} \simeq \frac{\pi_3}{\pi_2} = b \quad \Rightarrow \quad y_3 \simeq b\, x_3 \,, \tag{4}$$

where we have made use of equation (2) to conclude $\frac{\pi_3}{\pi_2} = b$. Thus, the total number of signaling units, $S_5(t)$, obeys the following differential equation

$$\dot{S}_5 = \dot{x}_5 + \dot{y}_5 = k_2\,(1+2b)\,x_3 - 2\,k_{-2}\,S_5 \,. \tag{5}$$

Finally, in the low ligand concentration limit as above, let us introduce $S_3 \equiv x_3 + y_3$. It is easy to show that equation (5) reduces to

$$\dot{S}_5 = k_2 \frac{1+2b}{1+b} S_3 - 2\,k_{-2}\,S_5 \,, \tag{6}$$

which is identical to the differential equation for x_5 above, but with $S_{5,3}$ replaced by $x_{5,3}$, respectively. This means that, except for a pre-factor $\frac{1+2b}{1+b}$ [which, for $b \in (0,1)$, is between 1 and 3/2], the study of dimeric and trimeric clusters is reduced to the dimeric case.

5.3. A SIMPLE FORMULA FOR THE MTSI

The basic idea behind the stochastic criterion is to count the cumulative number of events that may contribute to signaling (26). Here, we calculate the mean number of cross-linking events up to time t, $C(t)$, as the integral,

$$C(t) = k_2 \int_0^t x_3(s)\, ds \,. \tag{7}$$

It is possible to obtain an expression for $x_3(t)$ with the approximation that the product $x_1(t)x_2(t)$ is constant, so that the pair of equations for $x_3(t)$ and $x_5(t)$ can be solved exactly. This yields (69):

$$\begin{aligned}
C(t) = k_2 \Bigg[&\frac{c_1}{\lambda_1}(\lambda_1 + 2k_{-2})(e^{\lambda_1 t} - 1) \\
&+ \frac{c_2}{\lambda_2}(\lambda_2 + 2k_{-2})(e^{\lambda_2 t} - 1) + a_1 t \Bigg] \,,
\end{aligned} \tag{8}$$

where

$$\begin{aligned}
c_1 &= \frac{-4\lambda_2 k_{\text{on}} \rho N_B}{(\lambda_2 - \lambda_1)(4k_{\text{on}}\rho k_2 + 2k_{\text{off}} k_{-2} + 8k_{\text{on}}\rho k_{-2})}, \\
c_2 &= \frac{4\lambda_1 k_{\text{on}} \rho N_B}{(\lambda_2 - \lambda_1)(4k_{\text{on}}\rho k_2 + 2k_{\text{off}} k_{-2} + 8k_{\text{on}}\rho k_{-2})}, \\
\lambda_{1,2} &= \frac{1}{2}\Big(-4k_{\text{on}}\rho - k_{\text{off}} - k_2 - 2k_{-2} \\
&\quad \pm \big[(4k_{\text{on}}\rho + k_{\text{off}} - k_2 - 2k_{-2})^2 + 4k_{\text{off}} k_2\big]^{1/2}\Big), \\
a_1 &= \frac{8k_{-2} k_{\text{on}} \rho N_B}{4k_{\text{on}}\rho k_2 + 2k_{\text{off}} k_{-2} + 8k_{\text{on}}\rho k_{-2}}, \\
a_2 &= \frac{4k_2 k_{\text{on}} \rho N_B}{4k_{\text{on}}\rho k_2 + 2k_{\text{off}} k_{-2} + 8k_{\text{on}}\rho k_{-2}},
\end{aligned}$$

and N_B is the number of dimeric receptors. The MTSI is then given by the solution of the equation $C(T(N, \tau)-\tau) = N \exp(2k_{-2}\tau)$.

The expressions in equation (3) are obtained from equation (8) in the appropriate regimes. At low ligand concentration, $C(t)$ is simply proportional to time: $C(t) \simeq k_2 a_1 t$, so that $C(T-\tau) = k_2 a_1 (T-\tau) = N \exp(2k_{-2}\tau)$. When $\lambda_{1,2}\tau \ll 1$, on the other hand, the first non-zero term in a Taylor expansion of $C(t)$ in time is quadratic: $C(t) \propto t^2$. This provides the exponent 1/2 in the second line of equation (3).

ACKNOWLEDGMENTS

We thank Ed Palmer, Wolfgang Schamel, and Thomas Höfer for helpful discussions. We also thank the Max Planck Institute for the Physics of Complex Systems (Dresden) and the International Centre for Mathematical Sciences (Edinburgh), where part of this work was discussed and presented, for their hospitality. This work has been partially supported through Grants No. FIS2009-12964-C05-03 (Mario Castro, Grant Lythe, Carmen Molina-París), BFU2009-08009 from the Ministerio de Ciencia e Innovación (Hisse M. van Santen), FP7 PIRSES-GA-2008-230665 and PIRSES-GA-2012-317893 (Mario Castro, Grant Lythe, and Carmen Molina-París), BBSRC BB/F003811/1 (Grant Lythe and Carmen Molina-París), and BBSRC BB/G023395/1 (Carmen Molina-París).

REFERENCES

1. Huppa JB, Davis MM. T-cell-antigen recognition and the immunological synapse. *Nat Rev Immunol* (2003) **3**(12):973–83. doi:10.1038/nri1245
2. Batista FD, Dustin ML. Cell: cell interactions in the immune system. *Immunol Rev* (2013) **251**(1):7–12. doi:10.1111/imr.12025
3. Schamel WW, Alarcón B. Organization of the resting TCR in nanoscale oligomers. *Immunol Rev* (2013) **251**(1):13–20. doi:10.1111/imr.12019
4. Allard JF, Dushek O, Coombs D, van der Merwe PA. Mechanical modulation of receptor-ligand interactions at cell-cell interfaces. *Biophys J* (2012) **102**(6):1265–73. doi:10.1016/j.bpj.2012.02.006
5. Lillemeier BF, Mörtelmaier MA, Forstner MB, Huppa JB, Groves JT, Davis MM. TCR and Lat are expressed on separate protein islands on T cell membranes and concatenate during activation. *Nat Immunol* (2009) **11**(1):90–6. doi:10.1038/ni.1832
6. Edwards LJ, Zarnitsyna VI, Hood JD, Evavold BD, Zhu C. Insights into t cell recognition of antigen: significance of two-dimensional kinetic parameters. *Front Immunol* (2012) **3**:86. doi:10.3389/fimmu.2012.00086
7. Zarnitsyna V, Zhu C. T cell triggering: insights from 2D kinetics analysis of molecular interactions. *Phys Biol* (2012) **9**(4):045005. doi:10.1088/1478-3975/9/4/045005
8. McKeithan T. Kinetic proofreading in T-cell receptor signal transduction. *Proc Natl Acad Sci U S A* (1995) **92**(11):5042. doi:10.1073/pnas.92.11.5042
9. Kalergis AM, Boucheron N, Doucey M-A, Palmieri E, Goyarts EC, Vegh Z, et al. Efficient T cell activation requires an optimal dwell-time of interaction between the TCR and the pMHC complex. *Nat Immunol* (2001) **2**(3):229–34. doi:10.1038/85286
10. Matis LA, Glimcher LH, Paul WE, Schwartz RH. Magnitude of response of histocompatibility-restricted T-cell clones is a function of the product of the concentrations of antigen and IA molecules. *Proc Natl Acad Sci U S A* (1983) **80**(19):6019–23. doi:10.1073/pnas.80.19.6019
11. Valitutti S, Müller S, Cella M, Padovan E, Lanzavecchia A. Serial triggering of many T-cell receptors by a few peptide MHC complexes. *Nature* (1995) **375**(6527):148–51. doi:10.1038/375148a0
12. Friedl P, Gunzer M. Interaction of T cells with APCS: the serial encounter model. *Trends Immunol* (2001) **22**(4):187–91. doi:10.1016/S1471-4906(01)01869-5
13. Dushek O, Das R, Coombs D. A role for rebinding in rapid and reliable T cell responses to antigen. *PLoS Comput Biol* (2009) **5**(11):e1000578. doi:10.1371/journal.pcbi.1000578
14. Daniels MA, Teixeiro E, Gill J, Hausmann B, Roubaty D, Holmberg K, et al. Thymic selection threshold defined by compartmentalization of RAS/MAPK signalling. *Nature* (2006) **444**(7120):724–9. doi:10.1038/nature05269
15. Valitutti S, Coombs D, Dupré L. The space and time frames of T cell activation at the immunological synapse. *FEBS Lett* (2010) **584**(24):4851–7. doi:10.1016/j.febslet.2010.10.010
16. Smith-Garvin JE, Koretzky GA, Jordan MS. T cell activation. *Annu Rev Immunol* (2009) **27**:591. doi:10.1146/annurev.immunol.021908.132706
17. Kumar R, Ferez M, Swamy M, Arechaga I, Rejas MT, Valpuesta JM, et al. Increased sensitivity of antigen-experienced T cells through the enrichment of oligomeric T cell receptor complexes. *Immunity* (2011) **35**(3):375–87. doi:10.1016/j.immuni.2011.08.010
18. Schamel WW, Arechaga I, Risueño RM, van Santen HM, Cabezas P, Risco C, et al. Coexistence of multivalent and monovalent TCRs explains high sensitivity and wide range of response. *J Exp Med* (2005) **202**(4):493–503. doi:10.1084/jem.20042155
19. Lu X, Gibbs JS, Hickman HD, David A, Dolan BP, Jin Y, et al. Endogenous viral antigen processing generates peptide-specific MHC class I cell-surface clusters. *Proc Natl Acad Sci U S A* (2012) **109**(38):15407–12. doi:10.1073/pnas.1208696109
20. Ferez M, Castro M, Alarcon B, van Santen HM. Cognate peptide-MHC complexes are expressed as tightly apposed nanoclusters in virus-infected cells to allow tcr crosslinking. *J Immunol* (2014) **192**(1):52–8. doi:10.4049/jimmunol.1301224
21. Bosch B, Heipertz EL, Drake JR, Roche PA. Major histocompatibility complex (MHC) class II-peptide complexes arrive at the plasma membrane in cholesterol-rich microclusters. *J Biol Chem* (2013) **288**(19):13236–42. doi:10.1074/jbc.M112.442640
22. Goldstein B, Faeder JR, Hlavacek WS. Mathematical and computational models of immune-receptor signalling. *Nat Rev Immunol* (2004) **4**(6):445–56. doi:10.1038/nri1374
23. Alarcón B, Swamy M, van Santen HM, Schamel WW. T-cell antigen-receptor stoichiometry: pre-clustering for sensitivity. *EMBO Rep* (2006) **7**(5):490–5. doi:10.1038/sj.embor.7400682
24. Bray D, Levin MD, Morton-Firth CJ. Receptor clustering as a cellular mechanism to control sensitivity. *Nature* (1998) **393**(6680):85–8. doi:10.1038/30018
25. Slifka MK, Whitton JL. Functional avidity maturation of CD8+ T cells without selection of higher affinity TCR. *Nat Immunol* (2001) **2**(8):711–7. doi:10.1038/90650
26. Currie J, Castro M, Lythe G, Palmer E, Molina-París C. A stochastic T cell response criterion. *J R Soc Interface* (2012) **9**(76):2856–70. doi:10.1098/rsif.2012.0205
27. van der Merwe P, Dushek O. Mechanisms for T cell receptor triggering. *Nat Rev Immunol* (2010) **11**(1):47–55. doi:10.1038/nri2887
28. Yewdell JW. Drips solidify: progress in understanding endogenous MHC class I antigen processing. *Trends Immunol* (2011) **32**(11):548–58. doi:10.1016/j.it.2011.08.001
29. Rock KL, Farfán-Arribas DJ, Colbert JD, Goldberg AL. Re-examining class-I presentation and the DRiP hypothesis. *Trends Immunol* (2014). doi:10.1016/j.it.2014.01.002
30. Antón LC, Yewdell JW. Translating DRiPs: MHC class I immunosurveillance of pathogens and tumors. *J Leukoc Biol* (2014). doi:10.1189/jlb.1113599
31. Stone J, Cochran J, Stern L. T-cell activation by soluble MHC oligomers can be described by a two-parameter binding model. *Biophys J* (2001) **81**(5):2547–57. doi:10.1016/S0006-3495(01)75899-7
32. Stone J, Chervin A, Kranz D. T-cell receptor binding affinities and kinetics: impact on T-cell activity and specificity. *Immunology* (2009) **126**(2):165–76. doi:10.1111/j.1365-2567.2008.03015.x
33. Coombs D, Dushek O, Merwe P. A review of mathematical models for T cell receptor triggering and antigen discrimination. In: Molina-París C, Lythe G, editors. *Mathematical Models and Immune Cell Biology.* New York: Springer (2011). p. 25–45.
34. Coombs D, Kalergis AM, Nathenson SG, Wofsy C, Goldstein B. Activated TCRs remain marked for internalization after dissociation from pMHC. *Nat Immunol* (2002) **3**(10):926–31. doi:10.1038/ni838
35. Choudhuri K, Dustin ML. Signaling microdomains in T cells. *FEBS Lett* (2010) **584**(24):4823–31. doi:10.1016/j.febslet.2010.10.015

36. Yokosuka T, Saito T. The immunological synapse, TCR microclusters, and T cell activation. In: Saito T, Batista FD, editors. *Immunological Synapse.* Berlin Heidelberg: Springer (2010). p. 81–107.
37. Torres J, Briggs JA, Arkin IT. Multiple site-specific infrared dichroism of CD3-ζ, a transmembrane helix bundle. *J Mol Biol* (2002) **316**(2):365–74. doi:10.1006/jmbi.2001.5267
38. Kuhns MS, Girvin AT, Klein LO, Chen R, Jensen KD, Newell EW, et al. Evidence for a functional sidedness to the $\alpha\beta$TCR. *Proc Natl Acad Sci U S A* (2010) **107**(11):5094–9. doi:10.1073/pnas.1000925107
39. Norris JR. *Markov Chains.* Cambridge University Press (1998).
40. Taylor H, Karlin S. *An Introduction to Stochastic Modeling.* San Diego: Academic Press (1998).
41. Janeway CA Jr. Ligands for the T-cell receptor: hard times for avidity models. *Immunol Today* (1995) **16**(5):223–5. doi:10.1016/0167-5699(95)80163-4
42. Ma Z, Sharp KA, Janmey PA, Finkel TH. Surface-anchored monomeric agonist pMHCs alone trigger TCR with high sensitivity. *PLoS Biol* (2008) **6**(2):e43. doi:10.1371/journal.pbio.0060043
43. Huang J, Brameshuber M, Zeng X, Xie J, Li QJ, Chien YH, et al. A single peptide-major histocompatibility complex ligand triggers digital cytokine secretion in CD4+ T cells. *Immunity* (2013) **39**:846–57. doi:10.1016/j.immuni.2013.08.036
44. Stone J, Artyomov M, Chervin A, Chakraborty A, Eisen H, Kranz D. Interaction of streptavidin-based peptide-MHC oligomers (tetramers) with cell-surface TCRs. *J Immunol* (2011) **187**(12):6281–90. doi:10.4049/jimmunol.1101734
45. Abastado J-P, Lone Y-C, Casrouge A, Boulot G, Kourilsky P. Dimerization of soluble major histocompatibility complex-peptide complexes is sufficient for activation of T cell hybridoma and induction of unresponsiveness. *J Exp Med* (1995) **182**(2):439–47. doi:10.1084/jem.182.2.439
46. Cochran JR, Cameron TO, Stern LJ. The relationship of MHC-peptide binding and T cell activation probed using chemically defined MHC class II oligomers. *Immunity* (2000) **12**(3):241–50. doi:10.1016/S1074-7613(00)80177-6
47. Boniface JJ, Rabinowitz JD, Wülfing C, Hampl J, Reich Z, Altman JD, et al. Initiation of signal transduction through the T cell receptor requires the multivalent engagement of peptide/MHC ligands. *Immunity* (1998) **9**(4):459–66. doi:10.1016/S1074-7613(00)80629-9
48. Palmer E, Naeher D. Affinity threshold for thymic selection through a T-cell receptor-co-receptor zipper. *Nat Rev Immunol* (2009) **9**(3):207–13. doi:10.1038/nri2469
49. Gillespie D. Exact stochastic simulation of coupled chemical reactions. *J Phys Chem* (1977) **81**:2340–61. doi:10.1021/j100540a008
50. Brumeanu T-D, Preda-Pais A, Stoica C, Bona C, Casares S. Differential partitioning and trafficking of GM gangliosides and cholesterol-rich lipid rafts in thymic and splenic CD4 T cells. *Mol Immunol* (2007) **44**(4):530–40. doi:10.1016/j.molimm.2006.02.008
51. Kersh EN, Kaech SM, Onami TM, Moran M, Wherry EJ, Miceli MC, et al. TCR signal transduction in antigen-specific memory CD8 T cells. *J Immunol* (2003) **170**(11):5455–63.
52. Lingwood D, Simons K. Lipid rafts as a membrane-organizing principle. *Science* (2010) **327**(5961):46–50. doi:10.1126/science.1174621
53. Robert P, Aleksic M, Dushek O, Cerundolo V, Bongrand P, van der Merwe P. Kinetics and mechanics of two-dimensional interactions between T cell receptors and different activating ligands. *Biophys J* (2012) **102**(2):248–57. doi:10.1016/j.bpj.2011.11.4018
54. Cochran JR, Stern LJ. A diverse set of oligomeric class II MHC-peptide complexes for probing T-cell receptor interactions. *Chem Biol* (2000) **7**(9):683–96. doi:10.1016/S1074-5521(00)00019-3
55. Dushek O, Goyette J, Merwe PA. Non-catalytic tyrosine-phosphorylated receptors. *Immunol Rev* (2012) **250**(1):258–76. doi:10.1111/imr.12008
56. Stone JD, Stern LJ. CD8 T cells, like CD4 T cells, are triggered by multivalent engagement of TCRs by MHC-peptide ligands but not by monovalent engagement. *J Immunol* (2006) **176**(3):1498–505.
57. Day M, Lythe G. Timescales of the adaptive immune response. In: Molina-París C, Lythe G, editors. *Mathematical Models and Immune Cell Biology.* New York: Springer (2011). p. 351–61.
58. Minguet S, Swamy M, Alarcón B, Luescher IF, Schamel WW. Full activation of the T cell receptor requires both clustering and conformational changes at CD3. *Immunity* (2007) **26**(1):43–54. doi:10.1016/j.immuni.2006.10.019
59. Marks F, Klingmüller U, Müller-Decker K. *Cellular Signal Processing: An Introduction to the Molecular Mechanisms of Signal Transduction.* New York, NY: Garland Science (2009).
60. Blanco R, Alarcón B. TCR nanoclusters as the framework for transmission of conformational changes and cooperativity. *Front Immunol* (2012) **3**:115. doi:10.3389/fimmu.2012.00115
61. Mac Gabhann F, Popel AS. Dimerization of VEGF receptors and implications for signal transduction: a computational study. *Biophys Chem* (2007) **128**(2–3):125–39. doi:10.1016/j.bpc.2007.03.010
62. Bachmann MF, Salzmann M, Oxenius A, Ohashi PS. Formation of TCR dimers/trimers as a crucial step for T cell activation. *Eur J Immunol* (1998) **28**(8):2571–9. doi:10.1002/(SICI)1521-4141(199808)28:08<2571::AID-IMMU2571>3.0.CO;2-T
63. Bachmann MF, Ohashi PS. The role of T-cell receptor dimerization in T-cell activation. *Immunol Today* (1999) **20**(12):568–76. doi:10.1016/S0167-5699(99)01543-1
64. Sousa J, Carneiro J. A mathematical analysis of tcr serial triggering and down-regulation. *Eur J Immunol* (2000) **30**:3219–27. doi:10.1002/1521-4141(200011)30:11<3219::AID-IMMU3219>3.0.CO;2-7
65. Davis SJ, van der Merwe PA. The kinetic-segregation model: TCR triggering and beyond. *Nat Immunol* (2006) **7**(8):803–9. doi:10.1038/ni1369
66. Mukhopadhyay H, Cordoba S-P, Maini PK, van der Merwe PA, Dushek O. Systems model of T cell receptor proximal signaling reveals emergent ultrasensitivity. *PLoS Comput Biol* (2013) **9**(3):e1003004. doi:10.1371/journal.pcbi.1003004
67. Hogquist KA, Jameson SC, Heath WR, Howard JL, Bevan MJ, Carbone FR. T cell receptor antagonist peptides induce positive selection. *Cell* (1994) **76**(1):17–27. doi:10.1016/0092-8674(94)90169-4
68. El-Gogo S, Staib C, Meyr M, Erfle V, Sutter G, Adler H. Recombinant murine gammaherpesvirus 68 (MHV-68) as challenge virus to test efficacy of vaccination against chronic virus infections in the mouse model. *Vaccine* (2007) **25**(20):3934–45. doi:10.1016/j.vaccine.2007.02.054
69. Currie J. *Stochastic Modelling of TCR Binding.* Ph.D. thesis, Leeds: University of Leeds (2012).

12

The effects of cocoa on the immune system

Francisco J. Pérez-Cano[1,2], Malen Massot-Cladera[1,2], Àngels Franch[1,2], Cristina Castellote[1,2] and Margarida Castell[1,2]*

[1] Departament de Fisiologia, Facultat de Farmàcia, Universitat de Barcelona, Barcelona, Spain
[2] Institut de Recerca en Nutrició i Seguretat Alimentària, Universitat de Barcelona, Barcelona, Spain

Edited by:
Rabia Latif, University of Dammam, Saudi Arabia

Reviewed by:
Rabia Latif, University of Dammam, Saudi Arabia
Luis Goya, Consejo Superior de Investigaciones Científicas, Spain

***Correspondence:**
Margarida Castell, Departament de Fisiologia, Facultat de Farmàcia, Universitat de Barcelona, Av Joan XXIII s/n, Barcelona E-08028, Spain
e-mail: margaridacastell@ub.edu

Cocoa is a food relatively rich in polyphenols, which makes it a potent antioxidant. Due to its activity as an antioxidant, as well as through other mechanisms, cocoa consumption has been reported to be beneficial for cardiovascular health, brain functions, and cancer prevention. Furthermore, cocoa influences the immune system, in particular the inflammatory innate response and the systemic and intestinal adaptive immune response. Preclinical studies have demonstrated that a cocoa-enriched diet modifies T cell functions that conduce to a modulation of the synthesis of systemic and gut antibodies. In this regard, it seems that a cocoa diet in rats produces changes in the lymphocyte composition of secondary lymphoid tissues and the cytokines secreted by T cells. These results suggest that it is possible that cocoa could inhibit the function of T helper type 2 cells, and in line with this, the preventive effect of cocoa on IgE synthesis in a rat allergy model has been reported, which opens up new perspectives when considering the beneficial effects of cocoa compounds. On the other hand, cocoa intake modifies the functionality of gut-associated lymphoid tissue by means of modulating IgA secretion and intestinal microbiota. The mechanisms involved in these influences are discussed here. Further research may elucidate the cocoa compounds involved in such an effect and also the possible medical approaches to these repercussions.

Keywords: cocoa, lymphocyte, macrophage, antibody, cytokine, gut-associated lymphoid tissue, thymus, spleen

INTRODUCTION

In addition to the beneficial effects on oxidative stress, cardiovascular health, nervous system diseases, aging, and cancer prevention, cocoa has been revealed as a food with immunoregulatory properties. In the following sections, the influence of cocoa or its flavonoids on the innate and adaptive immunity are reviewed. Firstly, the anti-inflammatory properties of cocoa are briefly summarized, and secondly, the effects of cocoa on the adaptive immune system and intestinal immunity are reported.

To achieve this objective, a systematic search in SCOPUS-V.4 (Elsevier) – SciVerse was conducted for the following key terms: "cocoa" AND "lymphocyte" OR "immun*" OR "inflammation" OR "microbiota." In order to prevent potential misclassification of relevant articles no exclusion criteria were used. The search included the period from January 1990 to March 2013.

ANTI-INFLAMMATORY POTENTIAL OF COCOA

Inflammation is the response of tissues to an aggression caused by pathogens, chemicals or wounding. Inflammation involves a complex network of reactions initially designed to protect the host from injury and to heal damaged tissue. The activation and migration of leukocytes to the site of the lesion and the release of growth factors, cytokines, reactive oxygen species (ROS), and nitric oxide (NO) are known to play a crucial role in the inflammatory response. Constant overproduction of pro-inflammatory molecules leads to chronic inflammation.

In general, flavonoids are associated with anti-inflammatory properties. In this regard, the flavanols contained in cocoa have been the subject of both *in vitro* and *in vivo* studies (reviewed in Pérez-Cano et al., 2010). Many studies have reported cocoa's ability to reduce cytokines, chemokines, ROS, NO, etc. involved in inflammatory response. However, few studies have focused on the *in vivo* anti-inflammatory activity of cocoa.

COCOA EFFECTS ON INFLAMMATORY CELLS

Cocoa extracts or single flavonoids, both as monomers (epicatechin, catechin) or polymers (procyanidins) have demonstrated *in vitro* their anti-inflammatory potential, although there have been some controversial results.

A cocoa flavonoid-enriched extract and the monomers epicatechin and isoquercitrin were able to decrease the production of inflammatory molecules such as tumor necrosis factor (TNF)-α and monocyte chemoattractant protein (MCP)-1 by macrophages under stimulation with lipopolysaccharide (LPS; Ramiro et al., 2005a). Similarly, epicatechin in stimulated whole blood cells culture suppressed the production of interleukin (IL)-6 and IL-8 (Al-Hanbali et al., 2009). However, monomer to pentamer units and longer chain fractions of cocoa flavanols increased the secretion of TNF-α, IL-1, and IL-6 in LPS-stimulated peripheral blood mononuclear cells (PBMC; Mao et al., 2002; Kenny et al., 2007; Wisman et al., 2008).

Aside from cytokines, other inflammatory molecules can be influenced by cocoa. Epicatechin, procyanidin B_1, procyanidin B_2, and a cocoa extract reduced NO release by stimulated macrophages (Ono et al., 2003; Ramiro et al., 2005a; Hämäläinen et al., 2007). Likewise, the *in vitro* treatment with cocoa fractions or flavonoids alone decreased the production of ROS from several kinds of cells (Sanbongi et al., 1997; Erlejman et al., 2006; Granado-Serrano et al., 2007; Ramiro-Puig et al., 2009).

Neutrophils also play an important role during inflammation. It has been demonstrated that cocoa has the potential to positively modulate the neutrophil inflammatory activity. In this sense, certain flavanols and procyanidins isolated from cocoa moderated some signaling pathways induced by LPS on neutrophils, particularly those of oxidative bursts and activation markers, and cocoa could influence selected apoptosis mechanisms (Kenny et al., 2009).

Regarding the mechanisms of action, it has been reported that hexameric cocoa procyanidins have the capacity to modulate TNF-α-induced NF-κB (nuclear factor kappa-light-chain-enhancer of activated B cells) activation in intestinal epithelial cells (Erlejman et al., 2008). NF-κB is a transcription factor involved in the regulation of genes encoding cytokines (IL-1, IL-2, IL-6, IL-8, TNF-α, among others), adhesion molecules (e.g., intercellular adhesion molecule 1, vascular cell adhesion molecule 1, and endothelial leukocyte adhesion molecule 1), acute phase proteins, inducible enzymes [inducible NO synthase (iNOS) and cyxlooxygenase 2 (COX-2)], etc. (Pahl, 1999).

ANTI-INFLAMMATORY POTENTIAL OF COCOA IN HEALTHY CONDITIONS

In a more physiological approach, using cells isolated from humans or animals fed with diets containing cocoa, the *in vitro* ability to produce inflammatory mediators and the serum concentrations of inflammatory molecules has been studied.

Some studies have focused on the *in vitro* response of macrophages isolated from rats fed cocoa. It has been demonstrated that these cells produced lower amounts of TNF-α, IL-6, NO, and ROS (Ramiro-Puig et al., 2007a; Castell et al., 2009). Similarly, serum concentration of MCP-1 decreased after a cocoa diet in rats (Ramos-Romero et al., 2012a).

With regard to studies in humans, it has been reported that a supplementation with cocoa products in healthy humans did not affect inflammation markers (Mathur et al., 2002); however, a cross-sectional analysis showed that the regular intake of dark chocolate by a healthy population in Southern Italy was inversely related to serum C-reactive protein concentration (di Giuseppe et al., 2008). In addition, cocoa consumption for 4 weeks decreased some adhesion molecules involved in the recruitment of inflammatory cells (Monagas et al., 2009). More recently, leukocytes from healthy volunteers showed a decrease in the activation of NF-κB and also in the serum concentrations of some adhesion molecules, such as intercellular adhesion molecule 1 and E-selectin, 6 h after receiving 40 g of cocoa powder (Vázquez-Agell et al., 2013).

COCOA DIET AND INFLAMMATORY DISEASES

Although at present no human intervention studies applying cocoa treatment in inflammatory conditions have been reported, some studies in animal models of diseases suggest the anti-inflammatory effect of cocoa. In this context, the oral administration of a cocoa polyphenolic fraction to mice has seen to inhibit ear edema in a dose-dependent manner (Lee et al., 2006a). Moreover, rats that received cocoa for a week (4.8 g/kg/day) developed a lower paw edema induced by carrageenan and by bradykinin (Ramos-Romero et al., 2008; Castell et al., 2009).

The anti-inflammatory activity of cocoa has been extended to inflammatory bowel disease (IBD). Using IBD models, a number of flavonoids, such as quercitrin, rutin, diosmin, hesperidin, morin, and silymarin have demonstrated anti-inflammatory activity (reviewed in Comalada et al., 2013). However, a study using a cocoa diet in a dextran sodium sulfate (DSS) model demonstrated that cocoa intake did not improve clinical colitis, although it certainly contributed to reducing colonic oxidative activity and serum inflammatory mediator concentrations (Pérez-Berezo et al., 2012a). These results agree with those obtained with luteolin and with a lemon verbena infusion rich in polyphenolic compounds (Karrasch et al., 2007; Lenoir et al., 2011). More interestingly, it has recently been reported that a polyphenol-enriched cocoa extract was able to decrease acute DSS colitis in mice (Andújar et al., 2011), thus evidencing the need for a high polyphenol content in the cocoa to achieve anti-inflammatory activity in the IBD.

The effect of a cocoa diet on *in vivo* models of neuronal inflammation and systemic chronic inflammation such as adjuvant arthritis (AA) and collagen-induced arthritis (CIA) has also been reported. Rats fed a diet enriched with cocoa produced a decrease in the inflammatory response to an acute and chronic noxious stimulus of trigeminal ganglion neurons (Cady and Durham, 2010).

In AA, a cocoa-enriched diet was able to decrease the synthesis of antibodies against the pathology inducer, and to reduce the proportion of Th lymphocytes in blood and regional lymphoid tissues, but the cocoa diet produced only a tendency to modulate hind-paw swelling (Ramos-Romero et al., 2012b). It must be added that the oral administration of some flavonoids such as quercetin and hesperidin were only able to partially reduce AA swelling (Mamani-Matsuda et al., 2006; Li et al., 2010) or only slightly decreased this chronic inflammatory model (Rovenský et al., 2009). However, a cocoa diet was able to reduce the oxidative stress associated with AA (Ramos-Romero et al., 2012c).

Concerning the CIA model in rats, a diet enriched in cocoa beginning 2 weeks before CIA induction and given throughout the process, has been applied. Although arthritic cocoa-fed rats decreased specific autoantibody titers, the production of pro-inflammatory mediators from peritoneal macrophages, and the Th proportion in lymph nodes, they developed a similar hind-paw swelling as the reference arthritic animals (Ramos-Romero et al., 2012a). On the contrary, Miyake et al. (2008) reported that the oral administration of highly oligomeric procyanidins isolated from Jatoba (*Hymenaea courbaril*) ameliorated CIA in mice and also decreased the serum concentrations of some specific autoantibodies. Similarly, the oral consumption of an extract of green tea polyphenols reduced the incidence, the arthritis index and the autoantibody concentration of CIA in mice (Haqqi et al., 1999). Similarly, single flavonoids administered orally, such as hesperidin, resulted in preventive and therapeutic effects in mice CIA (Kawaguchi et al., 2006).

COCOA AND LYMPHOID TISSUES

Primary and secondary lymphoid tissues constitute two major categories of lymphoid organs. The formation of the primary

as thymus and bone marrow. Secondary lymphoid tissues are responsible for the coordination of immune responses by spatially organizing the interaction of immune effector cells (Drayton et al., 2006). By means of preclinical studies in rats, it has been evidenced that a cocoa diet can induce changes in the cell composition of both primary and secondary lymphoid organs. In particular, a cocoa diet has an influence on the proportion of B lymphocytes and T cell subsets, i.e., T cell receptor (TCR) $\alpha\beta^+$ cells, TCR$\gamma\delta^+$ cells, T helper (Th), cells and T cytotoxic (Tc) cells (**Figure 1**).

A cocoa diet influences antioxidant status and the cell composition of rat thymus. A diet containing 10% cocoa in rats increased the thymic content of catalase and superoxide dismutase and promoted the progression of immature thymocytes (double negative TCR$\alpha\beta^{low}$ and double positive TCR$\alpha\beta^{low}$ cells) toward more mature T cell stages ($CD4^+CD8^-$ TCR$\alpha\beta^{high}$ cells; Ramiro-Puig et al., 2007b). Similarly, a diet with 10% cocoa was able to influence a secondary lymphoid tissue such as the rat spleen and lymph nodes (**Figure 1**). Young rats fed cocoa decreased the spleen percentage of Th cells while increasing that of B cells (Ramiro-Puig et al., 2007a). Additionally, adult Louvain rats fed 10% cocoa for 6 weeks reduced the proportion of TCR$\alpha\beta^+$ cells in inguinal lymph nodes (Ramos-Romero et al., 2012a). Likewise, the percentage of Th cells was reduced in mesenteric lymph nodes (MLNs) at the expense of Tc cells that increased in young Wistar rats fed 10% cocoa for 3 weeks, but not 4% cocoa (Ramiro-Puig et al., 2008; **Figure 1**). A high-cocoa diet also affects the lymphocyte composition of intestinal Peyer's patches (PPs). In particular, cocoa intake reduced the TCR$\alpha\beta^+$ cell percentage, mainly due to a decrease in the Th cell proportion, and increased B cell and TCR$\gamma\delta^+$ cell percentages (Ramiro-Puig et al., 2008; **Figure 1**). The increase in TCR$\gamma\delta^+$ cell percentages in PPs and MLNs induced by cocoa is similar to the effects of apple polyphenol intake in healthy mice (Akiyama et al., 2005) and could be especially important during childhood, when the immune system is maturing (Pérez-Cano et al., 2005), or in the prevention of food allergies.

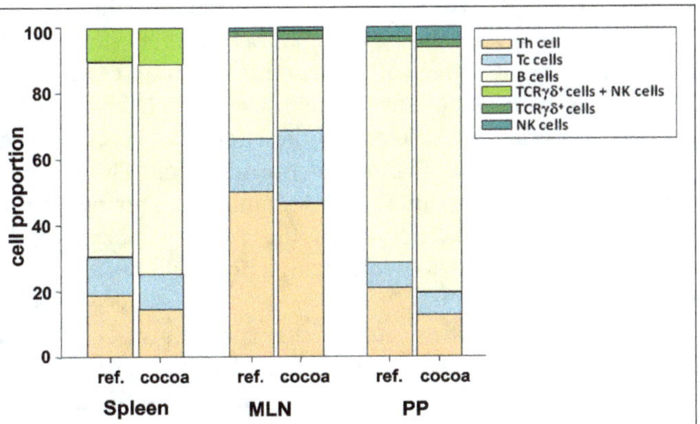

FIGURE 1 | Summary of the effects of a 10% cocoa diet in rats on lymphocyte proportion in secondary lymphoid tissues (based on Ramiro-Puig et al., 2007a, 2008). MLN, mesenteric lymph nodes; PP, Peyer's patches.

The adaptive immune response is an intricate reaction comprising a number of intracellular and intercellular events from the antigen entry until the development of effector mechanisms. Dendritic cells (DC), acting as antigen-presenting cells, take up, process and present antigen to TCR-specific Th lymphocytes. The interaction between DC and Th cells involves a lot of co-stimulatory molecules thus forming the immune synapses (Dustin and Groves, 2012). Next, Th lymphocytes proliferate and differentiate, becoming effector cells such as Th1, Th2, Th17, or regulatory T cells that produce cytokines. Some of these cytokines involve the activation of other antigen-specific cells such as Tc cells or B cells. Activated B cells differentiate into plasma cells, which synthesize antibodies that specifically bind the antigen that has triggered the adaptive immune response.

The first event in adaptive response refers to Th cell activation. Specific recognition of antigenic peptide by TCR together with co-stimulatory molecules causes production of IL-2 (Malek, 2008). IL-2 binds to a receptor consisting of the subunits α, β, and γ (CD25, CD122, and CD132, respectively) to produce cell proliferation (Boyman and Sprent, 2012). CD25 is expressed after Th cell activation. The binding of IL-2 to its receptor leads to the stimulation of complex transduction signals involving mitogen-activated protein kinase (MAPK), Janus kinase/signal transducer and activator of transcription (JAK/STAT), and phosphatidylinositide 3-kinase (PI3K)/Akt pathways that eventually mediates multiple biological processes including T cell and B cell growth and differentiation (Malek, 2008; Boyman and Sprent, 2012).

COCOA AND Th CELL ACTIVATION

IL-2 and CD25 are markers of early lymphocyte T activation. Some *in vitro* studies have reported the effect of isolated cocoa flavonoids and cocoa extracts in the synthesis of IL-2. Sanbongi et al. (1997) found that cocoa liquor polyphenols inhibited both IL-2 gene expression and IL-2 secretion in human blood T cells. Likewise, Mao et al. (1999, 2000) showed that a crude cocoa extract and pentamer, hexamer and heptamer procyanidins from cocoa also reduced IL-2 transcription in phytohemagglutinin (PHA)-stimulated human PBMC. Similarly, in a lymphoid cell line activated with phorbol 12-myristate 13-acetate (PMA) and IL-1 and cultured in the presence of epicatechin or a cocoa extract, it has been established that cocoa flavonoids were able to decrease the expression of surface CD25 and to diminish IL-2 secretion (Ramiro et al., 2005b). The ability of the cocoa extract to decrease CD25 expression was higher than that of epicatechin alone, which may be due to the effect of other cocoa flavanols (Ramiro et al., 2005b). Overall, these *in vitro* studies agree that cocoa flavonoids can decrease IL-2 production in Th cells. These results are also in line with those described with other flavonoids, such as genistein (Atluru et al., 1991) and Pycnogenol® (Cho et al., 2001). How cocoa flavonoids modulate IL-2 gene is not known but it has been demonstrated that epicatechin and dimeric procyanidins decrease NF-κB activation on PMA-activated Jurkat cells, a lymphoid cell line (Mackenzie et al., 2004). The inhibition of NF-κB might mediate the downregulation of both IL-2 and CD25 in a similar way to that of the decrease in pro-inflammatory mediators.

It is interesting to note the effect of cocoa procyanidins on the plasma membrane of Jurkat T cells. After the adsorption of flavonoids, the plasma membrane became more fluid, and procyanidins prevented the leakage of small molecules from vesicles (Verstraeten et al., 2004). These effects could also influence the establishment of immune synapses thus attenuating the interaction between the Th cell and the antigen-presenting cell.

In spite of the *in vitro* results, *in vivo* studies do not confirm the downregulation of IL-2 by cocoa flavonoids. Some studies carried out in rats showed the effect of a diet containing cocoa on the functionality of immune cells isolated from spleen or lymph nodes. Splenocytes from rats fed cocoa (a diet with either 4 or 10% defatted cocoa) did not decrease IL-2 production or CD25 surface expression after stimulation with PMA plus ionomycin (Ramiro-Puig et al., 2007a; Pérez-Berezo et al., 2009). Likewise, these cells showed a similar or even higher proliferative response (Ramiro-Puig et al., 2007a). In the same way, lymphocytes from cocoa-fed rat MLN produced higher or equal amounts of IL-2 (Ramiro-Puig et al., 2008; Pérez-Berezo et al., 2009; Ramos-Romero et al., 2012b).

COCOA AND EFFECTOR T CELLS

After naïve Th cell activation and proliferation, effector Th lymphocytes appear. Depending on the cytokines released to the medium, which are eventually related to the antigen that trigger the immune response, activated Th1 cells, Th2 cells, Th17 cells, or regulatory T cells result (Nakayama and Yamashita, 2008; Amsen et al., 2009; Korn et al., 2009). Th1 cells direct cell-mediated immunity against intracellular pathogens by means of the synthesis and release of interferon (IFN)-γ, TNF-α, and TNF-β, among others. These cytokines promote phagocytosis and cytotoxicity recruiting macrophages, natural killer (NK) cells, Tc cells, and also the enhancement of complement-activating antibodies synthesis. Th1 activity is usually associated with inflammation (Nakayama and Yamashita, 2008). Th2 cells are designed to fight against extracellular pathogens, activating mast cells and eosinophils, and the production of antibodies which are not able to activate the complement system. Th2 cells are involved in the humoral immunity and allergic reactions (Nakayama and Yamashita, 2008). The Th2 subset produces cytokines such as IL-4 and IL-5 that help B cells to proliferate and differentiate, and IL-10 with anti-inflammatory properties. IL-4 is mainly produced by activated Th2 cells and plays an important role in regulating Th1/Th2 balance (Nakayama and Yamashita, 2008). Recently, the effectors Th cell family expanded with the discovery of Th17 cells. These cells produce IL-17 and exhibit effector functions distinct from Th1 and Th2 cells. The primary function of Th17 cells appears to be the clearance of pathogens that are not adequately handled by Th1 or Th2 cells and they are potent inducers of tissue inflammation (Korn et al., 2009).

The effect of cocoa diets in rats on the cytokine production by Th1 and Th2 cells has been reported. The secretion of IFN-γ, the main cytokine related to Th1 activity, has been quantified in cells isolated from the spleen and lymph nodes of rats fed a cocoa diet. No changes in the secretion of this cytokine were observed in splenocytes (Ramiro-Puig et al., 2007a; Ramos-Romero et al., 2012b), although others found increased values (Pérez-Berezo et al., 2009), and *in vitro* studies demonstrated a suppression of IFN-γ production by PHA-stimulated PBMC (Jenny et al., 2009).

More interestingly, a cocoa diet in rats produced a lower IL-4 secretion in isolated splenocytes (Ramiro-Puig et al., 2007a; Pérez-Berezo et al., 2009) and MLN cells (Ramiro-Puig et al., 2008). However, IL-10 secretion was not modified in rats fed a cocoa diet (Ramiro-Puig et al., 2007a, 2008). The results obtained in these *in vivo* experiments did not exactly fit with those obtained in *in vitro* studies with cocoa flavonoids. Thus, an increase in IL-4 secretion after epicatechin addition in a lymphoid cell line and PBMC has been reported (Mao et al., 2000; Ramiro et al., 2005b), whereas hexamer to octamer cocoa procyanidins presented an inhibitory effect on this cytokine (Mao et al., 2000).

COCOA AND HUMORAL IMMUNE RESPONSE

As stated before, an increase in the percentage of B cells in spleen was observed in rats fed cocoa (**Figure 1**). However, the antibody response of these cells has been found to be attenuated. Thus, the ability to produce IgG, IgM, and IgA by splenocytes from rats fed cocoa was depressed (Ramiro-Puig et al., 2007a). This effect was also reflected in serum immunoglobulin concentrations. Three-week-old rats fed with 10% cocoa for 3 weeks, but not those fed 4% cocoa, had lower serum IgG, IgM, and IgA concentrations (Ramiro-Puig et al., 2007a; Pérez-Berezo et al., 2012b). However, when the cocoa diet began later and the dose was lower, the effect was not so patent (Pérez-Berezo et al., 2011).

The influence of a 4 and 10% cocoa diet on the antibody synthesis in immunized rats has been reported. When animals were fed cocoa before and during an immunization process, the synthesis of specific antibodies and the number of IgG-secreting cells decreased, although the proliferation rate of lymph node and spleen cells was maintained (Pérez-Berezo et al., 2009). The analysis of antibodies demonstrated that the impact on humoral response did not affect all antibody isotypes equally. The most attenuated isotypes were specific IgM, IgG1, IgG2a, and IgG2c whereas anti-OVA IgG2b concentrations held steady or increased with the 10% cocoa diet. IgG isotypes can be associated with Th1 or Th2 immunity. In the rat, IgG1 and IgG2a are related to the Th2 response, while IgG2b depends on the Th1 response (Binder et al., 1995; Gracie and Bradley, 1996; Saoudi et al., 1999; Bridle et al., 2007). These results agree with others that evaluated certain food polyphenols, such as those from apple or soybean (Akiyama et al., 2005; Kogiso et al., 2006). From all these results, it has been suggested that a cocoa diet mainly downregulates the Th2 immune response, whereas it maintains Th1 immunity. This hypothesis was supported by a lower IL-4 secretion from splenocytes and a higher production of IFN-γ from lymph node cells (Pérez-Berezo et al., 2009).

Because of a cocoa diet seems to attenuate antibody synthesis, it has been tested in experimental disease models in which antibodies play a pathogenic role, such as autoimmune diseases and allergic processes.

Rheumatoid arthritis (RA) is a systemic autoimmune disease in which chronic inflammation of synovial joints results in joint destruction, pain, disability, and a reduced life expectancy (Wegner et al., 2010). The pathology of the RA is mediated by specific autoantibodies, mainly against citrullinated proteins such as collagen type II (Wegner et al., 2010). In consequence, CIA in rats or mice is the gold standard *in vivo* model for RA studies (Asquith et al., 2009). In such rat experimental model, the influence of a cocoa diet on joint inflammation and autoantibody titers has been reported (Ramos-Romero et al., 2012a). Louvain rats fed cocoa from 2 weeks before arthritis induction, and during the disease period studied (4 weeks), reduced the synthesis of specific antibodies against type-II collagen, but this effect was not enough to mitigate the hind-paw swelling in arthritic animals during the study period (Ramos-Romero et al., 2012a).

Allergic reactions are mainly caused by IgE-mediated hypersensitivity. In allergic patients, the immune system reacts to innocuous substances by producing IgE. These antibodies bind to mast cells and, after allergen reaction, produce degranulation of mast cell mediators with a subsequent generation of allergic manifestations (Amim, 2012). The effect of cocoa in an allergy model has been preclinically studied. A diet containing 10% cocoa prevented the synthesis of antibodies involved in allergic reaction in young rats, in particular, rats fed a cocoa diet showed lower titers of specific IgG1, IgG2a and a decrease of specific IgE of about 60–70% (Abril-Gil et al., 2012). The effect of a cocoa diet on allergic manifestations has not yet been established. However, it is noteworthy that the modulation of specific IgE was also observed in allergy models after treatment with flavonoids, and in these studies the effect on IgE synthesis was associated with lower allergy signs. This is the case in treatment with luteolin (Das et al., 2003), baicalin (Won Jung et al., 2012), biochanin A (Ko et al., 2011), quercetin (Cruz et al., 2012), myricetin (Medeiros et al., 2008), and hesperidin (Rogerio et al., 2007; Joskova et al., 2011). In addition, it can be added that clinical trials applying a treatment with Pycnogenol®, an extract of *Pinus maritime* containing procyanidins, demonstrated the efficacy of such intervention in reducing some signs of allergic asthma (Hosseini et al., 2001; Lau et al., 2004; Belcaro et al., 2011). From all these studies it can be concluded that foods enriched in flavonoids, such as cocoa, open a new perspective in their use as a nutraceutical in allergic diseases.

EFFECTS OF COCOA ON INTESTINAL IMMUNITY

The digestive system is the first compartment reached by dietary compounds. Bacteria, epithelial cells, and immune cells in the intestine are the first ones to be affected by diet. Every day, the gut-associated lymphoid tissue (GALT), which constitutes the most extensive and complex part of the immune system in the body, receives a huge antigenic load and has to distinguish between invasive pathogens and innocuous antigens from food and commensal bacteria. Briefly, the intestinal immune response is initiated in the M cells from PPs which uptake luminal antigens and transport them toward DC, which interact with interfollicular T lymphocytes or migrate toward MLN (Cerutti and Rescigno, 2008). This process induces differentiation and maturation of B cells, which become IgA^{+} cells and later IgA-secreting cells (Kunisawa and Kiyono, 2005). The main resulting product of the GALT is the secretory-IgA (S-IgA; Mora and von Andrian, 2008; Brandtzaeg, 2010). This immunoglobulin constitutes the first line of non-inflammatory immune protection at mucosal surfaces by neutralizing microbial pathogens and exotoxins and by interacting with innocuous dietary antigens and commensal microbes (Corthésy, 2007; MacPherson et al., 2008).

Few studies addressing the dietary effects of cocoa on GALT function in healthy animals or humans have been reported to date. Dietary intervention with cocoa did not morphologically affect the intestinal structure (Ramiro-Puig et al., 2008), but is capable of modifying some important aspects of the GALT composition and functionality in rats as next detailed (Ramiro-Puig et al., 2008; Pérez-Berezo et al., 2011, 2012b; **Figure 2**).

COCOA DIET AND MESENTERIC LYMPH NODE LYMPHOCYTE ACTIVATION

Rat interventional nutrition with a cocoa diet modulates MLN lymphocyte activation in certain conditions. Isolated MLN cells from young rats fed 10% cocoa for 3 weeks strongly enhanced IL-2 secretion; nevertheless, the proliferation rate did not increase after 48 h of cell culture (Ramiro-Puig et al., 2008). On the other hand, isolated MLN lymphocytes from rats fed a long-term cocoa diet (9 weeks) did not change IL-2 production after *in vitro* mitogen activation nor their proliferative ability after *in vitro*-specific activation (Pérez-Berezo et al., 2009).

To ascertain whether cocoa modified Th effector cell functionality in the GALT, IFNγ, IL-4, and IL-10 cytokine production was studied in stimulated MLN cells isolated from animals fed a cocoa diet (Ramiro-Puig et al., 2008). The nutritional 10% cocoa intervention for 3 weeks resulted in a lower IL-4 secretion, IL-10 secretion tended to decrease whereas that of IFN-γ tended to increase. A 4% cocoa intake for 3 weeks did not produce any significant modification (Ramiro-Puig et al., 2008). These results suggest that high-cocoa diets, similarly to the results found in the systemic compartment, downregulate Th2 responses, and therefore, may downregulate B cell differentiation and immunoglobulin production even at mucosal sites.

COCOA AND SECRETORY-IgA

Secretory-IgA plays a key role in the maintenance of gut homeostasis and oral tolerance and its function and production are tightly regulated (Cerutti and Rescigno, 2008). The relationship between a cocoa diet and S-IgA has been demonstrated in different experimental designs using rats, where the effect of varied proportions of cocoa diets (2, 4, 5, and 10%), different age at the beginning of the dietary nutritional (3 or 6 weeks of age) and length of diet (3, 6, or 9 weeks) have been analyzed. As demonstrated next, cocoa reduces S-IgA protein and gene expression which conduces a different pattern of IgA-coating bacteria. The effect of cocoa on S-IgA might be due to the influence of cocoa on genes related to Th maturation, Th–B cell interactions, and IgA^{+} B cell gut-homing, among others (Pérez-Berezo et al., 2011, 2012b).

First data showing a downmodulatory effect of cocoa on S-IgA were established in fecal samples after 2 weeks of both 4 and 10% cocoa intake in young rats. However, this effect only remained for 3 weeks in the 10% cocoa diet. The decrease in fecal IgA correlated with a lower concentration of S-IgA and S-IgM in gut washes (Ramiro-Puig et al., 2008). These results were confirmed in a study that extended the dietary intervention with a 10% cocoa diet up to 6 weeks (Pérez-Berezo et al., 2012b). If dietary intervention began later in rat age (6-week-old animals), the attenuating effect of

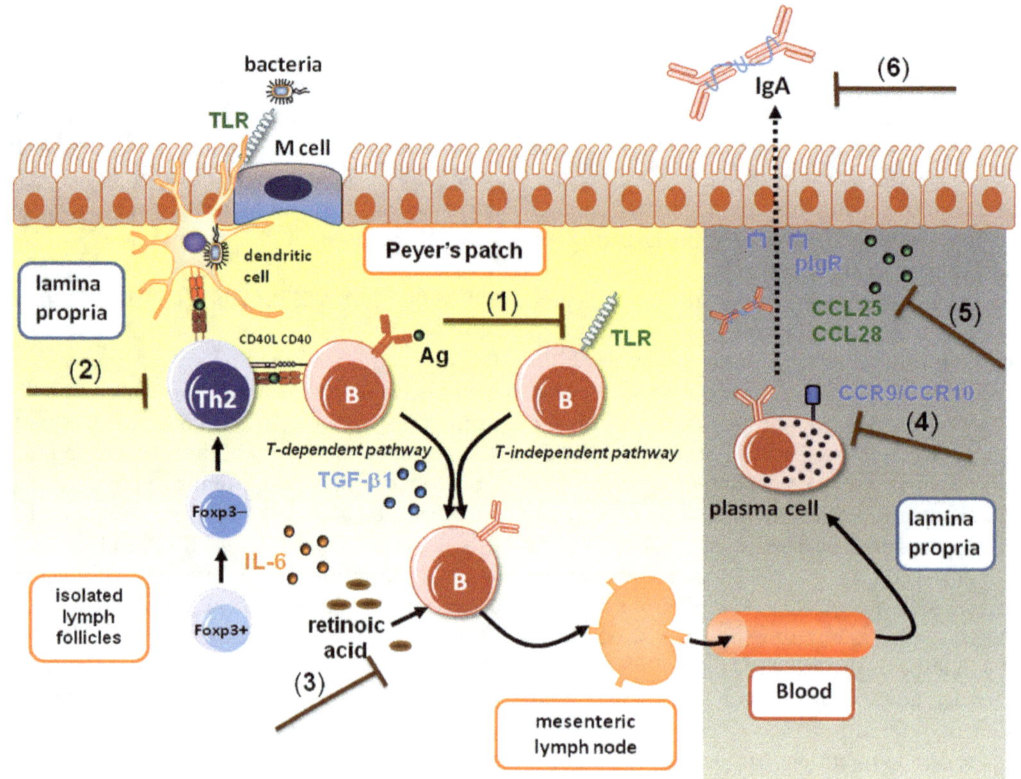

FIGURE 2 | Summary of the effects of a 10% cocoa diet in rat's gut-associated lymphoid tissue (Ramiro-Puig et al., 2008; Fagarasan et al., 2010; Pérez-Berezo et al., 2011; Pérez-Berezo et al., 2012b). Generation of S-IgA can be developed by a T cell-dependent process initiated in Peyer's patches or by a T cell-independent mechanism in isolated lymphoid follicles and lamina propria. Both mechanisms lead to the induction of IgA^+ B cells which migrate to blood and come back to the gut lamina propria where they differentiate into plasma cells and produce S-IgA. The mechanisms showing how cocoa modulates immune response are shown in the figure with numbers in brackets, and as follows: cocoa induces a differential pattern of Toll-like receptor (TLR) gene expression (1) which may interfere with both dependent and independent pathways. Moreover, Th2 development and conventional B–T cell interactions through major histocompatibility complex (MHC)-TCR and CD40–CD40L are also modulated by cocoa (2). The preferential generation of IgA^+ B cells is caused by the abundant production of activated TGF-β1. Cocoa compounds also influence the migration of IgA^+ B cells into the gut lamina propria, by modifying the expression of some chemokines (CCL25, CCL28) (5) or their receptors (CCR9) (4) whose expression depends on retinoic acid (3). As a result, the amount of S-IgA in the intestinal lumen in cocoa-fed animals is markedly reduced (6).

cocoa remained for 5 and 10% cocoa diet, showing a rapid effect even 1 week after the diet start (Pérez-Berezo et al., 2011). However, a lower cocoa proportion (2%) tended to reduce fecal IgA levels after only 3 weeks of diet. Therefore, cocoa diets, especially those with a higher cocoa proportion, decreased S-IgA concentration in the intestinal lumen of rats (Ramiro-Puig et al., 2008). This effect was associated with a lower number of PP cells with a high capacity to secrete IgA (Ramiro-Puig et al., 2008), and with a downregulation of IgA gene expression in PP cells and in the wall of the small intestine and colon (Pérez-Berezo et al., 2011, 2012b; Massot-Cladera et al., 2012).

Some commensal intestinal bacteria in humans and rodents coat S-IgA by an apparent non-random immunological phenomenon (Tsuruta et al., 2010). In fecal samples from rats collected before and after a cocoa diet, the IgA-coating bacteria were enumerated. After 6 weeks, reference animals showed an increase in the percentage of IgA-coating bacteria that was avoided with the 10% cocoa diet (Massot-Cladera et al., 2012).

In order to look further into the downregulation of S-IgA through a cocoa diet in rats, the gene expression of several molecules involved in intestinal immune response was established using different cocoa proportions (2, 5, and 10%), supplementation periods (3 or 6 weeks) and initial age of rats (3 or 6 weeks; Pérez-Berezo et al., 2011, 2012b). A pathway for B cells to become IgA-secretory cells is a T cell-dependent process located in either PPs or MLNs, inductive sites of the intestinal immune system (Kunisawa and Kiyono, 2005; Mora and von Andrian, 2008). The maturation of mucosal Th cells depends on IL-6, among others; the interaction between activated Th cells and B cells requires the interaction of CD40 ligand with CD40 (Islam et al., 1991; Cerutti, 2008), and the differentiation of B cells into IgA^+ B cells involves transforming growth factor-β1 (TGF-β1), IL-5, IL-6, IL-10, and IL-21 (Schoenbeck et al., 1989; Brière et al., 1994; Ramsay et al., 1994; Dullaers et al., 2009). The study of a 10% cocoa diet for 3 or 6 weeks in rats on the mechanisms of S-IgA secretion revealed that the cocoa diet did not modify TGF-β1 gene expression in PPs, MLNs, or the small intestine; however, IL-6 gene expression was reduced ~95% in MLNs after 6 weeks of a 10% cocoa diet (Pérez-Berezo et al., 2012b) but not earlier (Pérez-Berezo et al., 2011). Likewise, cocoa intake did not modify CD40 gene expression either in PPs or in MLNs (Pérez-Berezo et al., 2012b), which is in accordance with previous studies that have shown that a cocoa diet increased the proportion of B cells in PPs (Ramiro-Puig et al., 2008); however, a 10% cocoa diet (but not lower proportions) for 6 weeks (but not in a shorter period), reduced CD40 gene expression in the small intestine (Pérez-Berezo et al., 2011, 2012b).

When IgA^+ B cells become activated they leave PPs, go to the bloodstream and come back to the intestine or other mucosa (MacPherson et al., 2008; Brandtzaeg, 2010). The gut-homing system requires the integrin $\alpha4\beta7$ and some chemokine receptors on activated gut lymphocytes (Mora and von Andrian, 2008). Chemokines produced by epithelial cells such as CCL25 and CCL28 interact with the chemokine receptors CCR9 and CCR10 respectively, to recruit IgA^+ B cells (Hieshima et al., 2004). The CCR9 expression on IgA^+ B cells is induced by retinoic acid (Mora et al., 2006) through its ligation to nuclear retinoic acid receptors (RAR; Ross et al., 2009). Diets containing 2, 5, or 10% cocoa for 3 weeks in 6-week-old animals did not affect the gene expression of CCR9, CCL25, RARα, or RARβ but increased the CCL28 gene expression in the small intestine wall (Pérez-Berezo et al., 2011). The increase in the CCL28 gene expression could reflect a "rescue mechanism" to strongly attract the IgA^+ B cells to the gut, in an attempt to compensate the S-IgA downregulation. When the cocoa diet began earlier and lasted longer (3-week-old animals fed 10% cocoa for 6 weeks), the gene expression of gut-homing molecules such as RAR, CCR9, and CCL28, but not CCL25, was downregulated in the small intestine (Pérez-Berezo et al., 2012b). Overall, these results demonstrate the longer the cocoa intake the greater the sensitivity of gut-homing mechanisms in the intestine.

Finally, when IgA^+ B cells reach the intestine, they differentiate into IgA-secreting cells mainly releasing dimers of IgA. This immunoglobulin is actively secreted to the apical surface of epithelial cells by a polymeric immunoglobulin receptor (pIgR) expressed on the basolateral surface of epithelial cells (Cerutti and Rescigno, 2008). The gene expression of pIgR was not modified by any cocoa diet given for 3 or 6 weeks (Pérez-Berezo et al., 2011, 2012b).

In summary, a high-cocoa diet induces a lower number of IgA^+ B cells reaching the intestinal lamina propria by downregulating either the expression of chemokine or that of their receptors (**Figure 2**). However, in the gut lamina propria some other mechanisms remain working efficiently.

COCOA AND BACTERIA RECOGNITION

The GALT maintains mucosal homeostasis by inducing a state of non-responsiveness to innocuous antigens, such as commensal bacteria, or by responding actively to counteract pathogens (Fagarasan et al., 2010). In this regard, toll-like receptors (TLRs), through the recognition of conserved molecular motifs on microorganisms, are important molecules involved in the cross-talk between microorganisms and gut epithelial and immune cells (Abreu, 2010). It has been reported that the generation of IgA^+ B cells can be independent of Th cells and involve TLR non-specific recognition (Fagarasan et al., 2010). In this context, cocoa diets in rats have shown differential TLR expression patterns for TLR2, TLR4, TLR7, and TLR9 in PPs, MLNs, the small intestine and colon (Pérez-Berezo et al., 2011, 2012b; Massot-Cladera et al., 2012).

A high (10%) and continuous cocoa diet produced an upregulation of TLR4 and TLR9 and a downregulation of TLR2 and TLR7 in PPs and MLNs (inductor sites of intestinal immune response; Pérez-Berezo et al., 2011, 2012b). Conversely, in the small intestine and the colon, cocoa-fed animals showed lower TLR4 and TLR9 and higher TLR2 and TLR7 gene expression (Massot-Cladera et al., 2012; Pérez-Berezo et al., 2012b). TLR4 expression is positively correlated to the number of IgA-secreting cells in the lamina propria and their recruitment through CCL28 (Shang et al., 2008; Abreu, 2010). In consequence, the downregulation of TLR4 through a cocoa diet in the intestine (as effector site) could be associated with the decrease in S-IgA in feces.

Toll-like receptors are expressed preferentially in tissues that are in constant contact with microorganisms (Cario, 2005; Abreu, 2010). Therefore, changes in the TLR expression could reflect changes in the intestinal microbiota and/or its relation to intestinal immune cells (Shibolet and Podolsky, 2007).

INFLUENCE OF COCOA ON GUT MICROBIOTA

The above data demonstrate that cocoa-enriched diets in rats influence the intestinal immune system either through a direct effect on intestinal immune cells and/or an indirect effect mediated by changes in microbiota which would influence the cross-talk with the host (i.e., through TLR). Therefore, it remained to be seen whether cocoa diets modulated microbiota composition and, consequently, the intestinal immune system. This is possible due that cocoa flavonoids reaching the colon can interact with intestinal microbiota through a bidirectional relationship. Thus, bacteria can be involved in the polyphenol metabolism, and flavonoids can influence microbiota growth and composition (Hayek, 2013). In this context, changes in intestinal microbiota composition may influence the immune system as well as the compounds originated by the bacterial metabolism (**Figure 3**).

COCOA FLAVONOIDS METABOLISM

Cocoa flavonoids have a particular bacterial metabolism due to the high degree of polymerization of its flavanols. After cocoa intake, monomers (i.e., catechin and epicatechin) are rapidly absorbed in the small intestine, while the largest proportion of dietary polyphenols (90–95%) in the form of oligomers and polymers (i.e., cocoa procyanidins) pass intact through the gastrointestinal tract, reaching the colon (Monagas et al., 2010). This fact allows them to be metabolized by the intestinal microbiota (**Figure 3**). Colonic bacteria is composed of more than 500 species and a bacterial load of approximately 10^{11} to 10^{12} bacteria/g of colonic contents (O'Hara and Shanahan, 2006). It is known that microbiota has the ability to metabolize polyphenols to simpler metabolites and this conversion is often essential for absorption and modulates the biological activities of these compounds which are more beneficial than the original forms found in food (Clifford, 2004; Tzounis et al., 2008; Selma et al., 2009; Monagas et al., 2010; Neilson and Ferruzzi, 2011).

Cocoa polyphenols are extensively degraded in the colon by a broad range of reactions able to generate various phenolic

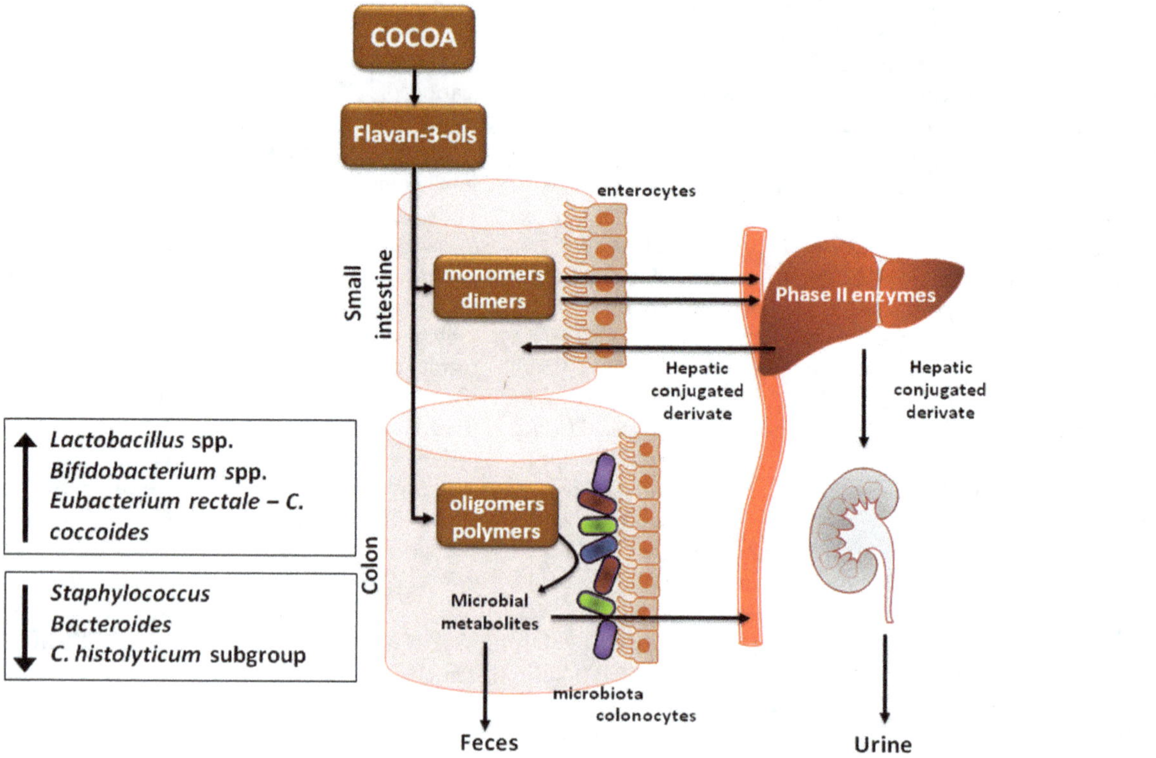

FIGURE 3 | Metabolic route of consumed cocoa flavonoids, and effect on intestinal microbiota (based on Tzounis et al., 2008, 2011; Monagas et al., 2010; Massot-Cladera et al., 2012). Flavanol monomers and dimers are absorbed in the small intestine, while procyanidins reach the colon and are metabolized by the intestinal microbiota into various phenolic acids that are later absorbed. Absorbed compounds are metabolized in the liver and subsequently eliminated in urine. A portion of microbial metabolites is eliminated in the feces. Cocoa flavonoids decrease the proportion of *Bacteroides*, *Staphylococcus* genus, and *C. histolyticum* subgroup whereas they enhance the growth of *Lactobacillus* spp. and *Bifidobacterium* spp., and *Eubacterium rectale–C. coccoides*.

acids, mainly including phenylpropionic, phenylacetic, and benzoic acid derivates (Déprez et al., 2000; Kohri et al., 2003; Aura, 2008; Tzounis et al., 2008; Fogliano et al., 2011). Later, colon bacterial metabolites are absorbed into the bloodstream, providing another source of potentially bioactive compounds (Rios et al., 2003). Once absorbed, the microbial metabolites from flavanols are mainly metabolized in the liver by phase-II enzymes as hepatic conjugated derivatives that are subsequently eliminated in urine (Neilson and Ferruzzi, 2011; **Figure 3**). In particular, the presence of 5-(3′,4′,5′-trihydroxyphenyl)-γ-valerolactone and 5-(3′,4′-dihydroxyphenyl)-γ-valerolactone in urine is considered to be a potential biomarker of flavan-3-ols consumption in humans after cocoa products intake (Urpi-Sarda et al., 2009). At the same time, a portion of microbial metabolites (non-conjugated microbial metabolites) is eliminated in the feces. The excretion of microbial metabolites varies markedly between subjects and, for some individuals, it may also vary with the substrate (Monagas et al., 2010).

Regarding the intestinal bacteria with the ability to catabolize flavanols, a limited number of bacterial species have been identified as being involved in the polyphenols catabolism. Interestingly, the majority of the bacteria characterized belong to the Clostridia group, which is a large component of the gut microbiota (Wang et al., 2001; Tzounis et al., 2008).

COCOA INFLUENCE ON GUT MICROBIOTA COMPOSITION

It is known that unabsorbed dietary phenolics and their metabolites can exert significant effects on the intestinal environment by modulation of the microbiota (Lee et al., 2006b). Although there is limited information concerning the ability of (+)-catechin and (−)-epicatechin, the main monomers present in cocoa, to promote or inhibit the growth of selected intestinal bacteria, there are some *in vitro*, preclinical and clinical studies regarding this subject (Tzounis et al., 2008, 2011; Massot-Cladera et al., 2012).

In vitro studies have shown the antimicrobial properties of some polyphenols (Puupponen-Pimiä et al., 2005; Lee et al., 2006b). To date, Tzounis et al. (2008) showed that (+)-catechin induced an inhibitory effect in the growth of the *Clostridium histolyticum* group using the batch culture approach, at the same time that both (+)-catechin and (−)-epicatechin enhanced the growth rate of the beneficial bacteria group, *Eubacterium rectale–C. coccoides*. Furthermore, there were increases in both *Lactobacillus* spp. and *Bifidobacterium* spp. genus following (+)-catechin exposure, as well as a small but significant increase in the growth of *E. coli* after (+)-catechin incubation (Tzounis et al., 2008; **Figure 3**).

The effects of cocoa polyphenols observed in animal models are partially in line with the above results. Young rats receiving a 10% cocoa intake for 6 weeks showed a significant decrease in the proportion of *Bacteroides*, *Staphylococcus* genus, and *C. histolyticum* subgroup (Massot-Cladera et al., 2012). The effect of this defatted cocoa powder on microbiota was also observed in rats fed for 4 weeks with diets based on cocoa polyphenols-enriched powders (Massot-Cladera et al., 2013).

With regard to human studies, evidence of the effects of cocoa or cocoa products intake on microbiota composition is scarce. A human intervention study evaluated the high-cocoa flavanol consumption effect on microbiota composition from healthy volunteers (Tzounis et al., 2011). The results showed that a 4 weeks daily ingestion of a high-cocoa flavanol beverage containing 494 mg flavanols increased the growth of *Lactobacillus* spp., and *Bifidobacterium* spp. in comparison with a control low-cocoa flavanol drink that contained only 29 mg flavanols (Tzounis et al., 2011). Although these results were not found in the preclinical interventions, it prompted the redefinition of cocoa polyphenols as prebiotics. It is important to mention that divergence between the animal and human data could be ascribed to several factors, such as the cocoa composition (fiber and flavonoids pattern), dose, and differential composition and distribution ecosystem (rats vs human gut). Overall, all these findings strengthen the evidence that cocoa polyphenols can have significant effects on the growth of select gut microbiota (**Figure 3**).

CONCLUDING REMARKS

A cocoa diet has been shown to influence the immune system: in the innate inflammatory response as well as in the adaptive immunity, and in both systemic and intestinal compartments.

From the results concerning the effects of cocoa on inflammatory reaction, it could be concluded that although cocoa demonstrates clear anti-inflammatory properties *in vitro*, when tested *in vivo* results are more controversial. To date, it can be concluded that if inflammation is mild and cocoa has a high polyphenol content, it could help in the resolution of inflammatory response, and, in any case, due to its antioxidant properties, cocoa can be a complementary anti-inflammatory therapy.

Concerning lymphocytes and adaptive immune response, cocoa diet in young rats influences lymphoid tissue composition mainly by decreasing the proportion of Th cells by unknown mechanisms. In addition, the influence of cocoa on the first phases of T lymphocyte activation is not clear. *In vitro* studies show the downregulatory effect of cocoa on IL-2 production, but is not confirmed *in vivo*. When studying effector Th cells, it seems clear that in rat, a diet containing 10% cocoa produces a downregulation of Th2 response. In addition, it is worth noting the effect of this diet in attenuating the synthesis of antibodies. The downregulatory effects of cocoa could then be applied to counteract immune-mediated diseases in which antibodies play a pathogenic role. In autoimmune inflammatory diseases, a cocoa diet does not potently reduce inflammation but counteracts concomitant oxidative stress. More interestingly, a cocoa diet in rats reduces IgE synthesis which could be useful in treating allergic diseases.

In addition to these effects, a cocoa diet also influences the functionality of gut-associated lymphoid tissue. Here, similarly to the results found in the systemic compartment, a cocoa diet in rats downregulates Th2 responses and also the intestinal immunoglobulin production. It has been demonstrated that a cocoa diet influences some intercellular reactions and the gut-homing process of activated cells, resulting, therefore, in an attenuation in the synthesis of S-IgA into the intestinal lumen. Moreover, a cocoa diet is able to modify intestinal microbiota and also the cross-talk between these bacteria and body cells.

All these results allow us to suggest that a cocoa diet could be beneficial in certain immune processes. Further research may elucidate the cocoa compounds involved in such an effect and also the possible medical approaches to these repercussions.

ACKNOWLEDGMENTS

This study was supported by the Ministerio de Ciencia y Tecnología (AGL2008-02790) and the Ministerio de Economía y Competitividad (AGL2011-24279). MM is the recipient of a fellowship from the Generalitat de Catalunya (FI-DGR-401).

REFERENCES

1. Abreu, M. T. (2010). Toll-like recep- tor signaling in the intestinal epithelium: how bacterial recognition shapes intestinal function. *Nat. Rev. Immunol.* 10, 131–144. doi: 10.1038/nri2707
2. Abril-Gil, M., Massot-Cladera, M., Pérez-Cano, F. J., Castellote, C., Franch, A., and Castell, M. (2012). A diet enriched with cocoa prevents IgE synthesis in a rat allergy model. *Pharmacol. Res.* 65, 603–608. doi: 10.1016/j.phrs.2012.02.001
3. Akiyama, H., Sato, Y., Watanabe, T., Nagaoka, M. H., Yoshioka, Y., Shoji, T., et al. (2005). Dietary unripe apple polyphenol inhibits the development of food allergies in murine mod- els. *FEBS Lett.* 579, 4485–4491. doi: 10.1016/j.febslet.2005.07.019
4. Al-Hanbali, M., Ali, D., Bustami, M., Abdel-Malek, S., Al-Hanbali, R., Alhussainy, T., Qadan, F., et al. (2009). Epicatechin suppresses IL-6, IL-8 and enhances IL-10 production with NF-κB nuclear translocation in whole blood stimulated system. *Neuro Endocrinol. Lett.* 30, 131–138.
5. Amim, K. (2012). The role of mast cells in allergic inflamma- tion. *Respir. Med.* 106, 9–14. doi: 10.1016/j.rmed.2011.09.007
6. Amsen, D., Spilianakis, C. G., and Flavell, R. A. (2009). How are TH 1 and TH 2 effector cells made? *Curr. Opin. Immunol.* 21, 153–160. doi: 10.1016/j.coi.2009.03.010
7. Andújar, I., Recio, M. C., Giner, R. M., Cienfuegos-Jovellanos, E., Laghi, S., Muguerza, B., et al. (2011). Inhibi- tion of ulcerative colitis in mice after oral administration of a polyphenol- enriched cocoa extract is mediated by the inhibition of STAT1 and STAT3 phosphorylation in colon cells. *J. Agric. Food Chem.* 59, 6474–6483. doi: 10.1021/jf2008925
8. Asquith, D. L., Miller, A. M., McInnes, I. B., and Liew, F. Y. (2009). Animal models of rheumatoid arthritis. *Eur. J. Immunol.* 39, 2040–2044. doi: 10.1002/eji.200939578
9. Atluru, D., Jackson, T. M., and Atluru, S. (1991). Genistein, a selective protein tyrosine kinase inhibitor, inhibits interleukin-2 and leukotriene B4 production from human mononuclear cells. *Clin. Immunol. Immunopathol.* 59, 379–387. doi: 10.1016/0090- 1229(91)90033-7
10. Aura, A. M. (2008). Microbial metabolism of dietary phenolic com- pounds in the colon. *Phytochem. Rev.* 7, 407–429. doi: 10.1007/s11101-008- 9095-3
11. Belcaro, G., Luzzi, R., Cesinaro Di Rocco, P., Cesarone, M. R., Dugall, M., Feragalli, B., et al. (2011). Pycnogenol® improvements in asthma management. *Panminerva Med.* 53, S57–S64.
12. Binder, J., Graser, E., Hancock, W. W., Wasowaska, B., Sayegh, M. H., Volk, H. D., et al. (1995). Downregulation of intragraft IFN-γ expression cor- relates with increased IgG1 alloanti- body response following intrathymic immunomodulation of sensitized rat recipients. *Transplantation* 60, 1516–1524. doi: 10.1097/00007890- 199560120-00025
13. Boyman, O., and Sprent, J. (2012). The role of interleukin-2 during homeostasis and activation of the immune system. *Nat. Rev. Immunol.* 12, 180–190. doi: 10.1038/nri3156 Brandtzaeg, P. (2010). The mucosal immune system and its integra- tion with the mammary glands. *J. Pedriatr.* 156, S8–S15. doi: 10.1016/j.jpeds.2009.11.014
14. Bridle, B. W., Wilkie, B. N., Jevnikar, A. M., and Mallard, B. A. (2007). Devia- tion of xenogeneic immune response and bystander suppression in rats fed porcine blood mononuclear cells. *Transpl. Immunol.* 17, 262–270. doi: 10.1016/j.trim.2007.01.010
15. Brière, F., Bridon, J. M., Chevet, D., Souillet, G., Bienvenu, F., Guret, C., et al. (1994). Interleukin 10 induces B lymphocytes from IgA-deficient patients to secrete IgA. *J. Clin. Invest.* 94, 97–104. doi: 10.1172/JCI117354

16. Cady, R. J., and Durham, P. L. (2010). Cocoa enriched diets enhance expression of phosphatases and decrease expression of inflamma- tory molecules in trigeminal ganglion neurons. *Brain Res.* 1323, 18–32. doi: 10.1016/j.brainres.2010.01.081
17. Cario, E. (2005). Bacterial inter- actions with cells of the intesti- nal mucosa: Toll-like receptors and NOD2. *Gut.* 54, 1182–1193. doi: 10.1136/gut.2004.062794
18. Castell, M., Franch, A., Ramos- Romero, S., Ramiro-Puig, E., Pérez- Cano, F. J., and Castellote, C. (2009). "Effect of a diet rich in cocoa flavonoids on experimental acute inflammation," in *Flavonoids: Biosynthesis, Biological Effects and Dietary Sources*, ed. R. B. Keller (New York: Nova Science Publishers), 213–229.
19. Cerutti, A. (2008). The regulation of IgA class switching. *Nat. Rev. Immunol.* 8, 421–434. doi: 10.1038/nri2322
20. Cerutti, A., and Rescigno, M. (2008). The biology of intesti- nal immunoglobulin A responses. *Immunity* 28, 740–750. doi: 10.1016/ j.immuni.2008.05.001
21. Cho, K. J., Yun, C. H., Packer, L., and Chung, A. S. (2001). Inhibi- tion mechanisms of bioflavonoids extracted from the bark of *Pinus maritima* on the expression of proin- flammatory cytokines. *Ann. N. Y. Acad. Sci.* 928, 141–156. doi: 10.1111/j.1749-6632.2001.tb05644.x
22. Clifford, M. N. (2004). Diet-derived phenols in plasma and tissues and their implications. *Planta Med.* 70, 1103–1114. doi: 10.1055/s-2004- 835835
23. Comalada, M., Xaus, J., and Gálvez, J. (2013). "Flavonoids and immunomodulation" in *Bioactive Food as Interventions for Arthritis and Related Inflammatory Diseases*, eds R. R. Watson and V. R. Preedy (San Diego, CA: Elsevier), 555–579. doi: 10.1016/B978-0-12-397156-2. 00162-9
24. Corthésy, B. (2007). Roundtrip ticket for secretory IgA: role in mucosal homeostasis? *J. Immunol.* 178, 27–32.
25. Cruz, E. A., Reuter, S., Martin, H., Dehzad, N., Muzitano, M. F., Costa, S. S., et al. (2012). *Kalanchoe pinnata* inhibits mast cell activa- tion and prevents allergic airway dis- ease. *Phytomedicine* 19, 115–121. doi: 10.1016/j.phymed.2011.06.030
26. Das, M., Ram, A., and Ghosh, B. (2003). Luteolin alleviates bron- choconstriction and airway hyperre- activity in ovalbumin sensitized mice. *Inflamm. Res.* 52, 101–106. doi: 10.1007/s000110300021
27. Déprez, S., Brezillon, C., Rabot, S., Philippe, C., Mila, I., Lapierre, C., et al. (2000). Polymeric proan- thocyanidins are catabolized by human colonic microflora into low- molecular-weight phenolic acids. *J. Nutr.* 130, 2733–2738.
28. di Giuseppe, R., Di Castelnuovo, A., Centritto, F., Zito, F., De Curtis, A., Costanzo, S., et al. (2008). Regu- lar consumption of dark chocolate is associated with low serum concen- trations of C reactive protein in a healthy Italian population. *J. Nutr.* 138, 1939–1945.
29. Drayton, D. L., Liao, S., Mounzer, R. H., and Ruddle, N. H. (2006). Lymphoid organ development: from ontogeny to neogenesis. *Nat. Immunol.* 7, 344- 353. doi: 10.1038/ni1330
30. Dullaers, M., Li, D., Xue, Y., Ni, L., Gayet, I., Morita, R., et al. (2009). A T cell-dependent mechanism for the induction of human mucosal homing immunoglobulin A-secreting plas- mablasts. *Immunity.* 30, 120–129. doi: 10.1016/j.immuni.2008.11.008
31. Dustin, M. L., and Groves, J. T. (2012). Receptor signaling clusters in the immune synapse. *Annu. Rev. Biophys.* 41, 543–556. doi: 10.1146/annurev-biophys-042910-155238
32. Erlejman, A. G., Fraga, C. G., and Oteiza, P. I. (2006). Procyanidins protect Caco-2 cells from bile acid- and oxidant-induced damage. *Free Radic. Biol. Med.* 41, 1247–1256. doi: 10.1016/j.freeradbiomed.2006.07.002
33. Erlejman, A. G., Jaggers, G., Fraga, C. G., and Oteiza, P. I. (2008). TNF-Fα-induced NF-κB activation and cell oxidant production are modu- lated by hexameric procyanidins in Caco-2 cells. *Arch. Biochem. Bio- phys.* 476, 186–195. doi: 10.1016/ j.abb.2008.01.024
34. Fagarasan, S., Kawamoto, S., Kanagawa, O., and Sukuzi, K. (2010). Adaptive immune regulation in the gut: T cell- dependent and T cell-independent IgA synthesis. *Annu. Rev. Immunol.* 28, 243–273. doi: 10.1146/annurev- immunol-030409-101314
35. Fogliano, V., Corollaro, M. L., Vitaglione, P., Napolitano, A., Ferracane, R., Travaglia, F., et al. (2011). *In vitro* bioaccessibil- ity and gut biotransformation of polyphenols present in the water- insoluble cocoa fraction. *Mol. Nutr. Food Res.* 55, S44–S55. doi: 10.1002/ mnfr.201000360
36. Gracie, J. A., and Bradley, J. A. (1996). Interleukin-12 induces interferon-gamma-dependent switching of IgG alloantibody subclass. *Eur. J. Immunol.* 26, 1217–1221. doi: 10.1002/eji.1830260605
37. Granado-Serrano, A. B., Martín, M. A., Izquierdo-Pulido, M., Goya, L., Bravo, L., and Ramos, S. (2007). Molecular mechanisms of (–)-epicatechin and chlorogenic acid on the regulation of the apoptotic and survival/proliferation pathways in a human hepatoma cell line. *J. Agric. Food Chem.* 55, 2020–2027. doi: 10.1021/jf062556x
38. Hämäläinen, M., Nieminen, R., Vuorela, P., Heinonen, M., and Moila- nen, E. (2007). Anti-inflammatory effects of flavonoids: genistein, kaempferol, quercetin, and daidzein inhibit STAT-1 and NF-κB activa- tions, whereas flavone, isorham- netin, naringenin, and pelargoni- din inhibit only NF-κB activation along with their inhibitory effect on iNOS expression and NO produc- tion in activated macrophages. *Medi- ators Inflamm.* 45673–45683. doi: 10.1155/2007/45673
39. Haqqi, T. M., Anthony, D. D., Gupta, S., Ahmad, N., Lee, M. S., Kumar, G. K., et al. (1999). Prevention of collagen- induced arthritis in mice by a polyphenolic fraction from green tea. *Proc. Natl. Acad. Sci. U.S.A.* 96, 4524–4529. doi: 10.1073/pnas.96.8.4524
40. Hayek, N. (2013). Chocolate, gut microbiota, and human health. *Front. Pharmacol.* 4:11. doi: 10.3389/fphar.2013.00011
41. Hieshima, K., Kawasaki, Y., Hanamoto, H., Nakayama, T., Nagakubo, D., Kanamaru, A., et al. (2004). CC chemokine ligands 25 and 28 play essential roles in intestinal extravasa- tion of IgA antibody-secreting cells. *J. Immunol.* 173, 3668–3675.
42. Hosseini, S., Pishnamazi, S., Sadrzadeh, S. M. H., Farid, F., Farid, R., and Watson, R. R. (2001). Pycnogenol® in the management of asthma. *J. Med. Food* 4, 201–209. doi: 10.1089/10966200152744472
43. Islam, N. K., Nilsson, L., Sideras, P., Hammarström, L., and Smith, C. I. (1991). TGF-β1 induces germ- line transcripts of both IgA sub- classes in human B lymphocytes. *Int. Immunol.* 3, 1099–1106. doi: 10.1093/intimm/3.11.1099
44. Jenny, M., Santer, E., Klein, A., Ledochowski, M., Schennach, H., Ueberall, F., et al. (2009). Cacao extracts suppress tryptophan degradation of mitogen-stimulated peripheral blood mononuclear cells. *J. Ethnopharmacol.* 122, 261–267. doi: 10.1016/j.jep.2009.01.011
45. Joskova, M., Franova, S., and Sadlonova, V. (2011). Acute bronchodilator effect of quercetin in experimental allergic asthma. *Bratisl. Lek. Listy* 112, 9–12.
46. Karrasch, T., Kim, J. S., Jang, B. I., and Verspaget, H. W. (2007). The flavonoid luteolin worsens chemical- induced colitis in NF-κBEGFP trans- genic mice through blockade of NF- κB-dependent protective molecules. *PLoS ONE* 2:e596. doi: 10.1371/jour- nal.pone.0000596
47. Kawaguchi, K., Maruyama, H., Kometani, T., and Kumazawa, Y. (2006). Suppression of collagen- induced arthritis by oral admin- istration of the citrus flavonoid hesperidin. *Planta Med.* 72, 477–479. doi: 10.1055/s-2005-916254
48. Kenny, T. P., Chu, S. A., Mori- toki, Y., Keen, C. L., and Gersh- win, M. E. (2009). Cocoa fla- vanols and procyanidins can mod- ulate the lipopolysaccharide activa- tion of polymorphonuclear cells in vitro. *J. Med. Food* 12, 1–7. doi: 10.1089/jmf.2007.0263
49. Kenny, T. P., Keen, C. L., Schmitz, H. H., and Gershwin, M. E. (2007). Immune effects of cocoa procyani- din oligomers on peripheral blood mononuclear cells. *Exp. Biol. Med. (Maywood)* 232, 293–300.
50. Ko, W. C., Lin, L. H., Shen, H. Y., Lai, C. Y., Chen, C. M., and Shih, C. H. (2011). Biochanin A, a phy- toestrogenic isoflavone with selec- tive inhibition of phosphodiesterase 4, suppresses ovalbumin-induced airway hyperresponsiveness. *Evid. Based Complement. Alternat. Med.* 2011, 635058. doi: 10.1155/2011/ 635058
51. Kogiso, M., Sakai, T., Mitsuya, K., Komatsu, T., and Yamamoto, S. (2006). Genistein suppresses antigen- specific immune responses through competition with 17beta-estradiol for estrogen receptors in ovalbumin- immunized BALB/c mice. *Nutri- tion* 22, 802–809. doi: 10.1016/ j.nut.2006.04.003
52. Kohri, T., Sukuzi, M., and Nanjo, F. (2003). Identification of metabolites of (–)-epicatechin gallate and their metabolic fate in the rat. *J. Agric. Food Chem.* 51, 5561–5566. doi: 10.1021/jf034450x
53. Korn, T., Bettelli, E., Oukka, M., and Kuchroo, V. K. (2009). IL- 17 and Th17 cells. *Annu. Rev. Immunol.* 27, 485–517. doi: 10.1146/ annurev.immunol.021908.132710
54. Kunisawa, J., and Kiyono, H. (2005). A marvel of mucosal T cells and secretory antibodies for the cre- ation of first lines of defense. *Cell. Mol. Life Sci.* 62, 1308–1321. doi: 10.1007/s00018-005-5035-1
55. Lau, B. H. S., Riesen, S. K., Truong, K. P., Lau, E. W., Rohdewald, P., and Bar- reta, R. A. (2004). Pycnogenol® as an adjunct in the management of child- hood asthma. *J. Asthma* 41, 25–32. doi: 10.1081/JAS-200038433
56. Lee, K. W., Kundu, J. K., Kim, S. O., Chun, K. S., Lee, H. J., and Surh, Y. J. (2006a). Cocoa polyphe- nols inhibit phorbol ester-induced superoxide anion formation in cul- tured HL-60 cells and expression of cyclooxygenase-2 and activation of NF-κB and MAPKs in mouse skin in vivo. *J. Nutr.* 136, 1150–1155.

57. Lee, H. C., Jenner, A. M., Low, C. S., and Lee, Y. K. (2006b). Effect of tea phe- nolics and their aromatic fecal bacte- rial metabolites on intestinal micro- biota. *Res. Microbiol.* 157, 876–884. doi: 10.1016/j.resmic.2006.07.004
58. Lenoir, L., Rossary, A., Joubert-Zakeyh, J., Vergnaud-Gauduchon, J., Farges, M. C., and Fraisse, D., et al. (2011). Lemon verbena infusion consump- tion attenuates oxidative stress in dextran sulfate sodium-induced col- itis in the rat. *Dig. Dis. Sci.* 56, 3534–45. doi: 10.1007/s10620-011- 1784-x
59. Li, R., Cai, L., Xie, X. F., Yang, F., and Li, J. (2010). Hesperidin sup- presses adjuvant arthritis in rats by inhibiting synoviocyte activity. *Phy- tother. Res.* 24 (Suppl. 1), S71–S76. doi: 10.1002/ptr.2906
60. Mackenzie, G. G., Carrasquedo, F., Delfino, J. M., Keen, C. L., Fraga, C. G., and Oteiza, P. I. (2004). Epi- catechin, catechin, and dimeric pro- cyanidins inhibit PMA-induced NF- κB activation at multiple steps in Jurkat T cells. *FASEB J.* 18, 167–169.
61. MacPherson, A. J., McCoy, K. D., Johansen, F. E., and Brandtzaeg, P. (2008). The immune geogra- phy of IgA induction and function. *Mucosal Immunol.* 1, 11–22. doi: 10.1038/mi.2007.6
62. Malek, T. R. (2008). The biol- ogy of interleukin-2. *Annu. Rev. Immunol.* 26, 453–479. doi: 10.1146/ annurev.immunol.26.021607.090357
63. Mamani-Matsuda, M., Kauss, T., Al- Kharrat, A., Rambert, J., Fawaz, F., Thiolat, D., et al. (2006). Thera- peutic and preventive properties of quercetin in experimental arthritis correlate with decreased macrophage inflammatory mediators. *Biochem. Pharmacol.* 72, 1304–1310. doi: 10.1016/j. bcp.2006.08.001
64. Mao, T. K., Powell, J. J., Van de Water, J., Keen, C. L., Schmitz, H. H., and Gershwin, M. E. (1999). The influence of cocoa procyanidins on the transcription of interleukin-2 in peripheral blood mononuclear cells. *Int. J. Immunother.* 15, 23–29.
65. Mao, T. K., Van de Water, J., Keen, C. L., Schmitz, H. H., and Gershwin, M. E. (2000). Cocoa procyanidins and human cytokine transcription and secretion. *J. Nutr.* 130(Suppl. 8), S2093–S2099.
66. Mao, T. K., Van de Water, J., Keen, C. L., Schmitz, H. H., and Gersh- win, M. E. (2002). Effect of cocoa flavanols and their related oligomers on the secretion of interleukin-5 in peripheral blood mononuclear cells. *J. Med. Food.* 5, 17–22. doi: 10.1089/109662002753723188
67. Massot-Cladera, M., Pérez-Berezo, T., Franch, A., Castell, M., and Pérez-Cano, F. J. (2012). Cocoa modu- latory effect on rat faecal micro- biota and colonic crosstalk. *Arch. Biochem. Biophys.* 527, 105–112. doi: 10.1016/j. abb.2012.05.015
68. Massot-Cladera, M., Torres, S., Abril- Gil, M., Pérez-Berezo, T., Franch, A., Castell, M., et al. (2013). Influence of different sources of cocoa polyphenols on intestinal microbiota and IgA of Wistar rats. *Nutr. Hosp.* 28, S26.
69. Mathur, S., Devaraj, S., Grundy, S. M., and Jialal, I. (2002). Cocoa prod- ucts decrease low density lipoprotein oxidative susceptibility but do not affect biomarkers of inflammation in humans. *J. Nutr.* 132, 3663–3667.
70. Medeiros, K. C., Figueiredo, C. A., Figueredo, T. B., Freire, K. R., Santos, F. A., Alcantara-Neves, N.M., et al. (2008). Anti-allergic effect of bee pollen phenolic extract and myricetin in ovalbumin-sensitized mice. *J. Ethnopharmacol.* 119, 41–46. doi: 10.1016/j.jep.2008.05.036
71. Miyake, M., Ide, K., Sasaki, K., Mat- sukura, Y., Shijima, K., and Fuji- wara, D. (2008). Oral administra- tion of highly oligomeric procyani- dins of Jatoba reduces the severity of collagen-induced arthritis. *Biosci. Biotechnol. Biochem.* 72, 1781–1788. doi: 10.1271/bbb.80074
72. Monagas, M., Khan, N., Andres- Lacueva, C., Casas, R., Urpí-Sardà, M., Llorach, R., et al. (2009). Effect of cocoa powder on the modulation of inflammatory biomarkers in patients at high risk of cardiovascular disease. *Am. J. Clin. Nutr.* 90, 1144–1150. doi: 10.3945/ajcn.2009.27716
73. Monagas, M., Urpi-Sarda, M., Sánchez- Patán, F., Llorach, R., Garrido, I., Gómez-Cordovés, C., et al. (2010). Insights into the metabolism and microbial biotransformation of dietary flavan-3-ols and the bioactiv- ity of their metabolites. *Food Funct.* 1, 233–253. doi: 10.1039/c0fo00132e
74. Mora, J. R., Iwata, M., Eksteen, B., Song, S. Y., Junt, T., Sen- man, B., et al. (2006). Generation of gut-homing IgA-secreting B cells by intestinal dendritic cells. *Science* 314, 1157–1160. doi: 10.1126/science. 1132742
75. Mora, J. R., and von Andrian, U. H. (2008). Differentiation and hom- ing of IgA-secreting cells. *Mucosal Immunol.* 1, 96–109. doi: 10.1038/ mi.2007.14
76. Nakayama, T., and Yamashita, M. (2008). Initiation and maintenance of Th2 cell identity. *Curr. Opin. Immunol.* 20, 265–271. doi: 10.1016/ j. coi.2008.03.011
77. Neilson, A. P., and Ferruzzi, M. G. (2011). Influence of formu- lation and processing on absorp- tion and metabolism of flavan-3- ols from tea and cocoa. *Annu. Rev. Food Sci. Technol.* 2, 125–151. doi: 10.1146/annurev-food-022510- 133725
78. O'Hara, A. M., and Shanahan, F. (2006). The gut flora as a forgotten organ. *EMBO Rep.* 7, 688–693. doi: 10.1038/sj.embor.7400731
79. Ono, K., Takahashi, T., Kamei, M., Mato, T., Hashizume, S., Kamiya, S., et al. (2003). Effects of an aqueous extract of cocoa on nitric oxide production of macrophages activated by lipopolysaccharide and interferon-γ. *Nutrition* 19, 681– 685. doi: 10.1016/S0899-9007(03) 00092-3
80. Pahl, H. L. (1999). Activators and tar- get genes of Rel/NF-κ B transcription factors. *Oncogene* 18, 6853–6866. doi: 10.1038/sj.onc.1203239
81. Pérez-Berezo, T., Ramírez-Santana, C., Franch, A., Ramos-Romero, S., Castellote, C., Pérez-Cano, F. J., et al. (2012a). Effects of a cocoa diet on an intestinal inflammation model in rats. *Exp. Biol. Med. (May- wood)* 237, 1181–1188. doi: 10.1258/ ebm.2012.012083
82. Pérez-Berezo, T., Franch, A., Caste- llote, C., Castell, M., and Pérez- Cano, F. J. (2012b). Mecha- nisms involved in down-regulation of intestinal IgA in rats by high cocoa intake. *J. Nutr. Biochem.* 23, 838–844. doi: 10.1016/j. jnutbio.2011. 04.008
83. Pérez-Berezo, T., Franch, A., Ramos- Romero, S., Castellote, C., Pérez-Cano, F. J., and Castell, M. (2011). Cocoa-enriched diets modu- late intestinal and systemic humoral immune response in young adult rats. *Mol. Nutr. Food Res.* 55, S56–S66. doi: 10.1002/mnfr.201000588
84. Pérez-Berezo, T., Ramiro-Puig, E., Pérez-Cano, F. J., Castellote, C., Permanyer, J., Franch, A., et al. (2009). Influence of cocoa-enriched diet on specific immune response in ovalbumin-sensitized rats. *Mol. Nutr. Food Res.* 53, 389–397. doi: 10.1002/mnfr.200700396
85. Pérez-Cano, F. J., Castellote, C., Marín- Gallén, S., Franch, A., and Castell, M. (2005). Neonatal immunoglob- ulin secretion and lymphocyte phe- notype in rat small intestine lamina propria. *Pedriatr. Res.* 58, 164–169. doi: 10.1203/01.PDR.0000156367. 60769.36
86. Pérez-Cano, F. J., Pérez-Berezo, T., Ramos-Romero, S., Ramiro-Puig, E., Castellote, C., Franch, A., et al. (2010). "Is there an anti- inflammatory potential beyond the antioxidant power of cocoa?" in *Chocolate, Fast Foods and Sweeten- ers: Consumption and Health*, ed. M. Bishop (New York: Nova Science Publishers), 85–104.
87. Puupponen-Pimiä, R., Nohynek, L., Hartmann-Schmidlin, S., Kähkö- nen, M., Heinonen, M., Määttä- Riihinen, K., et al. (2005). Berry phe- nolics selectively inhibit the growth of intestinal pathogens. *J. Appl. Microbiol.* 98, 991–1000. doi: 10.1111/j.1365-2672.2005.02547.x
88. Ramiro, E., Franch, A., Castellote, C., Pérez-Cano, F., Permanyer, J., Izquierdo-Pulido, M., et al. (2005a). Flavonoids from *Theobroma cacao* down-regulate inflammatory media- tors. *J. Agric. Food Chem.* 53, 8506– 8511. doi: 10.1021/jf0511042
89. Ramiro, E., Franch, A., Castellote, C., Andrés-Lacueva, C., Izquierdo- Pulido, M., and Castell M. (2005b). Effect of *Theobroma cacao* flavonoids on immune activation of a lymphoid cell line. *Br. J. Nutr.* 93, 859–866. doi: 10.1079/BJN20051443
90. Ramiro-Puig, E., Casadesús, G., Lee, H. G., Zhu, X., McShea, A., Perry, G., et al. (2009). Neuroprotective effect of cocoa flavonoids on in vitro oxida- tive stress. *Eur. J. Nutr.* 48, 54–61. doi: 10.1007/s00394-008-0761-4
91. Ramiro-Puig, E., Pérez-Cano, F. J., Ramírez-Santana, C., Castellote, C., Izquierdo-Pulido, M., Permanyer, J., et al. (2007a). Spleen lympho- cyte function modulated by a cocoa enriched diet. *Clin. Exp. Immunol.* 149, 535–542. doi: 10.1111/j.1365- 2249.2007.03430.x
92. Ramiro-Puig, E., Urpí-Sardà, M., Pérez- Cano, F. J., Franch, A., Castellote, C., Andrés-Lacueva, C., et al. (2007b). Cocoa-enriched diet enhances antioxidant enzyme activity and modulates lymphocyte composition in thymus from young rats. *J. Agric. Food Chem.* 55, 6431–6438. doi: 10.1021/ jf070487w
93. Ramiro-Puig, E., Pérez-Cano, F. J., Ramos-Romero, S., Pérez-Berezo, T., Castellote, C., Permanyer, J., et al. (2008). Intestinal immune system of young rats influenced by cocoa-enriched diet. *J. Nutr. Biochem.* 19, 555–565. doi: 10.1016/ j.jnutbio.2007.07.002
94. Ramos-Romero, S., Pérez-Cano, F. J., Pérez-Berezo, T., Castellote, C., Franch, A., and Castell, M. (2012a). Effect of a cocoa flavonoid-enriched diet on experimental autoimmune arthritis. *Br. J. Nutr.* 107, 523–532. doi: 10.1017/S000711451100328X
95. Ramos-Romero, S., Pérez-Cano, F. J., Castellote, C., Castell, M., and Franch, A. (2012b). Effect of cocoa-enriched diets on lymphocytes involved in adjuvant arthritis in rats. *Br. J. Nutr.* 107, 378–387. doi: 10.1017/ S0007114511003035
96. Ramos-Romero, S., Pérez-Cano, F. J., Ramiro-Puig, E., Franch, A., and Castell, M. (2012c). Cocoa intake attenuates oxidative stress associated with rat adjuvant arthritis. *Phar- macol. Res.* 66, 207–212. doi: 10.1016/j. phrs.2012.05.009

97. Ramos-Romero, S., Ramiro-Puig, E., Pérez-Cano, F. J., Castellote, C., Franch, A., and Castell, M. (2008). Anti-inflammatory effects of cocoa in rat carrageenin-induced paw oedema. *Proc. Nutr. Soc.* 67, E65. doi: 10.1017/S0029665108006745
98. Ramsay, A. J., Husband, A. J., Ramshaw, I. A., Baos, S., Matthaei, K. I., Koehler, G., et al. (1994). The role of interleukin-6 in mucosal IgA antibody responses *in vivo*. *Sci- ence* 264, 561–563. doi: 10.1126/sci- ence.8160012
99. Rios, L. Y., Gonthier, M. P., Rémésy, C., Mila, I., Lapierre, C., Lazarus, A., et al. (2003). Chocolate intake increases urinary excretion of polyphenol-derived phenolic acids in healthy human subjects. *Am. J. Clin. Nutr.* 77, 912–918.
100. Rogerio, A. P., Kanashiro, A., Fonta- nari, C., da Silva, E. V., Lucisano-Valim, Y. M., Soares, E. G., et al. (2007). Anti-inflammatory activity of quercetin and isoquercitrin in experimental murine allergic asthma. *Inflamm. Res.* 56, 402–408. doi: 10.1007/s00011-007-7005-6
101. Ross, A. C., Chen, Q., and Ma, Y. (2009). Augmentation of antibody responses by retinoic acid and costimulatory molecules. *Semin. Immunol.* 21, 42–50. doi: 10.1016/j.smim.2008. 08.004
102. Rovenský, J., Stancíková, M., Roven- ská, E., Stvrtina, S., Stvrtinová, V., and Svík, K. (2009). Treatment of rat adjuvant arthritis with flavonoid (Detralex), methotrexate, and their combination. *Ann. N. Y. Acad. Sci.* 1173, 798–804. doi: 10.1111/j.1749- 6632.2009.04618.x
103. Sanbongi, C., Suzuki, N., and Tsuyoshi, S. (1997). Polyphenols in chocolate, which have antiox- idant activity, modulate immune functions in humans *in vitro*. *Cell. Immunol.* 177, 129–136. doi: 10.1006/cimm.1997.1109
104. Saoudi, A., Bernard, I., Hoedemaek- ers, A., Cautain, B., Martinez, K., Druet, P., et al. (1999). Experimental autoimmune myasthenia gravis may occur in the context of a polarized Th1- or Th2-type immune response in rats. *J. Immunol.* 162, 7189–7197.
105. Schoenbeck, S., McKenzie, D. T., and Kagnoff, M. F. (1989). Interleukin 5 is a differentiation factor for IgA B cells. *Eur. J. Immunol.* 19, 965–969. doi: 10.1002/eji.1830190602
106. Selma, M. V., Espín, J. C., and Tomás- Barberán, F. A. (2009). Interaction between phenolics and gut micro- biota: role in human health. *J. Agric. Food Chem.* 57, 6485–6501. doi: 10.1021/jf902107d
107. Shang, L., Fukata, M., Thirunarayanan, N., Martin, A. P., Arnaboldi, P., Maussang, D., et al. (2008). Toll- like receptor signaling in small intestinal epithelium promotes B- cell recruitment and IgA produc- tion in lamina propria. *Gastroen- terology* 135, 529–538. doi: 10.1053/ j.gastro.2008.04.020
108. Shibolet, O., and Podolsky, D. K. (2007). TLRs in the Gut. IV. Negative regula- tion of Toll-like receptors and intesti- nal homeostasis: addition by sub- traction. *Am. J. Physiol. Gastrointest. Liver Physiol.* 292, G1469–G1473. doi: 10.1152/ajpgi.00531.2006
109. Tsuruta, T., Inoue, R., Iwanaga, T., Hara, H., and Yajima, T. (2010). Devel- opment of a method for the iden- tification of S-IgA-coated bacterial composition in mouse and human feces. *Biosci. Biotechnol. Biochem.* 74, 968–973. doi: 10.1271/bbb.90801
110. Tzounis, X., Rodríguez-Mateos, A., Vulevic, J., Gibson, G. R., Kwik- Uribe, C., and Spencer, J. P. (2011). Prebiotic evaluation of cocoa-derived flavanols in healthy humans by using a randomized, controlled, double- blind, crossover intervention study. *Am. J. Clin. Nutr.* 93, 62–72. doi: 10.3945/ajcn.110.000075
111. Tzounis, X., Vulevic, J., Kuhnle, G. G., George, T., Leonczak, J., Gibson, G. R., et al. (2008). Flavanol monomer- induced changes to the human faecal microflora. *Br. J. Nutr.* 99, 782–792. doi: 10.1017/S0007114507853384
112. Urpi-Sarda, M., Monagas, M., Khan, N., Lamuela-Raventos, R. M., Santos-Buelga, C., Sacanella, E., et al. (2009). Epicatechin, procyanidins, and phenolic microbial metabolites after cocoa intake in humans and rats. *Anal. Bioanal. Chem.* 394, 1545– 1556. doi: 10.1007/s00216-009- 2676-1
113. Vázquez-Agell, M., Urpi-Sarda, M., Sacanella, E., Camino-López, S., Chiva-Blanch, G., Llorente-Cortés, V., et al. (2013). Cocoa consump- tion reduces NF-κB activation in peripheral blood mononuclear cells in humans. *Nutr. Metab. Cardio- vasc. Dis.* 23, 257–263. doi: 10.1016/ j.numecd.2011.03.015
114. Verstraeten, S. V., Oteiza, P. I., and Fraga, C. G. (2004). Membrane effects of cocoa procyanidins in lipo- somes and Jurkat T cells. *Biol. Res.* 37, 293–300. doi: 10.4067/S0716- 97602004000200016
115. Wang, L. Q., Meselhy, M. R., Li, Y., Nakamura, N., Min, B. S., Qin, G. W., et al. (2001). The hetero- cyclic ring fission and dehydroxyla- tion of catechins and related com- pounds by *Eubacterium* sp. strain SDG-2, a human intestinal bac- terium. *Chem. Pharm. Bull. (Tokyo)* 49, 1640–1643. doi: 10.1248/cpb.49. 1640
116. Wegner, N., Lundberg, K., Kinloch, A., Fisher, B., Malmström, V., Feldmann, M., et al. (2010). Autoimmu- nity to specific citrullinated proteins gives the first clues to the etiology of rheumatoid arthritis. *Immunol. Rev.* 233, 34–54. doi: 10.1111/j.0105- 2896.2009.00850.x
117. Wisman, K. N., Perkins, A. A., Jef- fers, M. D., and Hagerman, A. E. (2008). Accurate assessment of the bioactivities of redox-active polyphe- nolics in cell culture. *J. Agric. Food Chem.* 56, 7831–7837. doi: 10.1021/ jf8011954
118. Won Jung, H., Jung, J. K., Weon Cho, C., Kang, J. S., and Park, Y. K. (2012). Antiallergic effect of KOB03, a polyherbal medicine, on mast cell-mediated allergic responses in ovalbumin-induced allergic rhini- tis mouse and human mast cells. *J. Ethnopharmacol.* 142, 684–693. doi: 10.1016/j.jep.2012.05.039

13

Rapid detection of dendritic cell and monocyte disorders using CD4 as a lineage marker of the human peripheral blood antigen-presenting cell compartment

Laura Jardine[1], Dawn Barge[2], Ashley Ames-Draycott[1], Sarah Pagan[1], Sharon Cookson[1], Gavin Spickett[2], Muzlifah Haniffa[1], Matthew Collin[1]* and Venetia Bigley[1]

[1] Human Dendritic Cell Laboratory, Institute of Cellular Medicine, Newcastle University, Newcastle upon Tyne, UK
[2] Clinical Immunology, Newcastle upon Tyne Hospitals NHS Foundation Trust, Newcastle upon Tyne, UK

Edited by:
Lisa Helene Butterfield, University of Pittsburgh, USA

Reviewed by:
Geanncarlo Lugo-Villarino, Centre national de la recherche scientifique, France
Allan B. Dietz, Mayo Clinic, USA
Sylvia Kiertscher, University of California Los Angeles, USA

***Correspondence:**
Matthew Collin, Human Dendritic Cell Laboratory, Institute of Cellular Medicine, Newcastle University, Framlington Place, Newcastle upon Tyne NE2 4HH, UK
e-mail: matthew.collin@ncl.ac.uk

Dendritic cells (DCs) and monocytes are critical regulators and effectors of innate and adaptive immune responses. Monocyte expansion has been described in many pathological states while monocyte and DC deficiency syndromes are relatively recent additions to the catalog of human primary immunodeficiency disorders. Clinically applicable screening tests to diagnose and monitor these conditions are lacking. Conventional strategies for identifying human DCs and monocytes have been based on the use of a lineage gate to exclude lymphocytes, thus preventing simultaneous detection of DCs, monocytes, and lymphocyte subsets. Here we demonstrate that CD4 is a reliable lineage marker for the human peripheral blood antigen-presenting cell compartment that can be used to identify DCs and monocytes in parallel with lymphocytes. Based on this principle, simple modification of a standard lymphocyte phenotyping assay permits simultaneous enumeration of four lymphocyte and five DC/monocyte populations from a single sample. This approach is applicable to clinical samples and facilitates the diagnosis of DC and monocyte disorders in a wide range of clinical settings, including genetic deficiency, neoplasia, and inflammation.

Keywords: dendritic cells, monocytes, flow cytometry, immunodeficiency, humans

INTRODUCTION

Dendritic cells (DCs) and monocytes are bone marrow derived mononuclear cells involved in a wide range of immune functions. Blood DCs comprise three subsets: plasmacytoid DCs (pDCs), CD1c$^+$ myeloid DCs (mDCs), and CD141$^+$ mDCs (1–5). pDCs typically lack the myeloid antigens CD13, CD33, and CD11b and express CD123 (IL-3 receptor), CD303 [CLEC4C; Blood DC antigens (BDCA)-2], and CD304 (neuropilin; BDCA-4) (1). They are specialized to produce a rapid type I interferon response to viral infections (6). mDCs share markers in common with monocytes and granulocytes including CD13, CD33, and CD11b and perform the classical functions of DCs in taking up and presenting antigen on HLA class II molecules. DCs resembling all three subsets are found in lymph nodes (7, 8) both mDC subsets have tissue counterparts (5).

Monocytes also comprise a number of distinct functional subsets delineated by expression of CD14 and CD16 in humans. CD14$^+$ CD16$^-$ "classical monocytes" perform inflammatory functions including phagocytosis, production of reactive oxygen species, nitric oxide, and TNFα (9). Two additional populations have been described: CD16$^+$ CD14^{low} "non-classical" monocytes and CD14$^+$ CD16$^+$ "intermediate" monocytes (3, 10). There is variation in how these cells are divided, with a position paper on nomenclature suggesting that intermediate monocytes may be grouped with non-classical monocytes (both linked by the expression of CD16) while more recent gene expression studies suggest that intermediate monocytes are more closely linked to classical monocytes (11). Both by flow cytometry and gene set enrichment analysis, intermediate monocytes appear to be part of a continuum (12). It is clear, however, that the non-classical pole of the spectrum contains cells with higher class II expression, allostimulatory capacity, and cytokine production that have led to their classification as a type of DC (2, 13). CD16$^+$ non-classical monocytes are also smaller and become closely associated with the endothelium upon adoptive transfer into mice (11). A wide range of studies show that non-classical monocytes are increased by exercise, autoimmune disease, bacterial sepsis, tuberculosis, and HIV infection, reviewed in Ref. (10).

Routine analysis of human blood DCs and monocytes is usually confined to the enumeration of classical monocytes by automated blood counters. The complexity of changes in DC and monocyte subsets is not visible in most clinical scenarios. Flow cytometry is frequently used to analyze lymphocyte subsets but simultaneous detection of DCs and monocytes is hampered by the lack of a positive lineage marker. Although robust platforms for DC counting have been described, these invariably depend upon identifying MHC class II (HLA-DR) expression by lineage (lin) negative cells, a population defined by the exclusion of T cells (CD3), B cells (CD19, CD20), NK cells (CD56), monocytes (CD14, CD16), and progenitors (CD34) (2, 14, 15). The exclusion of lin$^+$ lymphocytes and monocytes either precludes simultaneous measurement with DCs or demands large number of fluorescence channels (4, 15). Differential DC and monocyte counting is therefore rarely performed as a clinical test.

Blood DC antigens 1–4 are helpful for identifying human DC subsets (1) but are often used to define pDC and mDC subsets within the HLA-DR^{+} lin^{-} population (4, 16). This is especially true for CD1c (BDCA-1), which identifies the main population of mDCs but is also expressed on B cells (1). CD303 (BDCA-2; CLEC4C) and CD304 (BDCA-4; neuropilin) are relatively robust markers for pDCs and give reliable counting even from unselected peripheral blood mononuclear cells. CD141 (BDCA-3) defines a very small population of mDCs (1, 2).

Early reports demonstrated that DCs and monocytes both express CD4, but at lower levels than T helper cells (17–19). While the CD4 glycoprotein acts as a co-receptor for the T cell receptor on T helper cells, its role on myeloid cells is less clear. CD4 also functions as a receptor for IL-16 (lymphocyte chemoattractant factor), which is capable of both recruiting CD4^{+} immune cells and driving cell growth (20). Studies in HIV suggest that CD4 may augment Fc receptor signaling (21). Numerous studies report the presence of CD4 on myeloid hematopoietic precursors including myeloid malignancies (22). While in mice, expression of CD4 is retained by T lymphocyte and myeloid precursors but lost by B lymphocyte precursors (23), the function and fate of CD4 expressing precursors in humans has not been adequately mapped.

Here we show that CD4 has significant utility as positive lineage marker of human blood antigen-presenting cells, allowing delineation of all the currently recognized subsets of human blood monocytes and DCs. This allowed us to adapt a standard 6-color flow cytometry protocol for lymphocyte immunophenotyping to allow simultaneous quantification of DC and monocyte subsets.

MATERIALS AND METHODS

PARTICIPANTS

For assay development, blood was collected into EDTA from 33 patients and 5 healthy controls. Patients were randomly selected from the regional clinical immunology laboratory. Patients were aged 2–83 (median 44) and had unknown conditions for further investigation [11], immunodeficiency [7], autoimmunity [7], or atopy [3]. To test the assay in pathological states, fresh blood was obtained from a 33-year old man with DCML deficiency due to GATA-2 deficiency and a 77-year old man with blastic plasmacytoid dendritic cell neoplasm (BPDCN). To recapitulate septic conditions with left-shifted myelopoiesis, eight samples of cryopreserved G-CSF-mobilized peripheral blood stem cells (PBSC) were thawed and washed for analysis. Ethical approval was granted by Newcastle and North Tyneside Research Ethics Committee 1.

PROCESSING AND ANALYSIS

TruCount™ tubes (Becton Dickinson; BD) containing a defined number of polyfluorescent beads per test were used in a single step "lyse-no wash" method to enumerate blood cells, according to the manufacturer's instructions. Fifty microliters of blood was transferred directly to the TruCount™ tube. Antibodies were added directly and staining was performed at 4°C for 20 min. Red cell lysis was achieved by addition of 450 μl of the proprietary reagent at room temperature for 10 min. Samples were then directly analyzed by flow cytometry and the number of cells per microliters of blood was calculated from the number of events and the fraction of beads analyzed, according to the formula:

$$\text{Cells}/\mu\text{l of population x} = (\text{population x events}/\text{bead events}) \times (\text{beads per test}/50)$$

The TBNK reagent (BD catalog number 337166) contains six reagents as described in **Table 1** for the detection of CD45, CD3, CD4, CD8, CD19, and CD16/56. Combined with TruCount tubes this reagent allows the enumeration of CD4^{+} and CD8^{+} T cells, B cells, and NK cells. The modification for detecting DCs and monocytes was to add CD14-APC-Cy7 to the CD8 channel and CD304-APC to the CD19 channel.

Flow cytometry was performed on FACSCanto two or three laser instruments running DiVa version 6 (BD). Instrument PMTs were set using whole blood stained with single antibodies. FSC and SSC thresholds were set at zero to in order to capture TruCount™ bead events. A threshold was set on CD45, allowing detection of leukocytes, but discounting platelet and red cell debris. Thresholds were 1000 on 635 780/60 channel for the 8-color panel and 1000 on 488 760LP channel for the 6-color panel. Isotype controls were performed for all antibodies at the initial set up and are shown specifically for CD4. Automatic compensation was performed using compensation beads (BD). Approximately 200,000 CD45^{+} events were acquired per sample **(Table 2)**. Analysis was performed with FlowJo version 9.5.2 (TreeStar). Graphing and statistical analysis were performed with Prism version 6 (GraphPad).

Table 1 | Antibody panels used for flow cytometry analysis.

Fluorochrome	8-Color DC panel	Modified 6-color panel
FITC	CD3 [a](345763; BD) CD19 (345776; BD) CD20 (345792; BD) CD56 (345811; BD)	CD3
PE	CD16 (555407; BD)	CD16, CD56
PERCPCy5.5	CD123 (558714; BD)	CD45
PECy7	CD14 (557742; BD)	CD4
APC	CD141 (130-090-907; Miltenyi)	CD19 **CD304** (130-090-900; Miltenyi)
APCCy7	CD14 (557742; BD)	CD8 **CD14** (557831; BD)
V450	CD11c (560369; BD)	
V500	HLA-DR (561224; BD)	

[a](Catalog number; supplier).

CD4 V500 (560768; BD), CD4 PE (555347; BD), CD3 PE (345765; BD), CD19 PE (555413; BD), and CD56 PE (345812; BD) were used in additional experiments. Bold text indicates the antibodies added to modify the 6-colour TBNK(TM) panel (337166; BD).

Table 2 | Flow cytometry events recorded for analysis of monocyte and DC subsets.

Cell population	8-Color DC panel events collected median (IQ range)	Modified 6-color panel events collected median (IQ range)
DC PANEL COMPARISON ($N = 24$)		
Total	204634 (125021)	197925 (101726)
CD14 monocytes	24422 (13512)	9289 (5981)
CD16 monocytes	1590 (2973)	570 (934)
CD14 CD16 monocytes	1381 (1443)	633 (499)
DC	971 (697)	369 (327)
DC SUBSET DISCRIMINATION ($N = 14$)		
Total	112172 (39906)	130255 (116775)
mDC	408 (218)	239 (98)
pDC	154 (295)	81 (190)

RESULTS

CD4 IS A LINEAGE MARKER FOR BLOOD ANTIGEN-PRESENTING CELLS

We designed a flow cytometry panel to examine known subsets of monocytes and DCs. Working with whole blood, the standard approach of lineage exclusion and HLA-DR selection required a minimum of eight fluorescence channels to categorize all monocyte and DC subsets. Throughout the study we used this 8-color panel as the standard reference panel for DC and monocyte enumeration (**Figure 1A**). In the CD45^{+} SSC^{low} gate, we first gated on HLA-DR^{+} lineage negative cells (CD3, CD19, CD20, CD56) to obtain all the monocyte and blood DC populations. Monocytes were analyzed by CD14 vs. CD16 and the double negative cells further separated into pDCs and two subsets of mDCs. We then explored the expression of CD4 on different leukocytes. We used specific fluorophores to identify each lineage-positive fraction and the schema outlined in **Figure 1A** to identify DCs and monocytes. CD4^{+} T cells are seen in the CD3^{+} fraction but B cells and NK cells are CD4 negative (**Figure 1B**). Back-gating illustrates where each population lies on the HLA-DR vs. lineage plot. This indicates that NK cells are most likely to broach the lin-DR^{+} gate. As many NK cells express CD16, the gate must be placed sufficiently low on the lineage axis to prevent subsequent NK contamination of the CD16 monocyte gate. All monocyte and DC populations express CD4 above isotype control (**Figures 1C,D**). Back-gating shows the relative HLA-DR expression of these populations. The position of the HLA-DR vs. lineage gate is critical as some monocytes express low HLA-DR. The lower border of the gate on the HLA-DR axis was judged according to isotype controls for HLA-DR (not shown) and the inclusion of a maximum number of CD14^{+} monocytes, the cells with the lowest HLA-DR expression. To ensure that all monocytes and DCs were being captured by this strategy, the gate was also drawn simply as a lineage negative gate (Figure S1 in Supplementary Material). Although this results in the inclusion of HLA-DR negative myeloid precursors and basophils (4), these are subsequently excluded out by the down-stream gating on monocytes and DCs. This at least confirms that no cells are lost by the HLA-DR^{+} lineage negative gate as it was defined in **Figure 1A**.

CD4 EXPRESSION IDENTIFIES MONOCYTES AND DCs WITHIN A LYMPHOCYTE PHENOTYPING PANEL

Having established the expression of CD4 by different leukocytes, we explored the ability of this marker to capture DCs and monocytes. The previous results predicted that a 2D plot of CD4 vs. CD3 should display a population of CD4^{+} CD3^{-} cells containing DCs and monocytes, with slightly lower CD4 expression than CD4^{+} T cells. Both these markers are found within a standard lymphocyte phenotyping panel, offering the potential to enumerate DCs monocytes and lymphocytes simultaneously. We used the TBNK™ reagent (BD) containing six colors to detect T, B, and NK lymphocytes and provide CD4:CD8 ratios from a single tube. As with the previous panel, mononuclear cells are initially separated from granulocytes, beads and debris by FSC and SSC properties (**Figure 2A**) and CD45^{+} cells selected (not shown). The subsequent 2D plot of CD4 vs. CD3 shows the predicted population of CD4^{+} CD3^{-} cells (**Figure 2B**) that does not contain B cells (**Figure 2C**) or NK cells (**Figure 2D**).

To characterize these cells further, we modified the TBNK reagent by re-using fluorescence channels that had already been excluded by the gating, namely APC (conjugated to CD19) and APCCy7 (conjugated to CD8). CD14 APCCy7 in combination with CD16/56 thus allows resolution of monocyte subsets and the CD14^{-} CD16^{-} parameter space, containing DCs (**Figure 2E**). Note that the CD4^{+} CD16^{+} population identified in **Figure 2D** is confirmed as the CD16^{+} non-classical monocyte by low to medium expression of CD14. Further display of the CD14^{-} CD16^{-} population by CD4 vs. CD304-APC enabled the assay to differentiate between mDCs and pDCs (**Figures 2F,G**). This also confirms that pDCs have the highest CD4 expression among DCs and monocytes. The TBNK reagent and its modification are detailed in **Table 1**.

THE MODIFIED TBNK PANEL PROVIDES ACCURATE ENUMERATION OF MONOCYTES AND DCs

To provide a proof-of-concept that modification of the 6-color TBNK reagent with CD14 APCCy7 could reproduce the enumeration of DCs and monocytes, we ran 24 samples in parallel with the standard 8-color panel (using HLA-DR vs. lineage as an initial gate). A further 14 samples were run including both CD14 APCCy7 and CD304 APC with the TBNK reagent to evaluate the ability to split DCs into pDCs and mDCs. To reproduce the conditions of a clinical test as closely as possible, we took samples referred to the regional clinical immunology lab and prepared and analyzed them independently on separate machines.

Both panels were run using TruCount tubes to achieve absolute quantification per microliters of blood. Results from the modified TBNK reagent were highly correlated with those of the standard 8-color panel. The least correlated results were produced for total DCs and mDCs. This is probably due to the fact that the 6-color strategy did not include a positive marker of mDCs (except for CD4); they were defined by the exclusion of other populations so it is possible for a variable low level of contaminating cells to be included. Approximately 200,000 total events were recorded in order to collect at least 100 events for rare subsets of DCs (**Table 2**).

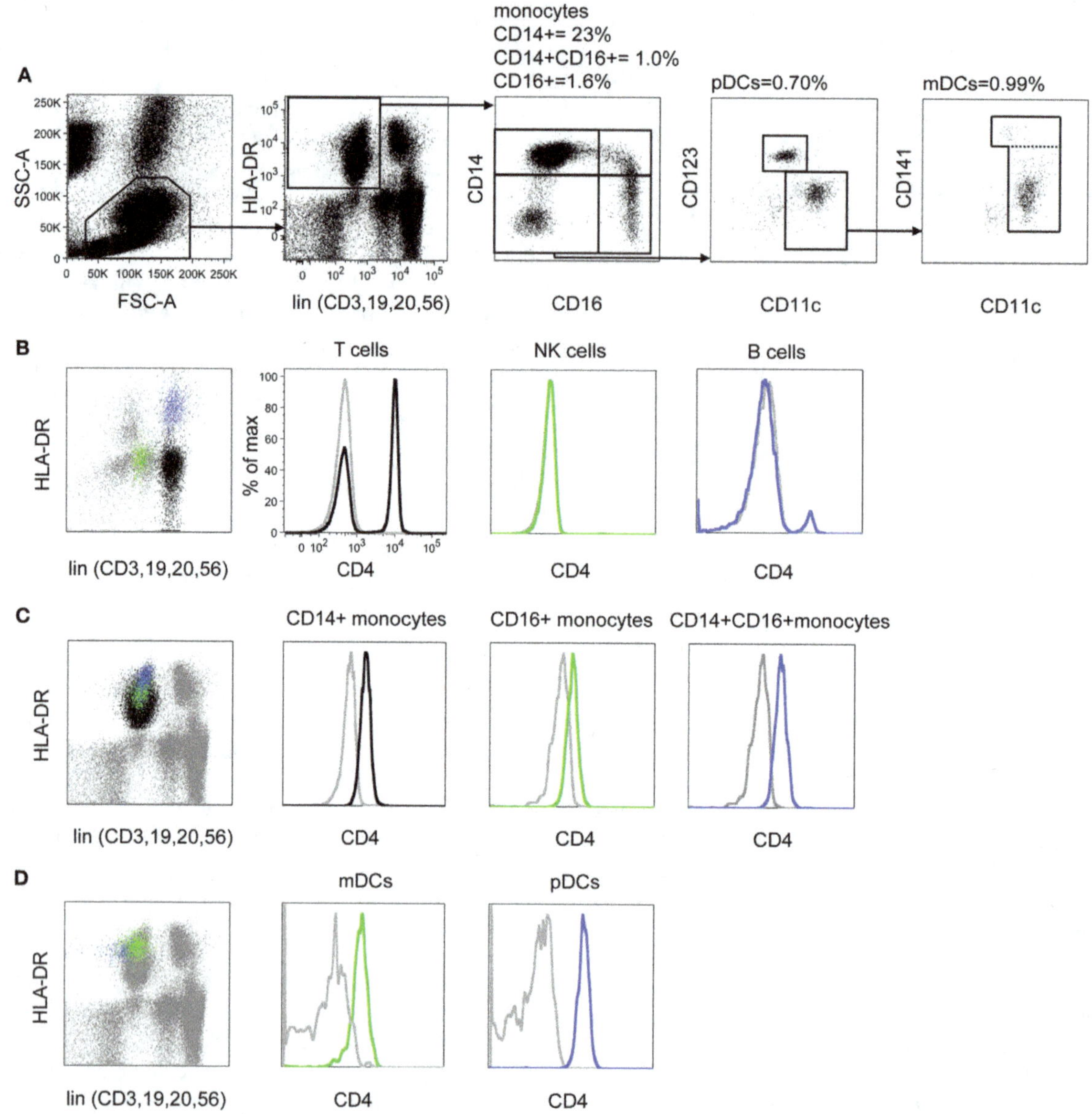

FIGURE 1 | CD4 is differentially expressed on monocytes and DCs. **(A)** In an 8-color DC profiling panel FSC and SSC parameters are used to distinguish mononuclear cells from granulocytes, counting beads, and debris. Mononuclear cells are confirmed as CD45⁺ SSC low (gate not shown). Lineage markers (CD3, 19, 20, 56) are used to remove T, B, and NK cells from analysis and DR⁺ monocytes and DCs are selected. The CD14 vs. CD16 plot reveals three subsets of monocytes and CD14⁻ CD16⁻ DCs. Plasmacytoid DCs are defined as $CD11c^{low}$ $CD123^{+}$. Two subsets of CD11c myeloid DC are split by CD141. Percentage values shown indicate the proportion of gated cells relative to $CD45^{+}$ SSC low cells. **(B)** $CD3^{+}$ T cells (black), $CD56^{+}$ NK cells (green), and $CD19^{+}$ B cells (blue) are back-gated onto the lineage vs. DR plot to demonstrate the locations of these populations. Expression of CD4 was then tested (colored histograms) relative to isotype control (gray). Note that a small population of activated DR^{+} $CD4^{+}$ T cells overlaps the B cell population. **(C)** $CD14^{+}$ monocytes (black), $CD16^{+}$ monocytes (green), and $CD14^{+}16^{+}$ monocytes (blue) are back-gated onto the lineage vs. DR plot. Expression of CD4 is shown (colored histograms), relative to isotype control (gray). **(D)** Myeloid DC (green) and plasmacytoid DC (blue) are back-gated onto the lineage vs. DR plot. Expression of CD4 is shown (colored histograms), relative to isotype control.

DETECTION OF DC AND MONOCYTE DISORDERS IN CLINICAL SPECIMENS

To further test the clinical utility of the modified TBNK reagent, we selected two cases where highly abnormal numbers of DC and monocytes were detected using the 8-color panel and re-examined them with the modified TBNK test. The results are plotted on **Figure 3**.

Case 1

A 33-year-old man presented to rheumatology with a history of pyogenic infections, chronic papillomatosis, and recurrent erythema nodosum. Automated blood counts were normal except for a monocyte count 0.03×10^9/l. DC, monocyte B, and NK lymphoid (DCML) deficiency was suspected and GATA-2 mutation subsequently confirmed by sequencing (24). A blood sample

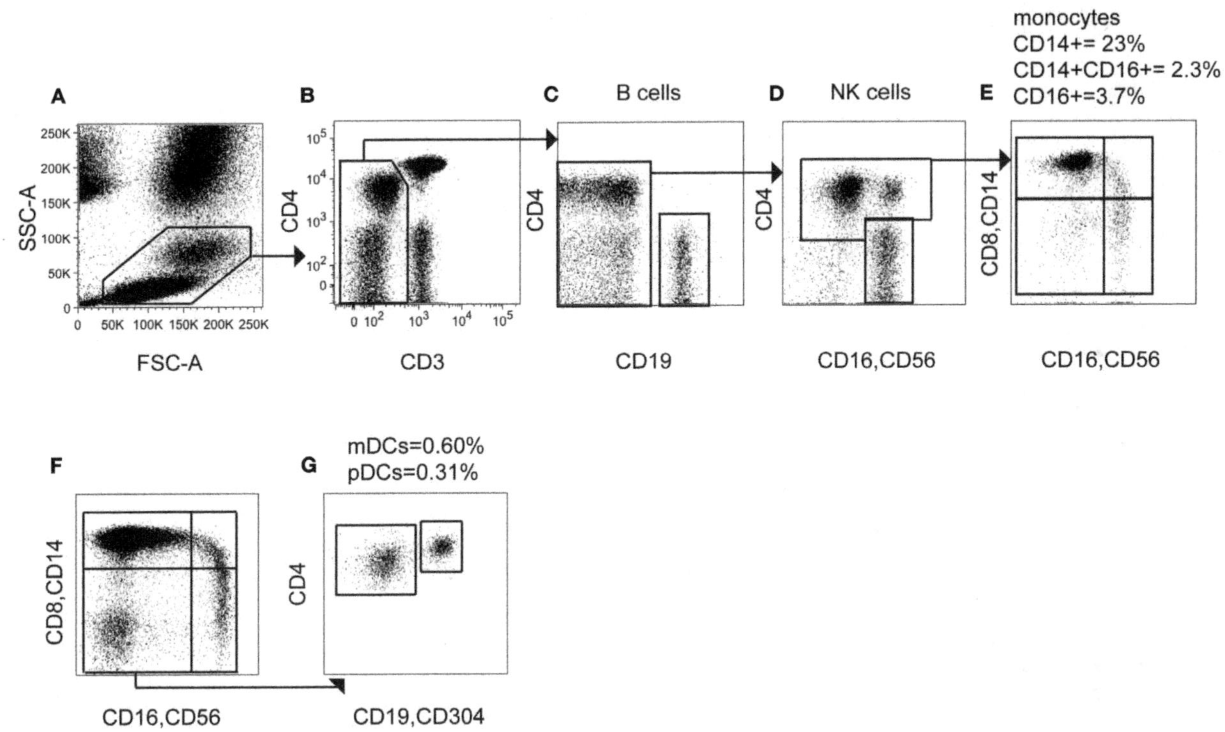

FIGURE 2 | Using CD4 as a lineage marker allows monocytes and DCs to be counted with a 6-color immunophenotyping panel. (A) In a 6-color immunophenotyping panel modified by addition of CD14 antibody, mononuclear cells are gated based on FSC and SSC parameters. **(B)** CD3 negative cells, including DCs and monocytes, B cells and NK cells are gated out from T cells. **(C)** CD19$^+$ B cells are removed from the CD3$^-$ population. **(D)** CD16$^+$ CD56$^+$ NK cells are removed from analysis and the CD4$^+$ population selected. **(E)** Visualized on a CD14 vs. CD16 plot, the CD4$^+$ population contains three subsets of monocytes and CD14$^-$ CD16$^-$ DC. **(F)** Adding CD304 antibody to the assay allows further separation of the CD14$^-$ CD16$^-$ DC population into **(G)** CD4$^+$ CD304$^-$ mDCs and CD4^{bright} CD304$^+$ pDCs.

obtained during routine clinical monitoring was analyzed with the modified TBNK panel (**Figure 3C**). Significant and parallel depletion of all monocyte and DC subsets was observed by both methods.

Case 2

A 77-year-old man presented to dermatology with progressive skin nodules and plaques. Immunohistochemistry of a skin biopsy revealed a dense infiltrate of mononuclear cells positive for CD4, CD56, and CD123 consistent with a diagnosis of BPDCN. The leukemic expansion of pDCs was evident with both 8-color and modified TBNK (**Figure 3D**) tests. In addition, a relative expansion of intermediate and non-classical monocytes was also found by both methods. In the pDC analysis, the 8-color method appeared to underestimate; we attribute this to the expression of CD56 by BPDCN which caused some cells to be lost from the HLA-DR$^+$ lineage$^-$ gate as they shifted into the lineage+ fraction. In this case, using CD4 as a positive DC marker proved to be a more reliable approach.

ENUMERATION OF DCs AND MONOCYTES IN INFLAMMATORY STATES

Septic shock and other inflammatory conditions are associated with an expansion of monocytes bearing lower HLA-DR. We therefore explored whether detecting monocytes and DCs by CD4 expression would circumvent the problem of counting cells with low HLA-DR expression in an HLA-DR$^+$ lineage$^-$ gate, or be subject to similar pitfalls. As a model of septic shock we took samples of G-CSF mobilized peripheral blood cells, which also show expanded monocytes with low HLA-DR, and compared counts derived from the two panels. The HLA-DR^{low} fraction of the DC/monocyte gate also expressed lower CD4 (**Figures 4A,B**) but as with the HLA-DR$^+$ lineage$^-$ gating approach (Figure S1 in Supplementary Material), it was possible to extend the lower limit of the gate to include the cells with lower expression of CD4 (**Figure 4C**) resulting in positively correlated results between the two methods (**Figure 4D**).

DISCUSSION

In this study we show that CD4 expression may be used within a lymphocyte typing panel to identify DCs and monocytes and that this has clinical utility in enabling the simultaneous detection of nine subsets of lymphocytes, monocytes, and DCs with only six flow cytometry channels.

Dendritic cells and monocytes have been known to express CD4 since the early descriptions of blood DCs and from studies of infectivity by HIV (17–19) but recent strategies for analysis of DCs and monocytes have typically relied upon resolving HLA-DR$^+$ lineage$^-$ cells (3, 4). CD4 has been used in combination with a lineage cocktail to identify DCs but lymphocytes are still excluded by this approach (16). The use of CD4 as a positive lineage

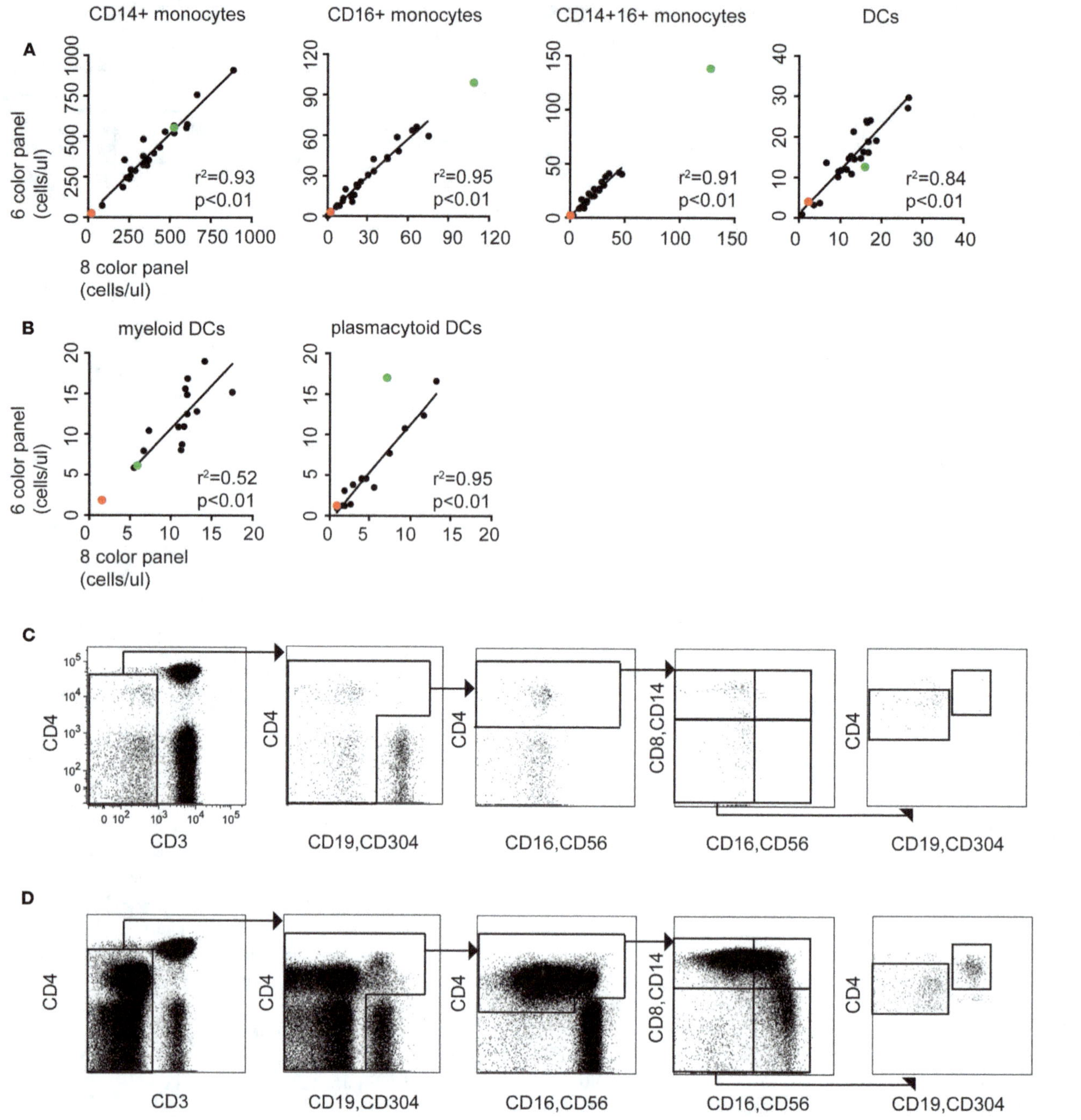

FIGURE 3 | The modified TBNK assay allows rapid quantitation of APC subsets, consistent with conventional methods. **(A)** Correlation between monocyte and DC counting performed using the 6-color immunophenotyping panel modified by addition of CD14 vs. the standard 8-color DC panel ($n = 24$). Red dots indicate results for case 1 (DCML deficiency). Green dots indicate case 2 (BPDCN). Linear regressions, r^2 and p values stated on the plots exclude these outlier cases. **(B)** Correlation between mDC and pDC counting using the 6-color panel modified with CD14 and CD304 vs. the standard 8-color DC panel ($n = 14$). **(C)** The modified TBNK assay applied to case 1 (DCML deficiency). Note the scarcity of $CD3^-$ cells relative to $CD3^+$ T cells. This arises from reduction in B cells, absence of NK cells, and virtual absence of all monocyte and DC subsets. The small population of $CD3^-$ $CD4^{bright}$ cells gated out in the initial plot are activated T cells with reduced CD3 expression. **(D)** The modified TBNK assay applied to case 2 (BPDCN).

marker, in combination with CD3, preserves the identification of lymphocyte subsets. Multiplexing fluorescence channels with more than one antibody appears to be a reliable means of expanding the number of parameters. Although we cannot exclude that aberrant expression of surface markers in some conditions may distort the analysis, this is true of any flow cytometry assay and our modified 6-color strategy actually enhanced the detection of the malignant $CD4^+$ $CD56^+$ pDC clone compared with an HLA-DR

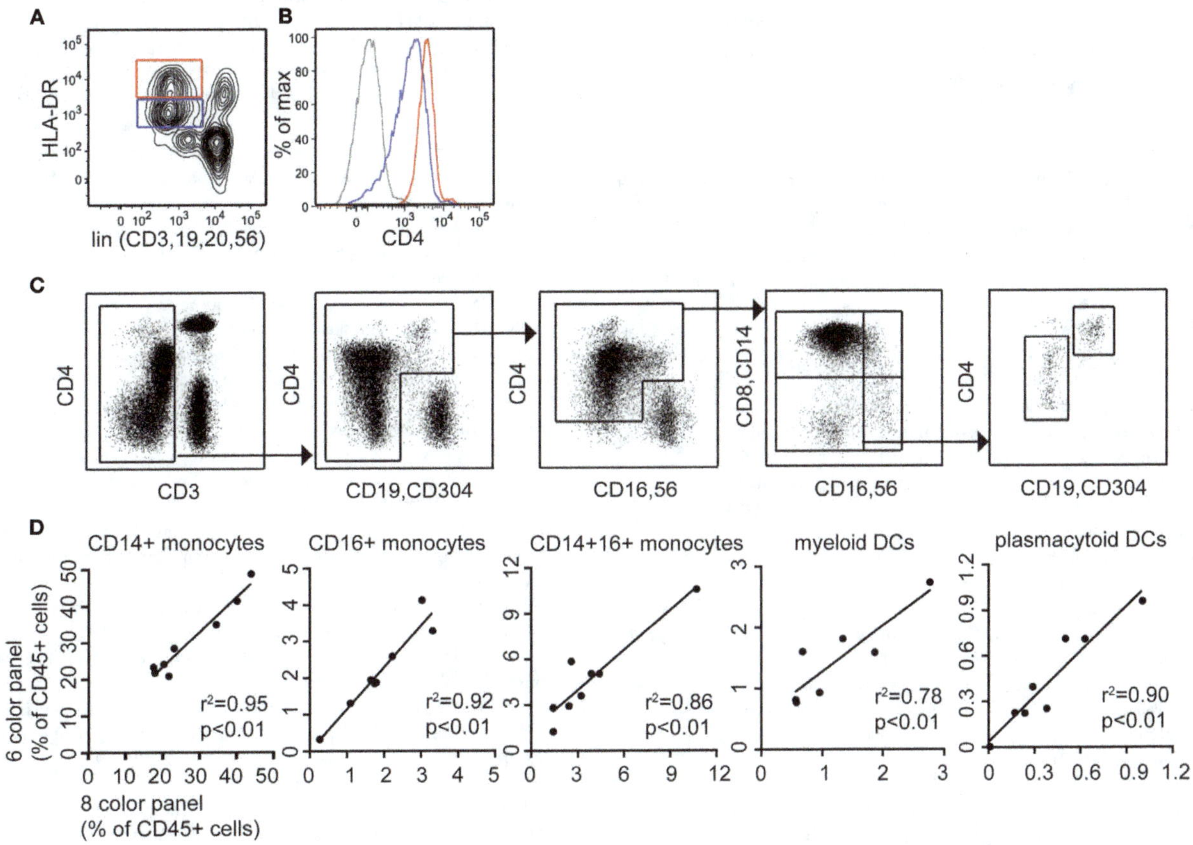

FIGURE 4 | CD4 is expressed on both DR low and DR bright populations following G-CSF mobilization. The modified TBNK assay allows clear discrimination of lymphocyte, monocyte, and DC populations in left-shifted blood. **(A)** The lineage DR plot used for 8-color DC profiling shows DR^{bright} and DR^{low} populations of monocytes and DCs in G-CSF mobilized blood. **(B)** CD4 expression is highest on lin^- DR^{bright} cells but also positive on lin^- DR^{low} cells. **(C)** The modified TBNK assay applied to G-CSF mobilized peripheral blood stem cells (PBSC) permits effective discrimination of lymphocyte, monocyte, and DC populations. **(D)** Correlation between 8-color and modified TBNK methods for DCs and monocytes in PBSC.

vs. lineage approach. Employing a single standard mononuclear cell profiling panel and multiplexing antibodies is likely to prove especially beneficial where resources and flow cytometry parameters are restricted, as in many clinical service laboratories. Here we provide proof-of-concept but additional validation and generation of local normal ranges will be required for clinical use.

This type of assay will be useful for identifying DC deficiency as recently described in a number of novel human syndromes (24–26). A typical approach to identifying immunodeficiency uses screening investigations to refine the differential diagnosis followed by more specialist investigations to specify the defect (27). The capacity to enumerate monocytes and DCs as part of an existing lymphocyte immunophenotyping platform, is an important addition to the screening repertoire. Between the 2009 and 2011 revision of the IUIS Primary Immunodeficiency Classification, 7 of the 15 new disease entities concerned the myeloid antigen-presenting cell compartment (28). The development of means to rapidly enumerate DCs and monocytes is therefore an unmet need of clinical importance (29).

Expansion of specific monocyte subsets has been observed in infection and inflammation in many clinical contexts. The delineation of monocytes is not always straightforward in relation to other cells such as NK cells through the expression of CD56 (30) or owing to the loss of HLA-DR expression during neoplasia or inflammation (31, 32). HLA^- DR^{low} monocytes also express less CD4. Rigorous comparison of gating strategies has shown that all monocytes may be collected using only HLA-DR, CD14, and CD16 (32); here we show that a CD4 gate with a lower threshold also captures the same events.

Bringing blood DC and monocyte subset analysis into routine clinical practice will most likely reveal even greater variety and subtlety of DC and monocyte deficiency states. New correlations between human disease and the behavior of this compartment are anticipated.

AUTHOR CONTRIBUTIONS

Laura Jardine performed experiments, analyzed data, and wrote the manuscript. Dawn Barge designed the study, performed experiments, and analyzed data. Ashley Ames-Draycott performed experiments, Sarah Pagan performed experiments. Sharon Cookson performed experiments. Gavin Spickett commented on the manuscript. Muzlifah Haniffa commented on the manuscript. Matthew Collin designed the study and wrote the manuscript. Venetia Bigley designed the study and wrote the manuscript.

ACKNOWLEDGMENTS

We thank all patients and volunteers who donated blood. This work was supported by grants from the Wellcome Trust (LEJ; WT097941) and Bright Red (www.brightred.org.uk).

REFERENCES

1. Dzionek A, Fuchs A, Schmidt P, Cremer S, Zysk M, Miltenyi S, et al. BDCA-2, BDCA-3, and BDCA-4: three markers for distinct subsets of dendritic cells in human peripheral blood. *J Immunol* (2000) **165**:6037–46.
2. MacDonald KP, Munster DJ, Clark GJ, Dzionek A, Schmitz J, Hart DN. Characterization of human blood dendritic cell subsets. *Blood* (2002) **100**:4512–20. doi:10.1182/blood-2001-11-0097
3. Ziegler-Heitbrock L, Ancuta P, Crowe S, Dalod M, Grau V, Hart DN, et al. Nomenclature of monocytes and dendritic cells in blood. *Blood* (2010) **116**:e74–80. doi:10.1182/blood-2010-02-258558
4. Autissier P, Soulas C, Burdo TH, Williams KC. Evaluation of a 12-color flow cytometry panel to study lymphocyte, monocyte, and dendritic cell subsets in humans. *Cytometry A* (2010) **77**:410–9. doi:10.1002/cyto.a.20859
5. Haniffa M, Collin M, Ginhoux F. Ontogeny and functional specialization of dendritic cells in human and mouse. *Adv Immunol* (2013) **120**:1–49. doi:10.1016/B978-0-12-417028-5.00001-6
6. Reizis B, Bunin A, Ghosh HS, Lewis KL, Sisirak V. Plasmacytoid dendritic cells: recent progress and open questions. *Annu Rev Immunol* (2011) **29**:163–83. doi:10.1146/annurev-immunol-031210-101345
7. Segura E, Durand M, Amigorena S. Similar antigen cross-presentation capacity and phagocytic functions in all freshly isolated human lymphoid organ-resident dendritic cells. *J Exp Med* (2013) **210**:1035–47. doi:10.1084/jem.20121103
8. Segura E, Valladeau-Guilemond J, Donnadieu MH, Sastre-Garau X, Soumelis V, Amigorena S. Characterization of resident and migratory dendritic cells in human lymph nodes. *J Exp Med* (2012) **209**:653–60. doi:10.1084/jem.20111457
9. Geissmann F, Gordon S, Hume DA, Mowat AM, Randolph GJ. Unravelling mononuclear phagocyte heterogeneity. *Nat Rev Immunol* (2010) **10**:453–60. doi:10.1038/nri2784
10. Ziegler-Heitbrock L. The CD14+ CD16+ blood monocytes: their role in infection and inflammation. *J Leukoc Biol* (2007) **81**:584–92. doi:10.1189/jlb.0806510
11. Cros J, Cagnard N, Woollard K, Patey N, Zhang SY, Senechal B, et al. Human CD14dim monocytes patrol and sense nucleic acids and viruses via TLR7 and TLR8 receptors. *Immunity* (2010) **33**:375–86. doi:10.1016/j.immuni.2010.08.012
12. Collin M, McGovern N, Haniffa M. Human dendritic cell subsets. *Immunology* (2013) **140**:22–30. doi:10.1111/imm.12117
13. Schäkel K, von Kietzell M, Hänsel A, Ebling A, Schulze L, Haase M, et al. Human 6-sulfo LacNAc-expressing dendritic cells are principal producers of early interleukin-12 and are controlled by erythrocytes. *Immunity* (2006) **24**:767–77. doi:10.1016/j.immuni.2006.03.020
14. Vuckovic S, Gardiner D, Field K, Chapman GV, Khalil D, Gill D, et al. Monitoring dendritic cells in clinical practice using a new whole blood single-platform TruCOUNT assay. *J Immunol Methods* (2004) **284**:73–87. doi:10.1016/j.jim.2003.10.006
15. Della Bella S, Giannelli S, Taddeo A, Presicce P, Villa ML. Application of six-color flow cytometry for the assessment of dendritic cell responses in whole blood assays. *J Immunol Methods* (2008) **339**:153–64. doi:10.1016/j.jim.2008.09.009
16. Wang JC, Kobie JJ, Zhang L, Cochran M, Mosmann TR, Ritchlin CT, et al. An 11-color flow cytometric assay for identifying, phenotyping, and assessing endocytic ability of peripheral blood dendritic cell subsets in a single platform. *J Immunol Methods* (2009) **341**:106–16. doi:10.1016/j.jim.2008.11.002
17. Crowe S, Mills J, McGrath MS. Quantitative immunocytofluorographic analysis of CD4 surface antigen expression and HIV infection of human peripheral blood monocyte/macrophages. *AIDS Res Hum Retroviruses* (1987) **3**:135–45. doi:10.1089/aid.1987.3.135
18. Collin M, Herbein G, Montaner L, Gordon S. PCR analysis of HIV1 infection of macrophages: virus entry is CD4-dependent. *Res Virol* (1993) **144**:13–9. doi:10.1016/S0923-2516(06)80006-3
19. Romani N, Gruner S, Brang D, Kämpgen E, Lenz A, Trockenbacher B, et al. Proliferating dendritic cell progenitors in human blood. *J Exp Med* (1994) **180**:83–93. doi:10.1084/jem.180.1.83
20. Center DM, Berman JS, Kornfeld H, Theodore AC, Cruikshank WW. The lymphocyte chemoattractant factor. *J Lab Clin Med* (1995) **125**:167–72.
21. Takeda A, Sweet RW, Ennis FA. Two receptors are required for antibody-dependent enhancement of human immunodeficiency virus type 1 infection: CD4 and Fc gamma R. *J Virol* (1990) **64**:5605–10.
22. Miwa H, Mizutani M, Mahmud N, Yamaguchi M, Takahashi T, Shikami M, et al. Biphasic expression of CD4 in acute myelocytic leukemia (AML) cells: AML of monocyte origin and hematopoietic precursor cell origin. *Leukemia* (1998) **12**:44–51. doi:10.1038/sj.leu.2400877
23. Wineman JP, Gilmore GL, Gritzmacher C, Torbett BE, Muller-Sieburg CE. CD4 is expressed on murine pluripotent hematopoietic stem cells. *Blood* (1992) **80**:1717–24.
24. Dickinson RE, Griffin H, Bigley V, Reynard LN, Hussain R, Haniffa M, et al. Exome sequencing identifies GATA-2 mutation as the cause of dendritic cell, monocyte, B and NK lymphoid deficiency. *Blood* (2011) **118**:2656–8. doi:10.1182/blood-2011-06-360313
25. Bigley V, Haniffa M, Doulatov S, Wang XN, Dickinson R, McGovern N, et al. The human syndrome of dendritic cell, monocyte, B and NK lymphoid deficiency. *J Exp Med* (2011) **208**:227–34. doi:10.1084/jem.20101459
26. Hambleton S, Salem S, Bustamante J, Bigley V, Boisson-Dupuis S, Azevedo J, et al. IRF8 mutations and human dendritic-cell immunodeficiency. *N Engl J Med* (2011) **365**:127–38. doi:10.1056/NEJMoa1100066
27. de Vries E. Patient-centred screening for primary immunodeficiency, a multi-stage diagnostic protocol designed for non-immunologists: 2011 update. *Clin Exp Immunol* (2012) **167**:108–19. doi:10.1111/j.1365-2249.2011.04461.x
28. Al-Herz W, Bousfiha A, Casanova JL, Chapel H, Conley ME, Cunningham-Rundles C, et al. Primary immunodeficiency diseases: an update on the classification from the international union of immunological societies expert committee for primary immunodeficiency. *Front Immunol* (2011) **2**:54. doi:10.3389/fimmu.2011.00054
29. Collin M, Bigley V, Haniffa M, Hambleton S. Human dendritic cell deficiency: the missing ID? *Nat Rev Immunol* (2011) **11**:575–83. doi:10.1038/nri3046
30. Bigley V, Spence LE, Collin M. Connecting the dots: monocyte/DC and NK subsets in human peripheral blood. *Blood* (2010) **116**:2859–60. doi:10.1182/blood-2010-05-285676
31. Lin Y, Gustafson MP, Bulur PA, Gastineau DA, Witzig TE, Dietz AB. Immunosuppressive CD14+HLA-DR(low)/- monocytes in B-cell non-Hodgkin lymphoma. *Blood* (2011) **117**:872–81. doi:10.1182/blood-2010-05-283820
32. Abeles RD, McPhail MJ, Sowter D, Antoniades CG, Vergis N, Vijay GK, et al. CD14, CD16 and HLA-DR reliably identifies human monocytes and their subsets in the context of pathologically reduced HLA-DR expression by CD14(hi)/CD16(neg) monocytes: expansion of CD14(hi)/CD16(pos) and contraction of CD14(lo)/CD16(pos) monocytes in acute liver failure. *Cytometry A* (2012) **81**:823–34. doi:10.1002/cyto.a.22104

A mathematical model of immune activation with a unified self-nonself concept

Sahamoddin Khailaie[1], Fariba Bahrami[2], Mahyar Janahmadi[3], Pedro Milanez-Almeida[4], Jochen Huehn[4] and Michael Meyer-Hermann[1,5]*

[1] Department of Systems Immunology, Helmholtz Centre for Infection Research, Braunschweig, Germany
[2] CIPCE, School of Electrical and Computer Engineering, College of Engineering, University of Tehran, Tehran, Iran
[3] Neuroscience Research Centre and Department of Physiology, Faculty of Medicine, Shahid Beheshti University of Medical Sciences, Tehran, Iran
[4] Department of Experimental Immunology, Helmholtz Centre for Infection Research, Braunschweig, Germany
[5] Bio Centre for Life Science, Technische Universität Braunschweig, Braunschweig, Germany

Edited by:
Rob J. De Boer, Utrecht University, Netherlands

Reviewed by:
Ichiro Taniuchi, RIKEN Research Center for Allergy and Immunology, Japan
Robin Callard, University College London, UK
Grant Lythe, University of Leeds, UK

***Correspondence:**
Michael Meyer-Hermann, Department of Systems Immunology, Helmholtz Centre for Infection Research, Inhoffenstr. 7, 38124 Braunschweig, Germany
e-mail: mmh@theoretical-biology.de

The adaptive immune system reacts against pathogenic nonself, whereas it normally remains tolerant to self. The initiation of an immune response requires a critical antigen(Ag)-stimulation and a critical number of Ag-specific T cells. Autoreactive T cells are not completely deleted by thymic selection and partially present in the periphery of healthy individuals that respond in certain physiological conditions. A number of experimental and theoretical models are based on the concept that structural differences discriminate self from nonself. In this article, we establish a mathematical model for immune activation in which self and nonself are not distinguished. The model considers the dynamic interplay of conventional T cells, regulatory T cells (Tregs), and IL-2 molecules and shows that the renewal rate ratio of resting Tregs to naïve T cells as well as the proliferation rate of activated T cells determine the probability of immune stimulation. The actual initiation of an immune response, however, relies on the absolute renewal rate of naïve T cells. This result suggests that thymic selection reduces the probability of autoimmunity by increasing the Ag-stimulation threshold of self reaction which is established by selection of a low number of low-avidity autoreactive T cells balanced with a proper number of Tregs. The stability analysis of the ordinary differential equation model reveals three different possible immune reactions depending on critical levels of Ag-stimulation: a subcritical stimulation, a threshold stimulation inducing a proper immune response, and an overcritical stimulation leading to chronic co-existence of Ag and immune activity. The model exhibits oscillatory solutions in the case of persistent but moderate Ag-stimulation, while the system returns to the homeostatic state upon Ag clearance. In this unifying concept, self and nonself appear as a result of shifted Ag-stimulation thresholds which delineate these three regimes of immune activation.

Keywords: Immune activation, autoimmunity, autoreactive T cells, regulatory T cells, central tolerance, peripheral tolerance

INTRODUCTION

The immune system is continuously exposed to a wide variety of disturbances. Such disturbances are recognized by T cells via antigen presentation. Antigen presentation is a process in which antigen presenting cells (APC) capture the antigens, break them into small peptides, couple them with MHC molecules, and present them on the cell surface, thus enabling their recognition by T cells (1–3). The majority of disturbances that the immune system deals with are pathogenic nonself-antigens. Since the APCs break down the nonself-antigens into smaller peptides and present them on their surface, presented peptide of nonself might have overlaps with self-peptides (4, 5).

In addition, rapidly evolving nonself pathogens, such as Hepatitis C virus, might acquire similarities to self-antigens (6). Apart from nonself, altered self such as cancer cells is also a disturbance that has to be recognized by the immune system. Therefore, an ideal immune system has to find a solution for dealing with nonself, self-similar nonself, and self-disturbances (**Figure 1**).

As a general solution, the immune system generates T cell clones with random specificities that could potentially recognize any peptides, including self-peptides. The classical idea that the T cell repertoire has to be self-tolerant and T cells should not react to self-peptides, assumes that self-reactive T cells should be eliminated. This assumption is partially true, as T cell clones which fully recognize self-peptides in the thymus undergo clonal deletion, in the so-called negative selection process (7, 8).

The self-tolerance resulting from negative selection is called central tolerance. A stringent central tolerance induction and deletion of all autoreactive T cells is believed to create holes in the specificity space of the T cell repertoire (9, 10) by prohibiting immune responses against self-similar nonself and altered self. Hence, a too stringent central tolerance does not seem beneficial.

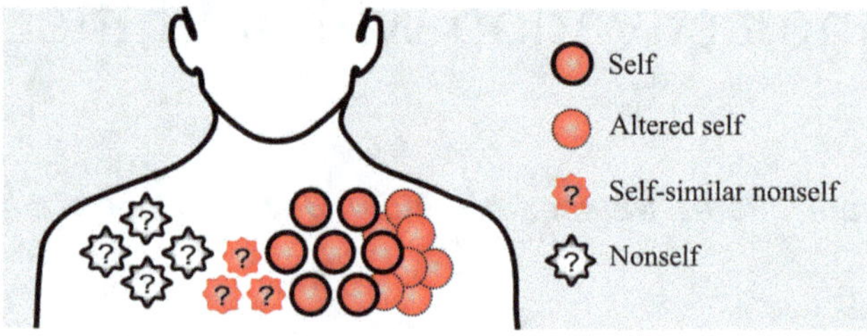

FIGURE 1 | Conceptual figure of different disturbances in the immune system. Pathogenic nonself-disturbances are recognized and attenuated by nonself-specific T cells. However, recognition and attenuation of altered self and self-similar nonself-disturbances is challenging for the immune system due to the existence of self-tolerance mechanisms; without self-specific immune cells, the immune system is not able to initiate an immune response against these disturbances.

In line with this idea, there is evidence that negative selection only partially deletes autoreactive T cells because availability of self-peptides required for negative selection in the thymus is limited and T cells spend only a limited time in the process of thymic selection (11–13). Autoreactive T cells escaping negative selection have been shown to be involved in autoimmunity (14). They normally exist in healthy individuals and are quiescent in steady state conditions in the presence of their cognate self-antigen (15).

Escaped autoreactive T cells are under the control of peripheral tolerance. A prominent mechanism of peripheral tolerance among others [reviewed in Ref. (16)] is induced by $CD4^+$ $Foxp3^+$ regulatory T cells (Tregs) (17). The majority of these cells, known as natural Tregs, are hypothesized to be selected from autoreactive T cells in thymus (18, 19). The main role of Tregs is the regulation of the immune response by suppression of the effector functions of conventional T cells (Tconv).

Despite the necessity of suppression by Tregs for avoiding autoimmunity (20, 21), production of too large numbers of Tregs in the thymus might prevent beneficial effector responses. Therefore, a too stringent peripheral tolerance induction by selection of large numbers of Tregs in the thymus does not seem favorable.

In view of this background, how does the immune system balance the tolerance mechanisms in order to ensure immune responses to any kind of disturbances including self-disturbances, yet staying tolerant to self in healthy homeostasis? Here, we address this question by using a mathematical model of immune activation that relies on identical components for self and nonself, i.e., using the same set of ordinary differential equations. The model considers the thymic production of Tregs and Tconvs as well as the dynamic interplay between Tregs, Tconvs, and IL-2 molecules in the presence of antigen(Ag)-stimulation in the periphery. The model is exploited to reveal the parametric regime of the immune system in which an immune response against self is restricted, but not impossible.

The interplay between Tregs and Tconvs during immune responses is a topic of extensive mathematical modeling (22–28). León and co-workers (22) proposed a series of models for studying immune tolerance by considering APCs, Tconvs, and Tregs. Their models rely on the assumption that regulatory interaction between Tregs and Tconvs takes place only in simultaneous conjugation with an APC. As a result of this assumption, efficient suppression of Tconvs requires a minimum population of Tregs per APC (29). As an extension, a crossregulation model is proposed by Carneiro and co-workers (26) in an attempt to incorporate Tregs in a coherent theory of the immune system. According to their model that shows a bistable behavior, immunity to a given Ag arises as competitive exclusion of Tregs by the expansion of Tconvs and tolerance results from limited APC availability or above threshold Treg numbers. Since the interactions between Tregs and Tconvs is assumed to depend on the density of the APCs, increasing the APC availability decreases the simultaneous conjugate formation of Tregs and Tconvs with the same APCs and hence, it is sufficient to break the immune tolerance.

An alternative concept was brought forward in a model proposed by Carneiro and co-workers (23) that assumes APC-independent interactions between Tconvs and Tregs for immune suppression which will be also used in our model. A direct interaction of Tconvs and Tregs was identified by experiments (30). The authors concluded that efficient immune suppression still requires a minimum population of Tregs regardless of the number of APCs.

In contrast to the aforementioned studies, we do not consider the conjugate formation of Tregs and Tconvs with APCs and therefore, there is not a competition between these cells for Ag. Instead, the role of APCs is indirectly captured by an Ag-stimulation factor which is the activation rate of naïve T cells and resting Tregs with identical Ag-specificity by APCs bearing their cognate Ag. In addition, we explicitly consider the dependency of Tregs on Tconvs through the growth factor IL-2.

Burroughs and co-workers (24) investigated Treg-induced inhibition of cytokine secretion by effector T cells. By assuming that Tregs are activated by self Ag and locally maintained by nonlinear competition for tissue-derived cytokines that are solely utilized by Tregs, the authors analyzed the role of local active Treg population size in the balance between suppressor and effector responses. Stimulation of Tregs and Tconvs is described by independent parameters. In contrast to their model, thymic output maintains the homeostatic population of Tregs in our model. Another essential difference is that Ag-stimulation of Tregs and Tconvs is described with a unified self-nonself concept and Tregs are assumed to also respond to nonself Ag-stimulation (31).

Parametric steady state analysis of the model provides insights about the physiological range of model parameters, and determines the overall conditions under which immune responses against self are possible. Furthermore, the impact of model parameters on the requirements for the initiation of immune reactions against self is analyzed. The model proposes that disturbed homeostatic balance between autoreactive T cells and Tregs increases the susceptibility to autoimmunity or cancer.

RESULTS

The mathematical model is constructed starting from a simple model of the immune response including essential components only. Then, additional complexity is incrementally added to the model to a degree allowing for validation and analysis of tolerance versus immunity. The scheme of the complete model is

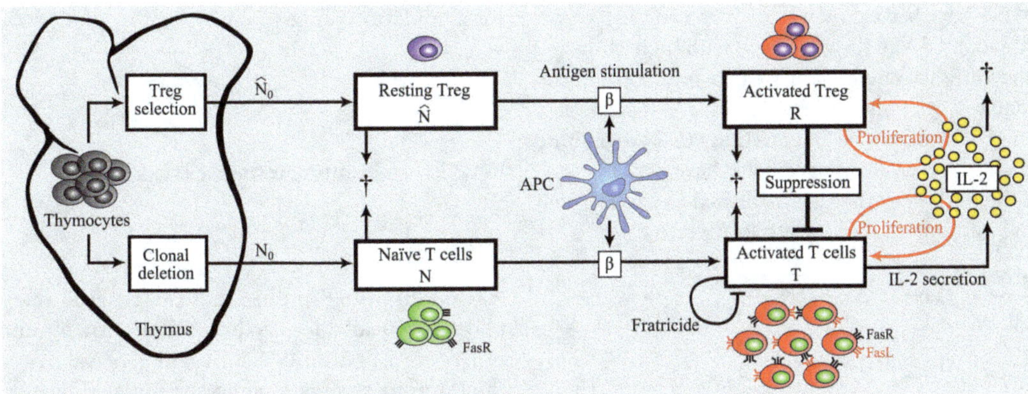

FIGURE 2 | Model of dynamic interplay between conventional T cells and regulatory T cells. Nonself-specific as well as some self-specific thymocytes that survived negative selection and were not selected as Tregs enter the periphery as naïve T cells. A part of detected autoreactive thymocytes differentiate into Tregs in the thymus and reside in the periphery in resting state. Upon Ag-stimulation by APCs, naïve T cells and resting Tregs become activated. In contrast to activated T cells, activated Tregs do not secrete IL-2, but both activated populations proliferate in dependence on the presence of IL-2 (46). Activated Tregs suppress activated T cells in a cell-contact-dependent and cytokine-driven manner. Activated T cells undergo Fas-induced apoptosis by interacting with each other (fratricide). In contrast, Tregs are resistant to Fas-induced apoptosis (68).

depicted in **Figure 2**. The model is conceptually independent of the self/nonself nature of the immune response, and differences of the immune responses against self versus nonself are reflected in different parameter values of the same model.

AN IMMUNE RESPONSE REQUIRES SUFFICIENT DIVISION AND IL-2 SECRETION RATE OF ACTIVATED T CELLS

Immune responses arise from massive proliferation of activated T cells and their subsequent effector function. Our simplest model attempts to capture the dynamic characteristics of an activated T cell population (T):

$$\begin{cases} \frac{dT}{dt} = aIT - bT \\ \frac{dI}{dt} = dT - eIT - fI \end{cases} \tag{1}$$

Activated T cells have a mean lifespan $1/b$ and secrete IL-2 (I) with rate d. Available IL-2 decays with rate f and is consumed by activated T cells with rate e. Activated T cells are able to proliferate (with rate aI) in the presence of IL-2. This IL-2 dependent proliferation rate is considered as a linear function of IL-2 in model (1). The impact of considering a nonlinear proliferation rate (a Hill-function of IL-2) instead of the linear term aIT is given in Section "Nonlinear Proliferation Rate of Conventional and Regulatory T Cells" in Appendix.

Steady state analysis of the model (1) is given in Section "Steady State Analysis of Model (1)" in Appendix. This model has two equilibrium points:

$$(T_1, I_1) = (0, 0), (T_2, I_2) = \left(\frac{bf}{ad - be}, \frac{b}{a}\right) \tag{2}$$

By assuming the biological range of parameters (all parameters are positive), the trivial equilibrium point (T_1, I_1) is stable and the nontrivial equilibrium (T_2, I_2) is unstable. T_2 is positive if and only if:

$$ad - be > 0 \tag{3}$$

The unstable equilibrium point imposes a threshold for initial conditions of the model in which the activated T cells proliferate unlimitedly, which in this simplest model, corresponds to an efficient immune response. This can be visualized by the phase portrait of the model as shown in **Figure 3A.** The condition (3) imposes a quality constraint on activated T cell clones to enter a highly proliferative state and implies that among T cell clones that are in the activated state, only the T cell clones with a sufficiently high proliferation rate (a) or IL-2 secretion rate (d) are able to contribute to the immune response against Ag. Since both, the proliferation and IL-2 secretion rate of activated T cells depend on the affinity/avidity of their TCR to the presented Ag (32–34), condition (3) implies that the existence of T cell clones with sufficiently high specificity for the presented Ag is required for induction of an immune response. Similar implications were derived from a model that considers a nonlinear IL-2 dependent proliferation rate of activated T cells (Nonlinear Proliferation Rate of Conventional and Regulatory T Cells in Appendix).

The major focus of central tolerance is to eliminate T cells that are self-specific. Therefore, it is unlikely that highly self-specific T cells escape from central tolerance, as they are more effectively detected and eliminated in the thymus (12, 34). It is thus expected that autoreactive T cells in the periphery are less aggressive than the ones that undergo clonal deletion in the thymus, and may not fulfill condition (3).

INITIATION OF AN IMMUNE RESPONSE REQUIRES A MINIMUM HOMEOSTATIC POPULATION OF NAÏVE T CELLS AND ANTIGEN STIMULATION

Continuous thymic production of naïve T cells maintains the peripheral number and diversity of mature naïve T cells (35), although other mechanisms such as stimulation of T cells with self-antigens and IL-7 have been shown to be involved (36). Upon Ag-stimulation by activated APCs, naïve T cells with high avidity to the presented Ag become activated. Here, we take into account the dynamics of the naïve T cell population (N) and T cell activation by Ag-stimulation (β), as described in equations (4). We assume that naïve T cells with identical Ag-specificity have a homeostatic population in the periphery that is established by naïve T cell renewal (by rate N_0) and natural cell death (with rate g):

$$\begin{cases} \frac{dN}{dt} = f(N) = N_0 - gN - \beta N \\ \frac{dT}{dt} = aIT - bT + \beta N \\ \frac{dI}{dt} = dT - eIT - fI \end{cases} \tag{4}$$

T cell activation $k(t)$ is defined as

$$k(t) = \beta N(t) \tag{5}$$

Steady state analysis of model (4) is given in Section "Steady State Analysis of Model (4)" in Appendix. This model has either 2 or no equilibrium points dependent on the steady state value of T cell activation (k). According to the bifurcation diagram of the model depicted in **Figure 3B**, which is obtained by treating k as bifurcation parameter, model (4) has no equilibrium points for:

$$k > k_{-} = \frac{adf}{e^2}\left(1 - \sqrt{1 - \frac{be}{ad}}\right)^2 \tag{6}$$

which corresponds to the unlimited proliferation state of activated T cells. Therefore, condition (6) has to be satisfied for initiation of an immune response. However, according to model (4), the steady state value of T cell activation (k) is limited by naïve T cell renewal (N_0) and Ag-stimulation (β):

$$k = \frac{\beta N_0}{g + \beta} \tag{7}$$

Therefore, according to equations (6) and (7), there exists an Ag-stimulation range

$$\beta > \frac{gk_{-}}{N_0 - k_{-}} \tag{8}$$

in which an immune response is initiated if:

$$N_0 > k_{-} \tag{9}$$

Condition (9) implies that the renewal rate of naïve T cells plays a critical role for the initiation of immune responses. In other words, without a sufficient renewal rate of naïve T cells, the immune response cannot be initiated by any Ag-stimulation. Instead, Ag-stimulation results in a subcritical immune response which is interpreted as insufficient for pathogen clearance. By increasing the proliferation rate or IL-2 secretion of activated T cells or the renewal rate of naïve T cells, the threshold of Ag-stimulation required for initiation of an immune response is decreased [equations (6) and (8)]. Therefore, central tolerance is able to tune the initiation criterion of self reaction not only by limiting the quality of autoreactive T cells, but additionally by restricting the renewal rate of autoreactive T cells. As central tolerance does not limit nonself-specific T cells, according to the model, these cells exhibit a lower threshold of activation by nonself Ag-stimulation.

FRATRICIDE: A MECHANISM TO LIMIT BUT NOT TO SUPPRESS IMMUNE RESPONSES

The immune response in model (4) is characterized by unlimited proliferation of activated T cells which is physiologically unrealistic. The linear death term of natural death of activated T cells in model (4) is not sufficient to limit proliferation, and requires a nonlinear limiting factor. A potential mechanism of limiting the immune response is activation-induced cell death (AICD) in activated T cells, known as fratricide (37). Upon T cell activation, death ligand (FasL) and receptor (Fas) proteins are expressed on

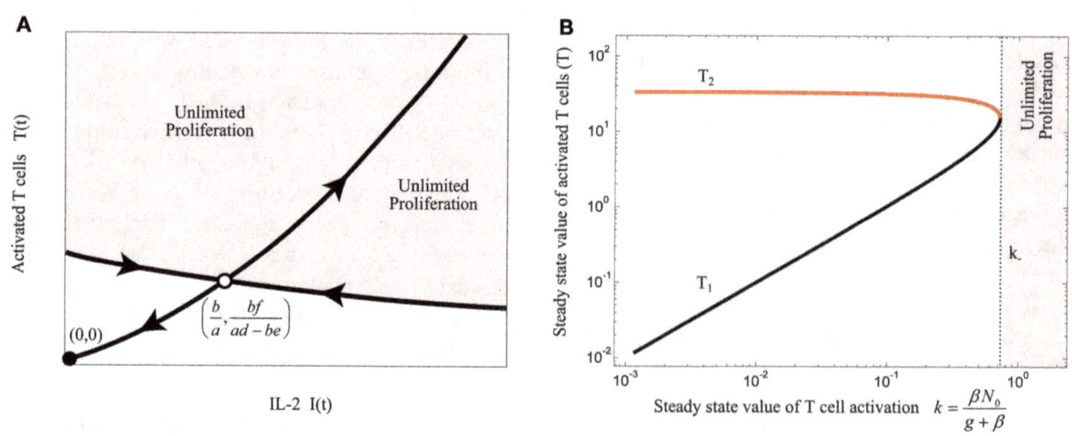

FIGURE 3 | (A) Qualitative phase portrait of model (1): the stable manifold of saddle node defines a threshold for the initial conditions that allow for unlimited proliferation of activated T cells. **(B)** Bifurcation diagram of model (4) by treating k as bifurcation parameter. Stable and unstable equilibrium points are shown by black and red lines, respectively. For $k > k_{-}$, the immune response enters the regime of unlimited proliferation.

the surface of T cells. Followed by expression of these proteins, T cells eliminate themselves in a cell-contact-dependent manner. The fratricide mechanism is modeled by a nonlinear death term (cT^2), as proposed by Callard et al. (37):

$$\begin{cases} \frac{\mathrm{d}N}{\mathrm{d}t} = f(N) = N_0 - gN - \beta N \\ \frac{\mathrm{d}T}{\mathrm{d}t} = aIT - bT - cT^2 + \beta N \\ \frac{\mathrm{d}I}{\mathrm{d}t} = dT - eIT - fI \end{cases} \tag{10}$$

The steady state analysis of model (10) is provided in Section "Steady State Analysis of Model (10)" in Appendix. This model has either 3 or 1 equilibrium points, depending on the value of fratricide death rate c. The bifurcation diagram of the model (10) with respect to c is depicted in **Figure 4A** for ($\beta = 0$). When c satisfies

$$c < c_{-} = f^{-1}\left(\sqrt{ad} - \sqrt{be}\right)^2 \tag{11}$$

the stable equilibrium point (T_3) exists and corresponds to a saturated population of activated T cell. When the conditions (3) and (11) are fulfilled, the model (10) exhibits the bifurcation diagram plotted in **Figure 4B** with respect to the steady state value of T cell activation (k). The fratricide mechanism added a large stable equilibrium point (T_3) to the model which imposes a saturation level to the activated T cell population. The larger the c, the smaller the saturated population of activated T cells is. Similar to model (4), model (10) shows an initiation threshold of the immune response ($k > k_i$). Despite solving the issue of unlimited proliferation of activated T cells by the fratricide mechanism, model (10) bears a hysteresis characteristic so that the immune response cannot be suppressed when Ag-stimulation (β) is removed.

DYNAMIC INTERPLAY OF ACTIVATED T CELLS AND TREGS

Tregs are essential in maintaining self-tolerance and immune homeostasis by preventing autoimmunity and limiting chronic inflammation in the periphery. However, they might also limit beneficial responses by inducing tolerance to pathogens (38, 39) or limiting anti-tumor immunity (40, 41). One functional role of Tregs is to shut down the cell-mediated immune response via cell-contact-dependent and inhibitory cytokine-driven suppression of activated T cells (42). Two different subsets of Tregs were identified. Natural Tregs are the dominant subset of peripheral Tregs (43) and are selected in the thymus. In our model, we consider only natural Tregs and neglect the induced Treg subset that differentiates from naïve T cells. Like for naïve T cells, the thymus contributes to the renewal of resting Tregs ($\widehat{N}$) by continuously selecting them from thymocytes. The renewal of resting Tregs is assumed to occur by rate $\widehat{N}_0$. Since we are interested in the relative renewal of resting Tregs and naïve T cells, we assume that:

$$\widehat{N}_0 = \lambda N_0 \tag{12}$$

Tregs remain in the resting state until they are stimulated by Ag (β) and become activated in a TCR-dependent manner. The dynamic population of the resting Treg compartment is assumed to be the same as the naïve T cell compartment in (4) and (10) ($\mathrm{d}\widehat{N}/\mathrm{d}t = f(\widehat{N})$). Activated Tregs ($R$) are assumed to suppress activated T cells (by rate γ). Survival and proliferation of activated Tregs depends strictly on IL-2, produced by activated non-Tregs (44–46). The IL-2 dependent proliferation rate of Tregs is considered as a linear function of IL-2 (see Nonlinear Proliferation Rate of Conventional and Regulatory T Cells in Appendix for a nonlinear case). In contrast to activated T cells, activated Tregs

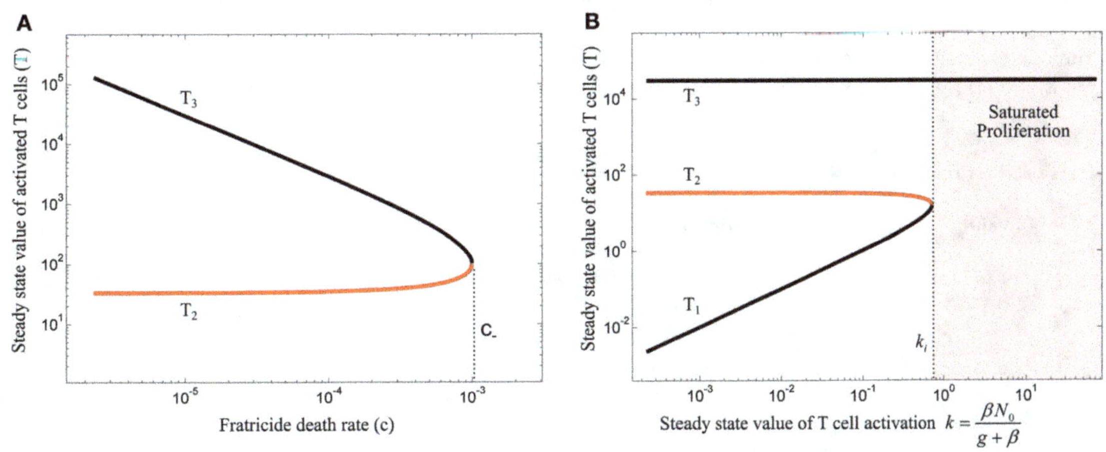

FIGURE 4 | (A) Bifurcation diagram of model (10) with $\beta = 0$ using the fratricide death rate c as bifurcation parameter. No immune response exists for fratricide death rates larger than c_{-} due to extensive activation-induced cell death. The trivial equilibrium point is omitted in this figure. **(B)** Bifurcation diagram of model (10) using k as bifurcation parameter: an immune response can be initiated for large values of k. However, due to hysteresis characteristic in this model, the immune response is not suppressed after decreasing T cell activation (k). Stable and unstable equilibrium points are shown by black and red lines, respectively.

lack the ability to secrete IL-2 (47). The relative proliferation rate of activated Tregs and activated T cells is controlled by the parameter ϵ:

$$\begin{cases} \dfrac{dT}{dt} = aIT - bT - cT^2 - \gamma RT + \beta N \\ \dfrac{dR}{dt} = \epsilon aIR - bR + \beta \widehat{N} \\ \dfrac{dI}{dt} = dT - eI(T+R) - fI \end{cases} \tag{13}$$

The parameters are given in **Table 1** and the model components are illustrated in **Figure 2**. Treg activation $\widehat{k}(t)$ is defined as

$$\widehat{k}(t) = \beta \widehat{N}(t) \tag{14}$$

According to equations (7) and (12), the steady state value of Treg activation $(\widehat{k})$ is given by

$$\widehat{k} = \lambda \frac{\beta N_0}{g+\beta} = \lambda k \tag{15}$$

The equilibrium points of model (13) are given in Section "Steady State Analysis of Model (13)" in Appendix. By incorporating the Treg compartment to model (10), two additional equilibrium points (T_4 and T_5) emerged for $\beta = 0$. The equilibrium point of interest (T_4), which depends on the Treg-associated parameters (ϵ, γ), has an impact on the topological changes of the phase portraits of the model under variations of the bifurcation parameter k. The value of ϵ and γ are assumed to be in a range where the model does not inherit the hysteresis characteristics of immune responses from model (10) in which the immune response is not suppressed after resolving Ag-stimulation (β). Then, the bifurcation diagrams of model (13) for two different values of λ are obtained by treating k as the bifurcation parameter (**Figure 5**). Depending on the value of k, the model has either 5 or 3 equilibrium points.

By varying the relative renewal rates of resting Tregs and naïve T cells [λ in equation (12)] a λ_{th} can be found, so that no immune response can be initiated for any value of k, if $\lambda > \lambda_{th}$ (**Figure 5A**). For $\lambda < \lambda_{th}$ (**Figure 5B**), there exists a T cell activation threshold (k_i) such that for $k > k_i$ the immune response can be initiated. However, in contrast to model (10), the immune response is completely suppressed by activated Tregs if k decreases to a lower value than k_i (gray region in **Figure 5B**). For persistent Ag-stimulation with $k > k_i$, two scenarios are possible. An oscillating immune response is induced when k remains in the range of $k_i < k < k_s$ (red region in **Figure 5B**). For $k > k_s$ the immune response is suppressed after its initiation to a minor immune response with an activated T cell population T_4 due to over-suppression of activated T cells by over-activation of Tregs (magenta region in **Figure 5B**). In the latter case ($k > k_s$), despite proper T cell stimulation, only a minor immune response is induced (and antigen is not cleared). Instead a chronic co-existence of antigen and inefficient immune activity is established. Therefore, according to the model, a range of T cell and Treg activation ($k_i < k < k_s$) exists in which an efficient immune response is induced. Outside of this range, the antigen persists because of under-stimulation of naïve T cells, or over-stimulation of Tregs. According to equation (7), the existence of Ag-stimulation thresholds β_i and β_s which correspond to the values of k_i and k_s, respectively, depends on the renewal rate of naïve T cells (N_0); β_i exists if $N_0 > k_i$ and β_s exists if $N_0 > k_s$. Increasing the renewal rate of naïve T cells reduces the Ag-stimulation required for initiation(β_i)/over-suppression(β_s) of the immune response.

The peak immune response depends on the value of the Treg-associated equilibrium point (T_4) which in turn depends on Treg-associated parameters. However, the fratricide-associated equilibrium point (T_3) is a limiting factor for the maximum population of activated T cells if the fratricide death rate (c) is sufficiently high.

According to our model, sufficient activated Tregs are required to suppress the proliferative response of activated T cells. These are supplied by two processes: Treg activation $(\widehat{k})$ which depends on Ag-stimulation (β), and Treg proliferation which depends on the IL-2 secretion by activated T cells. With a low Ag-stimulation and insufficient Treg activation ($\widehat{k} = \beta \widehat{N}$), Treg proliferation has to account for immune suppression. Since Treg proliferation is

Table 1 | Parameters used for model analysis.

Parameter	Value	Description	Dimension
a	0.4	Proliferation rate of activated T cells	molecules^{-1}time^{-1}
b	0.1	Natural death rate of activated T cells and Tregs	mime^{-1}
c	10^{-5}	Fratricide death rate of activated T cells	cells^{-1}time^{-1}
d	0.01	IL-2 secretion rate by activated T cells	molecules cells^{-1}time^{-1}
e	0.01	IL-2 consumption rate by activated T cells and Tregs	cells^{-1}time^{-1}
f	1	IL-2 decay rate	time^{-1}
g	B	Natural death rate of naïve T cells and resting Tregs	time^{-1}
β	$[0,\infty)$	Ag-stimulation of naïve T cells and resting Tregs	time^{-1}
γ	0.1	Treg-mediated suppression rate	cells^{-1}time^{-1}
ϵ	0.6	Proliferation rate ratio Treg/Tconv	–
N_0	4	Renewal rate of naïve T cells	cells time^{-1}
λ	0.006, 0.02	Relative renewal rate of resting Tregs and naïve T cells $\widehat{N}_0/N_0$	–
$\widehat{N}_0$	$\lambda\ N_0$	Renewal rate of resting Tregs	cells time^{-1}

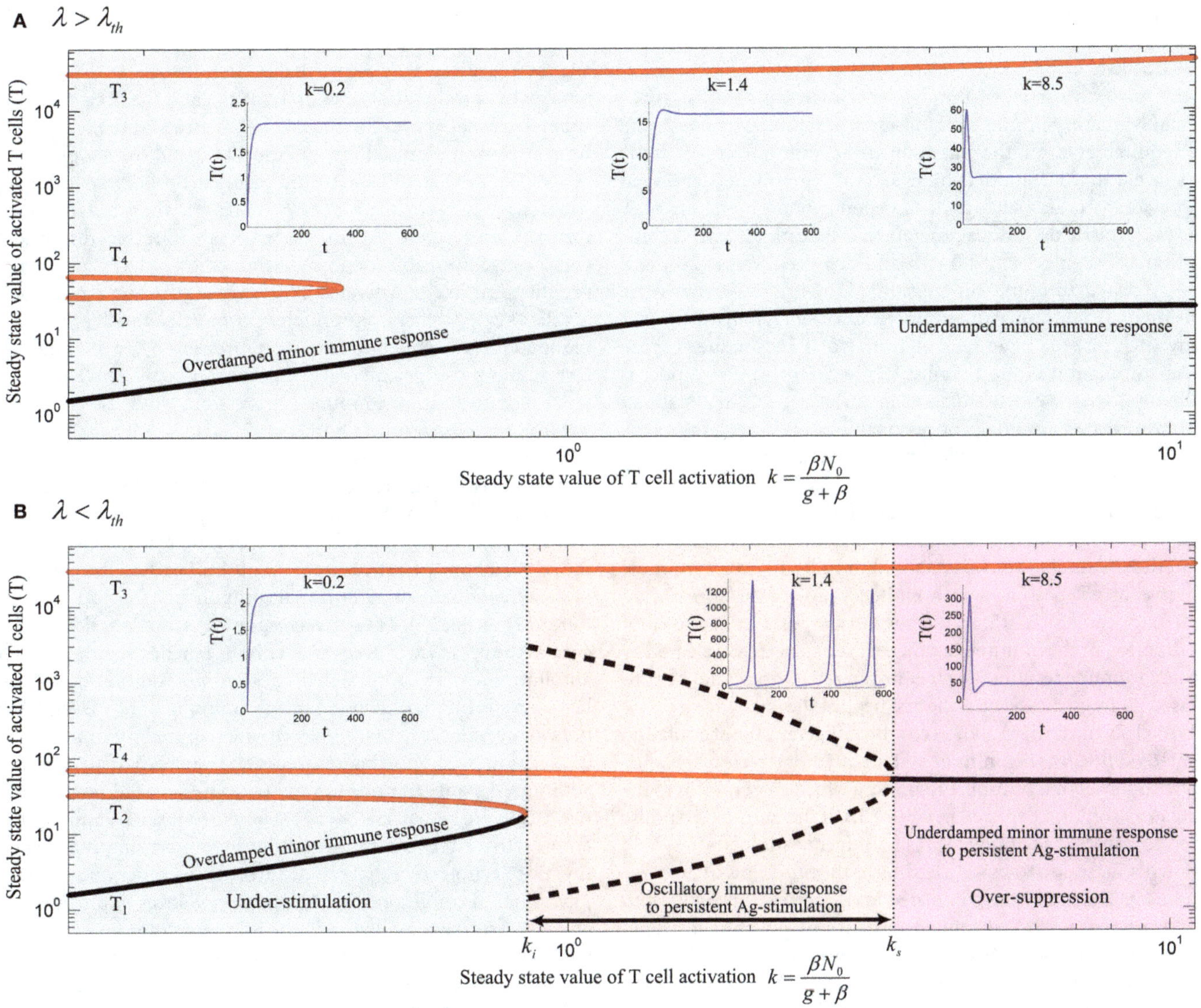

FIGURE 5 | Bifurcation diagram of model (13) using k as the bifurcation parameter with (A) $\lambda = 0.02$ and (B) $\lambda = 0.006$. Stable and unstable equilibrium points are drawn by black and red solid lines, respectively. Dashed black lines represent the stable limit cycles by showing the maximum and minimum populations of oscillating activated T cells for persistent k. Depending on the values of λ and k, an immune response is not initiated (gray), is initiated (red) or over-suppressed (magenta). With parameter values given in **Table 1**, the threshold becomes $\lambda_{th} = 0.01183$. The time-courses of the activated T cell population $T(t)$ were deduced from a numerical solution of model (13) with zero initial conditions and persistent β. The unstable negative equilibrium point (T_5) is not shown in the plots.

dependent on the availability of IL-2, sufficient activated T cells are required to secrete IL-2 and induce immune suppression. Therefore, activated T cells undergo the proliferation up to a level that sufficient IL-2 is available for Treg proliferation and subsequent immune suppression. In contrast, by facilitated Treg activation $(\widehat{k})$, less Treg proliferation is required for suppressing activated T cells which means that the dependency of immune suppression on proliferation of activated T cells decreases. Consequently, by increasing Ag-stimulation (β) in the range of $\beta_i < \beta < \beta_s$ (red region in **Figure 5B**), Treg activation $(\widehat{k})$ increases as well which results in a reduced maximum population of activated T cells (**Figure 5B**, dashed black line) and an increased frequency of oscillations. By further increasing Ag-stimulation to $\beta > \beta_s$ (magenta region in **Figure 5B**), Treg activation $(\widehat{k})$ completely prevent oscillating immune response.

In the same way, by increasing the relative homeostatic population of resting Tregs and naïve T cells ($\lambda > \lambda_{th}$), Treg activation increases up to a level that Treg suppression does not depend on the proliferative response of activated T cells. Thus, activated T cells are not able to enter the massive proliferation for any Ag-stimulation level, as shown in **Figure 5A**. Similar results were derived from a model that considers a nonlinear IL-2 dependent proliferation rate of activated T cells and Tregs (see Nonlinear Proliferation Rate of Conventional and Regulatory T Cells in Appendix).

DISCUSSION

In this study, a model of the dynamic interplay between effector and regulatory immune responses was examined to investigate the requirements for the initiation of an immune response by Ag-stimulation. The model unifies several components developed in previous studies, such as IL-2 dependent proliferation of T cells (48), fratricide-induce programed cell death (37), IL-2 competition between activated T cell and activated Tregs (24), and Treg-mediated immune suppression (23, 24, 28). Homeostatic division of T cell compartments was not considered in the present study, such that the main renewal source of T cells in the absence of Ag-stimulation is the thymus. While the presented model is still simplifying the real situation in many aspects, the stability analysis revealed a number of reasonable results matching many experimental findings and allowing for an analysis of reasons for immune failure and autoimmunity.

The model predicts three qualitatively different immune responses depending on the level of antigenic stimulation. At first, a threshold stimulation β_i is required in order to get an immune response at all. Secondly, in a limited range of Ag-stimulation $\beta \in (\beta_i, \beta_s)$ an efficient immune response is induced. Tregs limit the duration of the immune response. If the antigen was cleared by the first immune response, further immune activity would be suppressed by Tregs. However, if the first peak of the immune response fails to clear the antigen, but keeps the antigen in the stimulation range $\beta_i < \beta < \beta_s$, the immune system attempts to clear the antigen with subsequent immune responses, which corresponds to the oscillatory solution depicted in **Figure 5B**. If the immune response failed to control the antigen spread, antigenic stimulation would be further increased to $\beta > \beta_s$, leading to the third class of immune responses. Tregs are over-stimulated and suppress immune activity. In this situation, a chronic persistence of the antigen would develop. Treg-mediated over-suppression of immune responses in chronic infections is well-established (reviewed in Ref. (49)). According to our model, depletion of resting Tregs restores the immune response by transiently decreasing λ and by this increasing β_s. This notion is consistent with the experimental model of chronic infections according to which depletion of Tregs results in the restoration of effector immune response and restriction of antigen spread (50, 51). A key feature of our model is that the immune response does not rely on a stable equilibrium point with a dominant population of activated T cells which is typically derived from existing bistable models. It rather relies on a transient response (or stable limit cycles in the case of persistent Ag-stimulation) which originates from T-cell-mediated suppression and IL-2 consumption by Tregs. Moreover, the role of Tregs in the chronic state of the immune response is not represented by available models.

According to our model, the qualitatively different immune responses and their requirements are dependent on the quality and quantity of Tconv and Treg clones responding to the Ag-stimulation. The proliferation rate of activated T cells, which depends on their avidity to the stimulating antigen determines the existence of an Ag-stimulation threshold (β_i) which is required for the initiation of an immune response. The absolute renewal rate of naïve T cells (N_0) adjusts the Ag-stimulation threshold β_i, which exists when the renewal rate of resting Tregs remains below a threshold value ($\lambda < \lambda_{th}$). Further Treg-associated parameters, namely the proliferation rate of Tregs (ϵ) and the Treg-mediated suppression rate (γ), also affect the existence and the level of the Ag-stimulation required for initiation (β_i) and over-suppression (β_s) of immune responses. By increasing the proliferative (ϵ) and suppressive (γ) activity of Tregs, β_i increases, whereas β_s decreases up to a level where the initiation of an immune response is completely impossible for any Ag-stimulation. Interestingly, when proliferation rate of activated Tregs exceeds the one for activated T cells ($\epsilon > 1$) a massive proliferation of activated T cells is still required for subsequent immune suppression by Tregs. Thus, IL-2 secretion by sufficiently large numbers of activated T cells is a strict requirement for immune suppression. Note also that without Tregs, a return to the homeostatic state is not possible, even when the antigen was cleared.

Considering all aforementioned parameters controlling the initiation of an immune response, is it beneficial for the immune system to completely avoid self reaction, or is there a benefit in allowing self reaction? Clearly, autoreactive T cells exist in the periphery of healthy individuals as a normal component of the T cell repertoire (12, 14, 52, 53). These cells respond to self-tissue destruction even in the presence of Tregs and without genetic predisposition to autoimmunity (15). Although the activation of autoreactive T cells has been shown to be involved in autoimmunity (12), several lines of evidences indicate that these cells are required for limiting self-destruction by supporting self-regenerative processes (54–56). In addition, the anti-tumor immune responses evoked by autoreactive T cells are beneficial (34, 57). Therefore, it seems unlikely that autoreactive T cells escaping from the thymus are simply a result of thymic selection error that can disturb self-tolerance under certain physiological conditions. Instead, these evidences imply that beneficial self reaction is allowed in the immune system. According to the mathematical model, immune reactions against self are only possible with a critical homeostatic population of autoreactive T cells (or sufficient renewal rate N_0) which is balanced by a proper number of Tregs ($\lambda < \lambda_{th}$) which corresponds to region (C) or (D) in **Figure 6**. Since the T cell repertoire is normally stimulated with an endogenous level of self-antigens in the periphery which does not evoke any self reaction, the Ag-stimulation threshold for initiating an immune response (β_i) should be sufficiently high in comparison to a typical nonself Ag-stimulation. According to our model, this is achieved by ensuring a low renewal rate (N_0) of low-avidity autoreactive T cells and a high, but balanced renewal rate of Tregs (high λ but lower than λ_{th}). In other words, according to **Figure 6**, by choosing N_0 close to k_i and higher value of k_i which is obtained by higher λ, a large Ag-stimulation threshold (β_i) for the initiation of immunity against self can be achieved.

Aging of the immune system, the so-called immunosenescence, is characterized by involution of thymus, decreased number of thymic output, contraction in T cell diversity, and disturbed T cell homeostasis which all result in attenuated immune function and susceptibility to infectious diseases and cancer in the elderly (58, 59). By decreasing thymic output, the homeostatic population of some T cell clones diminishes which leads to the creation of holes

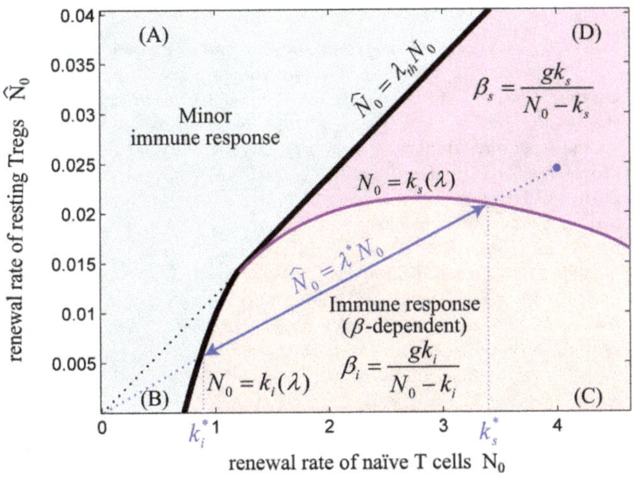

FIGURE 6 | The balance between renewal rate of naïve T cells and resting Tregs. The relative renewal rate of naïve T cells and resting Tregs ($\lambda = \widehat{N}_0/N_0$) determines the existence of an immune response. The initiation of an immune response requires a sufficient renewal rate of naïve T cells (N_0). **(A)** For $\lambda > \lambda_{th}$, the immune response does not exist for any value of N_0 and Ag-stimulation (β). **(B)** For $N_0 < k_i$, no immune response can be initiated for any value of β. **(C)** For $N_0 > k_i$, immune response can be initiated for $\beta > \beta_i$. In this regime, the Ag-stimulation that results in over-suppression of immune response (β_s) does not exist. **(D)** In this regime, immune response is initiated for $\beta > \beta_i$, and is over-suppressed for $\beta > \beta_s$. Note that k_i and k_s are dependent on the value of λ. For any point in the plane (e.g., blue point), the values of k_s^* and k_i^* are obtained by projecting the intersections of the line created by connecting the point to the origin (slope $= \lambda^*$) with the nonlinear curves $N_0 = k_i(\lambda)$ and $N_0 = k_s(\lambda)$ onto the N_0-axis. By decreasing λ^*, the effective range of T cell activation ($k_s^* - k_i^*$) or equivalently, the effective range of Ag-stimulation ($\beta_s^* - \beta_i^*$) which evoke immune response without over-suppression increases. We hypothesize that a healthy individual bears the potential to evoke self reaction and therefore its immune system is located in parametric regime **(C)** or **(D)**; however, higher self Ag-stimulation compared to nonself Ag-stimulation is required for initiating immune response due to low renewal rate of autoreactive T cells (N_0).

in the T cell repertoire (60). According to our model, a decreased renewal rate of a naïve T cell clone (N_0) *per se* could prevent an immune response or increase the Ag-stimulation level required for initiation of an immune response. In addition, as shown in many studies, the frequency of Tregs increases with age (61, 62) which results in a disturbed balance between the population of naïve T cells and resting Tregs (increased λ). In line with these results, in the mathematical model an increased λ prevents the initiation of an immune response corresponding to the age-related immune hyporesponsiveness in infection and cancer.

Based on the reasonable and physiologically realistic results that we could derive from the model, we dare to speculate about the self versus nonself concept emerging from the model. As mentioned before, the naïve T cells and resting Tregs are two major components of the immune reaction. The model does not distinguish self and nonself, but rather derives different responses to self and nonself from quantitative differences in the nature of Ag-stimulation. According to the model, by adjusting different parameters, different requirements in terms of Ag-stimulation level are found for the initiation of immune responses to self versus nonself. If the immune system responds according to a universal set of Ag-stimulation thresholds, regardless of whether the stimulus arises from self or nonself-antigens, a change of systemic parameters can lead to immune failure or autoimmunity. Self is no more considered as self if it exceeds an Ag-stimulation threshold determined by the stringency of central and peripheral tolerances. Similarly, nonself is considered as self if it does not properly stimulate the T cell repertoire. Autoimmunity might occur due to either a failure in tuning the Ag-stimulation threshold by the thymus that leads to unwanted self reaction in the periphery, or a chronic self Ag-stimulation in the periphery that leads to an oscillating self reaction and tissue destruction like in type 1 diabetes (63) and multiple sclerosis (64). Cancer or chronic infection would arise as the result of an imbalance in central and peripheral tolerances such as insufficient release of autoreactive T cells as well as high production or induction of Tregs that results in over-suppression of immune responses.

An early elegant mathematical modeling study analyzed a series of models to investigate self/nonself discrimination by T cells without explicitly considering suppressive Tregs (48). As a result of their critical assumption that memory cells accumulate in poor stimulatory conditions, the authors suggested that due to high stimulation by self antigens the lack of memory accumulation for T cell clones with high affinity to self accounts for self-tolerance. Also in our model, a high self Ag-stimulation ($\beta > \beta_s$ in **Figure 5B**) results in over-activation of Tregs and by this in over-suppression of self reaction. In both models an increased stimulation by self antigen would not lead to autoimmunity. The fact that autoreactive T cells do respond in the presence of Tregs when their stimulatory requirements are provided (15) makes it unlikely that this is the mechanism of self-tolerance induction. In the framework of our model, the view is supported that immune tolerance is induced by an increased stimulation threshold for self antigen and keeping self Ag-stimulation in a subcritical regime ($\beta < \beta_i$).

Undoubtedly, other mechanisms besides clonal deletion and Treg selection in the thymus also contribute to the fine tuning of the Ag-stimulation threshold required for initiation of immune reactions to self and nonself, such as anergy in the periphery (65) or activation threshold tuning in the thymus (66, 67). However, our simple model emphasizes the subtle balance between the generation of Tregs and autoreactive T cells which are both needed for beneficial autoimmunity. The model supports the view according to which self and nonself do not differ on a qualitative level. It is rather quantitative differences of the immune status and Ag-stimulation level that determine which molecule is treated as self or nonself.

ACKNOWLEDGMENTS

Michael Meyer-Hermann was supported by HFSP and BMBF within the GerontoSys initiative (projects GerontoMitoSys and GerontoShield). Sahamoddin Khailaie was supported by the Helmholtz International Graduate School for Infection Research.

REFERENCES

1. Babbitt BP, Allen PM, Matsueda G, Haber E, Unanue ER. Binding of immunogenic peptides to Ia histocompatibility molecules. *Nature* (1985) **317**:359–61. doi:10.1038/317359a0

2. Guermonprez P, Valladeau J, Zitvogel L, Théry C, Amigorena S. Antigen presentation and T cell stimulation by dendritic cells. *Annu Rev Immunol* (2002) **20**:621–67. doi:10.1146/annurev.immunol.20.100301.064828
3. Yewdell JW, Haeryfar SM. Understanding presentation of viral antigens to CD8+ T cells in vivo: the key to rational vaccine design. *Annu Rev Immunol* (2005) **23**:651–82. doi:10.1146/annurev.immunol.23.021704.115702
4. Kanduc D, Stufano A, Lucchese G, Kusalik A. Massive peptide sharing between viral and human proteomes. *Peptides* (2008) **29**(10):1755–66. doi:10.1016/j.peptides.2008.05.022
5. Trost B, Kusalik A, Lucchese G, Kanduc D. Bacterial peptides are intensively present throughout the human proteome. *Self Nonself* (2010) **1**(1):71–4. doi:10.4161/self.1.1.9588
6. Wolfl M, Rutebemberwa A, Mosbruger T, Mao Q, Li H, Netski D, et al. Hepatitis C virus immune escape via exploitation of a hole in the T cell repertoire. *J Immunol* (2008) **181**(9):6435–46.
7. McCaughtry T, Hogquist K. Central tolerance: what have we learned from mice? *Semin Immunopathol* (2008) **30**:399–409. doi:10.1007/s00281-008-0137-0
8. Palmer E, Naeher D. Affinity threshold for thymic selection through a T-cell receptor-co-receptor zipper. *Nat Rev Immunol* (2009) **9**:207–13. doi:10.1038/nri2469
9. Rolland M, Nickle DC, Deng W, Frahm N, Brander C, Learn GH, et al. Recognition of HIV-1 peptides by host CTL is related to HIV-1 similarity to human proteins. *PLoS One* (2007) **2**(9):e823. doi:10.1371/journal.pone.0000823
10. Frankild S, Boer RJD, Lund O, Nielsen M, Kesmir C. Amino acid similarity accounts for T cell cross-reactivity and for holes in the T cell repertoire. *PLoS One* (2008) **3**(3):e1831. doi:10.1371/journal.pone.0001831
11. Bouneaud C, Kourilsky P, Bousso P. Impact of negative selection on the T cell repertoire reactive to a self-peptide: a large fraction of T cell clones escapes clonal deletion. *Immunity* (2000) **13**:829–40. doi:10.1016/S1074-7613(00)00080-7
12. Zehn D, Bevan M. T cells with low avidity for a tissue-restricted antigen routinely evade central and peripheral tolerance and cause autoimmunity. *Immunity* (2006) **25**:261–70. doi:10.1016/j.immuni.2006.06.009
13. Derbinski J, Kyewski B. How thymic antigen presenting cells sample the body's self-antigens. *Curr Opin Immunol* (2010) **22**(5):592–600. doi:10.1016/j.coi.2010.08.003
14. Bulek AM, Cole DK, Skowera A, Dolton G, Gras S, Madura F, et al. Structural basis for the killing of human beta cells by CD8(+) T cells in type 1 diabetes. *Nat Immunol* (2012) **13**(3):283–9. doi:10.1038/ni.2206
15. Enouz S, Carrié L, Merkler D, Bevan MJ, Zehn D. Autoreactive T cells bypass negative selection and respond to self-antigen stimulation during infection. *J Exp Med* (2012) **209**(10):1769–79. doi:10.1084/jem.20120905
16. Mueller DL. Mechanisms maintaining peripheral tolerance. *Nat Immunol* (2010) **11**(12):21–7. doi:10.1038/ni.1817
17. Hsieh C-S, Lee H-M, Lio C-WJ. Selection of regulatory T cells in the thymus. *Nat Rev Immunol* (2012) **12**(3):157–67. doi:10.1038/nri3155
18. Jordan MS, Boesteanu A, Reed AJ, Petrone AL, Holenbeck AE, Lerman MA, et al. Thymic selection of CD4+CD25+ regulatory T cells induced by an agonist self-peptide. *Nat Immunol* (2001) **2**:301–6. doi:10.1038/86302
19. Killebrew JR, Perdue N, Kwan A, Thornton AM, Shevach EM, Campbell DJ. A self-reactive TCR drives the development of Foxp3+ regulatory T cells that prevent autoimmune disease. *J Immunol* (2011) **187**(2):861–9. doi:10.4049/jimmunol.1004009
20. Kim JM, Rasmussen JP, Rudensky AY. Regulatory T cells prevent catastrophic autoimmunity throughout the lifespan of mice. *Nat Immunol* (2006) **8**:191–7. doi:10.1038/ni1428
21. Lahl K, Loddenkemper C, Drouin C, Freyer J, Arnason J, Eberl G, et al. Selective depletion of Foxp3+ regulatory T cells induces a scurfy-like disease. *J Exp Med* (2007) **204**(1):57–63. doi:10.1084/jem.20061852
22. León K, Peréz R, Lage A, Carneiro J. Modelling T-cell-mediated suppression dependent on interactions in multicellular conjugates. *J Theor Biol* (2000) **207**(2):231–54. doi:10.1006/jtbi.2000.2169
23. Carneiro J, Paixão T, Milutinovic D, Sousaa J, León K, Gardner R, et al. Immunological self-tolerance: lessons from mathematical modeling. *J Comput Appl Math* (2005) **184**(1):77–100. doi:10.1016/j.cam.2004.10.025
24. Burroughs NJ, Miguel Paz Mendes de Oliveira B, Adrego Pinto A. Regulatory T cell adjustment of quorum growth thresholds and the control of local immune responses. *J Theor Biol* (2006) **241**(1):134–41. doi:10.1016/j.jtbi.2005.11.010
25. Kim PS, Lee PP, Levy D. Modeling regulation mechanisms in the immune system. *J Theor Biol* (2007) **246**(1):33–69. doi:10.1016/j.jtbi.2006.12.012
26. Carneiro J, León K, Caramalho I, Van Den Dool C, Gardner R, Oliveira V, et al. When three is not a crowd: a cross regulation model of the dynamics and repertoire selection of regulatory CD4+ T cells. *Immunol Rev* (2007) **216**(1):48–68. doi:10.1111/j.1600-065X.2007.00487.x
27. Burroughs NJ, Ferreira MF, Oliveira B, Pinto AA. Autoimmunity arising from bystander proliferation of T cells in an immune response model. *Math Comput Model* (2011) **53**(7):1389–93. doi:10.1016/j.mcm.2010.01.020
28. Almeida ARM, Amado IF, Reynolds J, Berges J, Lythe G, Molina-París C, et al. Quorum-sensing in CD4(+) T cell homeostasis: a hypothesis and a model. *Front Immunol* (2012) **3**:125. doi:10.3389/fimmu.2012.00125
29. León K, Peréz R, Lage A, Carneiro J. Three-cell interactions in T cell-mediated suppression? A mathematical analysis of its quantitative implications. *J Immunol* (2001) **166**(9):5356–65.
30. Thornton AM, Shevach EM. Suppressor effector function of CD4+CD25+ immunoregulatory T cells is antigen nonspecific. *J Immunol* (2000) **164**(1):183–90.
31. Pacholczyk R, Kern J, Singh N, Iwashima M, Kraj P, Ignatowicz L. Nonself-antigens are the cognate specificities of Foxp3+ regulatory T cells. *Immunity* (2007) **27**(3):493–504. doi:10.1016/j.immuni.2007.07.019
32. Hofmann M, Radsak M, Rechtsteiner G, Wiemann K, Günder M, Bien-Gräter U, et al. T cell avidity determines the level of CTL activation. *Eur J Immunol* (2004) **34**(7):1798–806. doi:10.1002/eji.200425088
33. Zehn D, Lee SY, Bevan MJ. Complete but curtailed T-cell response to very low-affinity antigen. *Nature* (2009) **458**(7235):211–4. doi:10.1038/nature07657
34. Hebeisen M, Rufer N, Oberle SG, Speiser DE, Zehn D. Signaling mechanisms that balance anti-viral, auto-reactive, and anti-tumor potential of low affinity T cells. *J Clin Cell Immunol* (2012) **S12**(3). doi:10.4172/2155-9899.S12-003
35. Bourgeois C, Hao Z, Rajewsky K, Potocnik AJ, Stockinger B. Ablation of thymic export causes accelerated decay of naïve CD4 T cells in the periphery because of activation by environmental antigen. *Proc Natl Acad Sci U S A* (2008) **105**(25):8691–6. doi:10.1073/pnas.0803732105
36. Takada K, Jameson SC. Naive T cell homeostasis: from awareness of space to a sense of place. *Nat Rev Immunol* (2009) **9**(12):823–32. doi:10.1038/nri2657
37. Callard RE, Stark J, Yates AJ. Fratricide: a mechanism for T memory-cell homeostasis. *Trends Immunol* (2003) **24**(7):370–5. doi:10.1016/S1471-4906(03)00164-9
38. Belkaid Y. Regulatory T cells and infection: a dangerous necessity. *Nat Rev Immunol* (2007) **7**:875–88. doi:10.1038/nri2189
39. Zhou Y. Regulatory T cells and viral infections. *Front Biosci* (2008) **13**:1152–70. doi:10.2741/2752
40. Kretschmer K, Apostolou I, Jaeckel E, Khazaie K, von Boehmer H. Making regulatory T cells with defined antigen specificity: role in autoimmunity and cancer. *Immunol. Rev* (2006) **212**:163–9. doi:10.1111/j.0105-2896.2006.00411.x
41. Klages K, Mayer CT, Lahl K, Loddenkemper C, Teng MW, Ngiow SF, et al. Selective depletion of Foxp3+ regulatory T cells improves effective therapeutic vaccination against established melanoma. *Cancer Res* (2010) **70**(20):7788–99. doi:10.1158/0008-5472.CAN-10-1736
42. Vignali DA, Collison LW, Workman CJ. How regulatory T cells work. *Nat Rev Immunol* (2008) **8**(7):523–32. doi:10.1038/nri2343
43. Thornton AM, Korty PE, Tran D, Wohlfert EA, Murray PE, Belkaid Y, et al. Expression of Helios, an Ikaros transcription factor family member, differentiates thymic-derived from peripherally induced Foxp3+ T regulatory cells. *J Immunol* (2010) **184**:3433–41. doi:10.4049/jimmunol.0904028
44. Fontenot JD, Rasmussen JP, Gavin MA, Rudensky AY. A function for interleukin 2 in Foxp3-expressing regulatory T cells. *Nat Immunol* (2005) **6**:1142–51. doi:10.1038/ni1263
45. Zou T, Caton AJ, Koretzky GA, Kambayashi T. Dendritic cells induce regulatory T cell proliferation through antigen-dependent and -independent interactions. *J Immunol* (2010) **185**(5):2790–9. doi:10.4049/jimmunol.0903740
46. Busse D, de la Rosa M, Hobiger K, Thurley K, Flossdorf M, Scheffold A, et al. Competing feedback loops shape IL-2 signaling between helper and regulatory T lymphocytes in cellular microenvironments. *Proc Natl Acad Sci U S A* (2010) **107**(7):3058–63. doi:10.1073/pnas.0812851107

47. Sakaguchi S. Naturally arising Foxp3-expressing CD25+CD4+ regulatory T cells in immunological tolerance to self and non-self. *Nat Immunol* (2005) **6**:345–52. doi:10.1038/ni1178
48. de Boer RJ, Hogeweg P. Self-nonself discrimination due to immunological nonlinearities: the analysis of a series of models by numerical methods. *Math Med Biol* (1987) **4**(1):1–32. doi:10.1093/imammb/4.1.1
49. Li S, Gowans EJ, Chougnet C, Plebanski M, Dittmer U. Natural regulatory T cells and persistent viral infection. *J Virol* (2008) **82**(1):21–30. doi:10.1128/JVI.01768-07
50. Dietze KK, Zelinskyy G, Gibbert K, Schimmer S, Francois S, Myers L, et al. Transient depletion of regulatory T cells in transgenic mice reactivates virus-specific CD8 + T cells and reduces chronic retroviral set points. *Proc Natl Acad Sci U S A* (2011) **108**(6):2420–5. doi:10.1073/pnas.1015148108
51. Keynan Y, Card CM, McLaren PJ, Dawood MR, Kasper K, Fowke KR. The role of regulatory T cells in chronic and acute viral infections. *Clin Infect Dis* (2008) **46**(7):1046–52. doi:10.1086/529379
52. von Herrath MG, Dockter J, Oldstone MB. How virus induces a rapid or slow onset insulin-dependent diabetes mellitus in a transgenic model. *Immunity* (1994) **1**:231–42. doi:10.1016/1074-7613(94)90101-5
53. Turner MJ, Jellison ER, Lingenheld EG, Puddington L, Lefrançois L. Avidity maturation of memory CD8 T cells is limited by self-antigen expression. *J Exp Med* (2008) **205**(8):1859–68. doi:10.1084/jem.20072390
54. Barouch R, Schwartz M. Autoreactive T cells induce neurotrophin production by immune and neural cells in injured rat optic nerve: implications for protective autoimmunity. *FASEB J* (2002) **16**(10):1304–6. doi:10.1096/fj.01-0467fje
55. Hofstetter HH, Sewell DL, Liu F, Sandor M, Forsthuber T, Lehmann PV, et al. Autoreactive T cells promote post-traumatic healing in the central nervous system. *J Neuroimmunol* (2003) **134**(1):25–34. doi:10.1016/S0165-5728(02)00358-2
56. Wekerle H, Hohlfeld R. Beneficial brain autoimmunity? *Brain* (2010) **133**(8):2182–4. doi:10.1093/brain/awq206
57. Baitsch L, Fuertes-Marraco SA, Legat A, Meyer C, Speiser DE. The three main stumbling blocks for anticancer T cells. *Trends Immunol* (2012) **33**(7):364–72. doi:10.1016/j.it.2012.02.006
58. Goronzy JJ, Weyand CM. Understanding immunosenescence to improve responses to vaccines. *Nat Immunol* (2013) **14**:428–36. doi:10.1038/ni.2588
59. Vadasz Z, Haj T, Kessel A, Toubi E. Age-related autoimmunity. *BMC Med* (2013) **11**:94. doi:10.1186/1741-7015-11-94
60. Yager EJ, Ahmed M, Lanzer K, Randall TD, Woodland DL, Blackman MA. Age-associated decline in T cell repertoire diversity leads to holes in the repertoire and impaired immunity to influenza virus. *J Exp Med* (2008) **205**(3):711–23. doi:10.1084/jem.20071140
61. Sakaguchi S, Miyara M, Costantino CM, Hafler DA. FOXP3+ regulatory T cells in the human immune system. *Nat Rev Immunol* (2010) **10**:490–500. doi:10.1038/nri2785
62. Raynor J, Lages CS, Shehata H, Hildeman DA, Chougnet CA. Homeostasis and function of regulatory T cells in aging. *Curr Opin Immunol* (2012) **24**(4):482–7. doi:10.1016/j.coi.2012.04.005
63. von Herrath M, Sanda S, Herold K. Type 1 diabetes as a relapsing-remitting disease? *Nat Rev Immunol* (2007) **7**(12):988–94. doi:10.1038/nri2192
64. Nylander A, Hafler DA. Multiple sclerosis. *J Clin Invest* (2012) **122**(4):1180–8. doi:10.1172/JCI58649
65. Lechler R, Chai JG, Marelli-Berg F, Lombardi G. The contributions of T-cell anergy to peripheral T-cell tolerance. *Immunology* (2001) **103**(3):262–9. doi:10.1046/j.1365-2567.2001.01250.x
66. Grossman Z, Singer A. Tuning of activation thresholds explains flexibility in the selection and development of T cells in the thymus. *Proc Natl Acad Sci U S A* (1996) **93**(25):14747–52. doi:10.1073/pnas.93.25.14747
67. Scherer A, Noest A, de Boer RJ. Activation-threshold tuning in an affinity model for the T-cell repertoire. *Proc Biol Sci* (2004) **271**:609–16. doi:10.1098/rspb.2003.2653
68. Banz A, Pontoux C, Papiernik M. Modulation of Fas-dependent apoptosis: a dynamic process controlling both the persistence and death of CD4 regulatory T cells and effector T cells. *J Immunol* (2002) **169**(2):750–7.

APPENDIX

A.1. STEADY STATE ANALYSIS OF MODEL (1)

The equilibrium points of model (1) can be obtained from the following:

$$\text{Equilibrium points} = \begin{cases} (T_1, I_1) = (0,0) \\ (T_2, I_2) = \left(\dfrac{bf}{ad-be}, \dfrac{b}{a}\right) \end{cases} \tag{A1}$$

For a positive nontrivial equilibrium point (T_2, I_2), we have to assume that:

$$ad - be > 0 \tag{A2}$$

The stability of equilibrium points can be determined from the sign of real part of eigenvalues of Jacobian matrix (J). An equilibrium point is stable if all the eigenvalues of J evaluated at the equilibrium point have negative real parts, and it is unstable if at least one of the eigenvalues has a positive real part.

$$\text{Jacobian Matrix J} = \begin{bmatrix} aI - b & aT \\ d - eI & -eT - f \end{bmatrix} \tag{A3}$$

$$\begin{aligned} \text{Characteristic Equation } Q(\lambda) &= det\left\{\begin{bmatrix} \lambda - aI + b & -aT \\ -d + eI & \lambda + eT + f \end{bmatrix}\right\} \\ &= \lambda^2 + \left[eT + f + b - aI\right]\lambda + \left[-afI + beT + bf - adT\right] = 0 \end{aligned} \tag{A4}$$

The eigenvalues ($\lambda_{1,2}$) of J for trivial equilibrium point (T_1, I_1) are obtained by solving the characteristic equation (A4):

$$\lambda_{1,2}|_{(T_1,I_1)} : Q(\lambda)|_{(T_1,I_1)} = \lambda^2 + (f + b)\lambda + bf = 0 \tag{A5}$$

By checking Routh–Hurwitz stability Criterion (RHC) it can be easily confirmed that the eigenvalues have negative real parts since all the coefficients of polynomial $Q(\lambda)$ are positive, and hence, the trivial equilibrium point (T_1, I_1) is locally stable. For stability of nontrivial equilibrium point, the characteristic equation (A4) is evaluated and solved in (T_2, I_2):

$$\lambda_{1,2}|_{(T_2,I_2)} : Q(\lambda)|_{(T_2,I_2)} = \lambda^2 + \left(\frac{afd}{ad - be}\right)\lambda - bf = 0 \tag{A6}$$

With the assumption (A2), the coefficient of λ is positive. The sign of $Q(\lambda)$ coefficients change only once and hence, there exists one positive eigenvalue. Therefore, the nontrivial equilibrium point (T_2, I_2) is a saddle point and unstable.

A.2. STEADY STATE ANALYSIS OF MODEL (4)

The equilibrium points of model (4) with definition of T cell activation ($k(t)$) given in equation (5) can be obtained from the following

$$N = \frac{N_0}{g + \beta} = \frac{k}{\beta} \tag{A7}$$

$$I = \frac{dT}{eT + f} = \frac{bT - k}{aT} \tag{A8}$$

$$(ad - be)\,T^2 + (ek - bf)\,T + fk = 0 \tag{A9}$$

By keeping the assumption (A2), if the coefficient of T in (A9) is negative, the equilibrium points (T), if exist, will be positive:

$$ek - bf < 0 \rightarrow k < \frac{bf}{e} \tag{A10}$$

Otherwise, the equilibrium points will be negative. According to equation (A8), for $T \geq 0, I \geq 0$. Now, let's check the condition for existence of equilibrium points:

$$\Delta = 0 \rightarrow (ek + bf)^2 - 4afdk = \underbrace{\left(ek + bf + 2\sqrt{afdk}\right)}_{>0} \underbrace{\left(ek + bf - 2\sqrt{afdk}\right)}_{=0} = 0 \tag{A11}$$

$$\left(ek + bf - 2\sqrt{afdk}\right) = 0 \rightarrow k_+ = \frac{adf}{e^2}\left(1 + \sqrt{1 - \frac{be}{ad}}\right)^2, k_- = \frac{adf}{e^2}\left(1 - \sqrt{1 - \frac{be}{ad}}\right)^2 \tag{A12}$$

The model does not have any equilibrium points for $k_- < k < k_+$, and two equilibrium points otherwise. It can be verified that by keeping assumption (A2), we always have:

$$0 < k_- < \frac{bf}{e} < k_+ \tag{A13}$$

Therefore, for $0 < k < k_-$, condition (A10) is satisfied and the model has two positive equilibrium points and for $k > k_+$, condition (A10) is not satisfied and model has two negative equilibrium points. Let's assume that the model has two positive equilibrium points ($\Delta > 0$ and $0 < k < k_-$). In the following, the linear stability of equilibrium points is analyzed:

$$\text{Jacobian Matrix J} = \begin{bmatrix} -g - \beta & 0 & 0 \\ \beta & aI - b & aT \\ 0 & d - eI & -eT - f \end{bmatrix} \tag{A14}$$

$$\begin{aligned} \text{Characteristic Equation } Q(\lambda) &= det\left\{\begin{bmatrix} \lambda + g + \beta & 0 & 0 \\ -\beta & \lambda - aI + b & -aT \\ 0 & -d + eI & \lambda + eT + f \end{bmatrix}\right\} \\ &= [\lambda + (g + \beta)]\underbrace{[(\lambda - aI + b)(\lambda + eT + f) + aT(eI - d)]}_{Q^*} = 0 \end{aligned} \tag{A15}$$

The model has one negative eigenvalue $\lambda = -(g + \beta)$ for all equilibrium points. For the other two remaining eigenvalues, polynomial Q^* has to be checked for existence of positive eigenvalue.

$$Q^* = \lambda^2 + \underbrace{[eT + f + b - aI]}_{U}\lambda + \underbrace{[-afI + beT + bf - adT]}_{V} = 0 \tag{A16}$$

From equation (A8) it can be easily verified that $b - aI > 0$ and hence, coefficient U is positive. Therefore, the stability depends on the sign of coefficient V.

$$V = -afI + beT + bf - adT \xrightarrow{I = \frac{dT}{eT+f}} V = -\frac{afd}{eT + f}T - (ad - be)T + bf \tag{A17}$$

$$V_1 = TV = -\frac{afd}{eT + f}T^2 - \underbrace{\left[(ad - be)T^2 + (ek - bf)T + fk\right]}_{\text{According to (A9)}\rightarrow=0} + k(eT + f) \tag{A18}$$

$$V_2 = \frac{1}{k(eT + f)}V_1 = -\frac{af}{kd}\left(\frac{dT}{eT + f}\right)^2 + 1 \xrightarrow{I = \frac{dT}{eT+f}} V_2 = -\frac{af}{kd}I^2 + 1 \tag{A19}$$

According to equations (A8) and (A9), the equilibrium values of I are:

$$I_2 = \frac{1}{2}\left(\frac{(ek + bf) + \sqrt{\Delta}}{af}\right), T_2 = \frac{k}{b - aI_2}, N_2 = \frac{N_0}{g + \beta} \tag{A20}$$

$$I_1 = \frac{1}{2}\left(\frac{(ek + bf) - \sqrt{\Delta}}{af}\right), T_1 = \frac{k}{b - aI_1}, N_1 = \frac{N_0}{g + \beta} \tag{A21}$$

where $I_2 > I_1$ and:

$$\Delta = (ek + bf)^2 - 4fkad = (ek - bf)^2 - 4fk(ad - be) \tag{A22}$$

Next, the sign of V_2, which is similar to V_1 and V, has to be checked in the equilibrium points. For the larger equilibrium point (T_2, I_2):

$$\begin{aligned} V_2\,|_{I_2} &= -\frac{1}{2fkad}\left[e^2k^2 + 2ekbf + ek\sqrt{\Delta} + b^2f^2 + bf\sqrt{\Delta} - 4fkad\right] \\ &= -\frac{1}{2fkad}\underbrace{\left[\Delta + (ek + bf)\sqrt{\Delta}\right]}_{+} < 0 \end{aligned} \tag{A23}$$

$V_2, V_1,$ and V are negative for (T_2, I_2). Therefore, the model in this equilibrium point has a positive eigenvalue and it is locally unstable. For (T_1, I_1),

$$V_2\,|_{I_1} = -\frac{\sqrt{\Delta}}{2fkad}\left[\sqrt{\Delta} - (ek + bf)\right] \overset{\text{According to (A22)}}{=\!=\!=} -\frac{\sqrt{\Delta}}{2fkad}\underbrace{\left[\sqrt{(ek + bf)^2 - 4fkad} - (ek + bf)\right]}_{-} > 0 \tag{A24}$$

$V_2, V_1,$ and V are positive for (T_1, I_1). Therefore, all the eigenvalues of the model in this equilibrium point are negative and it is locally stable.

Next, let's assume that $k > k_+$ which means that the equilibrium points exist and the steady state values of T are negative, whereas the equilibrium values of I is positive. According to equation (A8), coefficient U in equation (A16) is negative since:

$$T = \frac{k}{b - aI} < 0 \rightarrow b - aI < 0, I = \frac{dT}{eT + f} > 0 \xrightarrow{dT<0} eT + f < 0 \tag{A25}$$

Therefore, the model at least has one positive eigenvalue in the equilibrium points. Let's check the sign of coefficient V in the equilibrium points:

$$V = -afI + beT + bf - adT \overset{T=\frac{k}{b-aI}}{=\!=\!=} -f(aI - b) + (ad - be)\frac{k}{aI - b} \tag{A26}$$

$$\begin{aligned} V_2 &= (aI - b)\,V \overset{aI-b>0}{=\!=\!=} -f(aI - b)^2 + (ad - be)\,k \overset{aI-b=-\frac{k}{T}}{=\!=\!=} -f\frac{k^2}{T^2} + (ad - be)\,k \\ V_3 &= \frac{T^2}{fk^2}V_2 = -1 + \left(\frac{ad - be}{fk}\right)T^2 \end{aligned} \tag{A27}$$

The sign of V_3 in equation (A27) which is the same as the sign of V in equation (A16) can be determined by substituting T with its equilibrium values from equation (A9):

$$V_3\,|_{T_2} = \frac{1}{4(ad - be)fk}\underbrace{\left[2\Delta + 2\sqrt{\Delta}\,(bf - ek)\right]}_{\text{sign?}} \tag{A28}$$

According to equation (A13) and reminding that $k > k_+$, it can be verified that V_3 or equivalently V is positive. Therefore, the equilibrium point (T_2, I_2) has one positive eigenvalue and is unstable. For (T_1, I_1),

$$V_3\,|_{T_1} = \frac{1}{4(ad - be)fk}\underbrace{\left[2\Delta + 2\sqrt{\Delta}\,\underbrace{(ek - bf)}_{+}\right]}_{+} \tag{A29}$$

V_3 and equivalently, V are positive and therefore, the equilibrium point (T_1, I_1) has one positive eigenvalue and it is unstable.

A.3. STEADY STATE ANALYSIS OF MODEL (10)

The equilibrium points of model (10) for $\beta = 0$ can be obtained from the following

$$(T_1, I_1, N_1) = \left(0,\ 0,\ \frac{N_0}{g}\right) \tag{A30}$$

$$N_{2,3} : N_{2,3} = \frac{N_0}{g} \tag{A31}$$

$$T_{2,3} : ceT^2 + (cf + be - ad)T + bf = 0, \begin{cases} T_3 = -\frac{1}{2ce}\left[-\left(cf + be - ad\right) + \sqrt{\Delta}\right] \\ T_2 = -\frac{1}{2ce}\left[-\left(cf + be - ad\right) - \sqrt{\Delta}\right] \\ \Delta = (cf + be - ad)^2 - 4cfbe \end{cases} \tag{A32}$$

$$I_{2,3} : I_{2,3} = \frac{cT_{2,3} + b}{a} \tag{A33}$$

According to equation (A32), the nontrivial equilibrium points, if available, are positive only if:

$$cf + be - ad < 0 \tag{A34}$$

The condition of the existence of positive equilibrium points can be obtained from equation (A32):

$$\Delta = \left(cf + be - ad\right)^2 - 4cebf = f^2c^2 - 2f\,(ad + be)\,c + (ad - be)^2 \geq 0 \tag{A35}$$

According to equation (A35), the nontrivial equilibrium points exist only if:

$$\{c < c_-\} \cup \{c > c_+\} \tag{A36}$$

where

$$\left[c_- = \frac{\left(\sqrt{ad} - \sqrt{be}\right)^2}{f}\right] < \left[\frac{ad - be}{f} = \frac{\left(\sqrt{ad} + \sqrt{be}\right)\left(\sqrt{ad} - \sqrt{be}\right)}{f}\right] < \left[c_+ = \frac{\left(\sqrt{ad} + \sqrt{be}\right)^2}{f}\right] \tag{A37}$$

Therefore, according to conditions (A34) and (A36) and inequality (A37), the two positive equilibrium points exist only if:

$$0 < c < c_- \tag{A38}$$

Next, we assume that the condition (A38) is satisfied, and we analyze the stability of the equilibrium points:

$$\text{Jacobian Matrix J} = \begin{bmatrix} -g - \beta & 0 & 0 \\ \beta & aI - b - 2cT & aT \\ 0 & d - eI & -eT - f \end{bmatrix} \tag{A39}$$

Characteristic Equation:

$$\begin{aligned} Q(\lambda) &= det\left\{\begin{bmatrix} \lambda + g + \beta & 0 & 0 \\ -\beta & \lambda - aI + b + 2cT & -aT \\ 0 & -d + eI & \lambda + eT + f \end{bmatrix}\right\} \\ &= [\lambda + g + \beta]\left[\lambda^2 + \underbrace{\left[eT + f + b - aI + 2cT\right]}_{U}\lambda + \underbrace{\left[-afI + 2ceT^2 + beT + bf + 2cfT - adT\right]}_{V}\right] \end{aligned} \tag{A40}$$

All the equilibrium points have a negative eigenvalue $\lambda = -g - \beta$. For the sign of other eigenvalues, the sign of coefficients of the characteristic equation has to be checked in equilibrium points. These coefficients are positive for the trivial equilibrium point and therefore, all eigenvalues have negative real value. Hence, the trivial equilibrium point is stable. For stability analysis of nontrivial equilibrium points, the sign of U and V in equation (A40) has to be analyzed:

$$U = eT + f + 2cT + (b - aI) \xlongequal{(A33):\ b-aI=-cT} eT + f + cT > 0 \tag{A41}$$

Coefficient U is positive for the positive equilibrium points. Therefore, their stability depends on the sign of V in equation (A40):

$$V = f(b - aI) + 2ceT^2 + beT + 2cfT - adT \xlongequal{(A33):\ b-aI=-cT} 2ceT^2 + (be - ad)T + cfT \tag{A42}$$

$$= ceT^2 + \underbrace{\left[ceT^2 + (cf + be - ad)\,T + bf\right]}_{\text{According to (A32): =0}} - bf = ceT^2 - bf \tag{A43}$$

$$V\,|_{T_3} = \frac{1}{2ce}\left[\Delta - \underbrace{(cf + be - ad)}_{\text{According to (A34): <0}}\sqrt{\Delta}\right] > 0 \tag{A44}$$

The sign of V for the larger equilibrium point is positive and hence, this equilibrium point is stable.

$$V|_{T_2} = \frac{\sqrt{\Delta}}{2ce}\underbrace{\left[\sqrt{\Delta} + \underbrace{(cf + be - ad)}_{\text{According to (A34): <0}}\right]}_{\text{According to (A32):<0}} < 0 \tag{A45}$$

The sign of V for the smaller equilibrium point is negative and therefore, this equilibrium point is unstable. The equilibrium points of the model with $\beta > 0$ and by considering $\beta N(t) = k(t)$ are obtained by solving:

$$-\,ceT^3 - (cf + be - ad)\,T^2 + (ek - bf)\,T + kf = 0 \tag{A46a}$$

$$I = \frac{dT}{eT + f} \tag{A46b}$$

By keeping the assumptions (A2) and (A38), the equation (A46a) has either one positive real equilibrium point or three positive real equilibrium points depending on the value of k. The stability of equilibrium points that are obtained from (A46a) and (A46b) by varying the value of k is hard to be checked analytically; instead, it is analyzed numerically by solving equation (A40).

A.4. STEADY STATE ANALYSIS OF MODEL (13)

The equilibrium points of model (13) for $\beta N(t) = k(t) = 0$ can be obtained from the following

$$(T_1,\ I_1,\ R_1,\ N_1) = \left(0,\ 0,\ 0,\ \frac{N_0}{g}\right) \tag{A47}$$

$$T_{2,3} : ceT_{2,3}^2 + (cf - ad + be)T_{2,3} + bf = 0,\ I_{2,3} = \frac{dT_{2,3}}{eT_{2,3} + f},\ R_{2,3} = 0,\ N_{2,3} = \frac{N_0}{g} \tag{A48}$$

$$T_4 = \frac{b(eR_5 + f)}{\epsilon ad - be},\ I_4 = \frac{b}{\epsilon a},\ R_4 = \left(\frac{b}{\epsilon}\right)\left(\frac{-\epsilon(cf + be - ad) + be(\epsilon - 1) - \epsilon(\epsilon ad - be)}{cbe + \gamma(\epsilon ad - be)}\right),\ N_4 = \frac{N_0}{g} \tag{A49}$$

$$T_5 = 0,\ I_5 = \frac{b}{\epsilon a},\ R_5 = \frac{-f}{e},\ N_5 = \frac{N_0}{g} \tag{A50}$$

The sign of the equilibrium point T_4 changes by changing the Treg-associated parameters (ϵ, γ). T_4 is positive if

$$\epsilon ad - be > 0,\ R > -\frac{f}{e} \tag{A51}$$

or

$$\epsilon ad - be < 0,\ R < -\frac{f}{e} \tag{A52}$$

The physiologically relevant regime of the model occurs by satisfying the condition (A51) which means both T_4 and R_4 are positive. The equilibrium points of model (13) for $\beta\, N(t) = k(t) \neq 0$ can be obtained from the following

$$N = \frac{\beta N_0}{g+\beta} \tag{A53}$$

$$R = \frac{-\lambda k}{\epsilon a I - b} \tag{A54}$$

$$T = \frac{-I\left(-e\lambda k + f\epsilon a I - bf\right)}{(\epsilon a I - b)(-d + eI)} \tag{A55}$$

$$P_5 I^5 + P_4 I^4 + P_3 I^3 + P_2 I^2 + P_1 I + P_0 = 0 \tag{A56}$$

where

$$P_5 = a^3 f \epsilon^2 e \tag{A57}$$

$$P_4 = -bf\epsilon^2 a^2 e + cf^2\epsilon^2 a^2 - k\epsilon^2 a^2 e^2 - a^3 f\epsilon^2 d - 2\,a^2 f\epsilon\, be - a^2 e^2 \lambda\, k\epsilon \tag{A58}$$

$$\begin{aligned} P_3 = {} & be^2\lambda\, k\epsilon\, a - 2\, cf^2\epsilon\, ab + ae^2\lambda\, kb + 2\, a^2 f\epsilon\, bd + \gamma\,\lambda\, kf\epsilon\, ae + ab^2 fe + bf\epsilon^2 a^2 d \\ & + 2\, k\epsilon^2 a^2 de - 2\, ce\lambda\, kf\epsilon\, a + 2\, b^2 f\epsilon\, ae + a^2 e\lambda\, k\epsilon\, d + 2\, k\epsilon\, abe^2 \end{aligned} \tag{A59}$$

$$\begin{aligned} P_2 = {} & 2\, ce\lambda\, kbf - 4\, k\epsilon\, abde - \gamma\,\lambda\, kbfe - b^2 e^2\lambda\, k - kb^2 e^2 - be\lambda\, k\epsilon\, ad - b^3 fe - ae\lambda\, kbd + cb^2 f^2 \\ & + ce^2\lambda^2 k^2 - ab^2 fd - k\epsilon^2 a^2 d^2 - \gamma\,\lambda^2 k^2 e^2 - 2\, b^2 f\epsilon\, ad - \gamma\,\lambda\, kf\epsilon\, ad \end{aligned} \tag{A60}$$

$$P_1 = \gamma\,\lambda^2 k^2 ed + b^2 e\lambda\, kd + 2\, kb^2 de + 2\, k\epsilon\, abd^2 + b^3 fd + \gamma\,\lambda\, kbfd \tag{A61}$$

$$P_0 = -kb^2 d^2 \tag{A62}$$

A.5. NONLINEAR PROLIFERATION RATE OF CONVENTIONAL AND REGULATORY T CELLS

In the models (1), (4), (10) and (13) it is assumed that proliferation rate of Tconvs and Tregs is a linear function of IL-2. This simplifying assumption is made in order to allow parametric stability analysis of the model in a closed form and to find explicitly the dependency between parametric variations and topological changes of the model. Here, we show that the simplifying assumption does not affect the three regimes of qualitative immune responses that could be derived from the model. The linear IL-2-dependent proliferation rate is replaced with a nonlinear function of IL-2, named $\Phi\,(I)$ in models (1), (4), and (13):

$$\begin{cases} \dfrac{dT}{dt} = \Phi(I)T - bT + k \\ \dfrac{dI}{dt} = dT - eIT - fI \end{cases} \tag{A63}$$

where $\Phi\,(I)$ is considered as a Hill-function of IL-2

$$\Phi(I) = a\frac{I^n}{h^n + I^n} \tag{A64}$$

The models (1) and (A63) are compared by steady state analysis. The equilibrium points of the modified model (A63) (with $k = \frac{\beta N_0}{g+\beta} = 0$) are

$$(T_1,\, I_1) = (0,\, 0) \tag{A65}$$

$$(T_2, I_2) = \left(\frac{fI_2}{d - eI_2},\, h\left(\frac{b}{a-b}\right)^{\frac{1}{n}}\right) \tag{A66}$$

The nontrivial equilibrium point (T_2, I_2) is positive and biologically meaningful only if

$$(a-b)d^n - be^n h^n > 0 \tag{A67}$$

The local stability of the equilibrium points can be determined by obtaining the eigenvalues from the characteristic equation:

$$\text{Characteristic Equation } Q(\lambda) = det\left\{\begin{bmatrix} \lambda - a\frac{I^n}{h^n+I^n} + b & -aT\frac{nh^nI^{n-1}}{(h^n+I^n)^2} \\ -d+eI & \lambda + eT + f \end{bmatrix}\right\} \tag{A68}$$

$$= \lambda^2 + \left[eT + f - a\frac{I^n}{h^n+I^n} + b\right]\lambda + \left[\left(-a\frac{I^n}{h^n+I^n} + b\right)(eT+f) + aT\frac{nh^nI^{n-1}}{(h^n+I^n)^2}(-d+eI)\right] = 0 \tag{A69}$$

By checking Routh–Hurwitz stability Criterion (RHC) it can be easily confirmed that the eigenvalues have negative real parts for trivial equilibrium point since all the coefficients of polynomial $Q(\lambda)$ are positive, and hence, the trivial equilibrium point (T_1, I_1) is locally stable. For checking the stability of the nontrivial equilibrium point, the characteristic equation (A69) is evaluated in (T_2, I_2):

$$\lambda_{1,2}|_{(T_2,I_2)} : Q(\lambda)|_{(T_2,I_2)} = \lambda^2 + \underbrace{\left[eT_2 + f\right]}_{U}\lambda + \underbrace{\left[-\frac{nbh^nT_2}{I_2(h^n+I_2{}^n)}(d - eI_2)\right]}_{V} = 0 \tag{A70}$$

By assuming the condition (A67), the coefficients U and V are positive and negative respectively. Therefore, the sign of the coefficients of $Q(\lambda)$ (U and V) changes only once and hence, there exists an eigenvalue with positive real part. Therefore, the nontrivial equilibrium point (T_2, I_2) is a saddle node and unstable.

Similar to the model (1), the stable manifold of saddle node in the model (A63) defines a threshold for the initial conditions that allow for unlimited proliferation of activated T cells. By comparing the conditions (A67) and (3), the dependencies of these conditions to the model parameters, specifically the proliferation rate (a) and IL-2 secretion rate (d), are positively correlated. In other words, in both models, only T cell clones with sufficiently high proliferation rate (a) and/or high IL-2 secretion rate (d) are able to undergo major T cell proliferation.

For $k \neq 0$, the equilibrium points of the model (A63) are obtained from the following equations:

$$T = \frac{fI}{d - eI} \tag{A71}$$

$$I : \left[(a-b)f - ke\right]I^{n+1} + [kd]\,I^n - \left[h^n(bf + ke)\right]I + kdh^n = 0 \tag{A72}$$

The stability of equilibrium points is analyzed by evaluating the characteristic equation and is shown in **Figure A1** for parameter values given in **Table 1** and Hill-function parameters $n = 2$ and $h = 0.5$. By comparing the bifurcation diagram in **Figures A1** and **3B**, the qualitative similarity between model (4) and (A63) is evident. This qualitative similarity also holds true between model (13) and the following model:

$$\begin{cases} \dfrac{dT}{dt} = \Phi(I)T - bT - cT^2 - \gamma RT + k \\ \dfrac{dR}{dt} = \epsilon\Phi(I)R - bR + \beta\widehat{N} \\ \dfrac{dI}{dt} = dT - eI(T+R) - fI \end{cases} \tag{A73}$$

where $\Phi\ (I)$ is identical to (A64).

The equilibrium points of model (A73) are calculated and their stability is analyzed by deriving the characteristic equation of the model and obtaining the eigenvalues. By keeping assumption (12), the bifurcation diagrams of model (A73) for two different values of λ are obtained by treating $k = \frac{\beta N_0}{g+\beta} > 0$ as the bifurcation parameter (depicted in **Figure A2**). Depending on the value of k, the model has either 8 or 6 equilibrium points (4 or 2 equilibrium points with $T > 0$, identical to model (13)) with parameter values given in **Table 1** and Hill-function parameters $n = 4$ and $h = 1$. The additional equilibrium points resulted from considering the Hill-function nonlinearity are all in the negative space of the model variables. As it can be seen from **Figure A2**, similar to the model (13), the three qualitatively different responses still could be derived from the modified model. It is clear that the value of k_i, k_s, and λ_{th} are different from their corresponding values in the model (13).

In summary, imposing the nonlinear IL-2 dependent proliferation rate of cells results in a more restricted condition for initiation of an immune response in comparison to the linear IL-2 dependent proliferation rate, namely the requirement of higher T cell avidity (higher a and d), higher Ag-stimulation (increased β_i), and lower Treg/Tconv ratio (lower λ_{th}); but three qualitatively different immune reactions depending on the critical levels of Ag-stimulation could still be derived, very similar to model (13).

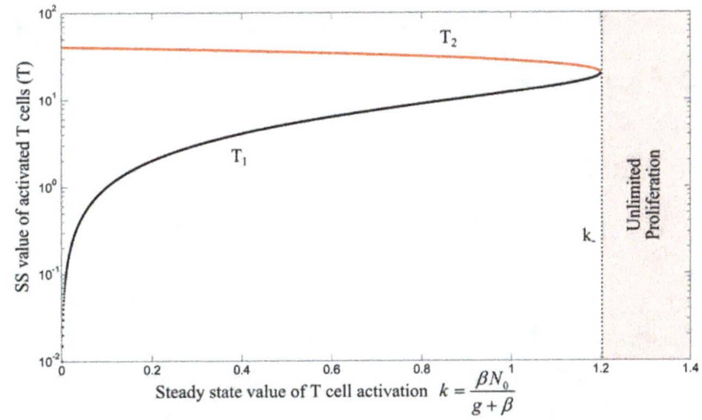

FIGURE A1 | Bifurcation diagram of model (A63) with Hill-function parameters $n = 2$ and h = 0.5 by treating k as bifurcation parameter. Stable and unstable equilibrium points are shown by black and red lines, respectively. For $k > k_{-}$, the immune response enters the regime of unlimited proliferation. The unstable negative equilibrium point is omitted in this figure.

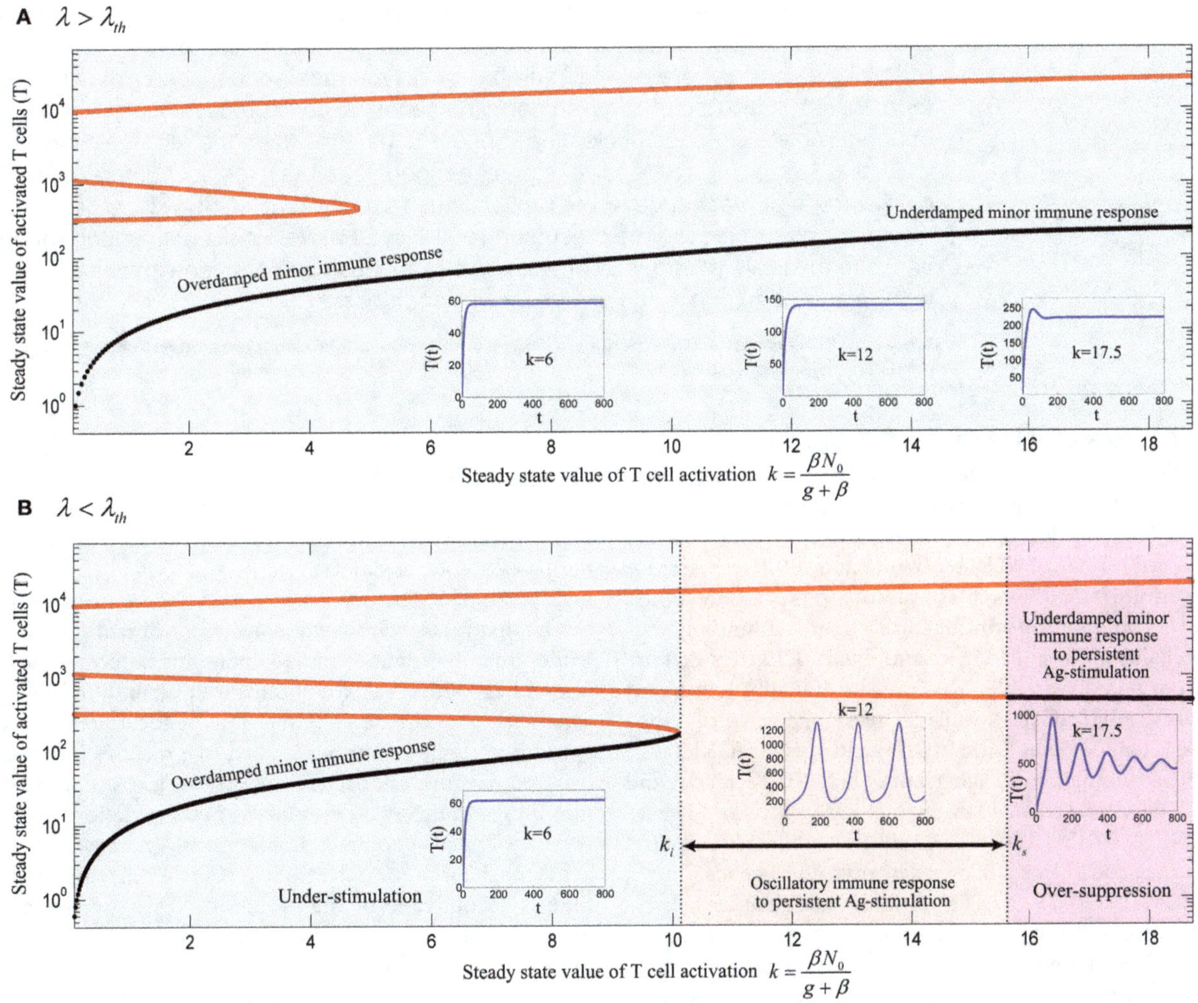

FIGURE A2 | Bifurcation diagram of model (A73) with Hill-function parameters $n = 4$ and h = 1 using k as the bifurcation parameter with (A) $\lambda = 0.0016$ and (B) $\lambda = 0.0008$. Stable and unstable equilibrium points are drawn by black and red solid lines, respectively. The stable limit cycles are not shown for all value of $k_i < k < k_s$ except for $k = 12$. Depending on the values of λ and k, an immune response is not initiated (gray), is initiated (red) or over-suppressed (magenta). With parameter values given in **Table 1** and Hill-function parameters $n = 4$ and h = 1, the threshold becomes $\lambda_{th} = 0.00111$. The time-courses of the activated T cell population $T(t)$ were deduced from a numerical solution of model (A73) with zero initial conditions and persistent β. The negative equilibrium points which are all unstable are not shown in the plots.

15

The shape of the lymphocyte receptor repertoire: lessons from the B cell receptor

Katherine J. L. Jackson*, Marie J. Kidd, Yan Wang and Andrew M. Collins

School of Biotechnology and Biomolecular Sciences, University of New South Wales, Sydney, NSW, Australia

Edited by:
Ramit Mehr, Bar-Ilan University, Israel

Reviewed by:
Ramit Mehr, Bar-Ilan University, Israel
Gur Yaari, Yale University, USA
Nir Friedman, Weizmann Institute of Science, Israel

***Correspondence:**
Katherine J. L. Jackson, School of Biotechnology and Biomolecular Sciences, University of New South Wales, Sydney, NSW 2052, Australia
e-mail: katherine.jackson@unsw.edu.au

Both the B cell receptor (BCR) and the T cell receptor (TCR) repertoires are generated through essentially identical processes of V(D)J recombination, exonuclease trimming of germline genes, and the random addition of non-template encoded nucleotides. The naïve TCR repertoire is constrained by thymic selection, and TCR repertoire studies have therefore focused strongly on the diversity of MHC-binding complementarity determining region (CDR) CDR3. The process of somatic point mutations has given B cell studies a major focus on variable (IGHV, IGLV, and IGKV) genes. This in turn has influenced how both the naïve and memory BCR repertoires have been studied. Diversity (D) genes are also more easily identified in BCR VDJ rearrangements than in TCR VDJ rearrangements, and this has allowed the processes and elements that contribute to the incredible diversity of the immunoglobulin heavy chain CDR3 to be analyzed in detail. This diversity can be contrasted with that of the light chain where a small number of polypeptide sequences dominate the repertoire. Biases in the use of different germline genes, in gene processing, and in the addition of non-template encoded nucleotides appear to be intrinsic to the recombination process, imparting "shape" to the repertoire of rearranged genes as a result of differences spanning many orders of magnitude in the probabilities that different BCRs will be generated. This may function to increase the precursor frequency of naïve B cells with important specificities, and the likely emergence of such B cell lineages upon antigen exposure is discussed with reference to public and private T cell clonotypes.

Keywords: BCR repertoire, TCR repertoire, V(D)J recombination, public clonotypes, private clonotypes, combinatorial diversity, junctional diversity

GERMLINE GENES AND LYMPHOCYTE DIVERSITY

The mammalian immune system has the ability to respond to almost any antigen to which it is exposed because of the incredible diversity of lymphocyte receptor molecules. The diversity of both the B cell receptor (BCR) repertoire and the T cell receptor (TCR) repertoire is made possible by multiple sets of highly similar genes that recombine to form functional genes. Immunoglobulin heavy chains are encoded by recombined VDJ genes that are formed from sets of Variable (V), Diversity (D), and Joining (J) genes (IGHV, IGHJ, IGHD), while VJ rearrangements of kappa and lambda chain V genes (IGKV, IGLV) and J genes (IGKJ, IGLJ) encode the immunoglobulin light chains (1, 2). TCR β-chains and δ-chains are similarly encoded by distinct sets of V, D, and J genes (TRBV, TRBD, TRBJ; TRDV, TRDD, TRDJ), while α-chains and γ-chains are encoded by additional sets of V and J genes (TRAV, TRAJ; TRGV, TRGJ) (3–5). The resulting combinatorial diversity is expanded still further by junctional diversification arising from exonuclease trimming of the recombining gene ends and from the essentially random addition of nucleotides, between the recombining genes, by the enzyme terminal deoxynucleotidyl transferase (TdT) (6). Together, combinatorial diversity and junctional diversity create the diversity of the naïve T cell and B cell repertoires. Limitations to diversity may however be a feature of V(D)J rearrangement that is as significant to immune function as the bewildering number of lymphocyte specificities that can theoretically be generated.

This review will present evidence that biases in the processes that generate combinatorial and junctional diversity are such that the probabilities of different BCRs and TCRs being generated is highly variable. This results in B and T cells of some specificities being present within the naïve repertoire at high frequency, while other specificities may or may not be present at all. The unevenness of the receptor abundance distribution can be said to give "shape" to the naïve B and T lymphocyte repertoires. This distribution may be further shaped by processes including positive and negative selection, clonal expansion and, in the case of immunoglobulin genes, by somatic hypermutation, however this review will focus upon recombination and gene processing.

As the shape of the naïve human B and T cell lymphocyte repertoire is an outcome of the evolution of genetically determined biases, this should ensure the presence of critical rearrangements in the repertoire of all individuals. It should also ensure that these critical rearrangements are carried by multiple naïve cells (see **Figure 1**). Such populations of specific naïve lymphocytes will have a competitive advantage during antigen-driven clonal selection, and any discussion of repertoire diversity that is limited to the size of the population of unique receptors will therefore be ignoring a parameter of likely biological significance. In this review, we

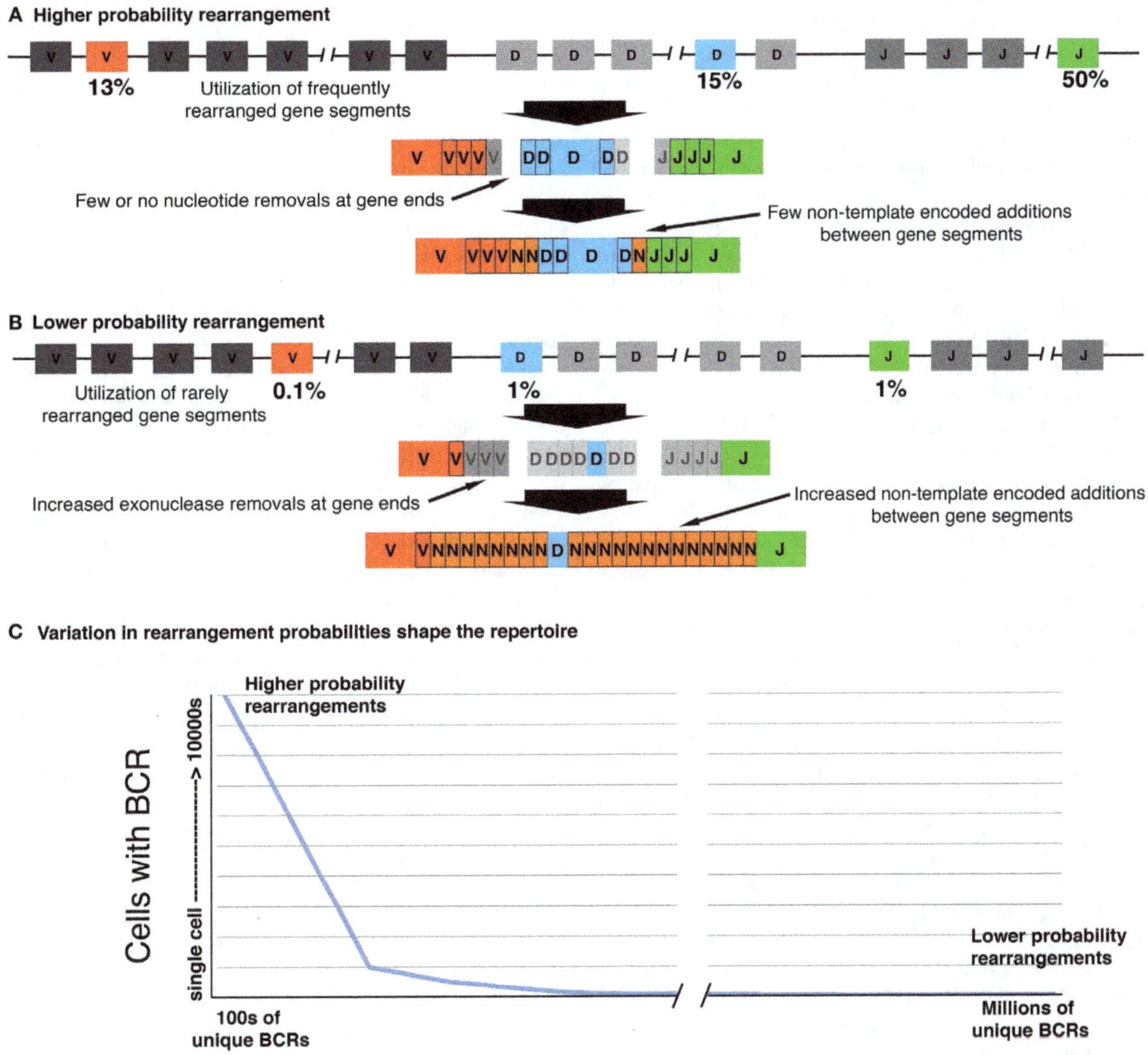

FIGURE 1 | The receptor repertoire has "shape," as biases and constraints in the recombination process vary the probabilities of generating particular V(D)J rearrangements. (A) Higher probability rearrangements are generated through utilization of more frequently rearranged gene segments. These segments are joined with minimal gene processing and N-addition, increasing the chance of independent rearrangements with identical or near identical CDR3s. **(B)** Lower probability rearrangements utilize rarely rearranged germline gene segments and the CDR3s are more diverse owing to increased nucleotide removals and additions at the joins. **(C)** The many order of magnitude differences in the likelihood of generating particular rearrangements shape the repertoire, with higher probability rearrangements being frequently generated and as a consequence being carried by many identical B-cells. Only a relatively small number of unique rearrangements will be generated with probabilities high enough to be carried by a large number of B cells, but this should ensure that they are always present in the repertoire at significant levels. Conversely, lower probability rearrangements may be so rare that they are carried only by a single B cell, or are entirely absent from the repertoire. The lower probability rearrangements that are carried by just one or at most a few B-cells likely represent many millions of unique rearrangements.

will use the term "repertoire" to refer to the complete set of receptors that are carried by an individual, including multiple copies of particular sequences. The number of unique sequences that are found within an individual's repertoire will be described as the "diversity" of the repertoire.

The size of the sets of germline genes make a major contribution to lymphocyte diversity, but surprisingly, our knowledge of these germline genes is far from complete. In part this is the result of the complexity of the loci, for they feature numerous highly similar genes that are thought to have evolved via gene conversion (7), and duplication and divergence (8). These genes are interspersed with many pseudogenes and repetitive elements (8). Sequencing and annotation of the loci is therefore challenging. These complexities also mean that SNPs arising from short read-length sequences generated in studies such as the HapMap and 1000 Genomes projects, cannot be used for the imputation of full-length allelic variants. In fact, these projects utilize polyclonal lymphoblastoid cells lines in which the immunoglobulin loci have undergone somatic recombination, and the rearranged genes may have been affected by somatic point mutation. This makes these cell lines unsuited to the study of immunoglobulin genes (9).

Arguably, it is the BCR germline genes that are best known, and paradoxically, this is because of their transformation through the process of somatic hypermutation, during an immune response. IGHV genes are by far the longest of the recombining IGH genes, and they are the principal targets of the mutational machinery (10, 11). Many studies of the immunogenetics of immunoglobulin have therefore concentrated upon the IGHV genes. As it is necessary to be certain of the germline origin of mutated sequences, if accurate studies of point mutations are to be conducted, the complete and accurate definition of the set of germline immunoglobulin IGHV genes and allelic variants has been and should remain a focus of research.

The official human IGHV germline gene dataset, curated by the ImMunoGeneTics (IMGT) group, includes 129 functional genes, open reading frames (ORF), and pseudogenes, as well as over 200 allelic variants (12). Interest in these germline genes has increased in recent years, resulting in 40 new allelic variants being reported since 2005 (13–17). Many additional IGHV allelic variants have also been identified in recent high-throughput sequencing studies, through analysis of cDNA-derived VDJ gene rearrangements (18, 19), but these have not been accepted as part of the official IGHV dataset. We have designated alleles identified in this way with unofficial allele names using an indicator ("p") of their "putative" nature (e.g., IGHV3-9*p03) (15), and these additional alleles can be found in the UNSWIg repertoire (http://www.ihmmune.unsw.edu.au/unswig.php).

The official human light chain V gene datasets appear to be relatively complete and accurate, though few allelic variants have been reported (20). Nevertheless these few variants appear to be of functional and clinical significance. For example, a variant kappa gene allele was identified within the Navajo population and has been reported to account for the susceptibility of this population to infections (21).

The human IGH germline genes receive continuing attention while the IMGT human TCR germline gene datasets have barely changed since the complete sequences of the TCR gene loci were first described (22, 23). The IMGT TRBV dataset includes 65 functional genes, ORFs and pseudogenes, and just 13 allelic variants, and no new TRBV sequence has been added to the dataset since the publication of the complete sequence of the TRB locus in 1996 (22). Only three TRAV/TRDV sequences (24) in the IMGT dataset are derived from studies published since the reporting of the complete sequence of the TRAV/TRDV locus (23), and some variants that were described soon afterward still remain officially unrecognized (25). The incomplete nature of the IMGT TRBV, and TRAV datasets in particular are clearly highlighted in the literature, for sequencing studies have reported many SNPs in the coding regions of these genes. Subramanyan and colleagues reported 279 SNPs in a study of 63 TRBV genes in 10 individuals from each of four human populations (26). Of these reported SNPs, 114 were located in coding regions of functional TRBV genes (26). A similar study of 57 TRAV/TRDV genes in the same 40 individuals resulted in the discovery of 284 SNPs, 51 of which encode amino acid changes in the coding regions of the gene sequences (27). The allelic variants associated with these TRAV/TRDV and TRBV SNPs have not been reported in the literature or in sequence databases, and they have not been incorporated into the official gene datasets. This is surprising because the SNPs were identified through amplification and sequencing of full-length genomic sequences. It is also unfortunate, for studies of TCR polymorphisms have shown that they can be of functional significance (28, 29).

The BCR and TCR D loci contribute differently to the generation of diversity, and the differences in the nature of the loci have influenced BCR and TCR research directions. The 27 human IGHD genes include 25 functional genes, 23 of which are unique (30). Although some IGHD genes, especially those of the IGHD1 gene family, are very similar, there is considerable sequence diversity amongst the genes. The lengths of the IGHD genes vary from 11 nucleotides to 37 nucleotides, and almost all of them are substantially longer than the TRBD and TRDD genes. This length and the IGHD gene variability have made improvement in the identification of IGHD genes within VDJ rearrangements a challenging but achievable research goal. Pursuit of this goal has driven the development of immunoglobulin gene alignment utilities including SODA2 (31), IgBLAST (32), and iHMMune-align (33). The objective measurement of the performance of these utilities is made difficult, however, by a lack of appropriate data sets. Ideally, performance would be measured using rearranged sequences of known composition. As such sets are unavailable, clonally related sequences can be used (32, 33). We have also compared the performance of different utilities using a set of long-read pyrosequenced (Roche 454) IGH rearrangements from an individual with a homozygous deletion of six IGHD genes (34). This test measures performance by the number of VDJ rearrangements in the dataset that are said to include the absent IGHD genes. Together these studies demonstrate that IGHD genes can now be identified with confidence, and as a consequence, analysis of the BCR heavy chain complementarity determining region (CDR) 3 can include detailed analysis of IGHD gene usage, gene processing, and N nucleotide addition.

Analysis of the TCR CDR3 is not so easy. The two human TRBD genes are both short (12 and 16 nucleotides) and highly similar at their 5′ ends (22). This makes their identification in VDJ rearrangements particularly difficult. The TRBD genes within a VDJ rearrangement are likely to be flanked by N-REGIONS of non-template encoded nucleotides. These nucleotides are introduced through the action of the TdT enzyme, which is biased to the addition of guanine (G) nucleotides (35) and to the addition of homopolymer tracts (36, 37). Distinguishing TRBD gene ends from G-rich N nucleotides is difficult because the TRBD genes are G-rich at both their 5′ and 3′ ends. A final complication is that the two alleles of TRBD2 differ by just a single nucleotide. This critical nucleotide is flanked on both sides, in both alleles, by GGG motifs. For these reasons, few TCR studies have included detailed analysis of TRBD genes and their processing, or of the N-REGIONS that can only be defined after the identification of a TRBD gene segment within the CDR3. Even the most recently developed TCR alignment utility excludes identification of TRBD genes from its output (38).

Analysis of the VDJ junction in TRD rearrangements is equally difficult. The three human TRDD genes are just 8, 9, and 13 nucleotides in length (4). This makes their reliable identification within VDJ rearrangements especially problematic if nucleotides have been lost through exonuclease activity. Application of an approach previously used in the analysis of BCR sequences (37) suggests that eight nucleotides is the minimum D gene length that will allow TRDD genes to be reliably distinguished from N-REGIONS within a junction of 12 or fewer nucleotides, while 9 nucleotides are needed for regions from 13 to 15 nucleotides and 10 nucleotides for junctions greater than 15 nucleotides (Jackson, unpublished data). It is therefore no surprise that few studies have reported the partitioning of TRD junctions as two of the three TRDD genes can only be confidently delineated from N-additions in their unprocessed form.

The J loci of the human BCR and TCR also include important differences. The IGHJ locus includes six functional genes, which are all found downstream of the IGHD locus in a single cluster. Allelic variants have been reported for IGHJ3, IGHJ4, IGHJ5, and IGHJ6, though there is reason to doubt the existence of the reported allelic variants of IGHJ3 and IGHJ5 (39). TCR J genes are more numerous and are differently organized. The TRBJ genes are found as a block of six genes located downstream from the TRDB1 gene, and a block of seven genes located downstream from the TRDB2 gene. The TRDB1 gene can pair with all J genes, but the TRDB2 gene is strongly biased toward pairing with its associated J genes (40). There are also four functional J genes in the TRDJ locus. Functional allelic variants have only been reported for the TRBJ1-6 gene.

BIASES IN COMBINATORIAL DIVERSITY AND THE SHAPING OF THE REPERTOIRE

Combinatorial diversity is that part of repertoire diversity that results from the fact that functional receptor genes form by the recombination of members of the sets of germline V, D, and J genes. This diversity is usually calculated by simply multiplying together the number of functional V, D, and J genes that are available within the genome. Such calculations, however, may promote misunderstandings, for they encourage the view that "all genes are equal," and that all combinations are equally likely. TCR studies have paid considerable attention to capturing an unbiased sampling of the repertoire, for example using 5′ RACE to amplify TCR transcripts from the constant region gene. Such studies have shown that TCR genes are highly biased in their usage (41–43). In contrast, many BCR repertoire studies have amplified both mRNA and genomic rearrangements, often using IGHV gene family-targeting primer sets that were developed for the detection of malignancies rather than for the investigation of the repertoire (44, 45). Such primers almost certainly lead to some distortions in the relative abundances of different sequences that are seen. Nevertheless, BCR studies utilizing different primer sets, and amplifying different source material are surprisingly consistent, and the B cell literature provides unequivocal evidence of strong gene utilization biases.

Different IGHV genes are used at frequencies that range from as little as 0.1% to more than 10% of all rearrangements in an individual's naïve B cell repertoire (18, 46). Utilization frequencies also vary between alleles. For example, analysis of VDJ recombination in different individuals has shown that IGHV1-2*02 is used approximately three times as often as IGHV1-2*04, in individuals who carry both these alleles (18). IGHV utilization frequencies are surprisingly constant between individuals (47). Examples of such consistency include IGHV1-46 which varies from 2 to 3.1% in different individuals (average 2.65%), IGHV3-21 which varies from 3.5 to 6.3% (average 4.59%), and IGHV3-49 which varies from 0.8 to 1.3% (average 1.0%) (18). This is not true for all genes, with different individuals utilizing IGHV1-69 at frequencies that range from 3.1 to 9.1% (average 6.2%) (18). IGHV3-23, which is typically the most utilized IGHV gene, was seen on average in 6.7% of all VDJ sequences, but its utilization frequency in one individual was 13.7% (18).

Biased gene usage is not confined to the IGHV genes. IGHD gene usage varies from less than 1% (IGHD4-4/11) to over 15% (IGHD3-22) of total rearrangements. Biases in the resulting amino acid sequences of the CDR3 junction are even greater. IGHD segments can be utilized in all three reading frames, and each IGHD gene is therefore able to encode three distinct amino acid sequences. Analysis of IGH rearrangements in which the IGHJ is out-of-frame, and which are therefore non-productive, shows each IGHD gene rearranges at equal frequency in each of the three RFs, however among productive rearrangements there is a strong skewing of the utilization of each gene toward a dominant RF (48). This dominance is constant between individuals, and the preferred RF is gene family dependent. Analysis of in-frame and out-of-frame IGH rearrangements sequenced using the Illumina platform suggests that the underlying rearrangement processes have no reading frame bias, but that bias emerges from stronger negative selection of sequences in certain reading frames (48). Such negative selection particularly focuses on non-productive sequences that result from the presence of stop codons within the junction region. These are seen when many IGHD genes are translated in the non-dominant reading frame, and such genes can only be utilized in those reading frames if the stop codons are removed by exonuclease trimming. When analysis of IGHD usage in the expressed repertoire factors in the three RFs, the IGHD gene utilization frequencies span three orders of magnitude. There is also considerable variation between the utilization frequencies of IGHJ genes. The IGHJ4 gene is present in approximately 45–50% of rearrangements, while IGHJ6 accounts for a further 20–25% of VDJ rearrangements (49, 50). IGHJ1, on the other hand, is utilized by only 1% of all rearrangements (39).

Biases in light chain gene usage are just as strong. For IGK rearrangements, preferential inclusion of IGKV3-20 was noted in early studies of the expressed IGK repertoire of both adults and neonates (51–53), while single cell PCR (54) and bioinformatics analysis of IGK rearrangements from sequence databases showed IGKV3-15, IGKV3-11, IGKV1-5, IGKV2-30, and IGKV1-30/IGKV1D-39 to also display preferential rearrangement (20). These biases were confirmed again recently in a high-throughput sequencing study which also highlighted similarities in usage between individuals, including similarities between individuals from geographically distant and ethnically distinct populations (55). Under-utilization and over-utilization of the J gene segments have been reported. IGKJ1 and IGKJ2 appear more frequently, while there is under-utilization of IGKJ3 and IGKJ5 (20, 53, 54). This skewing of IGKJ usage toward the genes located 5′ in the IGKJ locus is seen despite the necessity for selection of more 3′ IGKJ genes during secondary IGK rearrangements (56, 57). A similar bias toward 5′ IGKJ genes is also seen in the mouse, and modeling of mouse light chain rearrangement supports the strong underlying tendency toward the initial rearrangement of IGKJ1 or IGKJ2 (58). The IGLV usage is strongly skewed toward a limited number of the functional V segments with 3 of the 30 IGLVs accounting for more than 50% of expressed rearrangements, and with individual IGLV segment frequencies ranging from 0.02 to 27% (59). Only four of the seven IGLJ are considered functional (60). The four IGLJ range from almost 55% utilization in the expressed B cell repertoire for IGLJ7, to just 5.5% for IGLJ1 (61).

Although bias in the reading frame of the IGHD gene is the result of selection, other biases appear to be intrinsic to the recombination process, for when analysis is confined to non-productive rearrangements which carry an out-of-frame J-REGION, preferential gene usage is still seen (48). Such sequences are not subject to positive or negative selection. The same biases have been observed among transcripts generated from transgenic mice that carry a human heavy chain mini-locus (62), while in NOD-scid-IL2Rγ null mice that had been reconstituted with human hematopoietic stem cells, typical patterns of biased usage were seen amongst the expressed light chain genes (63). Recent studies in monozygotic twins show that they share utilization frequencies for both the heavy and light chain genes (46, 63), with correlations in a similar range to replicate biological samples. When one twin was investigated following lymphocyte ablation therapy, the reconstituted repertoire showed the same utilization patterns (46). Unrelated individuals did not share this degree of correlation. The biases in utilization frequencies of different V, D, and J genes therefore appear to be genetically determined, and when acted upon by the recombination machinery, the biases in that process give rise to an individual's distinct repertoire. Repertoire shape is therefore directly linked to the genotype of an individual's immunoglobulin gene loci. This has become even clearer since high-throughput sequencing has allowed analysis to focus upon individual chromosomes.

The large datasets that are now being generated by high-throughput sequencing from single individuals are facilitating analysis of the processes that shape the repertoire, but each dataset still represents a mixture of rearrangements from two independently recombining chromosomes. The fact that V(D)J rearrangement is an intra-chromosomal event, however, means that every V(D)J gene rearrangement provides information about the association of different genes on a chromosome. Any heterozygous locus allows each chromosome to be associated with one or the other allele at that gene locus, and large sets of V(D)J rearrangements can be analyzed to determine all the V, D, and J genes that rearrange on each chromosome. This allows the determination of inferred haplotypes (see **Figure 2**).

In practice, the complete inference of V, D, and J gene haplotypes by the analysis of V(D)J rearrangements is only likely to be possible in the case of the IGH locus. Approximately 40% of individuals are heterozygous at the IGHJ6 locus, and the IGHJ6 gene is present in nearly 25% of all rearrangements. It therefore provides an ideal "anchor-point" from which to haplotype the IGH locus. Using this approach, we recently investigated the IGH locus in nine individuals, and showed that all 18 IGH variable region gene

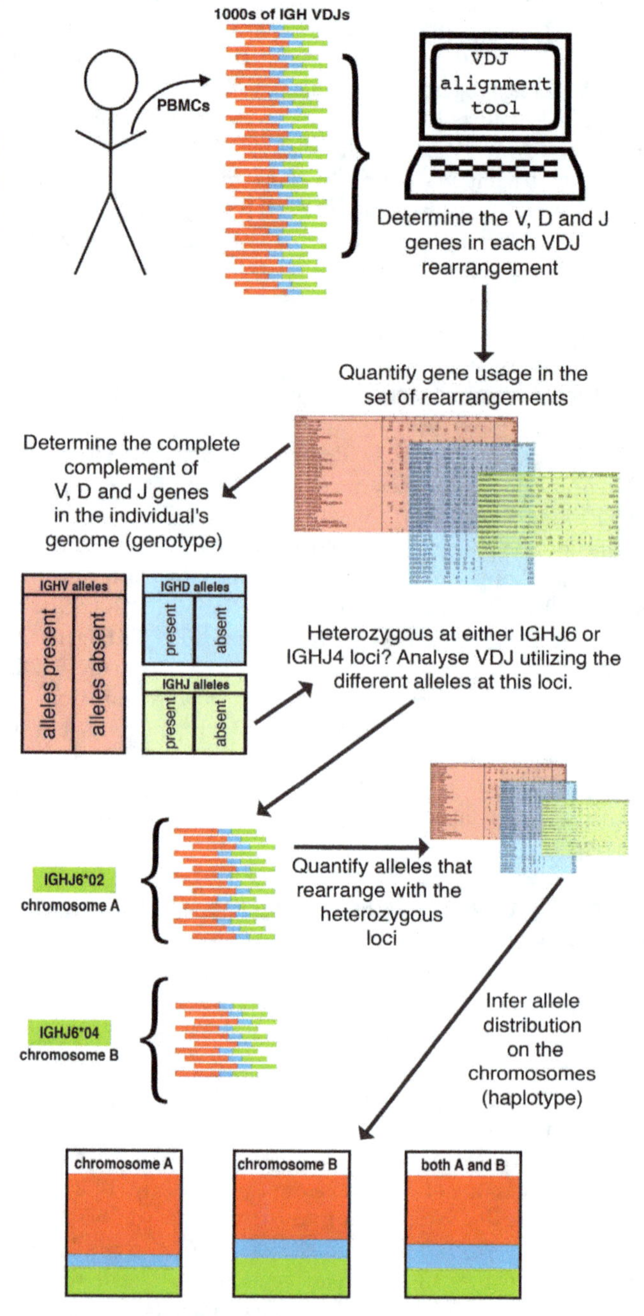

FIGURE 2 | Inference of IGH haplotypes from VDJ rearrangements. The availability of large datasets of VDJ rearrangements from single individuals permit the inference of all germline V, D, and J genes within the genome, from analysis of apparent gene utilization within a dataset. As IGH VDJ rearrangement is an intra-chromosomal event, gene pairing in VDJ rearrangements can be used to infer which gene segments are carried by the same chromosome. Leveraging the heterozygous IGHJ6 or IGHJ4 locus allows the reconstruction of IGH gene segments on each chromosome and for the IGH haplotype to be inferred.

haplotypes were unique (19). In addition to allelic variants, many IGHV and IGHD gene deletions and IGHV gene duplications were evident. The definition of haplotypes in this way is allowing IGH gene usage frequencies to be studied with unprecedented accuracy, but unfortunately no locus as appropriate as the IGHJ6 anchor-point exists amongst the light chain genes or amongst TCR genes. Limited investigations in the past have highlighted TCR haplotypic variation in the human population (64, 65), but the extent of variation within the IGH locus suggests that considerably more TCR variation may await discovery.

Many factors have been explored to explain biases in chromosomal recombination patterns. Variations in enhancers (66) have been implicated in biased murine TCR gene usage. Variations in recombination signal sequences (RSS) also influence utilization frequencies of both human BCR (67, 68) and TCR (69) genes. The IGKV polymorphism that has been linked to increased susceptibility to *Haemophilus influenzae* in the Navajo population includes a single nucleotide change in the heptamer sequence of the RSS, and it reduces recombination by 4.5-fold relative to the common allelic variant (21). The non-amer and heptamer sequences of the RSS are separated by either a 12 or 23 base pair spacer. Spacers also show sequence variation, and there has been debate about the impact this has on recombination efficiency. While some studies did not observe any impact when the regular spacer sequence was replaced with runs of GC pairs (70), competition assays using extra chromosomal substrates suggest differences in spacer sequence can result in differences in recombination efficiency that mirror differential gene usage in the V(D)J repertoire (67, 68). However, RSS variation cannot explain all differences in allele utilization. The recent re-sequencing of the complete IGH locus found that the IGHV-associated RSS were the same as those earlier reported by Matsuda (71) even where different alleles of the gene were present (17).

Some variation in the frequency with which particular gene sequences are seen in the repertoire may be explained by copy-number variations (CNV). The presence of CNV within the IG variable gene locus was first determined using sequence-specific RFLP analysis to determine gene copy-number (72), and the affect of CNV on expression levels was investigated through the examination of the binding of an anti-idiotypic monoclonal antibody (G6) to tonsillar IgD + B-cells (73). An examination of 35 individuals found that they carried between 0 and 4 copies of the IGHV1-69 gene. Linear regression determined that for each allele copy, approximately 3% of B-cells were G6 reactive. Individual differences in the IGHV1-69 copy-number could therefore result in the contribution that this single gene makes varying from being totally absent (0 copies) to being present in as many as 12% of rearrangements in individuals with four available copies.

Sequencing of single chromosomes of an individual's IGH locus has now demonstrated that insertions, deletions, and complex events have altered the copy-number of IGHV genes, including the IGHV1-69 and IGHV3-23 genes (17). The duplicate IGHV3-23 genes remain within the genome as absolutely identical sequences. The presence of these and other CNVs has also been highlighted in bioinformatic studies of immunoglobulin genotypes (18) and haplotypes (19), where sequence data from single individuals clearly demonstrated that some individuals had more than two "alleles" of a single IGHV gene. Genes were also found to be absent from the genome of some individuals. A limitation of these bioinformatics studies was that gene duplications could only be detected if two distinct "allelic variants" were carried on a single chromosome.

In addition to the underlying biases in utilization of germline genes, a final bias has been identified that affects the contribution of recombination frequencies to repertoire diversity. For reasons that are presently unclear, there appear to be pairing preferences for some IGHD and IGHJ genes that increase the frequency of particular IGHD-IGHJ pairs within the repertoire. Biases were first observed in a small set of 59 non-productive rearrangements (74). Later analysis of 6,500 IGH VDJ sequences collected from public databases led to the observation that 5′ IGHD genes paired with increased frequency to the most 3′ IGHJ (J5/J6) and with decreased frequency to the 5′ IGHJ (J1–J4) (50). In contrast, 3′ IGHD tended to preferentially pair with 5′ IGHJ rather than 3′ IGHJ (50). This observation is also supported by analysis of very large datasets generated by pyrosequencing of VDJ rearrangements from three healthy subjects (75). Significantly more pairings were seen of IGHD2-2 and IGHD3-3 with IGHJ6, and of IGHD3-22 and IGHJ3 than would be predicted from the frequencies of these genes in the overall dataset (75).

The bias in D-J pairing also extends to the TCRB loci where the application of HTS approaches to murine TCRB repertoires has revealed a pattern of TRBD to TRBJ pairing that correlates to the genomic distance between rearranged genes (40). The TRBV and TRBJ gene usage in the mice was biased toward particular genes, but the pairings of TRBV and TRBJ were independent. The physical chromatin structure of the TRBD and TRBJ loci was investigated using a biophysical model of the chromatin conformation. The biases in TRBD to TRBJ pairing appeared to be better explained by this mechanical model than previously proposed genetic models based on RSSs (40). The model was also extended to human TRBJ usage with favorable evidence that chromatin conformation determines TRJB gene usage.

Biases in the pairing of heavy and light chains have also been reported. The existence of forbidden or unfavorable pairings of germline heavy and light chain genes was described in the early literature (76). This was not supported by later studies (77, 78), nor was it supported by a recent study that applied high-throughput sequencing to generate thousands of linked heavy and light chain genes (79).

BIASES IN JUNCTIONAL DIVERSITY AND THE SHAPING OF THE REPERTOIRE

Both the naive B cell and T cell repertoires are limited in the periphery by processes of selection. However T cell selection within the thymus is a particularly rigorous process, and it leads to dramatic differences between the potential and the observed repertoire diversity. The idiosyncratic nature of TCR selection in a human population with abundant MHC diversity also means that analysis of the processes that contribute to TCR diversity will be difficult using datasets comprising sequences from multiple individuals. Sufficiently large datasets from single individuals with a specific MHC profile finally became available with the application of high-throughput sequencing to repertoire studies. However, the continuing difficulties involved with the identification of TCR

D genes and hence the other constituent elements within the TCR CDR3 still discourage analysis of the genetic elements and processes that contribute to this region. It is therefore studies of BCR genes that provide the clearest insights into the processes that contribute palindromic P nucleotides and non-template encoded N nucleotides to the V(D)J junction, and into the process of exonuclease trimming that depletes the ends of recombining genes. A recent study of BCR CDR3 suggested that as a result of these processes, the circulating B cell population in a typical adult human includes 3–9 × 10^6 unique heavy chain CDR3 (80).

Palindromic or P nucleotides are formed by the asymmetric opening of hairpin loops that form at gene ends during the rearrangement process (81). In the absence of exonuclease activity, the opening of the hairpins can add short, self-complementary single stranded extensions into the junctions. P nucleotide addition was first recognized as a process that can contribute to TCR CDR3 (82, 83), however the contributions of P nucleotides to the BCR repertoire have been more precisely quantified (84, 85). Similarly, it is recognized that N nucleotides make a major contribution to the diversity of both the TCR and BCR repertoire (86), but only BCR N-REGIONS have been subjected to detailed analysis (37). Where BCR studies have investigated the kinds of amino acids that are likely within N-REGIONS, studies of TCR N-REGIONS have focused upon analysis of the overall contribution of N-REGIONS to αβ TCR diversity. This has been studied in a comparison of wild-type mice with mice carrying homozygous null alleles for TdT (86). N-addition was estimated to contribute to 90% of the diversity of the αβ TCR repertoire (86). Diversity could be estimated in this and other studies because of the development of "spectratyping" techniques, which is the analysis of the CDR3 length distribution in PCR amplicons. It permitted some of the first explorations of the T cell repertoire, however it only allowed detailed analysis of N-REGIONS if further sequencing was undertaken. Until the advent of high-throughput sequencing, such analysis was usually compromised by the restricted number of sequences that could be generated from any individual, and by the challenges associated with D gene identification.

Non-template encoded N-additions are intrinsically biased owing to the preference of TdT toward the incorporation of G nucleotides. This is manifested in G/C-rich additions when viewing the N-REGIONS of the coding strand, as additions may be made to both the coding and non-coding strands during recombination. This has been demonstrated through analysis of extra-chromosomal substrates transfected into human cell lines (36), as well as by analysis of human BCR (37) and TCR (87) VDJ rearrangements. The G/C bias is coupled with an apparent inter-dependence of the additions, which leads to the formation of homopolymer tracts (36, 37, 87). Together these biases ensure that the germline gene-encoded regions of the CDR3 are frequently flanked by amino acids such as glycine, that are encoded by G-rich codons (88). It has been proposed that the inclusion of small amino acids such as glycine, which has only a single side chain, promotes flexibility of the CDR3 loop (88).

Exonuclease trimming is perhaps the least understood process that contributes to the BCR and TCR repertoires. The mechanisms responsible for the loss of nucleotides from the coding ends of the genes during rearrangement remains to be determined, but a number of features of the process have been described, and intrinsic biases have been identified. The extent of processing from each gene end involved in a join (VD or DJ) is independent (87). That is, we do not see more processing on one side of the join to compensate for reduced processing of the gene on the other side. The processing differs for V, D, and J genes and for gene families. Removals may therefore be impacted by the sequence of the gene ends. Sequences with high A/T content appear more susceptible to nucleotide loss, while sequences with high G/C content appear resistant to processing (36, 84, 89, 90). This bias is still seen after controlling for the G/C bias of N-REGIONS.

The gene sequence ends that remain after exonuclease processing provide a final bias that shapes the repertoire. The gene ends are constrained by the genetic code, to favor the formation of codons for a surprisingly limited number of amino acids. This is best illustrated in the case of the many IGHD genes that have the nucleotide sequence TAC at their 3′ end (see **Figure 3**). In the dominant reading frame, these nucleotides encode tyrosine. Removal of a single nucleotide creates a situation where only provision of a T or C (from N-addition or from the 5′ end of the IGHJ gene) will result in a functional sequence, for TAA and TAG are stop codons. Addition of C returns the sequence to its original state, while addition of T results in an alternative tyrosine codon. In this and other cases, the nucleotide sequences of the gene ends limit the diversity that results from exonuclease removals.

B CELL LINEAGES AND T CELL CLONOTYPES IN THE ANTIGEN-SPECIFIC RESPONSE

Biases that we have described in immunoglobulin V, D, and J gene usage mean that at least seven orders of magnitude separate the probabilities that the most likely and the least likely combinations of recombining genes will be generated in the bone marrow. Many additional orders of magnitude separate the most likely from the

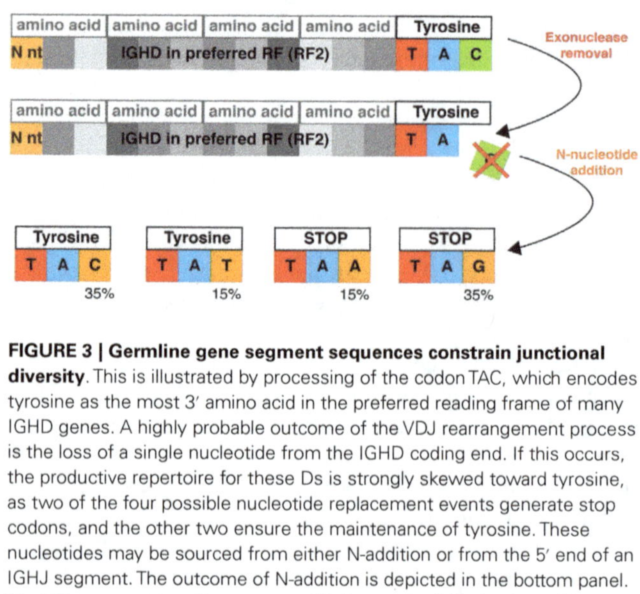

FIGURE 3 | Germline gene segment sequences constrain junctional diversity. This is illustrated by processing of the codon TAC, which encodes tyrosine as the most 3′ amino acid in the preferred reading frame of many IGHD genes. A highly probable outcome of the VDJ rearrangement process is the loss of a single nucleotide from the IGHD coding end. If this occurs, the productive repertoire for these Ds is strongly skewed toward tyrosine, as two of the four possible nucleotide replacement events generate stop codons, and the other two ensure the maintenance of tyrosine. These nucleotides may be sourced from either N-addition or from the 5′ end of an IGHJ segment. The outcome of N-addition is depicted in the bottom panel. N-additions are colored in orange and below each of the four possible outcomes is shown the likelihood of the enzyme TdT adding each nucleotide base.

least likely heavy and light chain pairs. The least likely BCRs are so unlikely to be generated in the bone marrow that they almost certainly will never be seen in an individual's lifetime. The most likely BCRs, on the other hand, may be so readily generated that they are always present within the repertoire at high copy number. These high copy-number sequences are likely to utilize a relative handful of the available germline genes, and to have been subject to minimal processing. TdT adds, on average, around 6 nucleotides between joining genes, and 30 or more nucleotides may occasionally be added to the VD, DJ, and VJ junctions, but it is highly likely that no more than two nucleotides will be added. Even long heavy chain CDR3 are likely to be the result of long germline sequences rather than the result of long N-REGIONS (47). Six or more nucleotides may be removed from the 3′ end of the IGHV gene, but most sequences lose no more than two or three IGHV nucleotides, and many sequences lose no nucleotides at all.

Without the added diversity that comes from D genes, the kappa and lambda repertoires are strongly shaped by biased gene usage and minimal processing and the diversity of the repertoires is surprisingly limited. The light chain repertoires are dominated by a very small number of amino acid sequences, and this dominance is so extreme that even in the days of Sanger sequencing, identical light chain gene rearrangements were reported by separate studies from independent laboratories (20). The theoretical diversity of the kappa repertoire has been estimated to be as high as 4×10^{24} unique nucleotide sequences (91). However analysis of kappa sequences generated from single individuals by high-throughput sequencing suggest the repertoire may include less than 10^4 unique amino acid sequences (55), and some of these sequences may be seen in over 1% of all kappa-bearing BCR (55). The diversity of the expressed lambda repertoire has recently been shown to be similarly restricted (63).

Although the heavy chain repertoire has much greater diversity then the light chain repertoire, repertoire shaping may be sufficiently extreme that some heavy chain sequences, and even some BCR will be present at high copy number in the repertoire of every individual. We are not aware of identical heavy chain sequences being amplified from multiple individuals, but highly similar "stereotypical" sequences have been found amongst leukemic clones of individuals with chronic lymphocytic leukemia (92). These stereotypical sequences differ through the stochastic processes of somatic hypermutation, but they appear to have evolved from cells expressing highly similar BCR within the naïve B cell repertoires of different individuals. Antigen selection, which may be associated with the pathogenesis of this condition (93), could be selecting and therefore revealing high copy-number heavy chain sequences.

The antigen specificity of most heavy and light chain sequences remain unclear, for it is only very recently that antigen-specific human B cells have been isolated and their BCRs investigated. The isolation of antigen-specific plasmablasts from the peripheral blood shortly after vaccination was first used to produce monoclonal human antibodies (94). These cells express BCR genes that are at once similar, as a consequence of their shared origins, yet highly divergent, as a result of the process of somatic point mutation. Together they make up a B cell clone lineage. High-throughput sequencing has since been used to identify clone lineages after booster shots with the influenza vaccine (95) and the pneumococcal vaccine (96). B cell lineages producing broadly neutralizing antibodies to HIV have also been identified using high-throughput sequencing (97). However this handful of studies of antigen-specific B cells in humans has not identified lineages that are shared between individuals. Highly similar BCR heavy chain sequences have recently been identified using high-throughput sequencing of PBMC from multiple individuals with acute symptomatic dengue (98). Although the specificities of these sequences were not determined, such lineages were not identified in uninfected individuals. These may therefore be the first antigen-specific heavy chain "public lineages" to be identified. The extent to which the response to specific antigen more generally involves such "public lineages" remains to be determined.

In contrast to the paucity of studies of antigen-specific B cells, antigen-specific TCRs have been investigated in the human repertoire for over 20 years. Early studies revealed that the immune response to specific antigen, in HLA-matched individuals, can include sets of T cells sharing identical or highly similar TCR α- and β-chains (99–101). The development of techniques for the creation of MHC peptide tetramer complexes has facilitated the identification of antigen-specific T cells by flow cytometry (102). This has allowed the detailed investigation of dominant sequence sets and these studies gave rise to the notions of public and private T cell "clonotypes." Public clonotypes are defined as VDJ amino acid sequences that are dominant and identical, or nearly identical, in multiple individuals. Private clonotypes, in contrast, are idiosyncratic. The apparently antigen-driven emergence of public B cell lineages in chronic lymphocytic B cell leukemia also has parallels amongst T cell leukemias. Studies of T cell large granular lymphocyte leukemias have identified a public clonotype in individuals with the shared DRB1*0701 HLA type (103). This same clonotype was independently identified in DRB1*0701$^+$ individuals who were infected with human cytomegalovirus (104), suggesting that antigen-driven pathogenesis may be expanding and revealing this public clonotype.

To understand the reasons for the emergence of particular clonotypes, the naïve repertoire must be better understood. Enrichment techniques have recently been developed which when combined with MHC peptide tetramer technology allows extremely rare peptide-specific naïve murine T cells to be identified (105). Using this approach in humans, naïve CD8$^+$ T cells specific for peptide-MHC have been shown to range from 0.6 to 500 cells per million cells (106, 107) and CD4+ T cells to range from 0.2 to 10 per million cells (107). Most of the cells within identified sets of antigen-specific murine T cells express unique TCRs (105), but clonal diversity within identified human cell populations remains unclear. It is likely though that in the much larger human T cell compartment, many circulating T cells could carry identical TCRs. This should ensure that early adaptive responses to these antigens are robust, for the strength of the response to antigen has been shown to reflect the size of the antigen-specific naïve T cell population (105).

The presence of particular public TCR clonotypes have not yet been reported within the naïve human TCR repertoire. Discussion of the emergence of such TCR clonotypes in an antigen-specific response has therefore been driven principally by analyses of their nucleotide and amino acid features, and the phenomenon of convergent recombination has been invoked to explain public clonotypes (108, 109). Many public TCR clonotypes are divergent at the nucleotide level, but identical at the amino acid level. This results from the fact that particular amino acid sequences can arise from multiple, variant nucleotide sequences, and that these nucleotide sequences in turn can sometimes be formed by different genes with varying levels of gene processing and nucleotide addition. Such convergent recombination will certainly contribute to the presence of multiple copies of particular amino acid clonotypes within an individual's repertoire, but arguably, it is unlikely to increase the likelihood of one clonotype over another by more than one or two orders of magnitude.

More recently the role of biases in gene usage and in the recombination process have been identified as an alternative source of public clonotypes (110). The biases in the usage of TCR V, D, and J genes are less pronounced than is the case for the BCR genes. This is the result of the lack of substantial germline diversity within the sets of TRBD and TRDD genes, and because the TRBJ and TRDJ genes lack the strong usage biases that are seen amongst the IGHJ genes. Nevertheless biases in the usage of TCR genes are still likely to ensure that the probabilities of the generation of the least likely and the most likely V(D)J combination seen in αβ and γδ TCR differ by many orders of magnitude. It has also been pointed out that many public clonotypes have short CDR3 loops that are mainly encoded by germline-derived nucleotides rather then TdT-derived nucleotides (110). The contribution this may make to the formation of T cell clonotypes is harder to judge, because of the lack of detailed analysis of these processes, in the context of the TCR repertoire. However lessons from analysis of the BCR repertoire give strong credence to this hypothesis.

Both the BCR and the TCR repertoires have been the subject of considerable study and even greater speculation over many decades. High-throughput sequencing is now revealing their separate secrets at a gratifying rate. Our understanding of the shaping of the BCR and TCR repertoires will now surely move faster if a greater dialog commences between researchers on the two sides of the lymphocyte divide. BCR repertoire studies will be transformed when greater attention is paid to antigen-specific lineages. TCR repertoire studies, in turn, could benefit from the lessons of the BCR repertoire, which suggest that the analysis of full-length V(D)J rearrangements, and detailed analysis of the nucleotide elements within the CDR3, can help explain the shaping of the repertoire.

ACKNOWLEDGMENTS

This work was made possible by a grant from the National Health and Medical Research Council.

REFERENCES

1. Tonegawa S. Somatic genera- tion of antibody diversity. *Nature* (1983) 302:575–81. doi:10.1038/ 302575a0
2. Schroeder HW Jr, Cavacini L. Structure and function of immunoglobulins. *J Allergy Clin Immunol* (2010) 125:S41–52. doi:10.1016/j.jaci.2009.09.046
3. Davis MM, Bjorkman PJ. T- cell antigen receptor genes and T-cell recognition. *Nature* (1988) 334:395–402. doi:10.1038/334395a0
4. Takihara Y, Tkachuk D, Michalopoulos E, Champagne E, Reimann J, Minden M, et al. Sequence and organization of the diversity, joining, and constant region genes of the human T-cell delta-chain locus. *Proc Natl Acad Sci U S A* (1988) 85:6097–101. doi:10.1073/pnas.85.16.6097
5. Nikolich-Zugich J, Slifka MK, Mes- saoudi I. The many important facets of T-cell repertoire diversity. *Nat Rev Immunol* (2004) 4:123–32. doi:10.1038/ nri1292
6. Desiderio SV, Yancopoulos GD, Paskind M, Thomas E, Boss MA, Landau N, et al. Insertion of N regions into heavy-chain genes is correlated with expression of ter- minal deoxytransferase in B cells. *Nature* (1984) 311:752–5.
7. Davies JM, Platts-Mills TA, Aal- berse RC. The enigma of IgE+ B-cell memory in human sub- jects. *J Allergy Clin Immunol* (2013) 131:972–6. doi:10.1016/j. jaci.2012.12.1569
8. Fukui K, Noma T, Takeuchi K, Kobayashi N, Hatanaka M, Honjo T. Origin of adult T-cell leukemia virus. Implication for its zoonosis. *Mol Biol Med* (1983) 1:447–56.
9. Watson CT, Breden F. The immunoglobulin heavy chain locus: genetic variation, miss- ing data, and implications for human disease. *Genes Immun* (2012) 13:363–73. doi:10.1038/gene.2012.12
10. Rada C, Milstein C. The intrin- sic hypermutability of antibody heavy and light chain genes decays exponentially. *EMBO J* (2001) 20:4570–6. doi:10.1093/emboj/20. 16.4570
11. Odegard VH, Schatz DG. Targeting of somatic hypermutation. *Nat Rev Immunol* (2006) 6:573–83. doi:10. 1038/nri1896
12. Pallares N, Lefebvre S, Contet V, Matsuda F, Lefranc MP. The human immunoglobulin heavy variable genes. *Exp Clin Immuno- genet* (1999) 16:36–60. doi:10. 1159/000019095
13. Ohm-Laursen L, Larsen SR, Barington T. Identification of two new alleles, IGHV3-23⊠04 and IGHJ6⊠04, and the com- plete sequence of the IGHV3-h pseudogene in the human immunoglobulin locus and their prevalences in Danish Caucasians. *Immunogenetics* (2005) 57: 621–7. doi:10.1007/s00251-005- 0035-8
14. Romo-Gonzalez T, Morales- Montor J, Rodriguez-Dorantes M, Vargas-Madrazo E. Novel substitution polymorphisms of human immunoglobulin VH genes in Mexicans. *Hum Immunol* (2005) 66:732–40. doi:10.1016/j. humimm.2005.03.002
15. Wang Y, Jackson KJ, Sewell WA, Collins AM. Many human immunoglobulin heavy-chain IGHV gene polymorphisms have been reported in error. *Immunol Cell Biol* (2008) 86:111–5.
16. Wang Y, Jackson KJ, Gaeta B, Pomat W, Siba P, Sewell WA, et al. Genomic screening by 454 pyrose- quencing identifies a new human IGHV gene and sixteen other new IGHV allelic variants. *Immuno- genetics* (2011) 63:259–65. doi:10. 1007/s00251-010-0510-8
17. Watson CT, Steinberg KM, Huddleston J, Warren RL, Malig M, Schein J, et al. Com- plete haplotype sequence of the human immunoglobulin heavy-chain variable, diver- sity, and joining genes and characterization of allelic and copy-number variation. *Am J Hum Genet* (2013) 92:530–46. doi:10.1016/j.ajhg.2013.03.004
18. Boyd SD, Gaeta BA, Jackson KJ, Fire AZ, Marshall EL, Merker JD, et al. Individual variation in the germline Ig gene reper- toire inferred from variable region gene rearrangements. *J Immunol* (2010) 184:6986–92. doi:10.4049/ jimmunol.1000445
19. Kidd MJ, Chen Z, Wang Y, Jackson KJ, Zhang L, Boyd SD, et al. The inference of phased haplotypes for the immunoglobulin H chain V region gene loci by analysis of VDJ gene rearrangements. *J Immunol* (2012) 188:1333–40. doi:10.4049/ jimmunol.1102097
20. Collins AM, Wang Y, Singh V, Yu P, Jackson KJ, Sewell WA. The reported germline repertoire of human immunoglobulin kappa chain genes is relatively com- plete and accurate. *Immunogenet- ics* (2008) 60:669–76. doi:10.1007/ s00251-008-0325-z
21. Feeney AJ, Atkinson MJ, Cowan MJ, Escuro G, Lugo G. A defective Vkappa A2 allele in Navajos which may play a role in increased sus- ceptibility to *Haemophilus influen- zae* type b disease. *J Clin Invest* (1996) 97:2277–82. doi:10.1172/ JCI118669
22. Rowen L, Koop BF, Hood L. The complete 685-kilobase DNA sequence of the human beta T cell receptor locus. *Science* (1996) 272:1755–62. doi:10.1126/science. 272.5269.1755
23. Boysen C, Simon MI, Hood L. Analysis of the 1.1-Mb human alpha/delta T-cell receptor locus with bacterial artificial chromo- some clones. *Genome Res* (1997) 7:330–8.
24. Ibberson MR, Copier JP, Llop E, Navarrete C, Hill AV, Cruickshank JK, et al. T-cell receptor variable alpha (TCRAV) polymorphisms in European, Chinese, South American, AfroCaribbean, and Gambian populations. *Immunogenetics* (1998) 47:124–30. doi:10.1007/ s002510050337

25. Moody AM, Reyburn H, Willcox N, Newsom-Davis J. New poly- morphism of the human T-cell receptor AV28S1 gene segment. *Immunogenetics* (1998) 48:62–4. doi:10.1007/s002510050401
26. Subrahmanyan L, Eberle MA, Clark AG, Kruglyak L, Nick- erson DA. Sequence variation and linkage disequilibrium in the human T-cell receptor beta (TCRB) locus. *Am J Hum Genet* (2001) 69:381–95. doi:10.1086/ 321297
27. Mackelprang R, Livingston RJ, Eberle MA, Carlson CS, Yi Q, Akey JM, et al. Sequence diversity, nat- ural selection and linkage dise- quilibrium in the human T cell receptor alpha/delta locus. *Hum Genet* (2006) 119:255–66. doi:10. 1007/s00439-005-0111-z
28. Vessey SJ, Bell JI, Jakobsen BK. A functionally significant allelic polymorphism in a T cell recep- tor V beta gene segment. *Eur J Immunol* (1996) 26:1660–3. doi: 10.1002/eji.1830260739
29. Gras S, Chen Z, Miles JJ, Liu YC, Bell MJ, Sullivan LC, et al. Allelic polymorphism in the T cell receptor and its impact on immune responses. *J Exp Med* (2010) 207:1555–67. doi:10.1084/ jem.20100603
30. Corbett SJ, Tomlinson IM, Sonnhammer EL, Buck D, Win- ter G. Sequence of the human immunoglobulin diversity (D) segment locus: a systematic analysis provides no evidence for the use of DIR segments, inverted D segments, "minor" D segments or D-D recombination. *J Mol Biol* (1997) 270:587–97. doi:10.1006/jmbi.1997.1141
31. Munshaw S, Kepler TB. SoDA2: a Hidden Markov Model approach for identification of immunoglob- ulin rearrangements. *Bioinformat- ics* (2010) 26:867–72. doi:10.1093/ bioinformatics/btq056
32. Ye J, Ma N, Madden TL, Ostell JM. IgBLAST: an immunoglobulin variable domain sequence analy- sis tool. *Nucleic Acids Res* (2013). doi:10.1093/nar/ gkt382
33. Gaeta BA, Malming HR, Jackson KJ, Bain ME, Wilson P, Collins AM. iHMMune-align: hidden Markov model-based alignment and identification of germline genes in rearranged immunoglobulin gene sequences. *Bioinformatics* (2007) 23:1580–7. doi:10.1093/ bioinformatics/btm147
34. Jackson KJ, Boyd S, Gaeta BA, Collins AM. Benchmarking the performance of human antibody gene alignment utilities using a 454 sequence dataset. *Bioinformatics* (2010) 26:3129–30. doi:10.1093/ bioinformatics/btq604
35. Basu M, Hegde MV, Modak MJ. Synthesis of composition- ally unique DNA by termi- nal deoxynucleotidyl transferase. *Biochem Biophys Res Commun* (1983) 111:1105–12. doi:10.1016/ 0006-291X(83)91413-4
36. Gauss GH, Lieber MR. Mecha- nistic constraints on diversity in human V(D)J recombination. *Mol Cell Biol* (1996) 16:258–69.
37. Jackson KJ, Gaeta BA, Collins AM. Identifying highly mutated IGHD genes in the junctions of rearranged human immunoglobu- lin heavy chain genes. *J Immunol Methods* (2007) 324:26–37. doi:10. 1016/j.jim.2007.04.011
38. Thomas N, Heather J, Ndifon W, Shawe-Taylor J, Chain B. Decombinator: a tool for fast, efficient gene assignment in T- cell receptor sequences using a finite state machine. *Bioinformat- ics* (2013) 29:542–50. doi:10.1093/ bioinformatics/btt004
39. Lee CE, Jackson KJ, Sewell WA, Collins AM. Use of IGHJ and IGHD gene mutations in analysis of immunoglobulin sequences for the prognosis of chronic lympho- cytic leukemia. *Leuk Res* (2007) 31:1247–52. doi:10.1016/j. leukres. 2006.10.013
40. Ndifon W, Gal H, Shifrut E, Aha- roni R, Yissachar N, Waysbort N, et al. Chromatin conformation gov- erns T-cell receptor Jbeta gene segment usage. *Proc Natl Acad Sci U S A* (2012) 109:15865–70. doi:10. 1073/ pnas.1203916109
41. Quiros Roldan E, Sottini A, Bet- tinardi A, Albertini A, Imberti L, Primi D. Different TCRBV genes generate biased patterns of V- D-J diversity in human T cells. *Immunogenetics* (1995) 41:91–100.
42. Livak F, Burtrum DB, Rowen L, Schatz DG, Petrie HT. Genetic modulation of T cell receptor gene segment usage during somatic recombination. *J Exp Med* (2000) 192:1191–6. doi:10.1084/jem.192. 8.1191
43. Warren RL, Freeman JD, Zeng T, Choe G, Munro S, Moore R, et al. Exhaustive T-cell repertoire sequencing of human peripheral blood samples reveals signatures of antigen selection and a directly measured repertoire size of at least 1 million clonotypes. *Genome Res* (2011) 21:790–7. doi:10.1101/gr. 115428.110
44. van Dongen JJ, Langerak AW, Bruggemann M, Evans PA, Hummel M, Lavender FL, et al. Design and standardization of PCR primers and pro- to- cols for detection of clonal immunoglobulin and T-cell receptor gene recombinations in suspect lymphoproliferations: report of the BIOMED-2 Con- certed Action BMH4-CT98-3936. *Leukemia* (2003) 17:2257–317. doi:10.1038/sj.leu.2403202
45. Matthews C, Catherwood M, Mor- ris TC, Alexander HD. Rou- tine analysis of IgVH mutational status in CLL patients using BIOMED-2 standardized primers and protocols. *Leuk Lymphoma* (2004) 45:1899–904. doi:10.1080/ 10428190410001710812
46. Glanville J, Kuo TC, Von Büdin- gen H-C, Guey L, Berka J, Sun- dar PD, et al. Naive antibody gene- segment frequencies are heritable and unaltered by chronic lympho- cyte ablation. *Proc Natl Acad Sci U S A* (2011) 108:20066–71. doi:10. 1073/pnas.1107498108
47. Briney BS, Willis JR, Mckin- ney BA, Crowe JE Jr. High- throughput antibody sequencing reveals genetic evidence of global regulation of the naive and mem- ory repertoires that extends across individuals. *Genes Immun* (2012) 13:469–73. doi:10.1038/gene.2012. 20
48. Benichou J, Glanville J, Prak ET, Azran R, Kuo TC, Pons J, et al. The restricted DH gene read- ing frame usage in the expressed human antibody repertoire is selected based upon its amino acid content. *J Immunol* (2013) 190: 5567–77. doi:10.4049/jimmunol. 1201929
49. Yamada M, Wasserman R, Reichard BA, Shane S, Caton AJ, Rovera G. Preferential utiliza- tion of specific immunoglobulin heavy chain diversity and join- ing segments in adult human peripheral blood B lymphocytes. *J Exp Med* (1991) 173:395–407. doi:10.1084/jem.173.2.395
50. Volpe JM, Kepler TB. Large- scale analysis of human heavy chain V(D)J recombination pat- terns. *Immunome Res* (2008) 4:3. doi:10.1186/1745-7580-4-3
51. Klein R, Jaenichen R, Zachau HG. Expressed human immunoglobulin kappa genes and their hypermutation. *Eur J Immunol* (1993) 23:3248–62. doi:10.1002/eji.1830231231
52. Cox JP, Tomlinson IM, Winter G. A directory of human germ-line V kappa segments reveals a strong bias in their usage. *Eur J Immunol* (1994) 24:827–36. doi:10.1002/eji. 1830240409
53. Weber JC, Blaison G, Martin T, Knapp AM, Pasquali JL. Evidence that the V kappa III gene usage is nonstochastic in both adult and newborn peripheral B cells and that peripheral CD5+ adult B cells are oligoclonal. *J Clin Invest* (1994) 93:2093–105. doi:10.1172/ JCI117204
54. Foster SJ, Brezinschek HP, Brezin- schek RI, Lipsky PE. Molecular mechanisms and selective influ- ences that shape the kappa gene repertoire of IgM+ B cells. *J Clin Invest* (1997) 99:1614–27. doi:10. 1172/JCI119324
55. Jackson KJ, Wang Y, Gaeta BA, Pomat W, Siba P, Rimmer J, et al. Divergent human pop- ulations show extensive shared IGK rearrangements in periph- eral blood B cells. *Immunogenet- ics* (2012) 64:3–14. doi:10.1007/ s00251-011-0559-z
56. Gay D, Saunders T, Camper S, Weigert M. Receptor editing: an approach by autoreactive B cells to escape tolerance. *J Exp Med* (1993) 177:999–1008. doi:10. 1084/jem.177.4.999
57. Tiegs SL, Russell DM, Nemazee D. Receptor editing in self-reactive bone marrow B cells. *J Exp Med* (1993) 177:1009–20. doi:10.1084/ jem.177.4.1009
58. Mehr R, Shannon M, Litwin S. Models for antigen receptor gene rearrangement. I. Biased receptor editing in B cells: implications for allelic exclusion. *J Immunol* (1999) 163:1793–8.
59. Ignatovich O, Tomlinson IM, Jones PT, Winter G. The creation of diversity in the human immunoglobu- lin V(lambda) repertoire. *J Mol Biol* (1997) 268:69–77. doi:10.1006/jmbi.1997.0956
60. Vasicek TJ, Leder P. Structure and expression of the human immunoglobulin lambda genes. *J Exp Med* (1990) 172:609–20. doi: 10.1084/jem.172.2.609
61. Farner NL, Dorner T, Lipsky PE. Molecular mechanisms and selection influence the genera- tion of the human V lambda J lambda repertoire. *J Immunol* (1999) 162:2137–45.
62. Tuaillon N, Taylor LD, Lon- berg N, Tucker PW, Capra JD. Human immunoglobulin heavy- chain minilocus recombination in transgenic mice: gene-segment use in mu and gamma transcripts *Proc Natl Acad Sci U S A* (1993) 90:3720–4. doi:10.1073/pnas.90.8. 3720
63. Hoi KH, Ippolito GC. Intrinsic bias and public rearrangements in the human immunoglobulin Vlambda light chain repertoire. *Genes Immun* (2013) 14:271–6. doi:10.1038/gene.2013.10
64. Craddock TP, Zumla AM, Ollier WE, Chintu CZ, Muyinda GP, Lan- caster FC, et al. Predominance of one T-cell antigen receptor BV haplotype in African populations. *Immunogenetics* (2000) 51:231–7. doi:10.1007/ s002510050036
65. Donaldson IJ, Shefta J, Lawson CA, Bushnell JR, Morgan AW, Isaacs JD, et al. Unique TCR beta-subunit variable gene haplo- types in Africans. *Immunogenet- ics* (2002) 53:884–93. doi:10.1007/ s00251-001-0406-8
66. McMurry MT, Hernandez- Munain C, Lauzurica P, Krangel MS. Enhancer control of local accessibility to V(D)J recombinase. *Mol Cell Biol* (1997) 17:4553–61.
67. Nadel B, Tang A, Escuro G, Lugo G, Feeney AJ. Sequence of the spacer in the recom- bination signal sequence affects V(D)J rearrangement frequency and correlates with nonrandom Vkappa usage in vivo. *J Exp Med* (1998) 187:1495–503. doi:10. 1084/jem.187.9.1495
68. Feeney AJ, Tang A, Ogwaro KM. B-cell repertoire formation: role of the recombination sig- nal sequence in non-random V segment utilization. *Im-*

munol Rev (2000) 175:59–69. doi:10.1111/j. 1600-065X.2000.imr017508.x

69. Posnett DN, Vissinga CS, Pam- buccian C, Wei S, Robinson MA, Kostyu D, et al. Level of human TCRBV3S1 (V beta 3) expression correlates with allelic polymorphism in the spacer region of the recombination signal sequence. *J Exp Med* (1994) 179: 1707–11. doi:10.1084/jem.179.5. 1707
70. Wei Z, Lieber MR. Lymphoid V(D)J recombination. Functional analysis of the spacer sequence within the recombination signal. *J Biol Chem* (1993) 268:3180–3.
71. Matsuda F, Ishii K, Bourvagnet P, Kuma K, Hayashida H, Miy- ata T, et al. The complete nucleotide sequence of the human immunoglobulin heavy chain vari- able region locus. *J Exp Med* (1998) 188:2151–62. doi:10.1084/ jem.188.11.2151
72. Sasso EH, Willems Van Dijk K, Bull A, Van Der Maarel SM, Milner EC. VH genes in tandem array com- prise a repeated germline motif. *J Immunol* (1992) 149:1230–6.
73. Sasso EH, Johnson T, Kipps TJ. Expression of the immunoglobu- lin VH gene 51p1 is proportional to its germline gene copy number. *J Clin Invest* (1996) 97:2074–80. doi:10.1172/JCI118644
74. Souto-Carneiro MM, Longo NS, Russ DE, Sun HW, Lipsky PE. Characterization of the human Ig heavy chain antigen binding com- plementarity determining region 3 using a newly developed soft- ware algorithm, JOINSOLVER. *J Immunol* (2004) 172:6790–802.
75. Boyd SD, Marshall EL, Merker JD, Maniar JM, Zhang LN, Sahaf B, et al. Measurement and clini- cal monitoring of human lympho- cyte clonality by massively paral- lel VDJ pyrosequencing. *Sci Transl Med* (2009) 1:12ra23. doi:10.1126/ scitranslmed.3000540
76. De Preval C, Fougereau M. Spe- cific interaction between VH and VL regions of human mono- clonal immunoglobulins. *J Mol Biol* (1976) 102:657–78. doi:10. 1016/0022-2836(76)90340-5
77. Brezinschek HP, Foster SJ, Dorner T, Brezinschek RI, Lipsky PE. Pair- ing of variable heavy and variable kappa chains in individual naive and memory B cells. *J Immunol* (1998) 160:4762–7.
78. de Wildt RM, Hoet RM, Van Ven- rooij WJ, Tomlinson IM, Winter G. Analysis of heavy and light chain pairings indicates that recep- tor editing shapes the human antibody repertoire. *J Mol Biol* (1999) 285:895–901. doi:10.1006/ jmbi.1998.2396
79. DeKosky BJ, Ippolito GC, Deschner RP, Lavinder JJ, Wine Y, Rawlings BM, et al. High-throughput sequencing of the paired human immuno- glob- ulin heavy and light chain repertoire. *Nat Biotechnol* (2013) 31:166–9. doi:10.1038/nbt.2492
80. Arnaout R, Lee W, Cahill P, Honan T, Sparrow T, Weiand M, et al. High-resolution description of antibody heavy-chain repertoires in humans. *PLoS ONE* (2011) 6:e22365. doi:10.1371/journal. pone.0022365
81. Roth DB, Menetski JP, Naka- jima PB, Bosma MJ, Gellert M. V(D)J recombination: bro- ken DNA molecules with cova- lently sealed (hairpin) coding ends in scid mouse thymocytes. *Cell* (1992) 70:983–91. doi:10.1016/ 0092-8674(92)90248-B
82. Lafaille JJ, Decloux A, Bonneville M, Takagaki Y, Tonegawa S. Junc- tional sequences of T cell recep- tor gamma delta genes: impli- cations for gamma delta T cell lineages and for a novel inter- mediate of V-(D)-J joining. *Cell* (1989) 59:859–70. doi:10.1016/ 0092-8674(89)90609-0
83. Tian C, Luskin GK, Dischert KM, Higginbotham JN, Shepherd BE, Crowe JE Jr. Evidence for pref- erential Ig gene usage and dif- ferential TdT and exonuclease activities in human naive and memory B cells. *Mol Immunol* (2007) 44:2173–83. doi:10.1016/j. molimm.2006.11.020
84. Jackson KJ, Gaeta B, Sewell W, Collins AM. Exonuclease activ- ity and P nucleotide addition in the generation of the expressed immunoglobulin repertoire. *BMC Immunol* (2004) 5:19. doi:10.1186/ 1471-2172-5-19
85. Lu H, Schwarz K, Lieber MR. Extent to which hairpin opening by the Artemis:DNA- PKcs complex can contribute to junctional diversity in V(D) J recombination. *Nucleic Acids Res* (2007) 35:6917–23. doi:10.1093/nar/gkm823
86. Cabaniols JP, Fazilleau N, Cas- rouge A, Kourilsky P, Kanel- lopoulos JM. Most alpha/beta T cell receptor diversity is due to terminal deoxynucleotidyl trans- ferase. *J Exp Med* (2001) 194: 1385–90. doi:10.1084/jem.194.9. 1385
87. Murugan A, Mora T, Walczak AM, Callan CG. Statistical inference of the generation probability of T- cell receptors from sequence reper- toires. *Proc Natl Acad Sci USA* (2012) 109:16161–6. doi:10.1073/ pnas.1212755109
88. Hofle M, Linthicum DS, Ioerger T. Analysis of diversity of nucleotide and amino acid distributions in the VD and DJ joining regions in Ig heavy chains. *Mol Immunol* (2000) 37:827–35. doi:10.1016/ S0161-5890(00)00110-3
89. Boubnov NV, Wills ZP, Weaver DT. V(D)J recombination coding junction formation without DNA homology: processing of coding termini. *Mol Cell Biol* (1993) 13:6957–68.
90. Nadel B, Feeney AJ. Influence of coding-end sequence on coding-end processing in V(D)J recombination. *J Immunol* (1995) 155:4322–9.
91. Saada R, Weinberger M, Shahaf G, Mehr R. Models for anti- gen receptor gene rearrangement: CDR3 length. *Immunol Cell Biol* (2007) 85:323–32. doi:10.1038/sj. icb.7100055
92. Agathangelidis A, Darzentas N, Hadzidimitriou A, Brochet X, Murray F, Yan XJ, et al. Stereo- typed B-cell receptors in one-third of chronic lymphocytic leukemia: a molecular classification with implications for targeted therapies. *Blood* (2012) 119:4467–75. doi:10. 1182/blood-2011-11-393694
93. Hoogeboom R, Van Kessel KP, Hochstenbach F, Wormhoudt TA, Reinten RJ, Wagner K, et al. A mutated B cell chronic lympho- cytic leukemia subset that recog- nizes and responds to fungi. *J Exp Med* (2013) 210:59–70. doi:10. 1084/jem.20121801
94. Smith K, Garman L, Wrammert J, Zheng NY, Capra JD, Ahmed R, et al. Rapid generation of fully human monoclonal antibod- ies specific to a vaccinating anti- gen. *Nat Protoc* (2009) 4:372–84. doi:10.1038/nprot.2009.3
95. Jiang N, He J, Weinstein JA, Pen- land L, Sasaki S, He XS, et al. Lineage structure of the human antibody repertoire in response to influenza vaccination. *Sci Transl Med* (2013) 5:171ra119. doi:10. 1126/scitranslmed.3004794
96. Wu YC, Kipling D, Dunn-Walters DK. Age-related changes in human peripheral blood IGH reper- toire following vaccination. *Front Immunol* (2012) 3:193. doi:10. 3389/fimmu.2012.00193
97. Wu X, Zhou T, Zhu J, Zhang B, Georgiev I, Wang C, et al. Focused evolution of HIV-1 neu- tralizing antibodies revealed by structures and deep sequencing. *Science* (2011) 333:1593–602. doi: 10.1126/science.1207532
98. Parameswaran P, Yi Liu Q, Roskin KM, Jackson KK, Dixit VP, Lee J- Y, et al. Coherent immune reper- toire signatures in human dengue. *Cell Host Microbe* (Forthcoming 2013).
99. Moss PA, Moots RJ, Rosenberg WM, Rowland-Jones SJ, Bodmer HC, Mcmichael AJ, et al. Exten- sive conservation of alpha and beta chains of the human T-cell anti- gen receptor recognizing HLA-A2 and influenza A matrix peptide. *Proc Natl Acad Sci U S A* (1991) 88:8987–90. doi:10.1073/ pnas.88. 20.8987
100. Argaet VP, Schmidt CW, Burrows SR, Silins SL, Kurilla MG, Doolan DL, et al. Dominant selection of an invariant T cell antigen receptor in response to persistent infection by Epstein-Barr virus. *J Exp Med* (1994) 180:2335–40. doi:10.1084/ jem.180.6.2335
101. Pannetier C, Even J, Kourilsky P. T-cell repertoire diversity and clonal expansions in normal and clinical samples. *Immunol Today* (1995) 16:176–81. doi:10.1016/ 0167-5699(95)80117-0
102. Altman JD, Moss PA, Goulder PJ, Barouch DH, Mcheyzer-Williams MG, Bell JI, et al. Phenotypic analysis of antigen-specific T lymphocytes. *Science* (1996) 274: 94–6. doi:10.1126/science.274. 5284.94
103. Garrido P, Ruiz-Cabello F, Barcena P, Sandberg Y, Canton J, Lima M, et al. Monoclonal TCR- Vbeta13.1+/CD4+/NKa+/CD8- /+dim T-LGL lymphocytosis: evidence for an antigen-driven chronic T-cell stimulation origin. *Blood* (2007) 109:4890–8. doi:10. 1182/blood-2006-05-022277
104. Crompton L, Khan N, Khanna R, Nayak L, Moss PA. CD4+ T cells specific for glycoprotein B from cytomegalovirus exhibit extreme conservation of T-cell receptor usage between different individ- uals. *Blood* (2008) 111:2053–61. doi:10.1182/blood-2007-04- 079863
105. Moon JJ, Chu HH, Pepper M, Mcsorley SJ, Jameson SC, Kedl RM, et al. Naive CD4(+) T cell fre- quency varies for different epitopes and predicts repertoire diversity and response magnitude. *Immu- nity* (2007) 27:203–13. doi:10. 1016/j.immuni.2007.07.007
106. Alanio C, Lemaitre F, Law HK, Hasan M, Albert ML. Enumera- tion of human antigen-specific naive CD8+ T cells reveals con- served precursor frequencies. *Blood* (2010) 115:3718–25. doi:10. 1182/ blood-2009-10-251124
107. Kwok WW, Tan V, Gillette L, Littell CT, Soltis MA, Lafond RB, et al. Frequency of epitope- specific naive CD4(+) T cells cor- relates with immunodominance in the human memory reper- toire. *J Immunol* (2012) 188: 2537–44. doi:10.4049/jimmunol. 1102190
108. Venturi V, Kedzierska K, Price DA, Doherty PC, Douek DC, Turner SJ, et al. Sharing of T cell recep- tors in antigen-specific responses is driven by convergent recombi- nation. *Proc Natl Acad Sci USA* (2006) 103:18691–6. doi:10.1073/ pnas.0608907103
109. Quigley MF, Greenaway HY, Ven- turi V, Lindsay R, Quinn KM, Seder RA, et al. Convergent recombina- tion shapes the clonotypic land- scape of the naive T-cell reper- toire. *Proc Natl Acad Sci USA* (2010) 107:19414–9. doi:10.1073/ pnas.1010586107
110. Miles JJ, Douek DC, Price DA. Bias in the alphabeta T-cell repertoire: implications for disease patho- genesis and vaccination. *Immunol Cell Biol* (2011) 89:375–87. doi:10. 1038/icb.2010.139

16

History of innate immunity in neurodegenerative disorders

Patrick L. McGeer* and Edith G. McGeer

Kinsmen Laboratory of Neurological Research, University of British Columbia, Vancouver, BC, Canada

Edited by:
Roger A. Barker, University of Cambridge and Addenbrooke' Hospital, UK

Reviewed by:
Jason B. Wu, Cedars-Sinai Medical Center, USA
Muzamil Ahmad, Indian Institute of Integrative Medicine, India

***Correspondence:**
Patrick L. McGeer, Kinsmen Laboratory of Neurological Research, University of British Columbia, 2255 Wesbrook Mall, Vancouver, BC, Canada V6T1Z3.
e-mail: mcgeerpl@interchange.ubc.ca

The foundations of innate immunity in neurodegenerative disorders were first laid by Del Rio Hortega (1919). He identified and named microglia, recognizing them as cells of mesodermal origin. Van Furth in 1969 elaborated the monocyte phagocytic system with microglia as the brain representatives. Validation of these concepts did not occur until 1987 when HLA-DR was identified on activated microglia in a spectrum of neurological disorders. HLA-DR had already been established as a definitive marker of immunocompetent cells of mesodermal origin. It was soon determined that the observed inflammatory reaction was an innate immune response. A rapid expansion of the field took place as other markers of an innate immune response were found that were made by neurons, astrocytes, oligodendroglia, and endothelial cells. The molecules included complement proteins and their regulators, inflammatory cytokines, chemokines, acute phase reactants, prostaglandins, proteases, protease inhibitors, coagulation factors, fibrinolytic factors, anaphylatoxins, integrins, free radical generators, and other unidentified neurotoxins. The Nimmerjahn movies demonstrated that resting microglia were constantly active, sampling the surround, and responding rapidly to brain damage. Ways of reducing the neurotoxic innate immune response and stimulating a healing response continue to be sought as a means for ameliorating the pathology in a spectrum of chronic degenerative disorders.

Keywords: HLA-DR, Alzheimer disease, Parkinson disease, complement, neuroinflammation

BACKGROUND

Pio Del Rio Hortega, one of the greatest of all neuroscientists, established the basic foundation of neuroinflammation with his classic 1919 paper "El tercer elemento de los centros nerviosis" (Del Rio Hortega, 1919). He had developed an ammoniacal silver carbonate modification of the Golgi technique. With this new method he was able to identify small spidery cells which he named microglia. He recognized that they were of mesodermal origin, and that they migrated to the brain in late embryonic life. He also recognized their phagocytic capacity by examining their reaction to stab wounds. He categorized their morphology as resting, ameboid, and reactive. By further modifying his technique, he later recognized another type of glial cell which was of epithelial origin and had a sparse cytoplasm. He named these cells oligodendroglia, perhaps because of the difficulty he encountered in staining them.

These two glial cell types made up "the third element" which had baffled Ramon y Cajal. Cajal, Hortega's mentor and employer, had clearly identified astrocytes with his methodology, and knew there were still unclassified glial cells. He thought the cells identified by Hortega might be another astrocytic type that was resistant to staining. He objected to Hortega's desire to publish his results on oligodendroglia, and when Hortega went ahead, believing others would make the same discovery, Cajal dismissed him. Hortega's own account of these travails, which he never published, were obtained after his death, later appearing in part in Haymaker and Adams treatise on the histopathology of the nervous system (Haymaker and Adams, 1980a, pp. 484–485).

Hortega's travails were not limited to his falling out with Cajal. The Madrid laboratory he had set up after his departure from Cajal was bombed out in the Spanish civil war. He moved for a time to Paris, and then to Oxford, but was uncomfortable in these locations. As a Spaniard opposed to Franco, he emigrated to Buenos Aires in 1938 where, in 1945, he died of cancer.

His findings and their interpretation were still being actively challenged long after his death. Some scientists supported his conclusions, others did not. Wilder Penfield was the first prominent investigator to uphold Hortega. He described, in the first issue of the American Journal of Pathology, the various stages of microglia, going from resting to reactive (Penfield, 1925). Numerous others did differing experiments, interpreting microglia cells as being of epithelial origin with unknown function. A detailed account of the continuing controversy, which extended for over six decades, appears in Haymaker and Adams (1980b, Chapter VI). This unjustified controversy may help to explain why Hortega never received a Nobel prize for his epic work.

The next giant step was taken by Ralph van Furth. He elaborated the concept of a monocyte phagocytic system to explain the origin and function of resident phagocytes throughout the body. The Memoranda endorsing the concept, which was introduced at the Conference on Mononuclear Phagocytes held in Lieden in 1969, is available on the web Chttp://www.ncbi.nlm.nih.gov/pmc/articles/PMC2480884/pdf/bullwho00193-0157.pdf. He and his colleagues had studied labeled monocytes and their marrow precursors and followed their appearance as typical macrophages in various organs, including brain (Van Furth and Cohn, 1968). This concept replaced the vague theory of a reticulo-endothelial system introduced by Aschoff (1924) which, despite its shortcomings, had become entrenched in medical teaching.

While van Furth's concept of a monocyte phagocytic system was widely accepted, its relationship to brain microglia was not.

Fujita in particular opposed the idea that microglia were the brain representatives of this system. He injected tritiated thymidine into chick embryos and identified labeled brain cells which he interpreted as glioblasts of subependymal origin (Fujita, 1965). He did later studies of human embryonic brain tissue and reached a similar conclusion, that brain microglia were of epithelial and not mesenchymal origin (Fujita, 1973; Fujita and Kitamura, 1973).

Oemichan et al. (1979) and Wood et al. (1979) also concluded that brain microglia could not be phagocytes of monocytic origin. The reason was that they could not detect the same surface antigens on microglial cells that they were able to detect on peripheral monocytes. The idea became established that inflammation of the brain did not involve microglia, and did not occur unless there was invasion of the brain by peripheral monocytes, which then became transformed into macrophages.

IDENTIFICATION OF HLA-DR POSITIVE MICROGLIA IN HUMAN BRAIN

The entry of our laboratory into the neuroinflammatory field was entirely serendipitous. Several researchers had suggested that AD might result from a herpes infection entering through the nasal passages because of involvement of the rhinencephalon (Ball, 1982). Our effort over some years to detect herpes virus in the CNS had failed, although we were able to detect it in some cases in the trigeminal nucleus, the source of herpes labialis (Walker et al., 1989). We sought the advice of local immunologists regarding what might be a broader indicator of a viral infection, and were counseled to look for HLA-DR since this class II glycoprotein would be responsible for presenting viral epitopes to T-cells. We were even presented with a gift of the HB-104 cell line, known to produce high levels of antibodies against HLA-DR.

The results astonished us. A plethora of cells was visible in AD tissue with a morphology that was completely unfamiliar to us. However we were able to confirm that they were microglia by showing them to the founder of our laboratory, Dr. William Gibson, who had been a student and biographer of Hortega (Prados and Gibson, 1946). The morphology was identical to that published by Del Rio Hortega (1919), permitting us to sense in a very small way the excitement he must have experienced.

As many frustrated investigators well know, peer reviewers, whether evaluating applications for research grants, or papers submitted to journals, are typically well versed in the dogmas of the day. Findings that radically conflict with established views are too often dismissed. Our data conflicted with two dogmas. The first was that microglia were of epithelial origin and were not immunocompetent cells. The second was that brain inflammation was not a characteristic of AD. A pathological journal rejected our initial manuscript, reasoning that the absence of a neuropathologist as an author explained the faulty conclusions. A peer reviewer for a renewal of our grant dismissed it with the comment "the hypothesis is ridiculous." Nevertheless, our first paper appeared as a brief report in Neuroscience Letters (McGeer et al., 1987).

This final validation of Hortega depended on the availability of HB-104, a powerful and highly specific monoclonal antibody. The field of immunohistochemistry had been opened by Cesar Milstein's work on the technique for producing monoclonal antibodies. He was a co-winner of the Nobel prize in 1984 for this accomplishment. Then, as now, the ability to visualize brain biochemistry through the eyes of immunohistochemistry depends on the strength and specificity of the antibodies employed. HB-104 was a particularly good antibody, permitting us to make a clear distinction, which had eluded other investigators, between HLA-DR positive microglia and GFAP positive astrocytes.

We were not the first to report class II staining of brain cells. Lampson and Hickey (1986) had reported class II activity in occasional cell bodies of human brain with the "morphologic appearance of microglia or astrocytes." Similarly deTribolet et al. (1984) reported HLA-DR positive cells in the white matter of normal brain which they interpreted as being astrocytes (deTribolet et al., 1984). Rogers et al. reported HLA-DR positive microglia and astrocytes in AD in an abstract at the Society of Neuroscience meeting in 1986 but, as in our case, formal publication was held up by disbelief in the findings. Their work finally appeared in 1988 (Luber-Narod and Rogers, 1988; Rogers et al., 1988).

These data led to a number of unanswered questions. What was the source of the inflammation in AD? Was it a special phenomenon or a general one that applied to many chronic neurological disorders? If it was a general phenomenon, was it localized to the brain or did it involve the peripheral immune system? Was it helpful or harmful to ongoing degenerative processes? What were the implications for treatment? Exploration of these questions led to the opening up of an important new field of neuroscience, namely neuroinflammation.

ESTABLISHMENT OF NEUROINFLAMMATION AS A DISTINCT FIELD OF NEUROSCIENCE RESEARCH

The question as to whether or not the presence of activated microglia in brain was a special one applying to AD, or a general phenomenon was quickly answered. HLA-DR activated microglia were observed in a variety of degenerative neurological conditions, including Parkinson disease (PD), Pick disease, ALS, Huntington disease, multiple sclerosis, AIDS encephalopathy, parkinsonism dementia of Guam, and the Shy–Drager syndrome (McGeer et al., 1988a). Their phagocytic function was easily demonstrated by melanin being observed within the HLA-DR positive microglia of the SN (McGeer et al., 1988b). Each of these diseases has a differing etiology, so the activated microglial response had to be the consequence of initiating factors in each condition and not the fundamental cause.

At this same time, the laboratory of Kreutzberg in Germany was carrying out work of a more fundamental nature. His team was utilizing the facial nerve axotomy model to examine the CNS reaction to a sterile lesion outside of the CNS. They found activated microglia enveloping damaged neurons of facial nerve cell bodies, with phagocytosis of dead cells taking place. They concluded that microglia might function as antigen presenting cells and thus be the effector cells responsible for recruitment of lymphocytes to the brain resulting in an inflammatory reaction. A review of their results appeared in the first volume of Glia (Streit et al., 1988) and a later review (Kreutzberg, 1996).

Further groundwork was laid by four key papers which appeared in a special issue of Glia in 1993 devoted to microglia. They were by Ling and Wong (1993) describing the origin and nature of microglia; Dickson et al. (1993) detailing cytokines and microglia in Alzheimer disease and AIDS; Banati et al. (1993)

on the cytotoxicity of microglia; and McGeer et al. (1993) on microglia in neurodegenerative diseases generally.

Since our laboratory and that of Joe Rogers, who had founded the Sun Health Research Institute, had identified HLA-DR activated microglia in AD, we joined forces for further investigation of the phenomenon, particularly the role of complement. The name complement was introduced by Paul Ehrlich in the 1890's to explain the heat labile factor in serum which helped antibodies to kill microorganisms. As a result, complement was considered to be a peripherally generated system for assisting the activity of antibodies. It was therefore believed that complement factors would only be found as an accompaniment to immunoglobulin antibodies.

Eikelenboom and Stam (1982) were the first to report the presence of complement factors in AD senile plaques. Previously it had been reported that immunoglobulins were associated with amyloid deposits, which was consistent with prevailing theory (Ishii and Haga, 1975). Our laboratory was able to detect the opsonizing components of the classical complement pathway in association with plaques, and the membrane attack complex in association with dystrophic neurites, consistent with bystander lysis occurring in AD (McGeer et al., 1989).

Working with Joseph Rogers, we were unable to detect immunoglobulins in AD tissue using a host of antibodies. Then Rogers explored the idea that beta amyloid protein itself might be an activator of complement. In a classic paper he and his colleagues demonstrated that immunoglobulin immunostaining did not colocalize with complement, and that beta amyloid protein and its N-terminal fragments bound to C1q directly, thus initiating the complement cascade independently of antibodies (Rogers et al., 1992). But what was the source of the complement proteins? It was soon determined from RNA studies that brain itself was the source (Johnson et al., 1992; Walker and McGeer, 1992). Meanwhile evolutionary studies were underway, establishing that the complement system could be traced back at least as far as horseshoe crabs and that it was the mainstay of innate immunity in most primitive organisms (Zhu et al., 2005). It far predated the antibody producing adaptive immune system which is an invention of higher vertebrates.

Two principles which had broad implications for the developing field of neuroinflammation emerged from this joint endeavor. The first was establishing that complement was part of the innate immune system and further that it had the potential of exacerbating the pathology through formation of the membrane attack complex. The second was showing that the inflammatory reaction in AD did exacerbate the pathology. We decided to explore whether patients on long term anti-inflammatory therapy were relatively spared from AD. We selected rheumatoid arthritic patients because onset of the disease typically appears at an earlier age than AD and involves aggressive anti-inflammatory therapy. The results showed an estimated sixfold sparing of AD in rheumatoid arthritic patients compared with age matched general populations (McGeer et al., 1990). Many subsequent epidemiological studies, in which consumption of NSAIDs in particular were targeted, confirmed these general findings (McGeer and McGeer, 1995).

Rogers was then motivated to establish a Neuroinflammation Working Group of 37 investigators to assemble the rapidly accumulating data on inflammation in AD. The conclusion of the group was that the data represented "a virtual textbook of inflammatory mediators." Included were complement proteins and their regulators, inflammatory cytokines, chemokines, acute phase reactants, prostaglandins, proteases, protease inhibitors, coagulation factors, fibrinolytic factors, integrins, anaphylatoxins, free radical generators, and other unidentified neurotoxins (Akiyama et al., 2000). All are products of the innate immune system of brain, with major contributions coming from neurons, astrocytes, microglia, and endothelial cells.

Parkinson disease was another chronic degenerative disorder where activated microglia were detected in association with the SN lesions (McGeer et al., 1988b). An accidental model of PD provided new insights into the consequences of chronic neuroinflammation. Langston et al. (1984) had identified a group of young drug users who suddenly developed a parkinsonian syndrome. The causative agent (MPP+) was a metabolite of 1-methyl-4-phenyl-1,2,3,6-tetrahydropyridine (MPTP), a contaminant in the street drug they were using. The condition was progressive, and autopsy studies on those who had died from this exposure years previously showed neuroinflammation of the SN similar to that observed in PD (Langston et al., 1999). We found a parallel situation in monkeys. They showed nigral degeneration and activated microglia in the SN 5.5–15 years after systemic exposure to MPTP (McGeer et al., 2003). These findings represent the clearest example of how neuroinflammation, once initiated, can persist, and cause continuing neurodegeneration.

Activated microglia are the pivotal cells. Their functioning *in vivo* has been remarkably demonstrated by the movies of Nimmerjahn et al. (2005). They developed mice transgenic for a green fluorescent protein in microglial cells and used two-photon microscopy through a window in the skull to observe their behavior. Microglial cells in the normal state were found not to be dormant, as implied by their traditional designation as resting, but were extremely active, continuously extending, and retracting their processes to sense their environment. When activated by a laser lesion of a capillary, they surrounded the lesion and phagocytosed the leaking blood.

The innate immune system is the body's first line of defense. As the Nimmerjahn movies demonstrate, it can act immediately. As shown in chronic degenerative diseases, as well as the MPTP model, it can maintain its activity indefinitely without significant engagement of the adaptive immune system. The adaptive immune system is slower to react but more powerful and specific in attacking targets. It depends upon appropriate presentation of epitopes to lymphatic organs so that lymphocytes can be cloned to attack targets where that epitope is exposed. There is a long list of diseases where the adaptive immune system directs self attack on healthy tissues. These conditions are known as autoimmune disorders. They differ from AD and other chronic neurodegenerative disorders where the adaptive immune system does not become significantly engaged. To distinguish between the two, we have suggested that such diseases be described as autotoxic disorders (McGeer and McGeer, 2000).

In theory, the self destruction in autotoxic disorders should be milder and more amenable to therapeutic intervention than the self destruction in autoimmune disorders. The question is how to ameliorate the autotoxic response? Anti-inflammatory and antioxidant approaches have been the most widely utilized to date. But another, and potentially more effective method may be possible. That is to transform microglia from the attack mode, which has been so well characterized, to a healing mode. Such a transformation might result in enhanced phagocytotic activity, coupled with a switch from expressing inflammatory cytokines such as IL-1 and TNF to expressing anti-inflammatory cytokines such as IL-4 and IL-10. In the process the beneficial effects of phagocytosis might be enhanced. For example, suppressing the CD-40/CD 40L interaction in transgenic mice enhances the phagocytic activity of microglia and increase Aβ clearance (Tan et al., 2002). Clearly there is much still to be learned. It can be said that, despite the huge expansion of activity that has taken place in recent years, it is still a field in its infancy.

SUMMARY

Our understanding of the innate immune system in brain commenced with recognition of a single marker, HLA-DR, on a single cell type, microglia, in a single disorder, Alzheimer disease. Twenty five years later, more than a thousand innate immune system markers have been identified which are associated with neurons, astrocytes, oligodendrocytes, and endothelial cells, as well as microglia.

They include, but are not limited to, complement proteins and their regulators, cytokines, chemokines, acute phase reactants, prostaglandins, proteases, protease inhibitors, coagulation factors, fibrinolytic factors, anaphylatoxins, integrins, and free radical generators. They are found in a spectrum of neurological diseases. Some stimulate inflammation, others inhibit it. Shifting the balance from a mode of attack to one of healing holds promise of having significant therapeutic benefit in a spectrum of degenerative diseases. Clearly there is much still to be learned. It can be said that, despite the huge expansion of activity that has taken place in the last 25 years, it is still a field in its infancy.

ACKNOWLEDGMENTS

This work was supported by the Pacific Alzheimer Research Foundation.

REFERENCES

1. Akiyama, H. Barger, S., Barnum, S., Bradt, B., Bauer, J., Cole, G. M., Cooper, N. R., Eikelenboom, P., Emmerling, M., Fiebich, B. L., Finch, C. E., Frautschy, S., Griffin, W. S., Hampel, H., Hull, M., Landreth, G., Lue, L., Mrak, R., Mackenzie, I. R., McGeer, P. L., O'Banion, M. K., Pachter, J., Pasinetti, G., Plata-Salaman, C., Rogers, J., Rydel, R., Shen, Y., Streit, W., Strohmeyer, R., Tooyoma, I., Van Muiswinkel, F. L., Veerhuis, R., Walker, D., Web- ster, S., Wegrzyniak, B., Wenk, G., Wyss-Coray, T, and Neuroinflammation Working Group. (2000). Inflammation and Alzheimer's disease. *Neurobiol. Aging* 21, 383–421.
2. Aschoff, L. (1924). Das reticulo- endotheliale system. *Ergeb. Inn. Med. Kinderheilkd.* 26, 1.
3. Ball, M. J. (1982). Limbic predilection in Alzheimer dementia: is reactivated herpes virus involved. *Can. J. Neurol. Sci.* 9, 303–306.
4. Banati, R. B., Gehrmann, J., Schubert, P., and Kreutzberg, G. W. (1993). Cytotoxicity of microglia. *Glia* 7, 111–118.
5. Del Rio Hortega, P. (1919). El tercer ele- mento de los centros nerviosis. *Bol. Soc. Esp. Biol.* 9, 69–129.
6. deTribolet, N., Hamou, M. F., Mach, J.-P., Carrel, S., and Schreyer, M. (1984). Demonstration of HLA-DR antigens in normal human brain. *J. Neurol. Neurosurg. Psychiatr.* 47, 417–418.
7. Dickson, D. W., Lee, S. C., Mattiace, L. A.,Yen, S. H. C., and Brosnan, C. (1993). Microglia and cytokines in neurological disease, with special reference to AIDS and Alzheimer's disease. *Glia* 7, 75–83.
8. Eikelenboom, P., and Stam, F. C. (1982). Immunoglobulins and complement factors in senile plaques. *Acta Neu- ropathol.* 57, 239–242.
9. Fujita, S. (1965). An autoradiographic study on the origin and fate of the sub-pial glioblast in the embryonic chick spinal cord. *J. Comp. Neurol.* 124, 51–59.
10. Fujita, S. (1973). Genesis of glioblasts in the human spinal cord as revealed by Feulgen cytophotometry. *J. Comp. Neurol.* 151, 25
11. Fujita, S., and Kitamura, T. (1973). Ori- gin of brain macrophages and the nature of so-called microglia. *Acta Neuropathol. Suppl.* 6, 291–296.
12. Haymaker, W., and Adams, R. D. (1980a). *Histology and Histopathol- ogy of the Nervous System.* Spring- field, IL: C. C. Thomas, 484–485.
13. Haymaker, W., and Adams, R. D. (1980b). *Histology and Histopathol- ogy of the Nervous System,* Chapter VI. Springfield, IL: C. C. Thomas, 481–559.
14. Ishii, T., and Haga, S. (1975). Iden- tificantion of components of immunoglobulins in senile plaques by means of fluorescent antibody technique. *Acta Neuropathol.* 32, 157–162.
15. Johnson, S. A., Lampert-Etchells, M., Pasinetti, G. M., Rozovsky, I., and Finch, C. E. (1992). Complement mRNA in the mammalian brain: responses to Alzheimer's disease and experimental brain lesioning. *Neu- robiol. Aging* 13, 641–648.
16. Kreutzberg, G. W. (1996). Microglia: a sensor for pathological events in the CNS. *Trends Neurosci.* 19, 312–318.
17. Lampson, L. A., and Hickey, W. (1986). Monoclonal antibody analysis of MHC expression in human brain biopsies: tissue rang- ing from "histologically normal" to that showing different levels of glial tumor involvement. *J. Immunol.* 136, 4054–4062.
18. Langston, J. W., Forno, L. S., and Tetrud, J., Reeves, A. G., Kaplan, J. A., and Karluk, D. (1999). Evidence of active nerve cell degeneration in the substantia nigra of humans years after 1-methyl-4-phenyl-1,2,3,6- tetrahydropyridine exposure. *Ann. Neurol.* 46, 598–605.
19. Langston, J. W., Irwin, I., Langston, E. B., and Forno, L. S. (1984). 1-Metyl-4-phenylpyridium ion (MPP+): iden- tification of a metabolite of MPTP, a toxin selective to the sub- stantia nigra. *Neurosci. Lett.* 48, 87–92.
20. Ling, E. A., and Wong, W. C. (1993). The origin and nature of ramified and ameboid microglia – a historical review and current concepts. *Glia* 7, 9–18.
21. Luber-Narod, J., and Rogers, J. (1988). Immune system associated antigens expressed by cells of the human cen- tral nervous system. *Neurosci. Lett.* 94, 17–22.
22. McGeer, P. L., Akiyama, H., Itagaki, S., and McGeer, E. (1989). Activation of the classical complement path- way in brain tissue of Alzheimer patients. *Neurosci. Lett.* 107, 341–346.
23. McGeer, P. L., Itagaki, S., and McGeer, E. (1988a). Expression of the histo- compatibility glycoprotein HLA-DR in neurological disease. *Acta Neuropathol.* 76, 550–557.
24. McGeer, P. L., Itagaki, S., Akiyama, H., and McGeer, E. G. (1988b). Rate of cell death in parkinsonism indicates active neuropathological process. *Ann. Neurol.* 24, 574–576.
25. McGeer, P. L., Itagaki, S., Tago, H., and McGeer, E. G. (1987). Reac- tive microglia in patients with senile dementia of the Alzheimer types are positive for the histocompatibil- ity glycoprotein HLA-DR. *Neurosci. Lett.* 79, 195–200.
26. McGeer, P. L., Kawamata, T, Walker, G., Akiyama, H, Tooyama, I., and McGeer, E. G. (1993). Microglia in degenerative neurological disease. *Glia* 7, 84–92.
27. McGeer, P. L., and McGeer, E. G. (1995). The inflammatory response system of brain: implications for therapy of Alzheimer and other neurodegenerative disorders. *Brain Res. Rev.* 21, 195–218.
28. McGeer, P. L., and McGeer, E. G. (2000). Autotoxicity and Alzheimer disease. *Arch. Neurol.* 57, 789–790.
29. McGeer, P. L., Rogers, J., McGeer, G., and Sibley, J. (1990). Does anti-inflammatory treatment pro- tect against Alzheimer disease? *Lancet* 335, 1037.
30. McGeer, P. L., Schwab, C., Parent, A., and Doudet, D. (2003). Presence of reac- tive microglia in monkey substantia nigra years after 1-methyl-4- phenyl-1,2,3,6-tetrahydropyridine administration. *Ann. Neurol.* 54, 599–604.
31. Nimmerjahn, A., Kirchhoff, F., and Helmchen, F. (2005). Rest- ing microglial cells are highly dynamic surveillants of brain parenchyma in vivo. *Science* 308, 1314–1318.

32. Oemichan, M., Wietholter, H., and Greaves, M. F. (1979). Immunoloical analysis of human microglia: lack of monocytic and lymphoid mem- brane differentiation antigens. *J. Neuropath. Exp. Neurol.* 38, 99–103.
33. Penfield, W. (1925). Microglia and the process of phagocytosis in gliomas. *Am. J. Pathol.* 1, 77–89.
34. Prados, M., and Gibson, W. C. (1946). *Pio del Rio Hortega*, 1882–1945. *J. Neurosurg.* 3, 275–284.
35. Rogers, J., Cooper, N. R., Webster, S., Schultz, J., McGeer, P. L., Styren, S. D., Civin, W. H., Brachova, L., Bradt, B., Ward, P., and Lieberburg, I. (1992). Complement activation by β-amyloid in Alzheimer disease. *Proc. Natl. Acad. Sci. U.S.A.* 89, 10016–10020.
36. Rogers, J., Luber-Narod, J., Sturen, C. D., and Civin, W. H. (1988). Expression of immune system-associated antigens by cells of the human cen- tral nervous system: relationship to the pathology of Alzheimer's disease. *Neurobiol. Aging* 9, 339–349.
37. Streit, W. J., Graeber, M. B., and Kreutzberg, G. W. (1988). Func- tional plasticity of microglia: a review. *Glia* 1, 301–307.
38. Tan, J., Town, T., Crawford, F., Mori, T., DelleDonne, A., Crescentini, R., Obregan, D., Flavelli, R. A., and Mul- lan, M. J. (2002). Role of CD40 ligand in amyloidosis in transgenic Alzeheimer's mice. *Nat. Neurosci.* 5, 1288–1293.
39. Van Furth, R., and Cohn, Z. A. (1968). The origin and kinetics of mononuclear phagocytes. *J. Exp. Med.* 128, 415–435.
40. Walker, D. G., and McGeer, P. L. (1992). Complement gene expres- sion in human brains: compari- son between normal and Alzheimer disease cases. *Brain Res. Mol. Brain Res.* 14, 109–116.
41. Walker, D. G., O'Kusky, J. R., and McGeer, P. L. (1989). In situ hybridization analysis for herpes simplex virus nucleic acids in Alzheimer disease. *Alzheimer Dis. Assoc. Disord.* 3, 123–131.
42. Wood, G. W., Gollahon, K. A., Tilzer, S. A., Vats, T., and Morantz, R. A. (1979). The failure of microglia in normal brain to exhibit mononu- clear phagocyte markers. *J. Neu- ropathol. Exp. Neurol.* 38, 369–376.
43. Zhu, Y., Thangamani, S., and Ho, B. And Ding, J. L. (2005). The ancient origin of the complement system. *EMBO J.* 24, 382–394.

17

Complementarity of binding motifs is a general property of HLA-A and HLA-B molecules and does not seem to effect HLA haplotype composition

Xiangyu Rao[1], Rob J. De Boer[1], Debbie van Baarle[2], Martin Maiers[3] and Can Kesmir[1]*

[1] Theoretical Biology and Bioinformatics, Utrecht University, Utrecht, Netherlands
[2] Immunology Department, Wilhelmina Children's Hospital, University Medical Center Utrecht, Utrecht, Netherlands
[3] National Marrow Donor Program, Minneapolis, MN, USA

Edited by:
Michal Or-Guil, Humboldt University Berlin, Germany

Reviewed by:
Edward John Collins, The University of North Carolina at Chapel Hill, USA
Fernando A. Arosa, University of Beira Interior, Portugal
Dmitriy M. Chudakov, M.M. Shemyakin and Yu.A. Ovchinnikov Institute of Bioorganic Chemistry of the Russian Academy of Sciences, Russia

***Correspondence:**
Can Kesmir, Theoretical Biology and Bioinformatics, Utrecht University, Padualaan 8, 3584 CH Utrecht, Netherlands
e-mail: c.kesmir@uu.nl

Different human leukocyte antigen (HLA) haplotypes (i.e., the specific combinations of HLA-A, -B, -DR alleles inherited together from one parent) are observed in different frequencies in human populations. Some haplotypes, like HLA-A1-B8, are very frequent, reaching up to 10% in the Caucasian population, while others are very rare. Numerous studies have identified associations between HLA haplotypes and diseases, and differences in haplotype frequencies can in part be explained by these associations: the stronger the association with a severe (autoimmune) disease, the lower the expected HLA haplotype frequency. The peptide repertoires of the HLA molecules composing a haplotype can also influence the frequency of a haplotype. For example, it would seem advantageous to have HLA molecules with non-overlapping binding specificities within a haplotype, as individuals expressing such an haplotype would present a diverse set of peptides from viruses and pathogenic bacteria on the cell surface. To test this hypothesis, we collect the proteome data from a set of common viruses, and estimate the total ligand repertoire of HLA class I haplotypes (HLA-A-B) using *in silico* predictions. We compare the size of these repertoires to the HLA haplotype frequencies reported in the National Marrow Donor Program (NMDP). We find that in most HLA-A and HLA-B pairs have fairly distinct binding motifs, and that the observed haplotypes do not contain HLA-A and -B molecules with more distinct binding motifs than random HLA-A and HLA-B pairs. In addition, the population frequency of a haplotype is not correlated to the distinctness of its HLA-A and HLA-B peptide binding motifs. These results suggest that there is a not a strong selection pressure on the haplotype level favoring haplotypes having HLA molecules with distinct binding motifs, which would result the largest possible presented peptide repertoires in the context of infectious diseases.

Keywords: haplotypes, HLA antigens, selection, genetic, peptide binding, bioinformatics, computational biology

INTRODUCTION

The human leukocyte antigen (HLA) genes are the most polymorphic coding loci known in humans. The HLA gene cluster is located on the major histocompatibility complex (MHC) on chromosome 6, and contains over 200 genes. The two groups of loci that contain the MHC class I and II genes dictating T cell responses are the most polymorphic. It is widely accepted that this variability is maintained by balancing selection, as individuals that are heterozygous in their HLA class I and II loci seem to have a better outcome in infections diseases [see e.g., for HIV-1 (1)]. In line with this, it has been demonstrated that in several species, and up to a certain extent in humans, females prefer to mate with males having a dissimilar HLA to increase the chance of their offspring to survive infectious diseases (2, 3). We have argued that the heterozygous advantage is on its own not enough to maintain such a large degree of polymorphism, and that the frequency dependent co-evolution with pathogens should also play a major role (4).

On the functional level the HLA polymorphism seems to be much smaller. It is well established that MHC class II molecules have largely overlapping peptide repertoires [see e.g., (5)]. In the last few years we and others showed this to be also true for class I alleles (6–9). This promiscuous peptide binding is not limited to the alleles within each locus, and extends to alleles from different MHC class I loci (7, 9). This property has important evolutionary consequences as heterozygous individuals carrying genetically different HLA molecules that nevertheless have overlapping peptide repertoires should have a diminished heterozygous advantage.

Recombinations occur frequently in the HLA region and they generate novel HLA haplotypes (10). However, the number of haplotypes found in human populations is far lower than the number of alleles observed (11), suggesting that not all the HLA haplotypes have the same chance of becoming established in human populations. Indeed, different haplotypes occur with very different frequencies in different ethnic groups/subpopulations[1,2].

[1]www.allelefrequencies.net
[2]www.nmdp.org

The "usefulness" of HLA molecules is expected to play a role in determining the haplotype frequencies: haplotypes carrying HLA molecules that are protective for certain diseases are expected to be present in relatively high frequencies in endemic areas. Indeed, several HLA haplotype disease associations have been established, e.g., in autoimmune diseases (12), squamous cell cervical cancer (13) and recurrent aphthous stomatitis (14). Along these lines, one can speculate that it should be advantageous to have MHC molecules with distinct binding specificities in a haplotype, because such haplotypes would provide an individual with more epitopes eliciting T cell responses during an infectious disease than haplotypes containing HLA molecules with similar binding motifs. This hypothesis is rather impossible to test experimentally, because one needs to determine the total set of peptides presented by a very large set of HLA molecules in cells infected by different viruses. Such experiments (e.g., eluting peptides from HLA molecules expressed by a cell) are typically done at small scales because they are time consuming. Therefore, we here study the peptide repertoires of HLA molecules that are estimated to be combined in a haplotype (i.e., the ones with a strong linkage disequilibrium) using an *in silico* approach. This approach unfortunately suffers of two main limitations. First, the quality of the peptide-HLA predictions differs between the loci. The quality of HLA-A and HLA-B peptide binding predictions is very reliable. For the other loci (HLA-C, HLA-DR, etc.) the predictions are of low quality (15), and are therefore left out of this analysis. Second, having distinct HLA binding motifs might also be important in the context of cancer or autoimmunity, however, it is very complicated to determine the role of HLA haplotypes in these diseases. Therefore, we perform our analysis explicitly for infectious diseases, and focus on the peptides that can be presented from common viruses only. Still, we think that our study is a first step to investigate the role of HLA binding motifs in the evolution of HLA haplotype frequencies.

MATERIALS AND METHODS

NMDP DATA

All estimated HLA-A-B haplotype frequencies were downloaded from the National Marrow Donor Program (NMDP) database, which was established to develop and maintain a registry of HLA-typed volunteer unrelated donors for patients requiring a hematopoietic stem cell transplant (16)[3]. Four predominant US ethnic and racial groups were included in this data set: European Americans, African Americans, Asians, and Hispanic (17). Haplotype frequencies were estimated separately for each ethnic group using an implementation of the expectation maximization (EM) algorithm (18, 19).

The linkage disequilibrium, D, between two alleles in each haplotype was expressed as the difference between the observed and expected haplotype frequency: $D = f_{AB} - f_A f_B$, where f_{AB} is the observed (estimated) haplotype frequency, f_A is the allele frequency of the HLA-A molecule in the haplotype and f_B is the allele frequency of the HLA-B molecule in this haplotype. D is easy to calculate, but has the disadvantage of depending on the frequency of the alleles. In order to overcome this drawback, the normalized measure, D′, was calculated a $D' = \frac{D}{D_{\max}}$, where $D_{\max}$ is the lesser of f_{AB} or $(1 - f_A)(1 - f_B)$ when $D < 0$ and is the lesser of $f_A(1 - f_B)$ or $f_B(1 - f_A)$ when $D > 0$. The advantage of this measure of disequilibrium is that it ranges between -1 and 1, regardless of the allelic frequencies in the sample. $|D'| = 1$ indicates complete LD and $D' = 0$ corresponds to total absence of LD.

Linkage disequilibrium statistics were calculated for each haplotype to identify the haplotypes that have a significantly positive D'.

HLA LIGAND PREDICTION

To be able to perform our analysis for as many as possible HLA molecules, we used NetMHCpan (15) to predict peptide-HLA binding affinity. NetMHCpan assigns to each peptide-HLA pair a predicted IC50 value, indicative of the predicted binding affinity. To assess whether a peptide binds to an HLA molecule depends on the choice of binding threshold, and the optimal threshold has been discussed (20). If one assumes that all HLA molecules use a fixed threshold, one can use the default threshold of 500 nM (21, 22), otherwise a 5000 nM threshold can be used to allow for the comparison of more weakly binding peptides. However, using a fixed threshold to define predicted binders result in large differences in the predicted repertoire sizes between HLA molecules. For instance using a fixed threshold of 500 nM, the HLA repertoire sizes range between 20 and 6574 peptides for the viral set listed in Table S2 in Supplementary Material. As such a variance could introduce large biases in our analysis, we defined the 1% top-ranking peptides as candidate binders for each HLA molecule. This gives each HLA molecule the same ligand repertoire size (i.e., 570 binders per HLA molecule for the viral set listed in Table S2 in Supplementary Material). To check the consistency of our results with respect to these parameters, we repeated every analysis with the fixed threshold of 500 nM. All results presented below were derived using the threshold of 1% to define candidate binders, and remain similar for a fixed threshold, unless mentioned otherwise. To test whether our results change if one were to use a much larger data set, we also generated predicted binders using a much larger set of viruses (see below), in which case each HLA molecule had 60-fold more binders.

VIRAL DATA

The proteomes of 17 common human viruses were downloaded from the European Bioinformatics Institute website[4] (downloads were made in October 2006, listed in Table S2 in Supplementary Material) as the source of potential HLA ligands. To extend this data set, we downloaded another set of proteomes (downloads were made in October 2008)[4] from viruses that are known to infect mammalians ($n = 904$). We used the HLA-peptide binding predictors (see above) to screen all possible unique virus-derived 9-mer peptides.

PEPTIDE REPERTOIRE OVERLAP

We define the peptide repertoire overlap between two HLA alleles in the same HLA-A-B haplotype, F_p, as the fraction of overlapping ligands between these two HLA class I molecules among

[3]http://bioinformatics.nmdp.org

[4]www.ebi.ac.uk

all of their ligands: $F_p = \frac{A \cap B}{A \cup B}$, where A and B are the ligand sets for HLA-A and -B molecule, respectively. $F_p = 1$ implies that the HLA-A and HLA-B molecules belonging to the same haplotype have the same epitope repertories while $F_p = 0$ indicates completely different peptide repertoires for two HLA molecules.

RESULTS AND DISCUSSION

DETERMINING HLA-A-B HAPLOTYPES

The "true" HLA haplotypes can be determined either by molecular haplotyping or family-based segregation studies (23–25). However, both approaches are expensive and laborious, and therefore, statistical methods are typically used to infer haplotypes from datasets covering large population of individuals with known HLA genotypes (26). Several methods have been proposed to infer HLA haplotypes from genotype data, and in recent studies the performance of two most commonly used approaches, EM algorithm based (implemented in Arlequin V3.0), and the Bayesian algorithm based (implemented in PHASE V2.1.1), have been compared (27, 28). Unfortunately, neither of the methods could infer all of the known haplotypes: incorrect haplotypes were estimated in more than 30% of the cases. However, once the sample size increases, the power of these statistical methods is expected to increase tremendously.

National marrow donor program[2] provides, to our knowledge, the largest repository of HLA-typed donors. Here use of statistical methods should become more reliable (16): for the HLA-A-B haplotype, the total chromosome counts (2N) for the four major ethnic groups exceeds 2000. On the NMDP webpage[3], the high-resolution allele and haplotype frequencies [estimated by EM method, (18, 19)] are available (17). Focusing on HLA-A-B haplotypes, the most common haplotypes found in US population (separated into four main ethnic groups) are summarized in **Table 1** (adopted from bioinformatics.nmdp.org, December 2007 version). Alternatively Allele frequencies web server[1], provides allele frequencies established in smaller, but probably better defined studies (29).

In the NMDP database 660 possible haplotypes are reported for European Americans. However, many of these haplotypes are bound to be falsely predicted, e.g., due to the limited number of individuals carrying particular combinations of specific HLA molecules. To decrease the amount of wrongly identified haplotypes in our analysis, we apply a rather strict criterion for considering a predicted haplotype as a "true" haplotype: we demand a positive LD value that is significantly different than zero ($p < 0.01$, see Materials and Methods). This criterion decreases the number of haplotypes to 60 for European Americans. These 60 haplotypes are estimated to cover 58% of the population (see **Table 2**), i.e., current statistical methods and data sets (even the large repositories like NMDP) remain rather limited in providing the HLA haplotype diversity of a population. For other ethnical groups, the number of reliable haplotypes drops to 30–40 per ethnic group, even though the number of possible haplotypes was the same or higher (see **Table 2** and footnote text 3). The population coverage in non-European groups was lower, 30–40% of their respective populations, possibly due to the lower number of individuals with known HLA-typing. All together we detected 120 reliable unique haplotypes by summing over these ethnical groups (the full list of haplotypes can be found in Table S1 in Supplementary Material).

Table 1 | Occurrences of the three most common HLA-A-B frequency ranked haplotypes in four major ethnic groups in US (adopted from bioinformatics.nmdp.org).

		EUR		AFA		API		HIS	
HLA-A	**HLA-B**	***F* (%)**	**Rank**	***F* (%)**	**Rank**	***F* (%)**	**Rank**	***F* (%)**	**Rank**
0101	0801	9.55	1	1.50	6	0.41	46	2.21	2
0201	4402	5.70	3	1.33	9	0.17	130	1.94	4
0201	4501	0.05	200	1.66	3	–	–	0.23	105
0201	5101	2.00	9	0.61	26	0.91	25	2.20	3
0207	4601	–	–	–	–	3.34	2	–	–
0301	0702	6.01	2	1.73	2	0.26	82	1.92	5
2902	4403	2.38	7	1.08	15	0.03	433	2.54	1
3001	4201	–	–	2.96	1	–	–	0.40	50
3303	4403	–	–	0.09	261	2.94	3	0.16	156
3303	5801	0.08	162	0.28	88	4.53	1	0.10	230

EUR, Caucasian; AFA, African; API, Asian; HIS, Hispanic. F stands for population frequency in percentages.

Table 2 | Numbers of different haplotypes with a significantly positive LD in four major US ethnic groups.

Ethnicity	Haplotype # (%)
EUR	60 (57.7)
API	34 (35.4)
HIS	43 (33.5)
AFA	43 (33.7)

Population coverage in percentages is given within parenthesis.

PEPTIDE REPERTOIRE OF AN HAPLOTYPE

Having identified the HLA-A-B haplotypes for the US population, we next estimated the overlaps between peptide repertoires of HLA-A and -B molecules that belong to the same haplotype.

We used an *in silico* approach and predicted the peptide repertoire of all HLA-A and HLA-B alleles that are part of the 120 predicted haplotypes, using the proteomes of common viruses (see Table S2 in Supplementary Material) and HLA-peptide binding predictor NetMHCpan (15, 30) (see Materials and Methods). NetMHCpan is the only prediction system available right now that can reliably predict the peptide binding affinities for the large set of HLA-A and HLA-B molecules we are taking into account in this study. The analysis of the 120 significant haplotypes demands predictions for 39 HLA-A and 63 HLA-B molecules. This predictor assigns an IC50 value to each peptide-HLA pair, which can be used as a predicted binding affinity. Using the widely accepted IC50 value of 500 nM as a threshold to distinguish binders from non-binders, generated a large variation in the predicted repertoire sizes of different HLA molecules (20–6574 peptides for the viral set listed in Table S2 in Supplementary Material), which could strongly bias our results. As the physiologically relevant IC50 values are difficult to estimate for each HLA molecule, we have chosen a simplified approach and define the peptide repertoire as the top 1% peptides with the highest HLA binding affinities for each HLA molecule. This approach removes the potential bias introduced by different repertoire sizes, but ignores the fact that some HLA molecules can be more specific than others, and therefore present much fewer peptides.

The unique haplotypes listed in Table S1 in Supplementary Material have an average peptide overlap of 1.1% (with a standard deviation of 1.8%, and a median of 0.44%) using top 1% threshold. The distribution of the overlaps is given in **Figure 1A**, and varies somewhat among the haplotypes. Out of 120 haplotypes, 36 (30%) have non-overlapping peptide repertoires, at least for the common viruses that we tested (see Table S1 in Supplementary Material). Only for five haplotypes is the repertoire overlap higher than 5%, and HLA-A0101-B1517 with an overlap of 11.8% is the highest. HLA-A0101-B1517 is a rare haplotype and occurs only in Asian Americans with a population frequency of 0.4%. To test whether or not rare haplotypes tend to have larger overlaps than common haplotypes, we weighted the overlaps found in **Figure 1A** with the population frequency of the HLA-A-B haplotypes (**Figure 1B**). Since the weighted overlaps remain very similar to the unweighted overlaps (**Figures 1A,B**), there is no evidence for a trend of rare haplotypes having the largest overlaps. In line with this, the frequency of a haplotype is only weakly correlated with the degree of peptide overlap between the haplotype's HLA-A and HLA-B molecules ($r = -0.08$, $p = 0.4$, Spearman rank correlation). Apparently, there is no selection pressure increasing the frequency of the haplotypes with a small peptide repertoire overlap.

These results were obtained using the top 1% peptides with the highest HLA binding affinities as the set of presented peptides per molecule. Using the set of common viruses listed in Table S2 in Supplementary Material, this threshold results in approximately 570 predicted binders per HLA molecule. To test whether the results presented in **Figure 1A** would be sensitive to the number of peptides, we collected proteomes for a much larger set of mammalian viruses ($n = 904$), which contains approximately three million unique peptides of nine amino acids. Using the same 1% threshold for this larger set, we predict for each HLA molecule the extended peptide repertoire and calculate the overlaps as explained before. The distribution of the overlaps hardly changes despite the fact that we enlarged the presented peptide repertoire 60-fold per molecule (see Figure S1 in Supplementary Material). As the results presented in **Figure 1A** seem fairly insensitive to the number of peptides used, we perform the rest of the analysis on the small data set of common viruses.

To test whether or not HLA binding motifs affect haplotype compositions requires comparison of the peptide overlaps of "true" haplotypes with those of "random" haplotypes. To do this, we reshuffled HLA-A and HLA-B molecules in the 120 "true" haplotypes to calculate an expected peptide repertoire overlap for randomly made haplotypes. Although the HLA molecules in random haplotypes can have overlaps up to 28% in their peptide repertoires (see **Figure 1C** and results not shown), the distribution of the overlaps is not significantly different from the distribution given in **Figure 1A**. The set of random haplotypes was generated 100 times, and in none of these cases was the distribution significantly different from the one given in **Figure 1A** (using a Kolmogorov–Smirnov test). Finally, we calculated a weighted peptide repertoire overlap for the random haplotypes by assuming that the frequency of a random haplotype is simply the multiplication of the frequency of their HLA-A and HLA-B alleles (i.e., assuming a complete lack of linkage disequilibrium). Again, the distribution of weighted overlap of random haplotypes (**Figure 1D**) is not different from that of the real haplotypes (**Figure 1B**). Taken together, these results suggest that HLA-A and -B in pairs in general have distinct peptide binding preferences, and that a small overlap is not a unique property of the HLA molecules having a strong linkage disequilibrium.

The overlap distribution presented in **Figure 1** seems to be in contradiction with earlier results, which estimated cross loci peptide overlaps of 23–44% (7, 9). However, this overlap was estimated at the population level, i.e., these percentages reflect the fraction of the peptide repertoire of an HLA-A molecule which is also expected to be presented by at least one HLA-B molecule in the population (and vice versa). Within an individual having maximally two different HLA-A and HLA-B molecules, the overlaps should remain much lower than the population based overlaps. In addition, one needs to realize that the low overlaps presented in **Figure 1** depend on the threshold used to define the peptide repertoire of an HLA molecule. When we use a higher threshold of 2 or 5% the average overlap increases to 2.3 and 5.9%, respectively (with the standard threshold of 1%, the average overlap was 1.1%, see above). However, the choice of the threshold hardly affects our main result, namely that the HLA-A and -B pairs that are in a linkage disequilibrium do not have more distinct binding motifs than random HLA-A/B pairs (**Figure 1**).

CONCLUSION

We hypothesized that it should be advantageous to have HLA molecules with distinct binding specificities combined in a haplotype, because during a viral infection such haplotypes would give an individual a larger epitope repertoire than haplotypes containing HLA molecules with similar binding motifs during a viral infection. To test this hypothesis, we used the high-resolution data available in the NMDP database on haplotype frequencies, and employed state of the art peptide-HLA binding prediction tools. We find that for all the haplotypes we could reliably identify in the US population, their HLA-A and HLA-B molecules present largely distinct set of peptides (**Figure 1A**). However, this turned out to be a generic property of HLA-A and HLA-B molecules: when we compared random HLA-A and -B pairs we find a very similar distribution of the presented peptide overlaps (**Figure 1C**). Moreover, there is no evidence for selection as there is no correlation between the population frequency of the HLA-A-B haplotypes and the overlap in the peptide repertoires of their HLA-A and HLA-B molecules. Taken together, these results suggest the complementarity of binding motifs is a general property of HLA-A and HLA-B molecules, and that complementarity does not affect the HLA haplotype composition. We were not able to specifically test the effect of complimentary binding motifs in the context of autoimmunity and cancer, as for both cases it remains unclear which set of human proteins should be taken as possible auto antigens. Complimentary binding motifs are expected to increase the

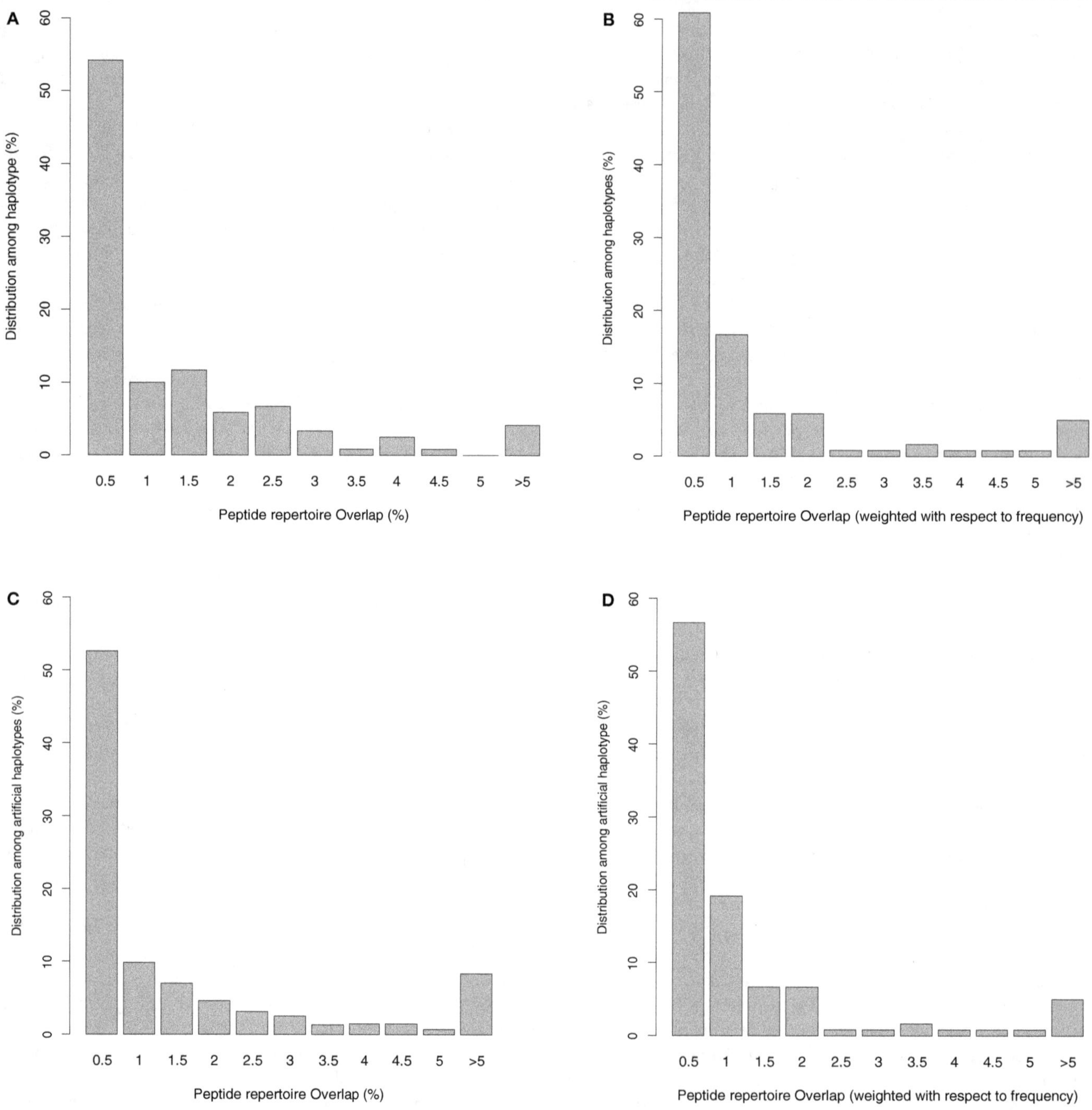

FIGURE 1 | Distribution of the presented peptide overlap (given in percentages, see Materials and Methods) between HLA-A and HLA-B molecules belonging to the same haplotype. (A) The distribution of the peptide overlaps for the 120 unique haplotypes we identified in the US population. **(B)** The distribution in A is weighted with the frequency of the haplotype in the population. If a haplotype was found in more than one ethnicity in US, we have taken the maximum frequency into account, normalizing the frequencies such that the sum remains one. In **(C)** we plot the overlaps found in artificially generated haplotypes (created by reshuffling the HLA-A and -B molecules from the 120 unique haplotypes). This plot is representative of 100 sets of artificially generated haplotypes. **(D)** The weighted peptide overlaps for the artificial haplotypes, where we estimate the frequency of the haplotype as the multiplication of the frequency of HLA-A and HLA-B molecule in the population (normalized to let the sum of the frequencies of the artificial haplotypes remain one).

number of potential self antigens, which could increase the risk of autoimmunity. Finally, the frequency of an HLA haplotype is determined by complex interactions with many different factors, one example is the correlation between birth weight and particular haplotypes (31). Our results suggest that complimentary binding motifs of HLA molecules during viral infections play a minor role, if any, compared to these other factors in the evolution of HLA haplotype frequencies.

ACKNOWLEDGMENTS

This study was financially supported by the University of Utrecht through a High Potential grant. The funders had no role in study design, data collection, and analysis, decision to publish or preparation of the manuscript.

REFERENCES

1. Carrington M, Nelson GW, Martin MP, Kissner T, Vlahov D, Goedert JJ, et al. HLA and HIV-1: heterozygote advantage and B*35-Cw*04 disadvantage. *Science* (1999) **283**:1748–52. doi:10.1126/science.283.5408.1748
2. Apanius V, Penn D, Slev PR, Ruff LR, Potts WK. The nature of selection on the major histocompatibility complex. *Crit Rev Immunol* (1997) **17**:179–224. doi:10.1615/CritRevImmunol.v17.i2.40
3. Boehm T, Zufall F. MHC peptides and the sensory evaluation of genotype. *Trends Neurosci* (2006) **29**:100–7. doi:10.1016/j.tins.2005.11.006
4. De Boer RJ, Borghans JAM, van Boven M, Kesmir C, Weissing FJ. Heterozygote advantage fails to explain the high degree of polymorphism of the MHC. *Immunogenetics* (2004) **55**:725–31. doi:10.1007/s00251-003-0629-y
5. O'Sullivan D, Arrhenius T, Sidney J, Del Guercio MF, Albertson M, Wall M, et al. On the interaction of promiscuous antigenic peptides with different DR alleles. Identification of common structural motifs. *J Immunol* (1991) **1950**(147):2663–9.
6. Axelsson-Robertson R, Weichold F, Sizemore D, Wulf M, Skeiky YA, Sadoff J, et al. Extensive major histocompatibility complex class I binding promiscuity for *Mycobacterium tuberculosis* TB10.4 peptides and immune dominance of human leucocyte antigen (HLA)-B*0702 and HLA-B*0801 alleles in TB10.4 CD8 T-cell responses. *Immunology* (2010) **129**:496–505. doi:10.1111/j.1365-2567.2009.03201.x
7. Frahm N, Yusim K, Suscovich TJ, Adams S, Sidney J, Hraber P, et al. Extensive HLA class I allele promiscuity among viral CTL epitopes. *Eur J Immunol* (2007) **37**:2419–33. doi:10.1002/eji.200737365
8. Nakagawa M, Kim KH, Gillam TM, Moscicki A-B. HLA class I binding promiscuity of the CD8 T-cell epitopes of human papillomavirus type 16 E6 protein. *J Virol* (2007) **81**:1412–23. doi:10.1128/JVI.01768-06
9. Rao X, Hoof I, Costa AI, van Baarle D, Kesmir C. HLA class I allele promiscuity revisited. *Immunogenetics* (2011) **63**:691–701. doi:10.1007/s00251-011-0552-6
10. Carrington M. Recombination within the human MHC. *Immunol Rev* (1999) **167**:245–56. doi:10.1111/j.1600-065X.1999.tb01397.x
11. Begovich AB, McClure GR, Suraj VC, Helmuth RC, Fildes N, Bugawan TL, et al. Polymorphism, recombination, and linkage disequilibrium within the HLA class II region. *J Immunol* (1992) **1950**(148):249–58.
12. Smith WP, Vu Q, Li SS, Hansen JA, Zhao LP, Geraghty DE. Toward understanding MHC disease associations: partial resequencing of 46 distinct HLA haplotypes. *Genomics* (2006) **87**:561–71. doi:10.1016/j.ygeno.2005.11.020
13. Madeleine MM, Johnson LG, Smith AG, Hansen JA, Nisperos BB, Li S, et al. Comprehensive analysis of HLA-A, HLA-B, HLA-C, HLA-DRB1, and HLA-DQB1 loci and squamous cell cervical cancer risk. *Cancer Res* (2008) **68**:3532–9. doi:10.1158/0008-5472.CAN-07-6471
14. Albanidou-Farmaki E, Deligiannidis A, Markopoulos AK, Katsares V, Farmakis K, Parapanissiou E. HLA haplotypes in recurrent aphthous stomatitis: a mode of inheritance? *Int J Immunogenet* (2008) **35**:427–32. doi:10.1111/j.1744-313X.2008.00801.x
15. Hoof I, Peters B, Sidney J, Pedersen LE, Sette A, Lund O, et al. NetMHCpan, a method for MHC class I binding prediction beyond humans. *Immunogenetics* (2009) **61**:1–13. doi:10.1007/s00251-008-0341-z
16. Maiers M, Gragert L, Klitz W. High-resolution HLA alleles and haplotypes in the United States population. *Hum Immunol* (2007) **68**:779–88. doi:10.1016/j.humimm.2007.04.005
17. Kollman C, Maiers M, Gragert L, Müller C, Setterholm M, Oudshoorn M, et al. Estimation of HLA-A, -B, -DRB1 haplotype frequencies using mixed resolution data from a National Registry with selective retyping of volunteers. *Hum Immunol* (2007) **68**:950–8. doi:10.1016/j.humimm.2007.10.009
18. Long JC, Williams RC, Urbanek M. An E-M algorithm and testing strategy for multiple-locus haplotypes. *Am J Hum Genet* (1995) **56**:799–810.
19. Excoffier L, Slatkin M. Maximum-likelihood estimation of molecular haplotype frequencies in a diploid population. *Mol Biol Evol* (1995) **12**:921–7.
20. MacNamara A, Kadolsky U, Bangham CR, Asquith B. T-cell epitope prediction: rescaling can mask biological variation between MHC molecules. *PLoS Comput Biol* (2009) **5**:e1000327. doi:10.1371/journal.pcbi.1000327
21. Buus S, Lauemoller SL, Worning P, Kesmir C, Frimurer T, Corbet S, et al. Sensitive quantitative predictions of peptide-MHC binding by a "Query by Committee" artificial neural network approach. *Tissue Antigens* (2003) **62**:378–84. doi:10.1034/j.1399-0039.2003.00112.x
22. Nielsen M, Lundegaard C, Worning P, Lauemoller SL, Lamberth K, Buus S, et al. Reliable prediction of T-cell epitopes using neural networks with novel sequence representations. *Protein Sci* (2003) **12**:1007–17. doi:10.1110/ps.0239403
23. Crawford DC, Nickerson DA. Definition and clinical importance of haplotypes. *Annu Rev Med* (2005) **56**:303–20. doi:10.1146/annurev.med.56.082103.104540
24. Yan H, Papadopoulos N, Marra G, Perrera C, Jiricny J, Boland CR, et al. Conversion of diploidy to haploidy. *Nature* (2000) **403**:723–4. doi:10.1038/35002251
25. Douglas JA, Boehnke M, Gillanders E, Trent JM, Gruber SB. Experimentally-derived haplotypes substantially increase the efficiency of linkage disequilibrium studies. *Nat Genet* (2001) **28**:361–4. doi:10.1038/ng582
26. Niu T. Algorithms for inferring haplotypes. *Genet Epidemiol* (2004) **27**:334–47. doi:10.1002/gepi.20024
27. Bettencourt BF, Santos MR, Fialho RN, Couto AR, Peixoto MJ, Pinheiro JP, et al. Evaluation of two methods for computational HLA haplotypes inference using a real dataset. *BMC Bioinformatics* (2008) **9**:68. doi:10.1186/1471-2105-9-68
28. Castelli EC, Mendes-Junior CT, Veiga-Castelli LC, Pereira NF, Petzl-Erler ML, Donadi EA. Evaluation of computational methods for the reconstruction of HLA haplotypes. *Tissue Antigens* (2010) **76**:459–66. doi:10.1111/j.1399-0039.2010.01539.x
29. Middleton D, Menchaca L, Rood H, Komerofsky R. New allele frequency database: http://www.allelefrequencies.net. *Tissue Antigens* (2003) **61**:403–7. doi:10.1034/j.1399-0039.2003.00062.x
30. Nielsen M, Lundegaard C, Blicher T, Lamberth K, Harndahl M, Justesen S, et al. NetMHCpan, a method for quantitative predictions of peptide binding to any HLA-A and -B locus protein of known sequence. *PLoS One* (2007) **2**:e796. doi:10.1371/journal.pone.0000796
31. Capittini C, Pasi A, Bergamaschi P, Tinelli C, De Silvestri A, Mercati MP, et al. HLA haplotypes and birth weight variation: is your future going to be light or heavy? *Tissue Antigens* (2009) **74**:156–63. doi:10.1111/j.1399-0039.2009.01282.x

18

Opposing roles for heat and heat shock proteins in macrophage functions during inflammation: a function of cell activation state?

Chen-Ting Lee[1] and Elizabeth A. Repasky[2]*

[1] Department of Radiation Oncology, Duke University Medical Center, Durham, NC, USA

[2] Department of Immunology, Roswell Park Cancer Institute, Buffalo, NY, USA

Edited by:
Willem van Eden, Utrecht University, Netherlands

Reviewed by:
Francesco Saverio Di Giovine, University of Sheffield, UK
Hiroki Yoshida, Saga University, Japan

***Correspondence:**
Elizabeth A. Repasky, Department of Immunology, Roswell Park Cancer Institute, Elm and Carlton Street, Buffalo, NY 14263, USA. e-mail: elizabeth.repasky@roswellpark.org

Macrophages function both under normothermia and during periods of body temperature elevation (fever). Whether macrophages sense and respond to thermal signals in a manner which regulates their function in a specific manner is still not clear. In this brief review, we highlight recent studies which have analyzed the effects of mild heating on macrophage cytokine production, and summarize thermally sensitive molecular mechanisms, such as heat shock protein (HSP) expression, which have been identified. Mild, physiologically achievable, hyperthermia has been shown to have *both pro- and anti-inflammatory effects on macrophage inflammatory cytokine production* and overall it is not clear how hyperthermia or HSPs can exert opposing roles on macrophage function. We propose here that the stage of activation of macrophages predicts how they respond to mild heating and the specific manner in which HSPs function. Continuing research in this area is needed which will help us to better understand the immunological role of body temperature shifts. Such studies could provide a scientific basis for the use of heat in treatment of inflammatory diseases.

Keywords: inflammation, hyperthermia, heat shock protein, fever, heat shock factor, cytokines, arthritis

INTRODUCTION

Inflammation is usually considered a beneficial event which helps to heighten the immune response initiated following tissue injury or infection. Molecular alarm signals generated from the damaged tissues or invading pathogens are recognized by antigen-presenting cells (APCs) such as macrophages. Macrophages are key players in innate immunity and respond rapidly to danger signals generated from inflamed sites. Recognition of these danger signals through specific cell surface pattern recognition receptors (PRRs) on macrophages results in the production of anti-microbial products as well as pro-inflammatory mediators (Depraetere, 2000; Fujiwara and Kobayashi, 2005).

Inflammation is a tightly regulated process with production of alarm signals sharply diminishing after the pathogens or cellular debris have been eliminated and tissue homeostasis restored. Many "stop signals" at appropriate checkpoints prevent further leukocyte infiltration into tissues if they are no longer needed (Serhan et al., 2007). If the balance between inflammation and resolution becomes dysregulated, excess macrophage responses will lead to chronic inflammation, and resultant disease states, which include atherosclerosis, rheumatoid arthritis (RA), asthma (Nathan, 2002), and cancer (Grivennikov et al., 2010). Therefore, understanding the regulation of inflammation and its resolution could help in the development of new therapeutic approaches for inflammatory disease management.

Macrophages are optimally activated by a combination of two macromolecular signals in their environment: antigen recognition by PRPs and IFN-γ (Mosser, 2003; O'Shea and Murray, 2008) and produce pro-inflammatory cytokines, TNF-α, IL-6, and IL-1β. These pro-inflammatory cytokines are important pyrogens capable of inducing the formation of the fever response and elevation of body temperature through complex neurological and behavioral changes (Kluger, 1991a,b; Cooper et al., 1994; Leon et al., 1997; Romanovsky et al., 1998, 2005). Fever is a highly conserved phenomenon in evolution (Kluger, 1979a, 1986; Mackowiak, 1981; Hasday et al., 2000). Although numerous human and animal studies reveal a positive correlation between the febrile response and a better survival rate, the mechanism by which increased core temperature improves host defense is still not clear. In addition, new studies suggest additional levels of complex interaction between macrophage function and body temperature. Nguyen et al. (2011) have shown that exposure to a cold environment induces alternative activation of adipose tissue macrophages. Thus, while it is likely that their function is responsive to thermal signals, the specific mechanisms by which macrophages sense and respond to temperature change in a way that specifically regulates their function has not been clarified.

To investigate the effect of febrile temperatures on macrophage activity, researchers often simply increase temperature in cell cultures, or elevate body temperature by external heat application in murine models. While these procedures do not reproduce critical features of actual fevers, several studies reveal both *positive* (Jiang et al., 2000b; Ostberg et al., 2000; Lee et al., 2012) and *negative* (Ensor et al., 1994; Fairchild et al., 2000; Hagiwara et al., 2007) effects on macrophage pro-inflammatory cytokine production. Both positive and negative effects of hyperthermia have been correlated with an induction of heat shock proteins (HSPs). The overall aim of this brief review is to present previous studies that have studied the impact of hyperthermia and HSPs on macrophage functions and to summarize available information regarding the underlying molecular mechanisms which may mediate this complex interaction of thermal signals.

FEVER-RANGE TEMPERATURES CAN ENHANCE MACROPHAGE PRO-INFLAMMATORY CYTOKINE PRODUCTION

Inducing hyperthermia has been used to study the role of febrile temperatures on the host defense system (Hasday et al., 2000; Jiang et al., 2000a). It was shown that increasing core body temperature has a protective role in the outcome of infection; the improved survival seen was determined not to be simply due to thermal suppression of bacterial growth. Data published by our laboratory (Ostberg et al., 2000) as well as by others (Jiang et al., 1999b) shows that mild, systemic heating at a target temperature of 39.5°C significantly enhances the concentration of TNF-α (3-fold increase in sera; 2.5-fold increase in liver) and IL-6 (4-fold increase in sera; 2.6-fold increase in spleen, 3.4-fold in lung, and 15-fold in liver) in the blood and tissues of BALB/c mice challenged with bacteria endotoxin (LPS). In addition, Jiang et al. (1999a) identified hepatic Kupffer cells as the predominant source of excess TNF-α secretion while multiple organs including lung, spleen, and liver could produce excess IL-6 in the warmer animals. These temperature-induced changes in cytokine expression are associated with an induction of HSP72 in the liver.

Our laboratory has recently observed that mild elevation of body temperature not only significantly enhances subsequent LPS-induced release of TNF-α (3-fold increase), but also reprograms macrophages, resulting in sustained subsequent responsiveness to LPS, i.e., this treatment reduces "endotoxin tolerance" *in vitro* and *in vivo* (Lee et al., 2012). Heat treatment results in an increase in LPS-induced downstream signaling including enhanced phosphorylation of IκB kinase (IKK) and IκB, NF-κB nuclear translocation and binding to the TNF-α promoter in macrophages upon secondary stimulation. The induction of HSP70 is important for mediation of thermal effects on macrophage function (Lee et al., 2012). Our *in vitro* experiments also show that the production of nitric oxide (NO) and inducible NO synthase (iNOS) by peritoneal macrophages is increased by exposure to febrile temperature together with LPS and IFN-γ stimulation. This result is correlated with the presence of HSP70 in the heat-treated macrophages (Pritchard et al., 2005). Collectively, these data suggest that fever-range hyperthermia can enhance macrophage cytokine expression and HSP70 expression, which in turn may help to improve host defense in response to infection.

FEVER-RANGE TEMPERATURES CAN ALSO SUPPRESS MACROPHAGE PRO-INFLAMMATORY CYTOKINE PRODUCTION

In contrast to the research summarized above, other studies using the macrophage cell lines RAW264.7 or human monocyte-derived macrophages have shown that hyperthermia has anti-inflammatory effects and suppresses activated macrophage pro-inflammatory cytokine expression (TNF-α, reduced by 50–98%; IL-6, reduced by 83–87%; and IL-1β, reduced by 50–94%; Ensor et al., 1994; Fairchild et al., 2000; Hagiwara et al., 2007). This inhibition is linked to a marked reduction in cytokine gene transcription and mRNA stability (Ensor et al., 1995). In addition, this thermally suppressed cytokine production is mediated by the binding of heat shock factor (HSF)-1, a transcriptional repressor, to the heat shock response element in the cytokine promoter region, including IL-1β and TNF-α (Cahill et al., 1996; Singh et al., 2002). Recently, Cooper et al. (2010a,b) have shown that fever-range temperatures selectively reduce LPS-induced recruitment of NF-κB and Sp-1 transcription factors to the TNF-α promoter regions.

Heat-induced suppression may involve high mobility group box 1 (HMGB1), an intra-nuclear protein that can be released by activated macrophages, necrotic or damaged cells during inflammation. HMGB1 helps immune cells to recognize damaged tissues and initiates intracellular signaling to activate NF-κB and pro-inflammatory cytokine production (Fiuza et al., 2003). Hyperthermia has been shown to inhibit macrophage HMGB1 secretion following LPS stimulation (Fairchild et al., 2000) and Hagiwara et al. (2007) found that high fever temperature (40°C) enhances HSF-1 and HSP70 expression. These increased levels of HSF-1 and HSP70 may reduce HMGB1 secretion and subsequent NF-κB activation and cytokine production. In general, these data support the concept that febrile temperatures can also have inhibitory effects on macrophage cytokine gene expression, an effect correlated with the activation of HSF-1 or induction of HSP70.

REGULATION OF HEAT SHOCK PROTEINS

Heat shock proteins are evolutionarily conserved proteins that can be induced by stress signals, including environmental stresses (e.g., heat shock), and pathophysiological states (e.g., fever, inflammation, and infection) as well as those induced by normal development stresses (Morimoto, 1993, 1998; Wu, 1995).

Heat shock proteins function as chaperones to assist with protein folding in order to protect cells from protein denaturation or cell death under stress conditions (Fink, 1999; Jaattela, 1999). Although HSPs are considered to be intracellular proteins, they can be mobilized to the plasma membrane or released into the extracellular environment and have immunomodulatory functions (Johnson and Fleshner, 2006). HSPs (e.g., HSP60, HSP70, HSP90, gp96, etc.) can be released from various cells through either a passive (during cell injury) or an active (translocation to the plasma membrane and then secretion) pathway. Previous studies have shown that HSP70 is released into the extracellular environment in a membrane-associated form after heat stress (Multhoff, 2007; Vega et al., 2008). HSPs are known to have both positive and negative effects in regulating macrophage function *and this may depend on the cellular location of these HSPs.* It is proposed that extracellular HSPs might serve as a danger signal to stimulate the immune response, whereas intracellular HSPs could serve as a negative regulator to control the inflammation (Schmitt et al., 2007).

PRO-INFLAMMATORY ROLE OF HEAT SHOCK PROTEINS ON MACROPHAGE FUNCTION

Previous studies have shown that extracellular HSPs exert immunostimulatory effects (Johnson and Fleshner, 2006). Wang et al. (2006) have shown that extracellular HSP70 binds to the lipid raft microdomain on the plasma membrane of macrophages and enhances their phagocytic ability. This HSP70-mediated phagocytosis enhances the processing and presentation of internalized antigens to CD4 T cells. Furthermore, extracellular HSPs can robustly stimulate the release of TNF-α, IL-6, IL-1β, IL-12, NO, as well as chemokines by monocytes/macrophages (Lehner et al., 2000; Asea et al., 2002; Panjwani et al., 2002; Vega et al., 2008). This effect is mediated through the CD14/TLR (both TLR2 and TLR4) complexes which lead to the activation of downstream NF-κB and MAPK pathway (Asea et al., 2000; Kol et al., 2000; Vabulas et al., 2002). In addition, HSPs are actively synthesized in peritoneal macrophages in mice which are administrated with LPS (Zhang et al., 1994). HSP70 and HSP90 have been shown to be involved in the innate recognition of bacterial products. These HSPs are able to bind LPS and form a cluster with TLR4–MD2 within lipid raft to deliver LPS to the complex. Following stimulation, these HSPs further assist the trafficking and targeting of this complex to the Golgi apparatus (Triantafilou et al., 2001; Triantafilou and Triantafilou, 2004). These results indicate that elevation of extracellular HSPs may serve as endogenous danger signals to alert the host defense system through their cytokine-like function.

ANTI-INFLAMMATORY ROLE OF HEAT SHOCK PROTEINS ON MACROPHAGE CYTOKINE EXPRESSION

On the other hand, intracellular HSPs have been shown to have anti-inflammatory roles in suppressing macrophage cytokine production. Intracellular HSPs are involved in protecting the organism from a variety of insults by directly interfering with cell death pathway and suppressing the expression of inflammatory genes (Yenari et al., 2005). The protect roles of stress-inducible intracellular HSPs (such as HSP72) in lethal sepsis and infection are well known. Induction of HSP70 *in vitro* by heat shock response or through overexpression can reduce mortality in experimental models of septic shock and endotoxemia as well as down-regulate inflammatory gene expression (Snyder et al., 1992; Hotchkiss et al., 1993; Villar et al., 1994; Van Molle et al., 2002; Shi et al., 2006). It has been shown that intracellular HSP70 can interact with IKK, prevent IκB phosphorylation, and NF-κB activation (Ran et al., 2004). In addition, HSP70 is actively synthesized in macrophages after exposure to endotoxin. Intracellular HSP70 inhibits LPS-induced NF-κB activation by binding with TRAF6, the important adaptor protein downstream of TLR4 and preventing its ubiquitination (Chen et al., 2006). These results suggest that intracellular HSP70 may act as a suppressor to interfere NF-κB signaling and downstream inflammatory cytokine production. Furthermore, HSP72 has been shown to inhibit LPS- and TNF-α-induced HMGB1 release and subsequent pro-inflammatory cytokine production in macrophages (Tang et al., 2007).

On the other hand, there is only one study by Bouchama et al. (2000) showing that hyperthermia (using target temperature 39, 41, and 43°C) inhibits LPS-stimulated IL-10 production by mononuclear cells isolated from healthy donor as compared to cells maintained at 43°C. In addition, by over-expressing HSP70 in human monocyte-derived macrophages, Ding et al. (2001) found that LPS-induced IL-10 production was significantly inhibited. In our unpublished data, we tried to address whether fever-range temperature affects macrophage IL-10 production at different activation stages. However, we found that temperature did not have any effect on IL-10 expression by either naïve macrophages or previously activated macrophages. Taken together, these studies suggest that intracellular HSPs may exert negative regulatory effects to dampen the inflammatory response in order to prevent tissue damage.

HEAT SHOCK PROTEINS AND INFLAMMATORY DISORDERS

There is some evidence that HSPs may play a role as immunological targets in chronic inflammatory diseases, such as RA (van Eden et al., 2005) and atherosclerosis (Xu, 2002). Increased HSP60 and HSP70 expression have been identified in the synovial tissues from animals with experimental induced arthritis and patients with RA (de Graeff-Meeder et al., 1990; Boog et al., 1992; Martin et al., 2003). Importantly, arthritis disease severity depends on the ability of human HSP60 and HSP70 to induce IL-10 production by monocytes/macrophages and fibroblast-like synoviocytes (MacHt et al., 2000; Luo et al., 2008). The production of IL-10 is negatively correlated with arthritis progression and joint destruction (Isomaki et al., 1996; Tanaka et al., 1996). Several clinical trials in RA patients using immunotherapies involving HSPs have shown to promote anti-inflammatory cytokine production and ameliorate disease severity, indicating that HSPs have immunoregulatory potential (Vischer, 1990; Rosenthal et al., 1991; Prakken et al., 2004).

On the other hand, HSP60 and HSP70 are also found in atherosclerotic lesions (Berberian et al., 1990; Kleindienst et al., 1993; Johnson et al., 1995). During the past decade, it has been noted that infections (e.g., chlamydiae infection) might contribute to the pathogenesis of atherosclerosis to directly stimulate cells of the arterial wall and/or other tissues to express high levels of HSPs (Kiechl et al., 2001). Chlamydial HSP60 (cHSP60) colocalizes with human HSP60 within macrophages in atherosclerotic lesions (Kol et al., 1998). Both chlamydial and human HSPs stimulate the expression of pro-inflammatory cytokines and adhesion molecules by macrophages through TLR4/MD2-dependent pathway (Bulut et al., 2002). Because of the high homology between chlamydial and human HSPs, it is possible that cross-reactions of antibodies and T cells against HSPs between microbes and humans contribute to the development of atherosclerosis (Xu, 2002). Taken together, a better understanding of the role of HSPs in the inflammatory process may lead to the development of new therapies to modify aberrant immune responses.

DOES THE MATURATION STATE OF MACROPHAGES INFLUENCE THE EFFECT OF HEAT AND HEAT SHOCK PROTEINS?

In this paper, we described previous studies revealing contrasting effects of febrile temperatures and HSPs on macrophage functions. Mild hyperthermia *enhances* macrophage TNF-α IL-6 as well as NO production in a HSP70/72-dependent mechanism.

On the other hand, mild hyperthermia *suppresses* macrophage pro-inflammatory cytokine production and this may involve an increase in HSF-1 and HSP70 expression. Thermally induced HSF-1 and HSP70 also play a role in blocking the transcription factors NF-κB and Sp-1 recruitment to the cytokine promoter and subsequent cytokine secretion (see **Figure 1**, for possible pathways by which thermal stress may result in both pro- and anti-inflammatory effects).

One possible explanation for these opposing results is that the resultant effect of heat is determined by the specific activation state of macrophages used for the analysis. For example, enhancing effects of heating were observed using cells freshly isolated from mice early after LPS injection (Jiang et al., 1999a,b; Lee et al., 2012). These cells express a naïve phenotype. On the other hand, the suppressing effects were obtained using RAW264.7 cells which express an activated phenotype (Ensor et al., 1994; Fairchild et al., 2000; Hagiwara et al., 2007). Therefore, we propose that in cells associated with the early activation stage of inflammation, febrile temperature may stimulate macrophage cytokine production, which helps to eliminate invading pathogens, whereas if heat is applied to cells associated with the resolution phase, a suppression of macrophage cytokine production occurs to prevent further tissue damage. This idea, if correct, would suggest that one of the functions of natural fever may be to help resolve inflammation. Furthermore, to our knowledge, there is no previous study addressing the role of heat/HSP on alternatively activated macrophage functions. This indicates that more research is needed to identify the mechanistic

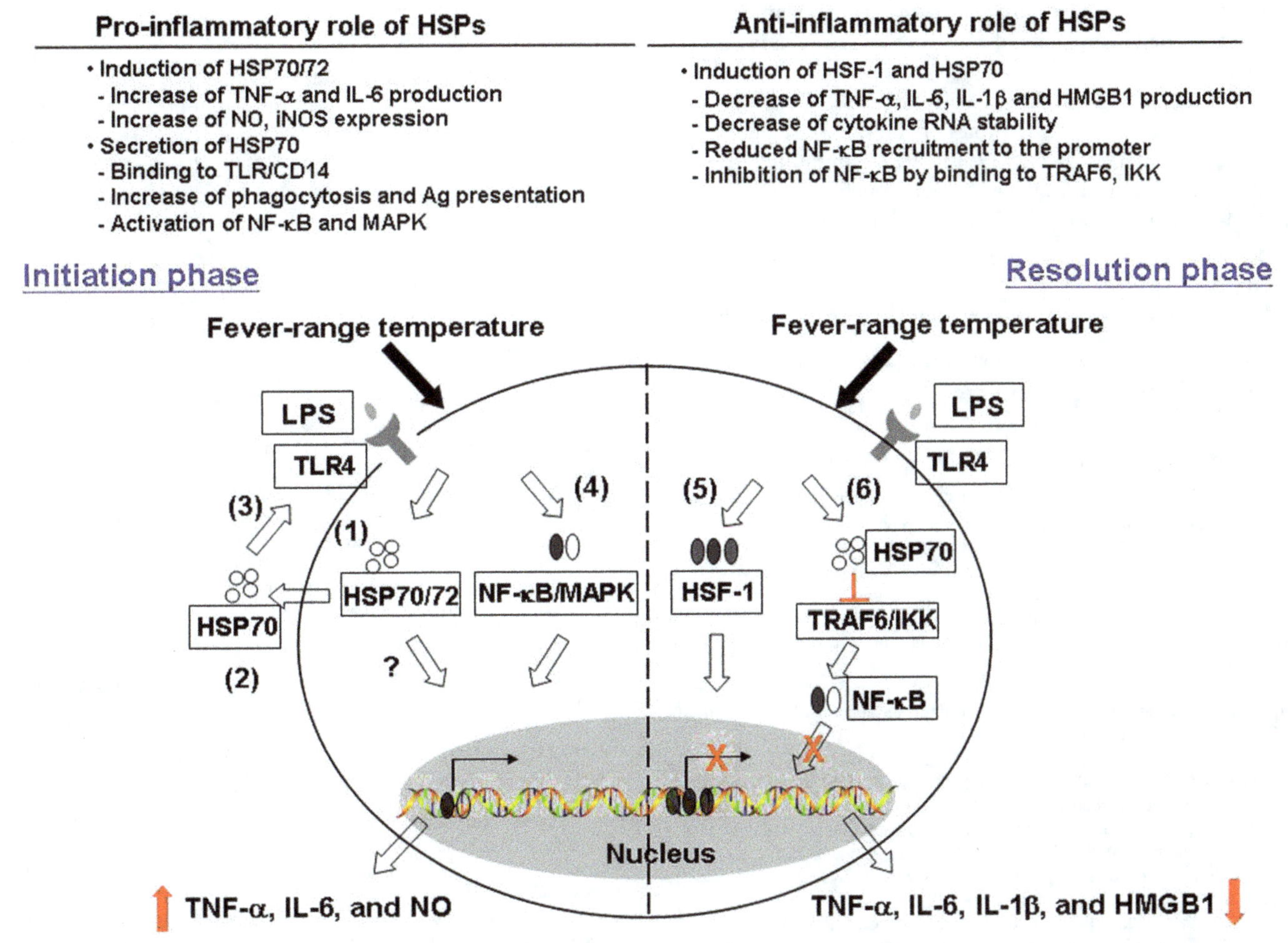

FIGURE 1 | Pro- and anti-inflammatory effects of heat and heat shock proteins. Fever range temperature exerts both positive and negative effects on macrophage pro-inflammatory cytokine production. We proposed that these opposing effects may depend on the activation stage of macrophages as well as the cellular location of heat shock proteins. First, in the initiation phase of macrophage activation, fever range temperature enhances the production of LPS-induced pro-inflammatory cytokines TNF-α, IL-6, and NO. (1) This thermally enhanced cytokine production is associated with an induction of HSP70/72 in these cells. (2) HSP70 can then be released into the extracellular environment, and (3) exerts its cytokine effect through the CD14/TLR pathway. (4) This leads to the activation of NF-κB and MAPK pathway and subsequent cytokine gene transcription. On the other hand, fever-range temperature can also suppress LPS-induced TNF-α, IL-6, and IL-1β production and HMGB-1 release. (5) This is due to thermally induced HSF-1 binding directly to the heat shock response element in the cytokine promoter region and functions as a transcriptional repressor. (6) In addition, LPS and heat treatment can also induce HSP70 expression. HSP70 then binds to TRAF6 or IKK and inhibits subsequent NF-κB activation and cytokine production.

basis of the contrasting effects of hyperthermia on macrophage function.

CONCLUSION

The host inflammatory response to injury or infection is clearly a complex process. Pro-inflammatory cytokines secreted by activated macrophages are essential for successful host defense. However, uncontrolled inflammatory cytokine production will also cause tissue damage. The febrile response is a well recognized component of inflammation and has been shown to provide a beneficial effect for the host but whether the thermal element of fever has a direct role in regulating macrophage function is still not clear. By using hyperthermia, many studies have reported that febrile temperatures can regulate macrophage pro-inflammatory cytokine production both *in vitro* and *in vivo*. These effects are associated with the induction of HSP. However, these effects can be either positive or negative and much more research is needed to understand how these two contrasting effects coincide.

In addition, we also summarized research which shows both the pro- and anti-inflammatory roles of HSPs. Extracellular HSPs might serve as a danger signal to stimulate the immune response, whereas intracellular HSPs could serve as a negative regulator to control the inflammation. Studies of the roles and mechanisms of heat as well as HSPs in inflammatory disorders could provide more information for therapeutic strategies targeting the molecular levels.

Finally, it is important to remember that most of the research on the role of elevated temperature on macrophage function does not actually use a physiological fever (i.e., induced by endoxin or other pyrogens), but instead, simply forces the elevation of body temperature using external heating. While some studies described above do include the addition of LPS, or use heat in the presence of infectious antigens, fever involves many biochemical, neurological, and vascular changes not seen in conditions of forced hyperthermia (Kluger, 1979b, 1991a; Gordon, 1993; Romanovsky et al., 1998, 2005). Therefore, it is possible that the elevated temperature associated with actual fever may have additional and more complex regulatory effects on macrophage function.

ACKNOWLEDGMENTS

The authors thank Lingwen Zhong, Thomas A. Mace, Nicholas Leigh, Bonnie Hylander and Maegan Capitano for their helpful discussions of the data summarized here. We also acknowledge grant support from NIH P01 CA094045, R01 CA135368-01A1, R01 CA071599-11, and the Roswell Park Cancer Institute Core Grant CA016056.

REFERENCES

Asea, A., Kraeft, S. K., Kurt-Jones, E. A., Stevenson, M. A., Chen, B., Finberg, R. W., Koo, G. C., and Calderwood, S. K. (2000). HSP70 stimulates cytokine produc- tion through a CD14-dependant pathway, demonstrating its dual role as a chaperone and cytokine. *Nat. Med.*6,435–442.

Asea, A., Rehli, M., Kabingu, E., Boch, J. A., Bare, O., Auron, P. E., Stevenson, A., and Calderwood, S. K. (2002). Novel signal transduction pathway utilized by extracellular HSP70: role of toll-like receptor (TLR) 2 and TLR4. *J. Biol. Chem.* 277, 15028– 15034.

Berberian, P. A., Myers, W., Tytell, M., Challa, V., and Bond, M. G. (1990). Immunohistochemical local- ization of heat shock protein-70 in normal-appearing and atheroscle- rotic specimens of human arteries. *Am. J. Pathol.* 136,71–80.

Boog, C. J., de Graeff-Meeder, E. R., Lucassen, M. A., Van Der Zee, R., Voorhorst-Ogink, M. M., Van Kooten, P. J., Geuze, H. J., and van Eden, W. (1992). Two monoclonal antibodies generated against human hsp60 show reactivity with synovial membranes of patients with juvenile chronic arthritis. *J. Exp. Med.* 175, 1805–1810.

Bouchama, A., Hammami, M. M., Al Shail, E., and De Vol, E. (2000). Dif- ferential effects of in vitro and in vivo hyperthermia on the production of interleukin-10. *Intensive Care Med.* 26, 1646–1651.

Bulut, Y., Faure, E., Thomas, L., Kara- hashi, H., Michelsen, K. S., Equils, O., Morrison, S. G., Morrison, R. P., and Arditi, M. (2002). Chlamy- dial heat shock protein 60 activates macrophages and endothelial cells through Toll-like receptor 4 and MD2 in a MyD88-dependent pathway. *J. Immunol.* 168, 1435–1440.

Cahill, C. M., Waterman, W. R., Xie, Y., Auron, P. E., and Calderwood, S. K. (1996). Transcriptional repression of the prointerleukin 1beta gene by heat shock factor 1. *J. Biol. Chem.* 271, 24874–24879.

Chen, H., Wu, Y., Zhang, Y., Jin, L., Luo, L., Xue, B., Lu, C., Zhang, X., and Yin, Z. (2006). Hsp70 inhibits lipopolysaccharide- induced NF-kappaB activation by interacting with TRAF6 and inhibit- ing its ubiquitination. *FEBS Lett.* 580, 3145–3152.

Cooper, A. L., Brouwer, S., Turnbull, A. V., Luheshi, G. N., Hopkins, S. J., Kunkel, S. L., and Rothwell, N. J. (1994). Tumor necrosis factor-alpha and fever after peripheral inflamma- tion in the rat. *Am. J. Physiol.* 267, R1431–R1436.

Cooper, Z. A., Ghosh, A., Gupta, A., Maity, T., Benjamin, I. J., Vogel, S. N., Hasday, J. D., and Singh, I. S. (2010a). Febrile- range temperature modifies cytokine gene expression in LPS-stimulated macrophages by differentially mod- ifying NF-{kappa}B recruitment to cytokine gene promoters. *Am. J. Physiol. Cell Physiol.* 298, C171–181.

Cooper, Z. A., Singh, I. S., and Hasday, J. D. (2010b). Febrile range temperature represses TNF-alpha gene expression in LPS-stimulated macrophages by selectively blocking recruitment of Sp1 to the TNF-alpha promoter. *Cell Stress Chaperones* 15, 665–673.

de Graeff-Meeder, E. R., Voorhorst, M., van Eden, W., Schuurman, H. J., Huber, J., Barkley, D., Maini, R. N., Kuis, W., Rijkers, G. T., and Zegers, B. J. (1990). Antibodies to the mycobacterial 65-kd heat-shock protein are reactive with synovial tis- sue of adjuvant arthritic rats and patients with rheumatoid arthritis and osteoarthritis. *Am. J. Pathol.* 137, 1013–1017.

Depraetere, V. (2000). "Eat me" signals of apoptotic bodies. *Nat. Cell Biol.* 2, E104.

Ding, X. Z., Fernandez-Prada, C. M., Bhattacharjee, A. K., and Hoover, D. L. (2001). Over-expression of hsp-70 inhibits bacterial lipopolysaccharide- induced production of cytokines in human monocyte-derived macro- phages. *Cytokine* 16,210–219.

Ensor, J. E., Crawford, E. K., and Hasday, D. (1995). Warming macrophages to febrile range destabilizes tumor necrosis factor-alpha mRNA without inducing heat shock. *Am. J. Physiol.* 269, C1140–C1146.

Ensor, J. E., Wiener, S. M., Mccrea, A., Viscardi, R. M., Crawford, E. K., and Hasday, J. D. (1994). Dif- ferential effects of hyperthermia on macrophage interleukin-6 and tumor necrosis factor-alpha expression. *Am. J. Physiol.* 266, C967–C974.

Fairchild, K. D., Viscardi, R. M., Hester, L., Singh, I. S., and Hasday, J. D. (2000). Effects of hypothermia and hyperthermia on cytokine pro- duction by cultured human mononu- clear phagocytes from adults and newborns. *J. Interferon Cytokine Res.* 20, 1049–1055.

Fink, A. L. (1999). Chaperone-mediated protein folding. *Physiol. Rev.* 79, 425–449.

Fiuza, C., Bustin, M., Talwar, S., Tropea, M., Gerstenberger, E., Shelhamer, J. H., and Suffredini, A. F. (2003). Inflammation-promoting activity of HMGB1 on human microvascular endothelial cells. *Blood* 101, 2652– 2660.

Fujiwara, N., and Kobayashi, K. (2005). Macrophages in inflammation. *Curr. Drug Targets Inflamm. Allergy* 4, 281–286.

Gordon, C. J. (ed.) (1993). "Fever," in *Temperature Regulation in Labora- tory Rodents* (Cambridge: Cambridge University Press), 41–45.

Grivennikov, S. I., Greten, F. R., and Karin, M. (2010). Immunity, inflammation, and cancer. *Cell* 140, 883–899.

Hagiwara, S., Iwasaka, H., Matsumoto, S., and Noguchi, T. (2007). Changes in cell culture temperature alter release of inflammatory mediators in murine macrophagic RAW264.7 cells. *Inflamm. Res.* 56,297–303.

Hasday, J. D., Fairchild, K. D., and Shanholtz, C. (2000). The role of fever in the infected host. *Microbes Infect.* 2, 1891–1904.

Hotchkiss, R., Nunnally, I., Lindquist, S., Taulien, J., Perdrizet, G., and Karl, I. (1993). Hyperthermia pro- tects mice against the lethal effects of endotoxin.

Am. J. Physiol. 265, R1447–R1457.

Isomaki, P., Luukkainen, R., Saario, R., Toivanen, P., and Punnonen, J. (1996). Interleukin-10 functions as an antiinflammatory cytokine in rheumatoid synovium. *Arthritis Rheum.* 39, 386–395.

Jaattela, M. (1999). Heat shock proteins as cellular lifeguards. *Ann. Med.* 31, 261–271.

Jiang, Q., Akashi, S., Miyake, K., and Petty, H. R. (2000a). Lipopolysac- charide induces physical proximity between CD14 and toll-like receptor 4 (TLR4) prior to nuclear transloca- tion of NF-kappa B. *J. Immunol.* 165, 3541–3544.

Jiang, Q., Cross, A. S., Singh, I. S., Chen, T. T., Viscardi, R. M., and Hasday, J. D. (2000b). Febrile core temperature is essential for optimal host defense in bacterial peritonitis. *Infect. Immun.* 68, 1265–1270.

Jiang, Q., Detolla, L., Singh, I. S., Gatdula, L., Fitzgerald, B., Van Rooi- jen, N., Cross, A. S., and Hasday,

J. D. (1999a). Exposure to febrile temperature upregulates expression of pyrogenic cytokines in endotoxin- challenged mice. *Am. J. Physiol.* 276, R1653–R1660.

Jiang, Q., Detolla, L., Van Rooijen, N., Singh, I. S., Fitzgerald, B., Lipsky, M. M., Kane, A. S., Cross, A. S., and Hasday, J. D. (1999b). Febrile-range temperature modifies early systemic tumor necrosis factor alpha expres- sion in mice challenged with bacte- rial endotoxin. *Infect. Immun.* 67, 1539–1546.

Johnson, A. D., Berberian, P. A., Tytell, M., and Bond, M. G. (1995). Dif- ferential distribution of 70-kD heat shock protein in atherosclerosis. Its potential role in arterial SMC sur- vival. *Arterioscler. Thromb. Vasc. Biol.* 15, 27–36.

Johnson, J. D., and Fleshner, M. (2006). Releasing signals, secretory pathways, and immune function of endogenous extracellular heat shock protein 72. *J. Leukoc. Biol.* 79, 425–434.

Kiechl, S., Egger, G., Mayr, M., Wieder- mann, C. J., Bonora, E., Oberhollen- zer, F., Muggeo, M., Xu, Q., Wick, G., Poewe, W., and Willeit, J. (2001). Chronic infections and the risk of carotid atherosclerosis: prospective results from a large population study. *Circulation* 103, 1064–1070.

Kleindienst, R., Xu, Q., Willeit, J., Waldenberger, F. R., Weimann, S., and Wick, G. (1993). Immunology of atherosclerosis. Demonstration of heat shock protein 60 expression and T lymphocytes bearing alpha/beta or gamma/delta receptor in human atherosclerotic lesions. *Am. J. Pathol.* 142, 1927–1937.

Kluger, M. J. (1979a). *Fever. Its biology, Evolution, and Function.* Princeton, NJ: Princeton University Press.

Kluger, M. J. (1979b). Temperature reg- ulation, fever, and disease. *Int. Rev. Physiol.* 20, 209–251.

Kluger, M. J. (1986). Is fever beneficial? *Yale J. Biol. Med.* 59, 89–95.

Kluger, M. J. (1991a). "The adaptive value of fever," ed. P. A. Mackowiak (New York: Raven Press), 105–124.

Kluger, M. J. (1991b). Fever: role of pyrogens and cryogens. *Physiol. Rev.* 71, 93–127.

Kol, A., Lichtman, A. H., Finberg, R. W., Libby, P., and Kurt-Jones, E. A. (2000). Cutting edge: heat shock pro- tein (HSP) 60 activates the innate immune response: CD14 is an essen- tial receptor for HSP60 activation of mononuclear cells. *J. Immunol.* 164, 13–17.

Kol, A., Sukhova, G. K., Lichtman, A. H., and Libby, P. (1998). Chlamy- dial heat shock protein 60 local- izes in human atheroma and reg- ulates macrophage tumor necrosis factor-alpha and matrix metallopro- teinase expression. *Circulation* 98, 300–307.

Lee, C.-T., Zhong, L., Mace, T. A., and Repasky, E. A. (2012). Eleva- tion in body temperature to Fever range enhances and prolongs subse- quent responsiveness of macrophages to endotoxin challenge. *PLoS ONE* 7, e30077. doi: 10.1371/ journal. pone.0030077

Lehner, T., Bergmeier, L. A., Wang, Y., Tao, L., Sing, M., Spallek, R., and Van Der Zee, R. (2000). Heat shock proteins generate beta-chemokines which function as innate adjuvants enhancing adaptive immunity. *Eur. J. Immunol.* 30, 594–603.

Leon, L. R., Kozak, W., Peschon, J., Glaccum, M., and Kluger, M. J. (1997). Altered acute phase responses to inflammation in IL-1 and TNF receptor knockout mice. *Ann. N. Y. Acad. Sci.* 813, 244–254.

Luo, X., Zuo, X., Zhang, B., Song, L., Wei, X., Zhou, Y., and Xiao, X. (2008). Release of heat shock protein 70 and the effects of extracellular heat shock protein 70 on the production of IL-10 in fibroblast-like synoviocytes. Cell Stress Chaperones 13, 365–373.

MacHt, L. M., Elson, C. J., Kirwan, J. R., Gaston, J. S., Lamont, A. G., Thompson, J. M., and Thompson, S. J. (2000). Relationship between dis- ease severity and responses by blood mononuclear cells from patients with rheumatoid arthritis to human heat- shock protein 60. *Immunology* 99, 208–214.

Mackowiak, P. A. (1981). Direct effects of hyperthermia on pathogenic microorganisms: teleologic implica- tions with regard to fever. *Rev. Infect. Dis.* 3, 508–520.

Martin, C. A., Carsons, S. E., Kowalewski, R., Bernstein, D., Valentino, M., and Santiago-Schwarz, F. (2003). Aberrant extracellular and dendritic cell (DC) surface expres- sion of heat shock protein (hsp)70 in the rheumatoid joint: possi- ble mechanisms of hsp/DC-mediated cross-priming. *J. Immunol.* 171, 5736–5742.

Morimoto, R. I. (1993). Cells in stress: transcriptional activation of heat shock genes. *Science* 259, 1409–1410.

Morimoto, R. I. (1998). Regulation of the heat shock transcriptional response: cross talk between a fam- ily of heat shock factors, molecular chaperones, and negative regulators. *Genes Dev.* 12, 3788–3796.

Mosser, D. M. (2003). The many faces of macrophage activation. *J. Leukoc. Biol.* 73, 209–212.

Multhoff, G. (2007). Heat shock pro- tein 70 (Hsp70): membrane location, export and immunological relevance. *Methods* 43, 229–237.

Nathan, C. (2002). Points of control in inflammation. *Nature* 420, 846–851.

Nguyen, K. D., Qiu, Y., Cui, X., Goh, Y. P., Mwangi, J., David, T., Mukundan, L., Brombacher, F., Lock- sley, R. M., and Chawla, A. (2011). Alternatively activated macrophages produce catecholamines to sustain adaptive thermogenesis. *Nature* 480, 104–108.

O'Shea, J. J., and Murray, P. J. (2008). Cytokine signaling modules in inflammatory responses. *Immu- nity* 28, 477–487.

Ostberg, J. R., Taylor, S. L., Bau- mann, H., and Repasky, E. A. (2000). Regulatory effects of fever- range whole-body hyperthermia on the LPS-induced acute inflamma- tory response. *J. Leukoc. Biol.* 68, 815–820.

Panjwani, N. N., Popova, L., and Srivas- tava, P.K. (2002). Heat shock proteins gp96 and hsp70 activate the release of nitric oxide by APCs. *J. Immunol.* 168, 2997–3003.

Prakken, B. J., Samodal, R., Le, T. D., Giannoni, F., Yung, G. P., Scavulli, J., Amox, D., Roord, S., DeKleer, I., Bonnin, D., Lanza, P., Berry, C., Massa, M., Billetta, R., and Albani, S. (2004). Epitope-specific immunotherapy induces immune deviation of proinflammatory T cells in rheumatoid arthritis. *Proc. Natl. Acad. Sci. U.S.A.* 101, 4228–4233.

Pritchard, M. T., Li, Z., and Repasky, A. (2005). Nitric oxide production is regulated by fever-range thermal stimulation of murine macrophages. *J. Leukoc. Biol.* 78, 630–638.

Ran, R., Lu, A., Zhang, L., Tang, Y., Zhu, H., Xu, H., Feng, Y., Han, C., Zhou, G., Rigby, A. C., and Sharp, R. (2004). Hsp70 promotes TNF- mediated apoptosis by binding IKK gamma and impairing NF-kappa B survival signaling. *Genes Dev.* 18, 1466–1481.

Romanovsky, A. A., Almeida, M. C., Aronoff, D. M., Ivanov, A. I., Kons- man, J. P., Steiner, A. A., and Turek, V. F. (2005). Fever and hypothermia in systemic inflammation: recent dis- coveries and revisions. *Front. Biosci.* 10, 2193–2216.

Romanovsky, A. A., Kulchitsky, V. A., Simons, C. T., and Sugimoto, N. (1998). Methodology of fever research: why are polyphasic fevers often thought to be biphasic? *Am. J. Physiol.* 275, R332–R338.

Rosenthal, M., Bahous, I., and Ambrosini, G. (1991). Longterm treatment of rheumatoid arthritis with OM-8980. A retrospective study. *J. Rheumatol.* 18, 1790–1793.

Schmitt, E., Gehrmann, M., Brunet, M., Multhoff, G., and Garrido, C. (2007). Intracellular and extracellu- lar functions of heat shock proteins: repercussions in cancer therapy. *J. Leukoc. Biol.* 81, 15–27.

Serhan, C. N., Brain, S. D., Buckley, C. D., Gilroy, D. W., Haslett, C., O'Neill, L. A., Perretti, M., Rossi, A. G., and Wallace, J. L. (2007). Reso- lution of inflammation: state of the art, definitions and terms. *FASEB J.* 21, 325–332.

Shi, Y., Tu, Z., Tang, D., Zhang, H., Liu, M., Wang, K., Calderwood, S. K., and Xiao, X. (2006). The inhibition of LPS-induced production of inflam- matory cytokines by HSP70 involves inactivation of the NF-kappaB path- way but not the MAPK pathways. *Shock* 26, 277–284.

Singh, I. S., He, J. R., Calderwood, S., and Hasday, J. D. (2002). A high affinity HSF-1 binding site in the 5'-untranslated region of the murine tumor necrosis factor-alpha gene is a transcriptional repressor. *J. Biol. Chem.* 277, 4981–4988.

Snyder, Y. M., Guthrie, L., Evans, G. F., and Zuckerman, S. H. (1992). Transcriptional inhibition of endotoxin-induced monokine syn- thesis following heat shock in murine peritoneal macrophages. *J. Leukoc. Biol.* 51, 181–187.

Tanaka, Y., Otsuka, T., Hotokebuchi, T., Miyahara, H., Nakashima, H., Kuga, S., Nemoto, Y., Niiro, H., and Niho, Y. (1996). Effect of IL-10 on collagen- induced arthritis in mice. *Inflamm. Res.* 45, 283–288.

Tang, D., Kang, R., Xiao, W., Wang, H., Calderwood, S. K., and Xiao, X. (2007). The anti- inflammatory effects of heat shock protein 72 involve inhibition of high-mobility-group box 1 release and proinflammatory function in macrophages. *J. Immunol.* 179, 1236–1244.

Triantafilou, K., Triantafilou, M., and Dedrick, R. L. (2001). A CD14- independent LPS receptor cluster. *Nat. Immunol.* 2,338–345.

Triantafilou, M., and Triantafilou, K. (2004). Heat-shock protein 70 and heat-shock protein 90 asso- ciate with Toll-like receptor 4 in response to bacterial lipopolysac- charide. *Biochem. Soc. Trans.* 32, 636–639.

Vabulas, R. M., Ahmad-Nejad, P., Ghose, S., Kirschning, C. J., Issels, R. D., and Wagner, H. (2002). HSP70 as endogenous stimulus of the Toll/interleukin-1 receptor sig- nal pathway. *J. Biol. Chem.* 277, 15107–15112.

van Eden, W., Van Der Zee, R., and Prakken, B. (2005). Heat-shock proteins induce T-cell regulation of chronic inflammation. *Nat. Rev. Immunol.* 5,318–330.

Van Molle, W., Wielockx, B., Mahieu, T., Takada, M., Taniguchi, T., Sekikawa, K., and Libert, C. (2002). HSP70 protects against TNF-induced lethal inflammatory shock. *Immunity* 16, 685–695.

Vega, V. L., Rodriguez-Silva, M., Frey, T., Gehrmann, M., Diaz, J. C., Steinem, C., Multhoff, G., Arispe, N., and De Maio, A. (2008). Hsp70 translocates into the plasma mem- brane after stress and is released into the extracellular environment in a membrane-associated form that acti- vates macrophages. *J. Immunol.* 180, 4299–4307.

Villar, J., Ribeiro, S. P., Mullen, J. B., Kuliszewski, M., Post, M., and Slutsky, A. S. (1994). Induction of the heat shock response reduces mortality rate and organ damage in a sepsis-induced acute lung injury model. *Crit. Care Med.* 22, 914–921.

Vischer, T. L. (1990). Follow-up with OM-8980 after a double-blind study of OM-8980 and auranofin in rheumatoid arthritis. *Clin. Rheuma- tol.* 9,356–361.

Wang, R., Kovalchin, J. T., Muh- lenkamp, P., and Chandawarkar, R. (2006). Exogenous heat shock pro- tein 70 binds macrophage lipid raft microdomain and stimulates phago- cytosis, processing, and MHC-II pre- sentation of antigens. *Blood* 107, 1636–1642.

Wu, C. (1995). Heat shock transcrip- tion factors: structure and regula- tion. *Annu. Rev. Cell Dev. Biol.* 11, 441–469.

Xu, Q. (2002). Role of heat shock pro- teins in atherosclerosis. *Arterioscler. Thromb. Vasc. Biol.* 22,1547–1559.

Yenari, M. A., Liu, J., Zheng, Z., Vexler, S., Lee, J. E., and Giffard, R. G. (2005). Antiapoptotic and anti- inflammatory mechanisms of heat- shock protein protection. *Ann. N. Y. Acad. Sci.* 1053, 74–83.

Zhang, Y. H., Takahashi, K., Jiang, G. Z., Zhang, X. M., Kawai, M., Fukada, M., and Yokochi, T. (1994). In vivo production of heat shock protein in mouse peritoneal macrophages by administration of lipopolysaccha- ride. *Infect. Immun.* 62, 4140–4144.

19

Large-scale analysis of B-cell epitopes on influenza virus hemagglutinin – implications for cross-reactivity of neutralizing antibodies

Jing Sun[1,2], Ulrich J. Kudahl[1,3], Christian Simon[1,3], Zhiwei Cao[4], Ellis L. Reinherz[1,2,5] and Vladimir Brusic[1,2]*

[1] Cancer Vaccine Center, Dana-Farber Cancer Institute, Harvard Medical School, Boston, MA, USA
[2] Department of Medicine, Harvard Medical School, Boston, MA, USA
[3] Center for Biological Sequence Analysis, Technical University of Denmark, Lyngby, Denmark
[4] School of Life Sciences and Technology, Tongji University, Shanghai, China
[5] Laboratory of Immunobiology, Department of Medical Oncology, Dana-Farber Cancer Institute, Harvard Medical School, Boston, MA, USA

Edited by:
Ramit Mehr, Bar-Ilan University, Israel

Reviewed by:
Juan C. Almagro, Pfizer, Inc., USA
Yanay Ofran, Bar-Ilan University, Israel

***Correspondence:**
Vladimir Brusic, Cancer Vaccine Center, Dana-Farber Cancer Institute, Harvard Medical School, 77 Avenue Louis Pasteur, HIM 401, Boston, MA 02115, USA
e-mail: vladimir_brusic@dfci.harvard.edu

Influenza viruses continue to cause substantial morbidity and mortality worldwide. Fast gene mutation on surface proteins of influenza virus result in increasing resistance to current vaccines and available antiviral drugs. Broadly neutralizing antibodies (bnAbs) represent targets for prophylactic and therapeutic treatments of influenza. We performed a systematic bioinformatics study of cross-reactivity of neutralizing antibodies (nAbs) against influenza virus surface glycoprotein hemagglutinin (HA). This study utilized the available crystal structures of HA complexed with the antibodies for the analysis of tens of thousands of HA sequences. The detailed description of B-cell epitopes, measurement of epitope area similarity among different strains, and estimation of antibody neutralizing coverage provide insights into cross-reactivity status of existing nAbs against influenza virus. We have developed a method to assess the likely cross-reactivity potential of bnAbs for influenza strains, either newly emerged or existing. Our method catalogs influenza strains by a new concept named discontinuous peptide, and then provide assessment of cross-reactivity. Potentially cross-reactive strains are those that share 100% identity with experimentally verified neutralized strains. By cataloging influenza strains and their B-cell epitopes for known bnAbs, our method provides guidance for selection of representative strains for further experimental design. The knowledge of sequences, their B-cell epitopes, and differences between historical influenza strains, we enhance our preparedness and the ability to respond to the emerging pandemic threats.

Keywords: influenza virus, neutralizing antibodies, B-cell epitope, cross-reactivity, discontinuous peptide

INTRODUCTION

Influenza epidemics result in substantial morbidity and mortality (1). The World Health Organization (WHO) Global Influenza Network provides annual recommendations on antigenic variants to be included in the influenza vaccine formulations. Influenza virus has low-fidelity polymerases that result in high mutation rates (2). As a consequence, seasonal influenza viruses efficiently escape from acquired immunity in the human population through antigenic drift increasing the impact of seasonal influenza. The antigenic shift in influenza A viruses – the reassortment of multiple viral genomes resulting in new strains with recombined antigens – leads to occasional worldwide pandemics that result in significant morbidity and, usually, high mortality. High transmissibility of influenza combined with rapid mutation rates makes the discovery of novel influenza therapeutics an imperative (3). The main challenge in developing antibody-based prophylactics and therapeutic vaccine against influenza is to understand the variation generated by the virus and developing means to elicit broadly neutralizing antibody responses.

The majority of neutralizing antibodies (nAbs) generated during a normal immune response target hemagglutinin (HA) and block viral entry into host cells (4). However, significant sequence diversity among HA genes limits the protective breadth of these nAbs (5). This sequence diversity of influenza A virus is high – there are 17 HA serotypes that belong into two major groups called group 1 (Grp1: H1, H2, H5, H6, H8, H9, H11, H12, H13, H16, and H17), and group 2 (Grp2: H3, H4, H7, H10, H14, and H15) (6). C179, the first neutralizing antibody reported to neutralize strains from H1 and H2 of influenza A virus, was isolated from mice immunized with the A/Okuda/57 (H2N2) strain (7). Later it was found that C179 was able to cross-neutralize H1, H2, H5, H6, and H9 subtypes (8–11). The next major advance in the field came about 15 years later (12), a novel class of human antibodies encoded by the V_H1–69 gene were discovered. Among these antibodies, a series of broadly neutralizing antibodies (bnAbs) have been described, such as CR6261 and F10 (13). Most bnAbs that neutralize influenza A virus have been reported to neutralize strains from either exclusively Grp1 or Grp2. FI6v3 (14) and 39.29 (5) are the only antibodies reported to neutralize human influenza isolates from both Grp1 and Grp2. Influenza B viruses are classified within a single influenza type, with two antigenically and genetically distinct lineages that co-circulate (15), represented by the prototype viruses B/Victoria/2/1987 (Victoria lineage) and B/Yamagata/16/1988 (Yamagata lineage) (16). Antibody CR8071 (17) is a bnAb against influenza B viruses, with neutralizing ability for both Victoria and Yamagata lineages. bnAb CR9114 (17) binds a conserved epitope on the HA stem and was shown to neutralize all tested influenza A viruses. However, it did not show *in vitro* neutralizing activity against influenza B viruses at the tested concentrations (17).

Generally, the neutralizing effectiveness of these bnAbs was evaluated using representative strains from the subtypes of influenza A virus or lineages of influenza B virus. Because of the high variability of HA genes, such evaluation might result in a conclusion that is limited to the tested viral variants. To determine the landscape of nAbs and better understand their cross-reactivity properties, we performed a systematic study of B-cell epitopes of a selection of nAbs against influenza virus. Antibodies recognize discrete sites on the surface of macromolecule called B-cell epitopes (antigenic determinants). Some 10% of B-cell epitopes are linear peptides while 90% are formed from discontinuous amino acids that create surface patches through the three dimensional (3D) conformation of proteins (18). We defined a novel way of describing discontinuous motifs, using virtual peptides, to represent B-cell epitopes and further used this representation to estimate potential cross-reactivity and neutralizing coverage of these nAbs.

Functional characterization of the increasing number of nAbs and known crystal structures of these nAbs complexed with HA proteins enables us to precisely define their B-cell epitopes. A large number of sequences of influenza variants are available in public databases (19) enabling systematic bioinformatics analysis of cross-reactivity of nAbs against influenza virus. Such systematic analysis improves our understanding of antibody/antigen interactions, facilitates mapping of the known universe of target antigens, and allows the prediction of cross-reactivity. These methods and tools are useful for the design of broadly protective vaccines against emerging pathogens. This article describes a study of influenza HA cross-reactivity, but the method is applicable to any viral pathogen where information about nAbs and a collection of variant sequences of the target antigen are available.

MATERIALS AND METHODS

NEUTRALIZING ANTIBODIES AGAINST HEMAGGLUTININ

The names and specificities of nAb against influenza virus HA were collected from published papers. Twenty-two nAbs against influenza virus with crystal structures available in PDB were collected from published articles (**Table 1**). Fifteen of these nAbs target at the globular head of HA, and for the other seven, the binding sites are located on HA stem region.

Table 1 | Summary of well-characterized neutralizing antibodies against influenza virus.

Location	Neutralizing antibodies	PDB ID	Neutralizing breadth	Reference
Head	1F1	4GXU	H1	(20)
	2D1	3LZF	H1	(21)
	2G1	4HG4	H2	(17)
	8F8	4HF5	H2	(17)
	8M2	4HFU	H2	(17)
	BH151	*1EO8*	*A/X-31 (H3N2)*	(22)
	C05	4FQR	H1, H2, H3, H9	(23)
	CH65	3SM5	H1	(24)
	CH67	4HKX	H1	(25)
	CR8059	4FQK	Influenza B virus	(17)
	CR8071	4FQJ	Influenza B virus: Yamagata and Victoria	(17)
	HC19	*2VIR*	*A/X-31 (H3N2)*	(26)
	HC45	*1QFU*	*A/X-31 (H3N2)*	(27)
	HC63	*1KEN*	*A/X-31 (H3N2)*	(28)
	S139/1	4GMS	H1, H2, H3, H13, H16	(8, 29)
Stem	39.29	4KVN	H1, H2, H3	(5)
	C179	4HLZ	Grp1: H1, H2, H5, H6, H9	(30)
	CR6261	3GBN/3GBM	Grp1: H1, H2, H5, H9	(31, 32)
	CR8020	3SDY	Grp2: H3, H7, H10	(33)
	CR9114	4FQI/4FQV/4FQY	Grp1: H1, H2, H5, H6, H8, H9, H12 Grp2: H3, H4, H7, H10	(17)
	F10	3FKU	Grp1: H1, H2, H5, H6, H8, H9, H11	(13)
	FI6v3	3ZTJ/3ZTN	H1, H3, H5, H7	(14)

The nAbs in underlined italics are nAbs specific for strain A/X-31 (H3N2). The designation of two groups (Grp1 and Grp2) of influenza A virus subtypes are shown in ***Figure 1****.*

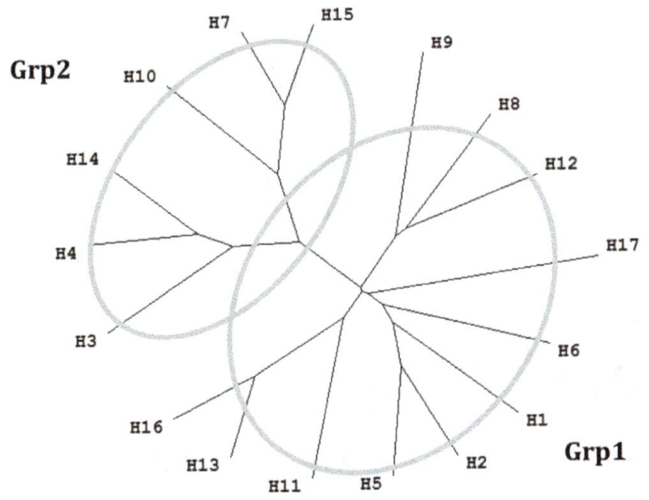

FIGURE 1 | Phylogenetic tree of 17 influenza A virus subtypes. Representative sequences were selected for each subtype (34) and the phylogenetic tree was made with ClustalX (35) and TreeView (36). H1: A/California/04/2009(H1N1); H2: A/Singapore/1/1957(H2N2); H3: A/Aichi/2/1968(H3N2); H4: A/duck/Czechoslovakia/1956(H4N6); H5: A/VietNam/1203/2004(H5N1); H6: A/chicken/California/431/2000(H6N2); H7: A/Turkey/Italy/8458/2002(H7N3); H8: A/Turkey/Ontario/6118/1968(H8N4); H9: A/Swine/Hong Kong/9/98(H9N2); H10: A/chicken/Germany/N/1949(H10N7); H11: A/duck/England/1/1956(H11N6); H12: A/duck/Alberta/60/1976(H12N5); H13: A/gull/Maryland/704/1977(H13N6); H14: A/Mallard/Astrakhan/263/1982(H14N5); H15: A/shearwater/West Australia/2576/79(H15N9); H16: A/black-headed gull/Sweden/2/99(H16N3); and H17: A/little yellow-shouldered bat/Guatemala/060/2010 (H17N10).

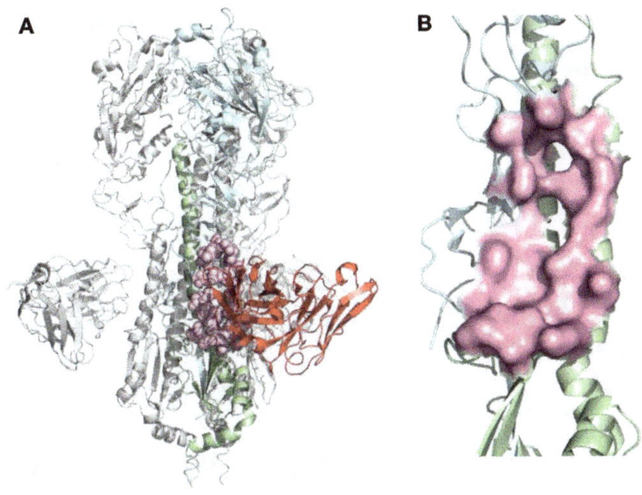

FIGURE 2 | B-cell epitope on the structure of neutralizing antibody F10 binding HA protein (PDB ID: 3FKU). (A) Complex of F10-HA [A/Vietnam/1203/04(H5N1)]. The structure is a HA trimer of three identical copies (one of them is colored as cyan and green; the other two are in gray). Each copy contains the HA1 (cyan) and HA2 (green) chain, also the heavy chain of F10 (red), the neutralized epitope is highlighted in pink; **(B)** Close-up view of neutralized epitope identified on the structure (highlighted as pink surface).

The majority of these nAbs were observed to bind or neutralize influenza A virus isolated either from Grp1 or Grp2. Antibodies FI6v3, CR9114, and 39.29 were shown to neutralize influenza strains within both Grp1 and Grp2 (5, 14, 27). Antibodies CR8059 and CR8071 (17) were the only two nAbs for influenza B virus. CR8059 is a light chain D95aN variant of CR8071. Since the mutation on CR8059 is not present at the binding interface and does not affect the binding, only CR8071 was used in the following study (17). The majority of these nAbs were shown to neutralize more than one strain, some of them are broadly neutralizing across subtypes of influenza A virus or lineages of influenza B virus. The Abs BH151, HC19, HC45, and HC63 were shown to specifically neutralize HA from the A/X-31(H3N2) strain. The available structures of nAb/HA complexes were downloaded from PDB (37).

VALIDATED INFLUENZA STRAINS BY NEUTRALIZING ANTIBODIES

Binding and neutralization assays were collected from published materials. Binding and non-binding strains were classified according to their affinity measurements. The thresholds used to discriminate binding and non-binding strains were inconsistent in different studies: the lowest affinity detectable values were set as 10^{-4} M (17), 10^{-5} M (33), and ~10^{-6} M (20). In some reports, nAbs showed positive binding results but did not display neutralization ability to the same strains [e.g., nAb CR9114 against strain B/Florida/4/2006 (Yamagata) (17)]. Because of the lack of standardized thresholds and ambiguous definition of binding, only results that indicate non-binding of antibodies were considered as useful information and were retained for the subsequent analysis as negatives.

Table 2 | B-cell epitope regions of the 22 neutralizing antibodies.

Binding site	Influenza A virus				Influenza B virus
	Sa site	Near RBS	F subdomain	Stem base	Head base
CROSS-REACTIVE NEUTRALIZING ANTIBODIES					
nAbs	**2D1**	**C05**	**CR6261**	**CR8020**	**CR8071**
		1F1	39.29		CR8059
		2G1	C179		
		8F8	CR9114		
		8M2	F10		
		CH65	FI6v3		
		CH67			
		S139/1			
Binding site	**Head base**	**RBS**	**Near RBS**		
X-31-SPECIFIC NEUTRALIZING ANTIBODIES					
nAbs	**BH151**	**HC19**	**HC63**		
	HC45				

*The nAbs are classified as cross-reactive or X-31-specific. For each binding region, a representative nAb was selected (shown in bold) and its B-cell epitope was mapped on the structures shown in **Figure 3**.*

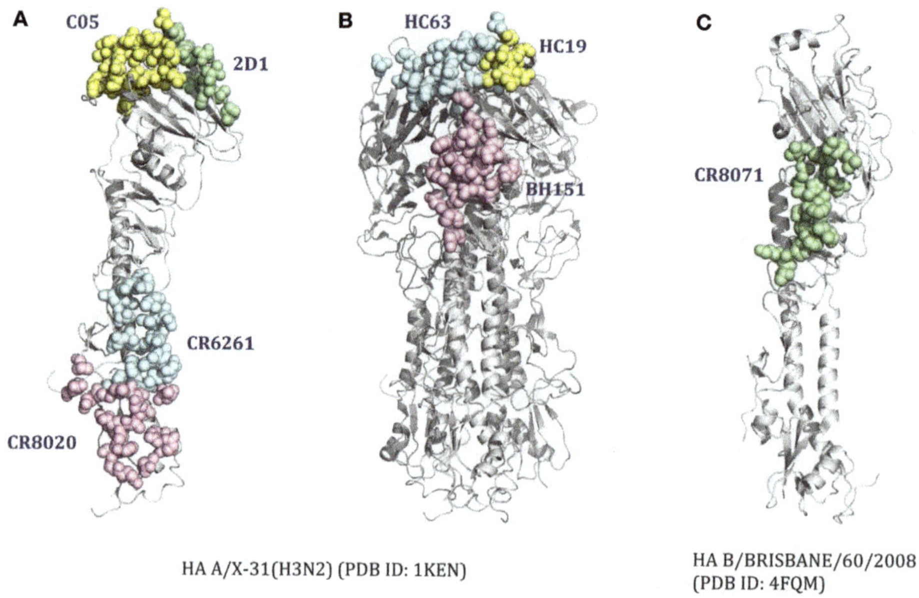

FIGURE 3 | The distinct B-cell epitope regions recognized by representative nAbs. The B-cell epitope regions of **(A)** represent cross-reactive nAbs against influenza A virus; **(B)** represent strain-specific nAbs against X-31(H3N2); **(C)** represent broadly nAb CR8071 against influenza B virus. The epitope regions of nAbs target influenza A virus were mapped on the monomer **(A)** or trimer **(B)** HA from A/X-31(H3N2) (PDB ID: 1KEN). The structure of B/Brisbane/60/2008 HA (PDB ID: 4FQM) was used as a template structure for influenza B virus. Different colors here were used for distinguishing B-cell epitope regions.

The neutralized and the escape strains were detected using the microneutralization assay (38) or HA inhibition assay (39). Several measurements were suggested in these studies:

1. The lowest concentration of nAb that displayed inhibition of hemagglutination or microneutralizing activity were set as either 2.5 μg/mL (40) or 5 μg/mL (41).
2. The 50% inhibitory concentration was set to $IC_{50} = 50$ μg/mL (17).
3. The effective concentration of antibody needed to inhibit at least 99% of viral infectivity was set as $EC_{99} = 100$ μg/mL (24, 25).

The HA sequences of strains that were experimentally validated for neutralization by studied antibodies ("validated strains") were retrieved from the literature. The influenza strains HA sequences were collected from the literature or, if absent, from the Influenza Knowledge Base (FLUKB)[1]. All experimentally validated strains were grouped into either neutralized strains or escape strains. The neutralized strains were selected based on reported experimental evidence. The escape strains included true escape strains as well as strains that were reported not to bind nAbs. We did not find any discrepancies in reported neutralizing properties across different studies used to collect functional data.

HEMAGGLUTININ SEQUENCES

All HA sequences were downloaded from the Influenza Knowledge Base (FLUKB[1], dated August 26th, 2013). After removing the incomplete sequences (fragments), 45,812 full-length HA sequences were left in the data set (HA sequence dataset) for further analysis.

GENERATION OF MULTIPLE SEQUENCE ALIGNMENT OF HEMAGGLUTININ SEQUENCES

The HA sequences of influenza strains from FLUKB were aligned using the MAFFT tool (42). The resulting multiple sequence alignment (MSA) results provided a consistent numbering scheme for all the further analyses. MSA were generated for both experimentally validated strains of HA and for all entries from FLUKB. For each nAb, every HA sequence from the crystal structure and from the experimentally validated strains were searched individually within the FLUKB database to find a strain with highest similarity using BLAST (43). This procedure was done to ensure that residue position mapping in following steps is consistent with the numbering scheme.

IDENTIFICATION OF B-CELL EPITOPES

B-cell epitope were identified from antigen–antibody structure, using a formula with the combination of the measurements of accessible surface area (ASA) and atom distance. For each residue from HA antigen, the ASA value was calculated using Naccess software (44) for both free HA and for HA coupled with an antibody. Residues r_i with ASA loss more than 20% were selected as epitope residues,

$$r_i \in \{\text{epitope residues}\} \text{ if } \frac{\text{ASA}_{\text{free}} - \text{ASA}_{\text{coupled}}}{\text{ASA}_{\text{free}}} > 0.2.$$

[1]http://research4.dfci.harvard.edu/cvc/flukb

Table 3 | B-cell epitope overlap for nAbs targeting HA head region.

	Sa	Near RBS							
	2D1	**1F1**	**2G1**	**8F8**	**8M2**	**C05**	**CH65**	**CH67**	**S139/1**
A98	–	+	–	+	+	+	+	+	+
A125	+	–	–	–	–	–	–	–	–
A126	+	–	–	–	–	–	–	–	–
A128	+	–	+	–	–	–	–	–	–
A130	+	–	+	+	+	–	–	+	–
A131	–	–	–	–	–	+	–	–	+
A132	–	–	+	+	+	–	–	–	–
A133	–	+	+	+	+	+	–	–	–
A134	–	–	+	+	+	+	+	+	+
A135	–	+	–	–	–	+	+	+	+
A136	–	–	+	+	+	+	+	+	+
A137	–	–	+	+	+	+	+	+	+
A140	–	–	–	+	–	–	–	–	–
A143	–	–	–	+	–	–	–	–	–
A144	–	–	–	+	–	–	–	–	–
A145	–		+	+	+	+	–	–	+
A153	–	+	+	+	+	+	+	+	+
A155	–	+	+	+	+	+	+	+	+
A156	–	+	+	+	+	+	+	+	+
A157	+	–	+	–	–	–	–	–	+
A158	+	–	+	+	+	+	+	+	+
A159	+	+	+	+	+	+	+	+	+
A160	+	–	–	–	–	–	+	+	+
A161	+	–	–	–	–	–	–	–	–
A162	+	–	–	–	–	–	–	–	–
A163	+	–	–	–	–	–	–	–	–
A165	+	–	–	–	–	–	–	–	–
A166	+	–	–	–	–	–	–	–	–
A167	+	–	–	–	–	–	–	–	–
A169	+	–	–	–	–	–	–	–	–
A183	–	+	–	–	–	+	+	–	+
A185	–	+	–	–	–	–	–	–	–
A186	–	+	–	–	+	+	–	–	+
A187	–	+	–	+	+	+	+	+	–
A188	–	–	–	–	+	–	–	–	–
A189	–	+	–	+	+	+	+	+	+
A190	–	+	+	+	+	+	+	+	+
A192	–	+	–	–	+	+	+	+	+
A193	–	+	+	+	+	+	+	+	+
A194	–	+	+	+	+	+	+	+	+
A196	–	+	–	–	–	–	+	+	+
A197	+	–	–	–	–	–	–	–	–
A219	–	+	–	–	–	–	–	+	–
A222	–	+	–	–	+	–	+	–	–
A225	–	+	–	–	+	+	+	+	+
A226	–	+	–	+	+	+	+	+	+
A227	–	+	–	–	+	+	+	–	–
A228	–	+	–	–	+	+	–	–	+
A246	+	–	–	–	–	–	–	–	–
A248	+	–	–	–	–	–	–	–	–

The epitope residue positions of nine nAbs were mapped to the 1EO8 structure chain A. The symbol "+" indicates a contact epitope residue by corresponding nAb, and the symbol "–" means it is not a epitope position. 2D1, with a different epitope area to other eight nAbs, is labeled in red.

The majority of contacts between two contacting atoms occur at distance smaller than 5 Å separation (45). Euclidean distance was calculated between atoms a_i and a_j using their coordinates $a_i(x_i, y_i, z_i)$ and $a_j(x_j, y_j, z_j)$ in PDB structure data,

$$d_{ij} = \sqrt{(x_i - x_j)^2 + (y_i - y_j)^2 + (z_i - z_j)^2}.$$

Hemagglutinin residues r_i whose minimum atom distance to the closest nAb atom was within 4 Å were also incorporated in the epitope. The minimal atom distance was defined as:

$$d_{\min} = \min\left\{d_{ij}\right\},\ a_i \in \text{antigen residue } r_i, a_j \in \text{antibody residue } r_j,$$
$$r_i \in \left\{\text{epitope residue}\right\} \text{ if } d_{\min} < 4\text{Å}.$$

The residues that satisfy either of these two conditions (ASA loss or minimum distance) are considered to constitute a B-cell epitope.

The specific residues on HA that form hydrogen bonds, salt bridges, disulfide bonds, and covalent bonds between the HA and nAb were considered to define a B-cell epitope. The antigen/antibody interaction was further analyzed using PISA tool (46). The analysis of HA structures showed that all the hydrogen bonds, salt bridges, disulfide bonds, and covalent bonds between HA and nAb in each studied structure were incorporated in B-cell epitopes defined in the previous step.

EXTRACTION OF DISCONTINUOUS MOTIFS FROM VALIDATED STRAINS

For each nAb, using the MSA result and the standardized numbering, the residue positions of B-cell epitope identified from the HA/antibody crystal structure were mapped onto all HA sequence of validated strains. Then discontinuous motifs composed of mapped residues were extracted from these sequences. These discontinuous motifs were classified as either "neutralized" or "escape" motifs according to the experimental validation status of the corresponding strain.

MAPPING OF DISCONTINUOUS MOTIFS TO HA SEQUENCE DATASET

For each nAb, based on the MSA result, the residue positions of B-cell epitope identified from the HA/antibody crystal structure were mapped onto the HA sequence dataset. A "discontinuous peptide" composed of amino acids that form B-cell epitope, in order that they appear in the sequence, was extracted from each HA sequence. By comparing the discontinuous peptides to all validated neutralized and escape motifs from experimentally validated strains, each discontinuous peptide was classified as neutralized (if 100%

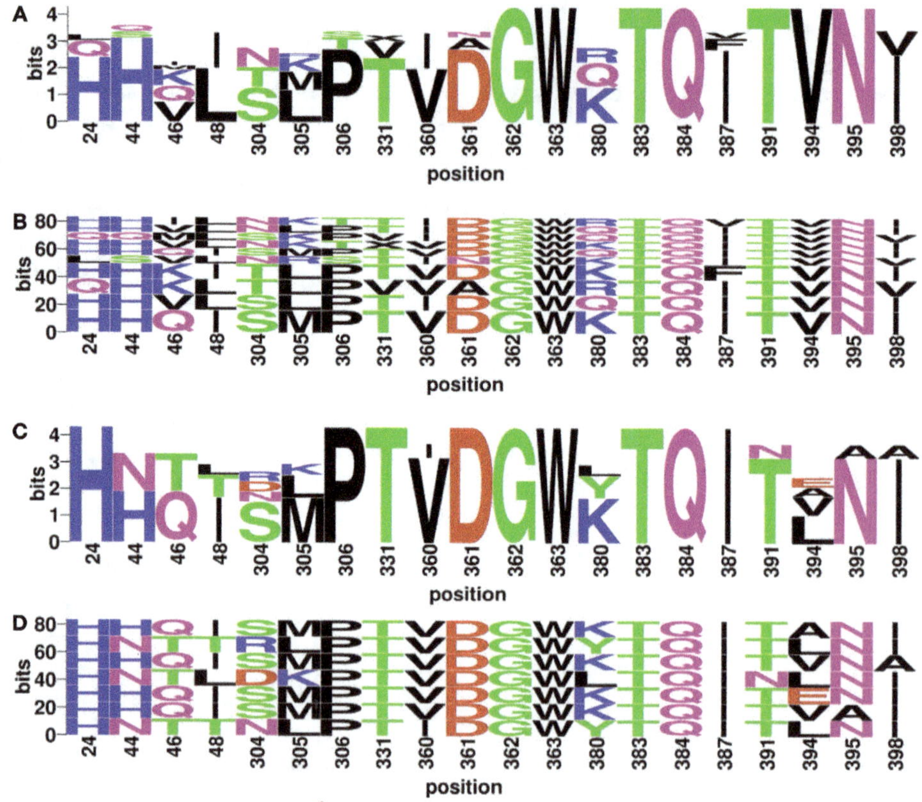

FIGURE 4 | Neutralized and escape discontinuous motifs from experimentally validated sequences with nAb F10. The WebLogo shows global **(A)** neutralized motifs, and **(C)** escape motifs and BlockLogo shows individual **(B)** neutralized motifs, and **(D)** escape motifs. The extracted discontinuous motif extracted from the structure (PDB ID: 3FKU, chain A and B), corresponds to the positions of reference sequence [FLU0293715, A/Viet Nam/1203/2004(H5N1)]: 24, 44, 46, 48, 304, 305, 306, 331, 360, 361, 362, 363, 380, 383, 384, 387, 391, 394, 395, and 398.

matching a neutralized epitope motif), escape (if 100% matching an escape epitope motif), or non-validated (if 100% matching validation data are missing). The term "discontinuous motif" indicates positions that define each B-cell epitope extracted from experimentally validated strains collected from publications, while term "discontinuous peptide" represents specific B-cell epitopes extracted from the HA sequence dataset.

RESULTS

B-CELL EPITOPE REGIONS

For each nAb, the B-cell epitope was identified from the crystal structure as described in Section "Materials and Methods." The structure of nAb F10-H5 (13) and identified epitope are illustrated in **Figure 2**. After B-cell epitopes of all studied nAbs were mapped to the same template structure, the overlapping of binding sites were found among different nAbs, particularly at the receptor-binding site (RBS), which is the necessary structure for binding to the sialic acid receptors during virus infection.

For cross-reactive nAbs against influenza A virus, four major binding locations on HA structure are apparent: two of them reside on the globular head of HA and the other two target the stem region of HA (**Table 2**; **Figure 3**). The RBS is a heavily targeted area, with overlapping epitopes defined by eight nAbs. The only nAb that binds HA head but not the RBS is 2D1 (21). The 2D1 recognizes the Sa site of A/South Carolina/1/1918(H1N1). Sa site is one of the earliest known antigenic sites (47), which is proximal to the receptor-binding pocket. The detailed comparison of epitope residue positions between 2D1 and the other HA head-targeted nAbs are listed in **Table 3**. In contrast to the Abs that interact with the HA head, a series of nAbs recognize another highly conserved helical region in the membrane-proximal HA stem. The epitopes on F subdomain (CR6261, 39.29, etc.) and stem base (CR8020) are adjacent to each other, with a small number of shared residues. The only broadly nAb neutralizing influenza B virus, CR8071 binds to the lower region of the globular head of HA – the "head base" (**Figure 3C**). All the remaining antibodies analyzed in our study bind specifically the HA on A/X-31(H3N2) strain. All X-31 specific nAbs complex with the membrane-distal domain of HA. NAbs BH151 and HC45 (22) recognize a single epitope located at the base of the eight-stranded antiparallel β-sheet structure. The HC19 binding site is adjacent to the RBS. The HC63 epitope shares several residues with HC19, thereby the antibody binding site overlaps the membrane-distal domains of two HA monomers.

EXPERIMENTALLY VALIDATED DISCONTINUOUS MOTIFS

Discontinuous motifs were extracted from the validated sequences as described in Section "Materials and Methods," and presented by WebLogo (48) and BlockLogo[2] [Ref. (49)]. WebLogo figures consist of stacks of amino acids, while the overall height of the stack indicates the sequence conservation at that position, and the height of symbols within the stack indicates the relative frequency of each amino or nucleic acid at that position. While BlockLogo is a web-based application for visualization of protein and nucleotide fragments, continuous protein sequence motifs, and discontinuous sequence motifs using calculation of block entropy from MSAs. The BlockLogo figures present the actual combinations of amino acids, and the height of each combination represents its relative frequency. In the nAb F10 as an example, the neutralized and escape discontinuous motifs are shown in **Figures 4A,C** (WebLogo figures), and **Figures 4B,D** (BlockLogo figures). WebLogos show a clear overall description of each residue conservation difference between individual neutralized and escape motifs. For example, 44N, 48T, 304R/D, 380L/Y, 391N, 394E/A/L on F10 epitope region are likely to contribute to the escape strains. In the BlockLogo figures, specific neutralized and escape B-cell epitopes of F10 were listed with their frequencies, which can be used for their direct comparison.

ANALYSIS OF VARIATION OF DISCONTINUOUS PEPTIDES IN HA SEQUENCES DATASET

For each nAb, the residue positions of their B-cell epitopes were mapped on the complete HA sequences dataset collected from the FLUKB. Amino acid strings representing discontinuous peptides were extracted from the HA sequence of each strain. The variability of discontinuous peptides and validated discontinuous motif coverage were analyzed for each nAb.

[2] http://research4.dfci.harvard.edu/cvc/blocklogo

For example, for the nAb F10, 589 different patterns of discontinuous peptides were generated among all 45,812 sequences in HA sequence dataset, using the F10 B-cell epitope identified from the crystal structure. In the next step, the discontinuous peptides were sorted according to their frequencies. The second most frequent peptide in FLUKB is identical an escape motif, while the 6th, 8th, and 19th are each identical to one of the neutralized motifs. However, the most frequent F10 discontinuous peptide in FLUKB (see text footnote 1) has not been experimentally tested (**Figure 5**), along with other 14 discontinuous peptides. The analysis of differences between the most frequent discontinuous peptide and neutralized or escape motifs was inconclusive. Therefore future experimental studies should include a representative sequence containing the discontinuous peptide HHVLSLPTVDGWLTQITVNI that is present in more than 10,000 entries in the FLUKB. We also recommend that motifs 1, 4, 5, 7, 9–18, and 20 are considered for the experimental validation. The remaining sequences are less common, each having <400 sequences in the data set.

The discontinuous peptides were generated and the variability was investigated for all cross-reactive nAbs (**Table 4**). The B-cell epitope regions on the HA stem are less variable as compared to the epitopes on the HA head. The specific result generated within each subtype in HA sequence dataset show similar patterns as for all subtypes (data not shown). This conclusion is consistent with our previous knowledge that the globular head of HA1 has a higher mutation rate than the stem (29), making the stem a more conserved region for bnAbs targeting.

DISCONTINUOUS MOTIFS COVERAGE IN HA SEQUENCES DATASET

The neutralized and escape discontinuous motifs of nAb F10 have covered 19 and 17% of FLUKB, respectively, while the discontinuous peptides from 64% of the strains have not been

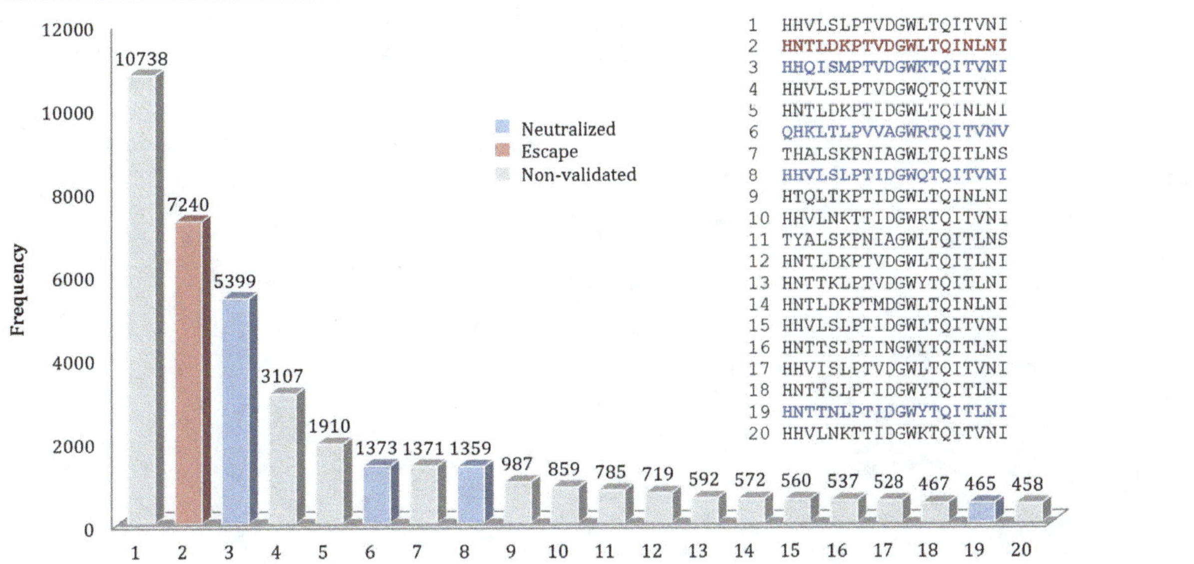

FIGURE 5 | Frequencies of top 20 discontinuous peptides (B-cell epitope of nAb F10) from the HA sequence dataset. FLU0243751 (A/Viet Nam/1203/2004) was used as reference HA sequence in the analysis of F10 B-cell epitopes. The corresponding positions of discontinuous peptides on FLU0243751 are: 24, 44, 46, 48, 304, 305, 306, 331, 360, 361, 362, 363, 380, 383, 384, 387, 391, 394, 395, and 398. Discontinuous peptides that were identical to neutralized motifs are shown in blue, while those identical to escape motifs are shown in red. The sequences of Top 20 most frequent discontinuous peptides are listed along with their validation status.

validated (**Figure 6A**). Viewed by the subtype, F10 neutralized coverage of subtypes H5, H8, H9, and H11 are higher (50–90%) than of H1 and H2 (5–20%), while the coverage of subtype H6 is negligible (8 in 1708 H6 sequences) (**Figure 6B**).

The motif coverage analysis within the 45,812 HA sequences was performed for all nAbs. For the nAbs with available cross-reactivity data, the motif coverages were different between the nAbs targeting the HA globular head and those targeting the stem part. The nAbs that bind stem normally have higher neutralized motif coverage than those that bind the globular head (**Figure 7**).

The motif coverage is shown as heat map for each subtype and each nAb (**Figure 8**). The nAbs (such as CR6261, CR9114, F10, and FI6v3) that target stem region are more cross-reactive – they cover more strains, and also more subtypes of influenza.

Table 4 | The number of different discontinuous peptides from B-cell epitopes of each nAb in the HA sequence dataset.

Neutralizing type	Neutralizing epitope regions		Neutralizing antibodies	Number of different discontinuous peptides
Influenza A virus				
	Head	Sa site	2D1	2,190
		Near RBS	1F1	2,887
			2G1	2,127
			8F8	2,885
			8M2	3,290
			C05	3,020
			CH65	2,727
			CH67	2,773
			S139/1	3,070
	Stem	F subdomain	39.29	983
			C179	755
			CR6261	658
			CR9114	663
			F10	589
			FI6v3	905
		Stem base	CR8020	620
Influenza B virus				
	Head base		CR8071	848

COMBINING OF NEUTRALIZING ANTIBODIES

For each sequence in the HA sequence dataset, 22 strings (discontinuous peptides) were extracted to represent 22 B-cell epitopes by all nAbs analyzed in this study. The majority (82.62%) of all strains in FLUKB have at least one discontinuous peptide that is identical to the validated neutralized motifs (**Table 5**). A small number (2.25%) of sequences can be neutralized by as many as seven nAbs.

Here, we propose a combination of nAbs, where a small number of nAbs can cover a large proportion of influenza strains. The nAbs FI6v3, F10, CR9114, and CR8071 (**Figure 9A**) were selected, and the neutralized coverage has increased from 18.91% (F10), 4.06% (CR8071), 43.89% (CR9114), and 58.44% (FI6v3) to 78.45% (**Figure 9B**) when these antibodies were combined. These nAbs also covered most subtypes of influenza A virus and both lineages in influenza B virus (**Figure 9C**).

DISCUSSION

This study presents an overview of binding specificities of reported nAbs, as well as an estimate of their neutralization and escape coverage (neutralization effectiveness) in more than 45,000 HA sequences available in FLUKB. The variety and frequency of discontinuous peptides within different B-cell epitopes have been analyzed in the HA data set. The results of the analysis of discontinuous peptides provide insights into further experimental design: strains with peptides that have high frequency among the strain populations should be given priority for experimental validation and their neutralizing status for specific nAbs.

Of note, additional sequence changes in HA outside the nAb epitope may result in either local or quaternary structural alterations that impacts antibody binding to the epitope *per se.*

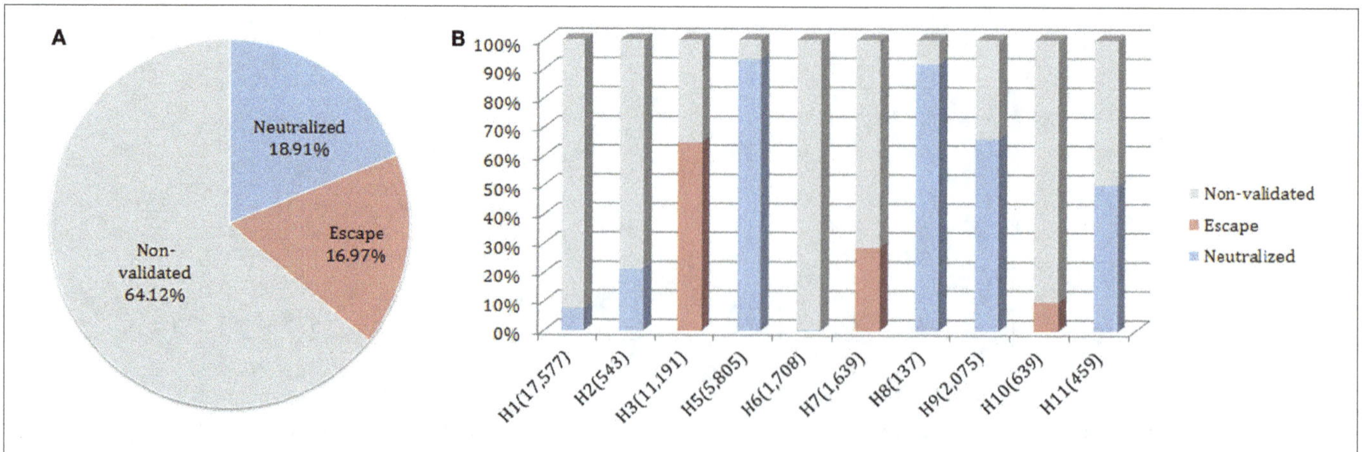

FIGURE 6 | Motif coverage for nAb F10. (A) The coverage of neutralized and escape discontinuous motifs, and non-validated discontinuous peptides within 45,812 HA sequences extracted from the FLUKB; **(B)** The motif coverage by subtype, the numbers in brackets indicate the number of sequence within the specific subtype (among 45,812 HA sequences).

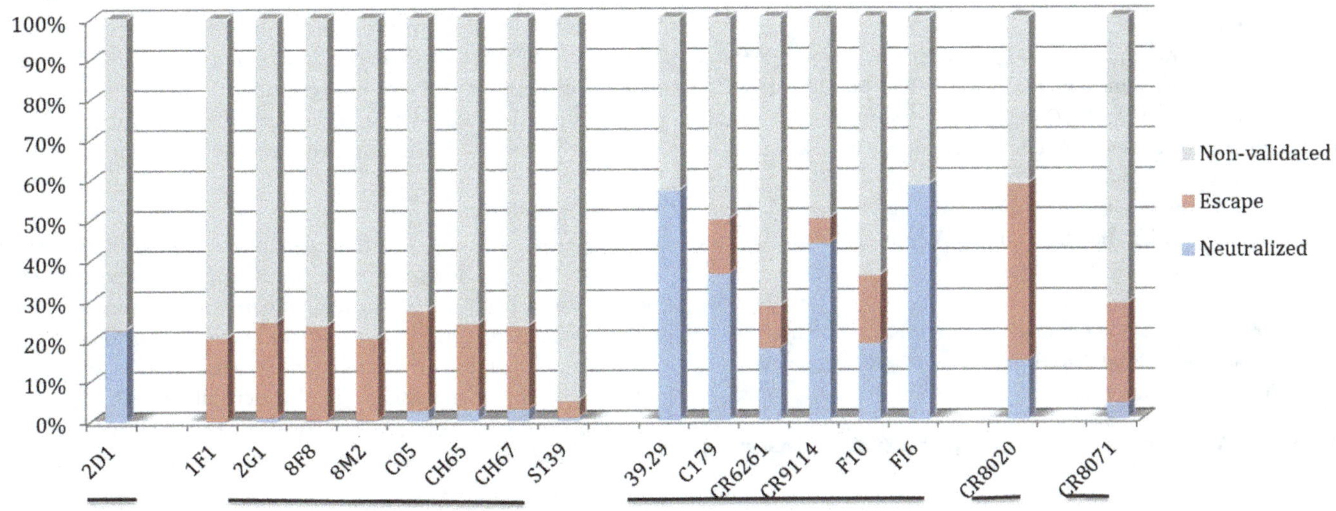

FIGURE 7 | Discontinuous motif coverage in the HA sequence dataset for cross-reactive nAbs. Only the coverage data for cross-reactive nAbs are shown here. The nAbs are grouped based on their binding locations and influenza types, from left to right: Sa site, near RBS, F subdomain, stem base on influenza A virus, and head base on influenza B virus.

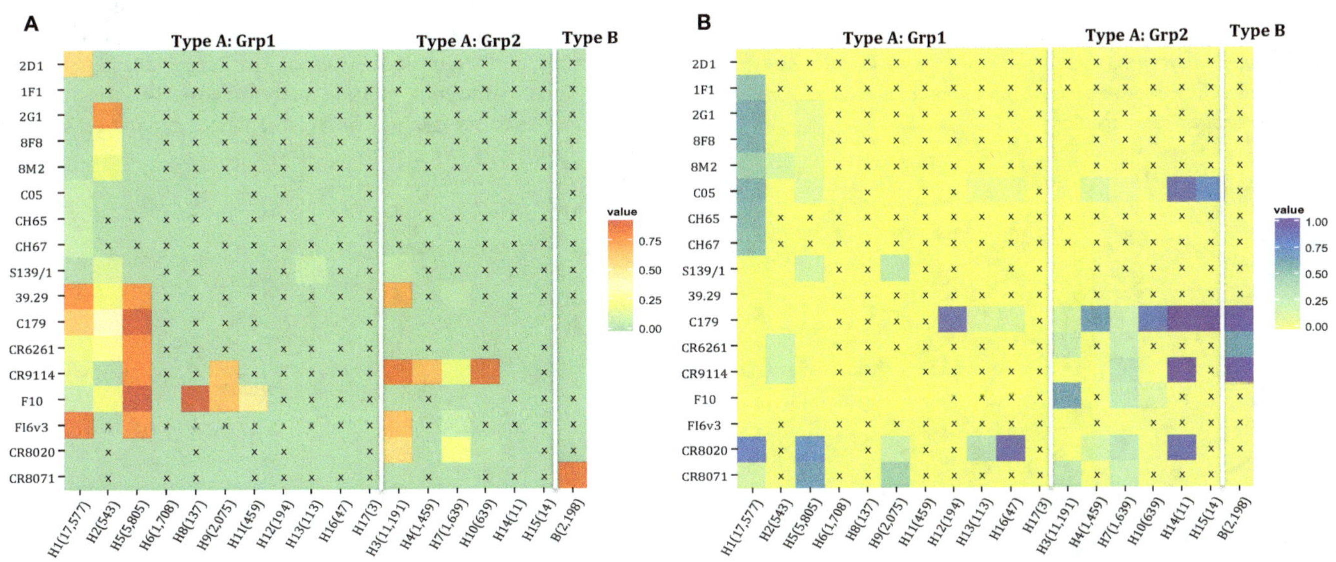

FIGURE 8 | The neutralized and escape motif coverage on each subtype within FLUKB of neutralizing antibodies. The heat map of **(A)** neutralized and **(B)** escape coverage are shown. Each cell on the grid represents coverage for a specific antibody (row name) on specific subtype (column name). The subtypes were sorted from Grp1 and Grp2 in influenza A virus, and influenza B virus. Different color schemes were used in order to differentiate neutralizing and escape coverage: from green to red/green to blue indicate rising neutralizing/escape coverage in HA sequence dataset. The boxes with symbol "X" indicate that no experimental validation data were available for this study.

Likewise, modification of glycosylation sites through sequence change may impact accessibility of antibodies to the neutralization site, creating discordance between sequence identity of binding site shown in BlockLogo and neutralization outcome between two strains of viruses sharing the same epitope sequence. The frequency of such occurrences will be important to determine. Neutralization assays of strains with discontinuous epitopes identical to validated B-cell epitopes will provide a proof of cross-neutralization. Since the experimental validation is time and money consuming, the introduction of extended B-cell epitope (see Supplementary Material) aims to help select representative sequences that differ in extended B-cell epitopes. For each proposed neutralizing or escape peptide (actual B-cell epitope), a small number of variants defined by changes in its environment (extended B-cell epitopes) constitute the majority of strains with the proposed peptide.

On the other hand, before more experimental data generated to fill the existing "non-validated gap," it will be meaningful to bring out some reasonable estimation. The assumption and methods in this paper are based on complete identity to discontinuous motifs on B-cell epitope (additionally extended B-cell epitope). To check the validity of this assumption, the similarity between discontinuous motifs and discontinuous peptides could be used to estimate and predict neutralization and binding results in the future. For example, a discontinuous peptide with mutated residues of similar feature to the neutralized motif would be considered as "possible neutralized peptide" against specific nAbs. These estimations could also be validated in experimental assays, and then be used to further experimental design iteratively.

Table 5 | Distribution of the number of neutralizing antibodies that share identical neutralized discontinuous motif with sequences within the HA sequence dataset.

Number of nAbs	Coverage in 45,812 HA dataset (%)
0	17.38
1	12.45
2	11.68
3	13.39
4	31.38
5	1.59
6	9.89
7	2.25

For each sequence within the 45,812 HA dataset, the number of nAbs that share identical neutralized motif was counted. The number of nAbs in our panel for any given influenza strain can range from 0 to 7.

CONCLUSION

Over the past few years, our understanding of nAbs and their responses against influenza HA have expanded tremendously. Besides the well-known HA head region interactions, an increasing number of characterized nAbs bind and neutralize influenza virus by targeting the more conserved stem regions. Among these stem-targeting nAbs, some show broadly neutralizing ability across subtypes/lineages, even across two groups in influenza A virus strains. However, the related experimental data for majority of nAbs are quite limited.

In sum, we have established a library of validated motifs (extracted from HA sequences in neutralized and escape strains) for each nAb. For any newly emerging strain, the cross-neutralization prediction can be made rapidly for existing nAbs and validation experiments can be designed judiciously. This study provides a method for investigation of cross-reactivity of nAbs against influenza viruses, but is directly applicable to any viral pathogen that has structurally characterized nAbs and a collection of variant sequences of the target antigen. Examples of such pathogens include orthomyxoviruses (influenza); flaviviruses such as dengue or West Nile; arenaviruses such as

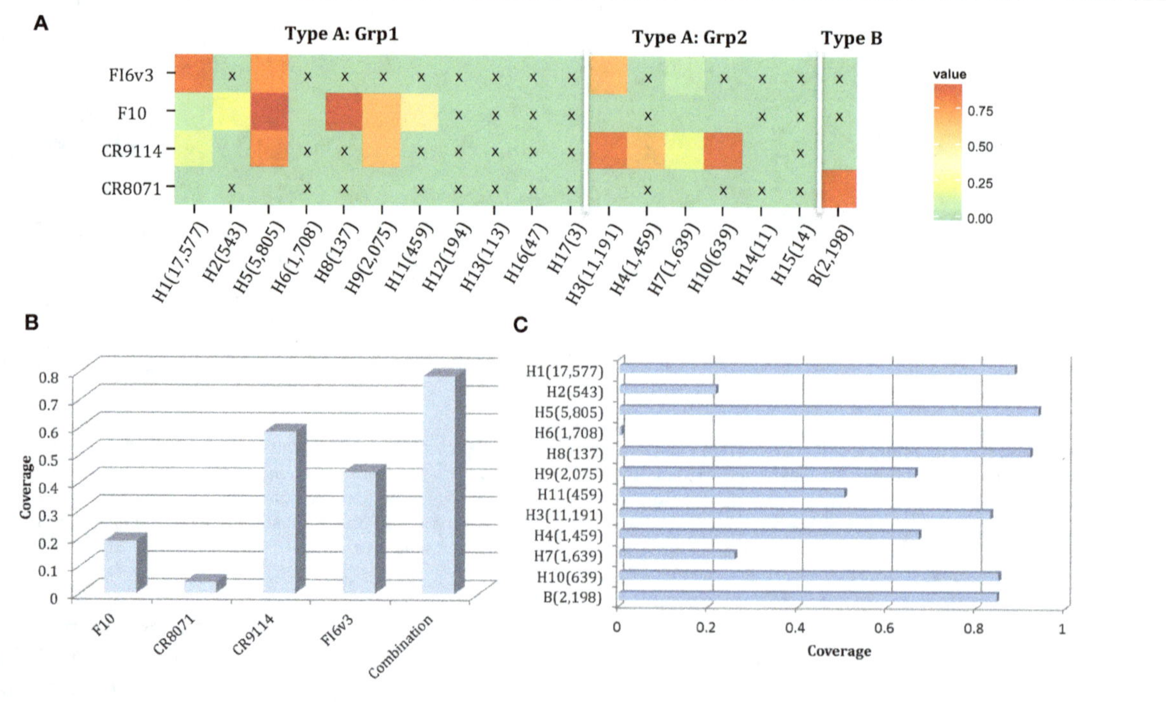

FIGURE 9 | A combination of four neutralizing subtype-diversified and potent neutralizing antibodies. (A) The heat map of the neutralized result for four nAbs, the color scheme is same as **Figure 8A**; **(B)** the neutralized coverage of four nAbs individually, and the combination of nAbs on HA dataset; and **(C)** the neutralizing result of combination of four nAbs by subtype. The subtypes were sorted from Grp1 and Grp2 in influenza A virus and influenza B virus. Only subtypes with neutralizing data are shown.

lymphocytic choriomeningitis virus and human immunodeficiency virus, among others. Insights from such bioinformatics analyses coupled with antibody antigenicity through crystallographic determinations will facilitate electronic neutralization profiling that can be tested empirically in subsequent laboratory neutralization assays.

ACKNOWLEDGMENTS

Jing Sun, Vladimir Brusic, and Ellis L. Reinherz acknowledge funding from NIH grant U01 AI 90043. Ulrich J. Kudahl was funded by Oticon Foundation, Otto Mønsted Foundation, Julie Dam's Stipend, Henry Shaws Stipend, and Reinholdt Jorcks Stipend. Christian Simon was funded by the Novo Scholarship Programme, Direktør Ib Henriksens Fond, and Augustinus Fonden.

REFERENCES

1. Thompson WW, Shay DK, Weintraub E, Brammer L, Cox N, Anderson LJ, et al. Mortality associated with influenza and respiratory syncytial virus in the United States. *JAMA* (2003) **289**(2):179–86. doi:10.1001/jama.289.2.179
2. Parvin JD, Moscona A, Pan WT, Leider JM, Palese P. Measurement of the mutation rates of animal viruses: influenza A virus and poliovirus type 1. *J Virol* (1986) **59**(2):377–83.
3. Fraser C, Donnelly CA, Cauchemez S, Hanage WP, Van Kerkhove MD, Hollingsworth TD, et al. Pandemic potential of a strain of influenza A (H1N1): early findings. *Science* (2009) **324**(5934):1557–61. doi:10.1126/science.1176062
4. Wiley DC, Skehel JJ. The structure and function of the hemagglutinin membrane glycoprotein of influenza virus. *Annu Rev Biochem* (1987) **56**:365–94. doi:10.1146/annurev.bi.56.070187.002053
5. Nakamura G, Chai N, Park S, Chiang N, Lin Z, Chiu H, et al. An in vivo human-plasmablast enrichment technique allows rapid identification of therapeutic influenza a antibodies. *Cell Host Microbe* (2013) **14**(1):93–103. doi:10.1016/j.chom.2013.06.004
6. Steel J, Lowen AC, Wang TT, Yondola M, Gao Q, Haye K, et al. Influenza virus vaccine based on the conserved hemagglutinin stalk domain. *MBio* (2010) **1**(1):e18–10. doi:10.1128/mBio.00018-10
7. Okuno Y, Isegawa Y, Sasao F, Ueda S. A common neutralizing epitope conserved between the hemagglutinins of influenza A virus H1 and H2 strains. *J Virol* (1993) **67**(5):2552–8.
8. Yoshida R, Igarashi M, Ozaki H, Kishida N, Tomabechi D, Kida H, et al. Cross-protective potential of a novel monoclonal antibody directed against antigenic site B of the hemagglutinin of influenza A viruses. *PLoS Pathog* (2009) **5**(3):e1000350. doi:10.1371/journal.ppat.1000350
9. Ueda M, Maeda A, Nakagawa N, Kase T, Kubota R, Takakura H, et al. Application of subtype-specific monoclonal antibodies for rapid detection and identification of influenza A and B viruses. *J Clin Microbiol* (1998) **36**(2):340–4.
10. Smirnov YA, Lipatov AS, Gitelman AK, Claas EC, Osterhaus AD. Prevention and treatment of bronchopneumonia in mice caused by mouse-adapted variant of avian H5N2 influenza A virus using monoclonal antibody against conserved epitope in the HA stem region. *Arch Virol* (2000) **145**(8):1733–41. doi:10.1007/s007050070088
11. Sakabe S, Iwatsuki-Horimoto K, Horimoto T, Nidom CA, Le M, Takano R, et al. A cross-reactive neutralizing monoclonal antibody protects mice from H5N1 and pandemic (H1N1) 2009 virus infection. *Antiviral Res* (2010) **88**(3):249–55. doi:10.1016/j.antiviral.2010.09.007
12. Ekiert DC, Wilson IA. Broadly neutralizing antibodies against influenza virus and prospects for universal therapies. *Curr Opin Virol* (2012) **2**(2):134–41. doi:10.1016/j.coviro.2012.02.005
13. Sui J, Hwang WC, Perez S, Wei G, Aird D, Chen LM, et al. Structural and functional bases for broad-spectrum neutralization of avian and human influenza A viruses. *Nat Struct Mol Biol* (2009) **16**(3):265–73. doi:10.1038/nsmb.1566
14. Corti D, Voss J, Gamblin SJ, Codoni G, Macagno A, Jarrossay D, et al. A neutralizing antibody selected from plasma cells that binds to group 1 and group 2 influenza A hemagglutinins. *Science* (2011) **333**(6044):850–6. doi:10.1126/science.1205669
15. Yamashita M, Krystal M, Fitch WM, Palese P. Influenza B virus evolution: co-circulating lineages and comparison of evolutionary pattern with those of influenza A and C viruses. *Virology* (1988) **163**(1):112–22. doi:10.1016/0042-6822(88)90238-3
16. Rota PA, Wallis TR, Harmon MW, Rota JS, Kendal AP, Nerome K. Cocirculation of two distinct evolutionary lineages of influenza type B virus since 1983. *Virology* (1990) **175**(1):59–68. doi:10.1016/0042-6822(90)90186-U
17. Dreyfus C, Laursen NS, Kwaks T, Zuijdgeest D, Khayat R, Ekiert DC, et al. Highly conserved protective epitopes on influenza B viruses. *Science* (2012) **337**(6100):1343–8. doi:10.1126/science.1222908
18. Huang J, Honda W. CED: a conformational epitope database. *BMC Immunol* (2006) **7**:7. doi:10.1186/1471-2172-7-7
19. Squires RB, Noronha J, Hunt V, Garcia-Sastre A, Macken C, Baumgarth N, et al. Influenza research database: an integrated bioinformatics resource for influenza research and surveillance. *Influenza Other Respir Viruses* (2012) **6**(6):404–16. doi:10.1111/j.1750-2659.2011.00331.x
20. Tsibane T, Ekiert DC, Krause JC, Martinez O, Crowe JE Jr, Wilson IA, et al. Influenza human monoclonal antibody 1F1 interacts with three major antigenic sites and residues mediating human receptor specificity in H1N1 viruses. *PLoS Pathog* (2012) **8**(12):e1003067. doi:10.1371/journal.ppat.1003067
21. Xu R, Ekiert DC, Krause JC, Hai R, Crowe JE Jr, Wilson IA. Structural basis of preexisting immunity to the 2009 H1N1 pandemic influenza virus. *Science* (2010) **328**(5976):357–60. doi:10.1126/science.1186430
22. Fleury D, Daniels RS, Skehel JJ, Knossow M, Bizebard T. Structural evidence for recognition of a single epitope by two distinct antibodies. *Proteins* (2000) **40**(4):572–8. doi:10.1002/1097-0134(20000901)40:4<572::AID-PROT30>3.3.CO;2-E
23. Ekiert DC, Kashyap AK, Steel J, Rubrum A, Bhabha G, Khayat R, et al. Cross-neutralization of influenza A viruses mediated by a single antibody loop. *Nature* (2012) **489**(7417):526–32. doi:10.1038/nature11414
24. Whittle JR, Zhang R, Khurana S, King LR, Manischewitz J, Golding H, et al. Broadly neutralizing human antibody that recognizes the receptor-binding pocket of influenza virus hemagglutinin. *Proc Natl Acad Sci U S A* (2011) **108**(34):14216–21. doi:10.1073/pnas.1111497108
25. Schmidt AG, Xu H, Khan AR, O'Donnell T, Khurana S, King LR, et al. Preconfiguration of the antigen-binding site during affinity maturation of a broadly neutralizing influenza virus antibody. *Proc Natl Acad Sci U S A* (2013) **110**(1):264–9. doi:10.1073/pnas.1218256109
26. Bizebard T, Gigant B, Rigolet P, Rasmussen B, Diat O, Bosecke P, et al. Structure of influenza virus haemagglutinin complexed with a neutralizing antibody. *Nature* (1995) **376**(6535):92–4. doi:10.1038/376092a0
27. Fleury D, Barrere B, Bizebard T, Daniels RS, Skehel JJ, Knossow M. A complex of influenza hemagglutinin with a neutralizing antibody that binds outside the virus receptor binding site. *Nat Struct Biol* (1999) **6**(6):530–4. doi:10.1038/9299
28. Barbey-Martin C, Gigant B, Bizebard T, Calder LJ, Wharton SA, Skehel JJ, et al. An antibody that prevents the hemagglutinin low pH fusogenic transition. *Virology* (2002) **294**(1):70–4. doi:10.1006/viro.2001.1320
29. Lee PS, Yoshida R, Ekiert DC, Sakai N, Suzuki Y, Takada A, et al. Heterosubtypic antibody recognition of the influenza virus hemagglutinin receptor binding site enhanced by avidity. *Proc Natl Acad Sci U S A* (2012) **109**(42):17040–5. doi:10.1073/pnas.1212371109
30. Dreyfus C, Ekiert DC, Wilson IA. Structure of a classical broadly neutralizing stem antibody in complex with a pandemic H2 influenza virus hemagglutinin. *J Virol* (2013) **87**(12):7149–54. doi:10.1128/JVI.02975-12
31. Throsby M, van den Brink E, Jongeneelen M, Poon LL, Alard P, Cornelissen L, et al. Heterosubtypic neutralizing monoclonal antibodies cross-protective against H5N1 and H1N1 recovered from human IgM+ memory B cells. *PLoS One* (2008) **3**(12):e3942. doi:10.1371/journal.pone.0003942
32. Ekiert DC, Bhabha G, Elsliger MA, Friesen RH, Jongeneelen M, Throsby M, et al. Antibody recognition of a highly conserved influenza virus epitope. *Science* (2009) **324**(5924):246–51. doi:10.1126/science.1171491

33. Ekiert DC, Friesen RH, Bhabha G, Kwaks T, Jongeneelen M, Yu W, et al. A highly conserved neutralizing epitope on group 2 influenza A viruses. *Science* (2011) **333**(6044):843–50. doi:10.1126/science.1204839
34. Sun X, Shi Y, Lu X, He J, Gao F, Yan J, et al. Bat-derived influenza hemagglutinin H17 does not bind canonical avian or human receptors and most likely uses a unique entry mechanism. *Cell Rep* (2013) **3**(3):769–78. doi:10.1016/j.celrep.2013.01.025
35. Larkin MA, Blackshields G, Brown NP, Chenna R, McGettigan PA, McWilliam H, et al. Clustal W and Clustal X version 2.0. *Bioinformatics* (2007) **23**(21):2947–8. doi:10.1093/bioinformatics/btm404
36. Page RD. TreeView: an application to display phylogenetic trees on personal computers. *Comput Appl Biosci* (1996) **12**(4):357–8.
37. Berman HM, Westbrook J, Feng Z, Gilliland G, Bhat TN, Weissig H, et al. The protein data bank. *Nucleic Acids Res* (2000) **28**(1):235–42. doi:10.1093/nar/28.1.235
38. Katz J, Hancock K, Veguilla V, Zhong W, Lu X, Sun H, et al. Serum cross-reactive antibody response to a novel influenza A (H1N1) virus after vaccination with seasonal influenza vaccine. *MMWR Morb Mortal Wkly Rep* (2009) **58**(19):521–4.
39. Stavitsky AB. Micromethods for the study of proteins and antibodies II. Specific applications of hemagglutination and hemagglutination-inhibition reactions with tannic acid and protein-treated red blood cells. *J Immunol* (1954) **72**(5):368–75.
40. Yu X, Tsibane T, McGraw PA, House FS, Keefer CJ, Hicar MD, et al. Neutralizing antibodies derived from the B cells of 1918 influenza pandemic survivors. *Nature* (2008) **455**(7212):532–6. doi:10.1038/nature07231
41. Krause JC, Tumpey TM, Huffman CJ, McGraw PA, Pearce MB, Tsibane T, et al. Naturally occurring human monoclonal antibodies neutralize both 1918 and 2009 pandemic influenza A (H1N1) viruses. *J Virol* (2010) **84**(6):3127–30. doi:10.1128/JVI.02184-09
42. Katoh K, Toh H. Recent developments in the MAFFT multiple sequence alignment program. *Brief Bioinform* (2008) **9**(4):286–98. doi:10.1093/bib/bbn013
43. Altschul SF, Madden TL, Schaffer AA, Zhang J, Zhang Z, Miller W, et al. Gapped BLAST and PSI-BLAST: a new generation of protein database search programs. *Nucleic Acids Res* (1997) **25**(17):3389–402. doi:10.1093/nar/25.17.3389
44. Hubbard SJ, Thornton JM. *Naccess. Computer Program.* (Vol. 2). London: Department of Biochemistry and Molecular Biology, University College London (1993).
45. McConkey BJ, Sobolev V, Edelman M. Discrimination of native protein structures using atom-atom contact scoring. *Proc Natl Acad Sci U S A* (2003) **100**(6):3215–20. doi:10.1073/pnas.0535768100
46. Krissinel E, Henrick K. Inference of macromolecular assemblies from crystalline state. *J Mol Biol* (2007) **372**(3):774–97. doi:10.1016/j.jmb.2007.05.022
47. Wilson IA, Skehel JJ, Wiley DC. Structure of the haemagglutinin membrane glycoprotein of influenza virus at 3 A resolution. *Nature* (1981) **289**(5796):366–73. doi:10.1038/289366a0
48. Crooks GE, Hon G, Chandonia JM, Brenner SE. WebLogo: a sequence logo generator. *Genome Res* (2004) **14**(6):1188–90. doi:10.1101/gr.849004
49. Olsen LR, Kudahl UJ, Simon C, Sun J, Schönbach C, Reinherz EL, et al. BlockLogo: Visualization of peptide and sequence motif conservation. *J Immunol Methods* (2013) **400**:37–44. doi:10.1016/j.jim.2013.08.014

20

The role of the innate immune system in ALS

Sudarshan Phani [1,2]**_, Diane Berengere Re_** [1,2] **_and Serge Przedborski_** [1,2]**_*_**

[1] *Department of Pathology and Cell Biology, Columbia University, New York, NY, USA*
[2] *Center for Motor Neuron Disease, Department of Neurology, Columbia University, New York, NY, USA*

Edited by:
Roger A. Barker, University of Cambridge and Addenbrooke' Hospital, UK

Reviewed by:
Raja S. Settivari, The Dow Chemical Company, USA
Kevin Talbot, Oxford University, UK

****Correspondence:***
Serge Przedborski, Department of Pathology, Cell Biology and Neurology, Center for Motor Neuron Disease, Columbia University, 630 West 168th Street, P&S 5-420 NY, USA.
e-mail: sp30@columbia.edu

Amyotrophic lateral sclerosis (ALS) is a fatal, adult-onset neurodegenerative disease that is characterized by the death of upper and lower motor neurons. Recent studies have made it clear that although motor neurons are the primary targets of the degenerative process, other cell types play key roles in the death of motor neurons. Most notably, cells of the immune system, including astrocytes and microglia have come under increasing scrutiny, after multiple lines of evidence have shown these cells to be deleterious to motor neurons. Both *in vitro* and *in vivo* experiments have shown that astrocytes and microglia containing mutated SOD1 are harmful to motor neurons. Several studies on ALS and other neurodegenerative diseases have revealed that reactive astrocytes and microglia are capable of releasing pro-inflammatory factors such as cytokines and chemokines, which are harmful to neighboring neurons. In addition, it is believed that diseased astrocytes can specifically kill motor neurons through the release of toxic factors. Furthermore, in an animal model of the disease, it has been shown that the reduction of SOD1 in microglia may be able to slow the progression of ALS symptoms. Although the exact pathways of motor neuron death in ALS have yet to be elucidated, studies have suggested that they die through aBax-dependent signaling pathway. Mounting evidence suggests that neuroinflammation plays an important role in the degeneration of motor neurons. Based on these findings, anti-inflammatory compounds are currently being tested for their potential to reduce disease severity; however, these studies are only in the preliminary stages. While we understand that astrocytes and microglia play a role in the death of motor neurons in ALS, much work needs to be done to fully understand ALS pathology and the role the immune system plays in disease onset and progression.

Keywords: amyotrophic lateral sclerosis, astrocyte, microglia, motor neuron, innate immune system

INTRODUCTION

Amyotrophic Lateral Sclerosis (ALS) is a fatal adult-onset neurodegenerative disorder that is characterized clinically by muscle weakness and wasting. Pathologically, it is identified by the degeneration of upper and lower motor neurons (Boillee et al., 2006a). Generally, death results from respiratory failure due to paralysis of the respiratory muscles. The incidence of ALS is reported to be between 1.5 and 3 per 100,000 in Europe and North America (Wijesekera and Leigh, 2009; Hardiman et al., 2011). ALS onset peaks between the ages of 50–75 and declines thereafter. These factors suggest that ALS may not be a disease of aging, but rather that age may be one of a multitude of contributing factors (Hardiman et al., 2011). Thus far, there are no effective treatments and no cure for ALS.

Amyotrophic lateral sclerosis is essentially a sporadic disorder, with greater than 90% of the cases originating from an unknown cause. However, approximately 10% of the cases are considered familial (FALS) and are generally inherited as a dominant disorder (Ince et al., 2011) due to mutations in a number of seemingly disparate genes. These include, but are not limited to, mutations in genes such as TAR DNA binding protein (TDP)-43 and Fused in Sarcoma (FUS) (Sreedharan et al., 2008; Kwiatkowski et al., 2009; Vance et al., 2009). Despite major enthusiasm by the research community about the recent discoveries of mutations in FUS and TDP-43, the best characterized form of FALS still remains that which is linked to mutations in the copper-zinc superoxide dismutase gene (SOD1) and which accounts for 10–20% of all FALS cases (Andersen, 2001). Myriad mutations in SOD1 all seem to give rise to an ALS phenotype via a toxic gain-of-function mechanism, which is clinically almost indistinguishable from sporadic cases. Histopathologically, however, recent studies have found TDP-43 to be a reliable marker for differentiating sALS from SOD1-related fALS. These studies have shown that all of the cases of sporadic ALS and SOD1-negative fALS had neural and glial inclusions which were immunoreactive for both ubiquitin and TDP-43, whereas fALS cases with mutations in SOD1 were universally absent of TDP-43 immunoreactivity (MacKenzie et al., 2007; Tan et al., 2007).

More recently, studies have identified an expanded GGGGCC hexanucleotide repeat in a non-coding region of C9ORF72. This expansion has been shown to be linked to chromosome 9p-linked FTD and ALS. Interestingly, this same repeat expansion was also identified in the majority of families with a combined FTD/ALS phenotype and TDP-43 pathology. Extended studies have identified the C9ORF72 expansion as the most common genetic abnormality in fALS (23.5%; DeJesus-Hernandez et al., 2011).

A number of studies have pointed to oxidative stress, protein aggregation, or mitochondrial dysfunction as mechanisms of mutant SOD1 toxicity. In addition, SOD1 toxicity has been shown to be linked to changes in the immune system, which has also been shown to contribute to the motor neuron pathology seen in ALS; however, the exact nature of the pathogenic mechanisms provoking motor neuron degeneration in mutant SOD1-linked ALS remains elusive (Ince et al., 2011). Interestingly, the repeat expansion in C9ORF72 results in the formation of nuclear RNA foci not seen in SOD1-linked pathology, suggesting multiple disease mechanisms (DeJesus-Hernandez et al., 2011).

While the discovery of the C9ORF72 repeat expansion has opened new avenues of ALS research, the abundance and well-studied nature of SOD1-mutant animals make them the *de facto* models of choice to study ALS pathology for the time being. Although imperfect, these models allow for a great deal of insight into potential mechanisms involved in ALS pathology, with the hope that the mechanisms elucidated through the use of these models may also provide understanding of sALS and non-SOD1-mediated fALS.

INFLAMMATION AND NEURODEGENERATION

Although ALS is a disease primarily affecting upper and lower motor neurons, it is increasingly recognized that the entire pathogenic process of ALS is not restricted to a set of cell-autonomous deleterious mechanisms taking place within motor neurons. Instead, it is now believed that non-cell autonomous mechanisms, such as neuroinflammation may also contribute to the disease process.

Germane to this issue is the fact that the immune system has been found to be altered in sporadic ALS. Studies have shown immunological differences in the blood of ALS patients compared to healthy controls. These include increased levels of CD4+ cells, and reduced CD8+ T-lymphocytes (Mantovani et al., 2009). Interestingly, blood samples analyzed from patients at an earlier and less severe stage of the disease also show altered expression of immune cells, such as significant reductions in CD4+CD25+ T-regulatory (T-reg) cells as well as CD14+ monocytes (Mantovani et al., 2009). Additionally, T-reg cells have been shown to play significant roles as neuroprotectants responsible for modulating the neuroinflammatory response in mouse models of neurodegeneration (Kipnis et al., 2004). It is therefore possible to hypothesize that the reduction of T-reg cells in the blood of sporadic ALS patients might represent a recruitment of these cells from the periphery into the CNS in order to activate resident innate immune cells such as microglia, as well as anti-inflammatory cytokines such as interleukin-10 and transforming growth factor-β in an effort to protect the area most affected by the early effects of ALS degeneration (Kipnis et al., 2004; Mantovani et al., 2009).

Markers for resident innate immune cells have also been found to be altered in the brains of ALS patients as well as in animal models of ALS. For instance, immunostaining for glial fibrillary acid protein (GFAP), a common marker for astrocytes, is markedly increased in all forms of ALS in the precentral gyrus of human samples (Kawamata et al., 1992). In addition, staining for leukocyte common antigen (LCA), lymphocyte function associate molecule-1 (LFA-1), and complement receptors CR3 (CD11b) and CR4 (CD11c) are increased, supporting the idea that microglia and macrophages are activated in the areas of ALS degeneration, such as the motor cortex, brainstem, and corticospinal tract (Kawamata et al., 1992; Papadimitriou et al., 2010). Remarkably, it is believed that the early site of pathological changes in ALS is the neuromuscular junction, and while this particular site of the lower motor neuron pathway has been extensively studied, very little information exists about the immune response at that level. Nonetheless, the data reviewed above provide compelling evidence that a robust neuroinflammatory response is part of the neuropathological changes that characterize ALS. However, none of the aforementioned studies address the actual role, if any, of neuroinflammation in ALS. Investigations in other neurodegenerative disorders have shown that neuroinflammation may exert dual effects, that it can be protective or harmful. In order to distinguish between these two possibilities, efforts have generally concentrated on studying animal models of ALS.

The blood brain barrier renders the brain as immune-privileged, therefore, the brain contains resident astrocytes and microglia that perform the duties of immune surveillance and act as an innate response system. Reactive astrocytes are most commonly recruited to the site of an injury, such as a spinal cord injury or ischemic events. Their main functions are to compact inflammatory cells, and to re-establish the blood brain barrier (Okada et al., 2006) they may also be involved in clearing CNS debris, such as amyloid plaques (Papadimitriou et al., 2010). Aside from astrocytes, the CNS immune system also consists of ramified resting microglial cells, whose processes play an active role in maintaining the homeostasis of the neural environment. Once activated by the presence of antigens and during times of distress, such as is the case during neurodegeneration, microglia, like other immune cells, become activated taking on an ameboid morphology. Once activated, microglia can secrete a myriad of neurotrophic factors and cytokines (Napoli and Neumann, 2009), and engage in the clearance of pathogens and debris through phagocytosis. However, unregulated activation of microglial activation may be harmful to neurons through the release of potentially harmful neurotoxins including quinolinic acid, reactive oxygen and nitrogen species (ROS; RNS), and pro-inflammatory cytokines. Although a large number of studies have shown that microglia and, to a lesser extent, astrocytes are activated in the affected areas of the CNS in ALS, thus far little attention has been paid to the determination of the actual phenotype of these cells. For instance, since activated resident immune cells can display either a pro-inflammatory or anti-inflammatory phenotype, sometimes referred to as M1 or M2, it will be critical to determine which phenotype they exhibit as a whole, and if possible as individual cells. It is also important to determine whether such profiles differ among the various affected structures of the CNS and stages of the disease. Aside from these outstanding questions, it is also critical to elucidate whether these inflammatory cells play a role in the pathogenesis of ALS. The use of animal models is greatly aiding in the attempts to answer the questions raised by the findings described above.

The most commonly studied animal models of ALS are rats and mice expressing mutant SOD1 (mSOD1). Although, as indicated above, SOD 1 mutations only account for a small percentage of human cases, animal models using mSOD1 are used with the hope that the mechanisms leading the disease are shared across cases, and knowledge gained from these models can be used to understand the development of the disease in humans. Notably, evidence for increases in astrocytes and microglia have also been found in transgenic mice expressing different forms of mutant SOD1 (mSOD1), supporting human pathology studies (Fischer et al., 2004). Specifically, GFAP and CD11b staining showed evidence for significant increases in reactive astrocytes and microglia in the motor regions of transgenic mice containing mSOD1 (Fischer et al., 2004). Although both astrocytosis and microgliosis have been observed in rodent models, the timing of events seems to be unclear. Some studies using mSOD1 mice have suggested astrocytosis to be an early stage event, with microgliosis as a late stage reaction (Yang et al., 2011). However, others have suggested that microglial response occurs at a much earlier stage of the disease (Sanagi et al., 2010). Nevertheless, it does appear that microglial activation starts after motor neuron degeneration, and initially tries to protect motor neurons from degeneration (Fischer et al., 2004; Henkel et al., 2009).

IMMUNE CELL MEDIATED NON-CELL AUTONOMY IN ALS

Motor neuron death and degeneration has been implicated in causing the debilitating symptoms characteristic of ALS, however, mounting evidence indicates that motor neuron death is, at least in part, non-cell autonomous. *In vivo* studies have shown that mSOD1 expressed only in motor neurons of transgenic mice is either not sufficient to cause neurodegeneration or causes only a mild ALS-like phenotype (Jaarsma et al., 2008). Support for non-cell autonomy comes from studies showing that when mSOD1 expression was reduced in microglia and macrophages in transgenic mice (Boillee et al., 2006b; Wang et al., 2009), motor neuron degeneration was decreased. Aside from microglia, evidence has shown that astrocytes may also play a role in motor neuron death. Early studies using transgenic mice expressing mSOD1 in astrocytes suggested the need for motor neurons to be impaired for a degenerative phenotype (Gong et al., 2000), however more recent studies have concluded that astrocytes expressing mSOD1 released toxic factor(s) which were sufficient to cause motor neuron degeneration in an *in vitro* model of ALS (Nagai et al., 2007).

THE ROLE OF ASTROCYTES IN ALS NON-CELL AUTONOMY

Astrocytes are one of the main cell types responsible for the clearance of potentially excitotoxic glutamate from the synaptic space, and as mentioned earlier, play a distinct role when they become activated by the immune system. Quite interestingly, glutamate handling has been reported to be modified in both sporadic and familial ALS (Boillee et al., 2006a). Studies have found that brain and spinal cord samples from ALS patients showed altered glutamate transport (Rothstein et al., 1992) resulting from changes in the glutamate transporter EAAT2 (Maragakis et al., 2004). Evidence suggests that EAAT2 is significantly decreased in the motor cortex and spinal cords of ALS patients (Fray et al., 1998), as well as in the spinal cords of mSOD1 transgenic mice (Bruijn et al., 1997) and rats (Howland et al., 2002). It should come as no coincidence then, that astrocytes were quickly targeted for their role in the ALS disease processes.

More interestingly in terms of inflammation, samples analyzed from the brains and spinal cords of ALS patients were found to contain greater numbers of activated or reactive astrocytes, a clear sign of an immune response (Sta et al., 2011). Of note, and useful for research purposes, increased reactive astrocyte expression has been found both in ALS patients and in animal models of ALS (Sta et al., 2011).

Although the main function of astrocytes in the synaptic space is the maintenance of a homeostatic environment for neurons though activities such as the clearance of neurotransmitters, reactive astrocytes gain properties that resting astrocytes do not exhibit. It has been shown that during and after injury, astrocytes have the ability to ameliorate symptoms by physically isolating the injured area through the formation of a glial scar, as well as release neurotrophins and growth factors such as IGF-1 which have been deemed beneficial to injured cells (Dong and Benveniste, 2001). Astrocytes have also been found to release NGF and induce additional sprouting both *in vitro* and *in vivo*, a key step in neuronal recovery (Chalmers et al., 1996; Wu et al., 1998).

Even though astrocytes do have the potential to be beneficial to neurons, the majority of evidence suggests that astrocytes actually contribute to neuronal degeneration during disease, with ALS being no exception. Interestingly, NGF release, which has generally been regarded as a positive attribute of reactive astrocytes, has been shown to directly lead to motor neuron apoptosis through the p75 pathway (Pehar et al., 2004). Notably, mSOD1-containing astrocytes have been found to be even more toxic to their environments than reactive astrocytes alone. Studies have found that reducing mSOD1 expressing astrocyte levels in an *in vivo* model of ALS decreased motor neuron degeneration and correspondingly increased the life span of the affected animals (Lepore et al., 2008; Barbeito et al., 2010). Although the exact mechanisms for astrocyte-mediated motor neuron toxicity is not known, several lines of evidence have pointed to the activation and release of toxic or harmful products such as pro-inflammatory cytokine oxidative stressors. These include, but are not limited to prostaglandins, leukotrienes, and RNS (Hensley et al., 2006a,b). In addition, *in vitro* models of ALS have shown that astrocytes containing mSOD1 release toxic factors that are preferentially toxic to motor neurons. Furthermore, it was noted that even wild-type motor neurons die in the presence of mSOD1-containing astrocytes. Moreover, wild-type motor neurons die when grown in media conditioned by mSOD1 containing astrocytes. These *in vitro* studies have suggested the pro-apoptotic Bax pathway as another mechanism through which astrocytes mediate motor neuron cell death (Nagai et al., 2007).

THE ROLE OF MICROGLIA IN ALS

Microglial cells perform the duties of immune surveillance in the CNS, and once activated, such as is the case during neurodegeneration, these cells secrete cytokines and neurotrophins in order to help restore homeostasis to the neuronal environment (Napoli and Neumann, 2009). However, just as astrocytes may play a deleterious role in ALS, microglia have also been found to exacerbate neuronal injury. *In vivo* studies have shown that microglial cells increase their expression and release of pro-inflammatory cytokines, such as TNF-α and IL-1β in a mouse model of ALS. Additionally, activated microglia have been shown to promote the generation of reactive oxidative species, causing more harm than good to motor neurons (Henkel et al., 2009).

In the case of ALS, a number of studies have looked at mSOD1 expression in microglia, and its effect on ALS disease progression and motor neuron degeneration. Recent studies have found that diminishing mSOD1 levels in microglia in a mouse model of ALS did not alter the age of onset of paralysis, however it was able to significantly slow the disease progression (Boillee et al., 2006b). Yet, the lack of effects on onset must be regarded with caution, as one cannot exclude that the reduction in mSOD1 in microglia was only at the time when some actual motor neuron degeneration has already occurred. Indeed, the technology used in this study to reduce mSOD1 expression was driven by the microglial specific promoter CD11b which only acquires significant driving forces in response to pathological stimuli such as motor neuron degeneration. Accordingly, it would not be surprising that the disease phenotype in these mice has only been modified after the onset of motor neuron degeneration. It has also been found that mSOD1 containing microglia produce and release greater levels of pro-inflammatory cytokines and free radicals than their wild-type counterparts (Henkel et al., 2009). While the presence of mSOD1 in microglia has been shown to be deleterious, new evidence has begun to pinpoint the mechanisms that may control ALS-related microglial toxicity. Specifically, increases in the pro-inflammatory cytokines and prostaglandin E_2 have been reported to be present in ALS patients (Papadimitriou et al., 2010). Additionally, *in vitro* data suggested that conditioned media obtained from activated microglia is sufficient to cause neuronal degeneration through the concurrent stimulation of TNF-α and NMDA receptors. These pathways are thought to up-regulate inducible nitric oxide synthase activity, thus causing oxidative stress which leads to cell death. Of note is the fact that activation of either the TNF-α or NMDA receptor alone was not found to cause cell death, and the blockade of either of these receptor pathways was found to alleviate cell death caused by microglial-conditioned media, suggesting that both of these receptors need to be activated for MN death to occur (Moisse and Strong, 2006).

Although there is compelling evidence supporting the notion that microglial activation could be sufficient to kill motor neurons in ALS, *in vivo* studies have cast doubt on this theory by showing that repopulating microglial-deficient mice with mSOD-containing microglia failed to cause motor neuron death. These studies have yet to be repeated (Boillee et al., 2006a,b). In addition, studies done in mSOD1 mice absent in TNF-α, a potent inflammatory signaling molecule, did not show any decrease in motor neuron death (Gowing et al., 2006). These data are perhaps suggestive of alternate inflammatory pathways, and may implicate inflammatory mechanisms as coincidental, but not causative.

When viewed together, mounting *in vitro* and *in vivo* evidence have given credence to the toxic effects of astrocytes and microglia on motor neurons and have suggested multiple mechanisms that may be involved. In addition to these, it must be noted that mSOD1 containing motor neurons are particularly vulnerable to Fas ligand and NO-triggered cell death (Moisse and Strong, 2006). Therefore, it is thought that the combined effects of mSOD1 in motor neurons as well as in neighboring astrocytes and microglia are what ultimately result in cell death and degeneration in ALS. While the discovery of the expansion repeat in C9ORF72 is too recent to know its relationship with the inflammatory system, it would be conceivable that the immune system response to such a widespread mutation would be equal to or greater than what has already been observed in other forms of ALS.

ANTI-INFLAMMATORY THERAPEUTICS IN ALS

With inflammation potentially playing a significant role in ALS pathogenesis and progression, it is logical to attempt anti-inflammatory drugs for use as therapeutics in combating ALS. Using SOD1 mice, a number of groups have attempted to administer COX2 inhibitors such as cyclosporine, thalidomide, and lenalidomide to COX2-deficient mice in order to attenuate the negative effects of inflammation. Interestingly, the use of these drugs in mSOD1 animal models was sufficient to prolong lifespan (Karlsson et al., 2004; Kiaei et al., 2006). Cyclosporine is currently in clinical trials. Initial double-blind, placebo-controlled clinical trials suggest that men may benefit from cyclosporine administration when given within 18 months of initial diagnosis (Appel et al., 1988). Based on these results, the group of Karlsson et al. are currently running Phase II clinical trials.

Another approach to anti-inflammatory therapy was the use of the drug Copaxone, which has most often been used to treat patients diagnosed with multiple sclerosis. The active ingredient, glatiramer acetate, was used both in animal models as well as clinical trials. While there was initial excitement for the drug, which increased survival in mSOD1 mouse models of ALS (Angelov et al., 2003), these results could not be replicated (Turner and Talbot, 2008). Clinical trials with glatiramer acetate were also unsuccessful (Meininger et al., 2009), suggesting the mouse strain or the delivery mechanism in the original study may have played a greater role than initially indicated.

Perhaps the most well-known of the anti-inflammatory compounds used against ALS is minocycline, a second-generation tetracycline which has been shown to have anti-inflammatory properties (Yrjanheikki et al., 1999). The use of minocycline was shown to delay motor neuron degeneration as well as increase survival in several different mSOD1 mouse models of ALS (Kriz et al., 2002; Zhu et al., 2002). These studies found that minocycline may have had a direct impact on motor neurons by decreasing apoptosis through a reduction in cytochrome *c* release (Zhu et al., 2002; Moisse and Strong, 2006). Furthermore, it may have decreased the level of microglial activation and proliferation in mSOD1 mouse models of ALS (Kriz et al., 2002; Moisse and Strong, 2006). Given these promising results, minocycline was moved into clinical trials, and thus far, no observable difference was found between placebo and drug cohorts in phase III trials (Barbeito et al., 2010).

It should be noted however, that the use of anti-inflammatory drugs in animal models does not lead to direct knowledge of drug dosing and further study may be needed in order to find correct dosing levels, and potentially more importantly, dosing schedules. The use of animal models allows researchers to administer therapeutics before, during, after, or any combination therein relative to symptom onset. Unfortunately, patients being treated for neurodegenerative disorders do not have the luxury of being pre-treated for ALS symptoms before they arise, thus vastly complicating any therapeutic regimen.

CONCLUSION

Recent lines of evidence have given strong support to the role of astrocytes and microglia in ALS disease pathology. Tissue samples from ALS patients have been found to contain increased inflammatory by-products, and animal models of ALS have corroborated these increases. There is some debate as to whether inflammation in ALS could potentially be protective, however most studies have found the activation of microglia and astrocytes to be more harmful than beneficial. These harmful effects may come through the up-regulation and increased release of pro-inflammatory cytokines and reactive oxidative species, as well as through decreased uptake of excitotoxic neurotransmitters such as glutamate from the synaptic space. One major unanswered question, however, is whether an external event causes neuroinflammatory activation leading to ALS, or whether an external event leads to ALS causing neuroinflammation. In either case, both ALS pathology and neuroinflammation seem to act concurrently to exacerbate the symptoms of neurodegeneration. Future therapies to combat motor neuron death may involve a combination of approaches which recognize the role of multiple mechanisms and cell types in the progression of ALS.

REFERENCES

1. Andersen, P. M. (2001). Genetics of sporadic ALS. *Amyotroph. Lateral Scler. Other Motor Neuron Disord.* 2(Suppl. 1), S37–S41.
2. Angelov, D. N., Waibel, S., Guntinas- Lichius, O., Lenzen, M., Neiss, W. F., Tomov, T. L., Yoles, E., Kipnis, J., Schori, H., Reuter, A., Ludolph, A., and Schwartz, M. (2003). Thera- peutic vaccine for acute and chronic motor neuron diseases: implications for amyotrophic lateral sclerosis. *Proc. Natl. Acad. Sci. U.S.A.* 100, 4790–4795.
3. Appel, S. H., Stewart, S. S., Appel, V., Harati, Y., Mietlowski, W., Weiss, W., and Belendiuk, G. W. (1988). A double-blind study of the effective- ness of cyclosporine in amyotrophic lateral sclerosis. *Arch. Neurol.* 45, 381–386.
4. Barbeito, A. G., Mesci, P., and Boillee, S. (2010). Motor neuron-immune interactions: the vicious circle of ALS. *J. Neural Transm.* 117, 981–1000.
5. Boillee, S., Vande Velde, C., and Cleve- land, D. W. (2006a). ALS: a dis- ease of motor neurons and their nonneuronal neighbors. *Neuron* 52, 39–59.
6. Boillee, S., Yamanaka, K., Lobsiger, C. S., Copeland, N. G., Jenkins, N. A., Kassiotis, G., Kollias, G., and Cleveland, D. W. (2006b). Onset and progres- sion in inherited ALS determined by motor neurons and microglia. *Science* 312, 1389–1392.
7. Bruijn, L. I., Becher, M. W., Lee, M. K., Anderson, K. L., Jenkins, N. A., Copeland, N. G., Sisodia, S. S., Roth- stein, J. D., Borchelt, D. R., Price, D. L., and Cleveland, D. W. (1997). ALS- linked SOD1 mutant G85R mediates damage to astrocytes and pro- motes rapidly progressive disease with SOD1-containing inclusions. *Neuron* 18, 327–338.
8. Chalmers, G. R., Peterson, D. A., and Gage, F. H. (1996). Sprouting adult CNS cholinergic axons express NILE and associate with astrocytic sur- faces expressing neural cell adhe- sion molecule. *J. Comp. Neurol.* 371, 287–299.
9. DeJesus-Hernandez, M., MacKenzie, I. R., Boeve, B. F., Boxer, A. L., Baker, M., Rutherford, N. J., Nicholson, A. M., Finch, N. A., Flynn, H., Adam- son, J., Kouri, N., Wojtas, A., Sengdy, P., Hsiung, G. Y., Karydas, A., Seeley, W. W., Josephs, K. A., Coppola, G., Geschwind, D. H., Wszolek, Z. K., Feldman, H., Knopman, D. S., Petersen, R. C., Miller, B. L., Dickson,
10. D. W., Boylan, K. B., Graff-Radford, N. R., and Rademakers, R. (2011). Expanded GGGGCC hexanu- cleotide repeat in noncoding region of C9ORF72 causes chromosome 9p-linked FTD and ALS. *Neuron* 72, 245–256.
11. Dong, Y., and Benveniste, E. N. (2001). Immune function of astrocytes. *Glia* 36, 180–190.
12. Fischer, L. R., Culver, D. G., Ten- nant, P., Davis, A. A., Wang, M., Castellano-Sanchez, A., Khan, J., Polak, M. A., and Glass, J. D. (2004). Amyotrophic lateral sclero- sis is a distal axonopathy: evidence in mice and man. *Exp. Neurol.* 185, 232–240.
13. Fray, A. E., Ince, P. G., Banner, S. J., Milton, I. D., Usher, P. A., Cook- son, M. R., and Shaw, P. J. (1998). The expression of the glial gluta- mate transporter protein EAAT2 in motor neuron disease: an immuno- histochemical study. *Eur. J. Neurosci.* 10, 2481–2489.
14. Gong, Y. H., Parsadanian, A. S., Andreeva, A., Snider, W. D., and Elliott, J. L. (2000). Restricted expression of G86R Cu/Zn superox- ide dismutase in astrocytes results in astrocytosis but does not cause motoneuron degeneration. *J. Neu- rosci.* 20, 660–665.
15. Gowing, G., Dequen, F., Soucy, G., and Julien, J. P. (2006). Absence of tumor necrosis factor-alpha does not affect motor neuron disease caused by superoxide dismutase 1 mutations. *J. Neurosci.* 26, 11397–11402.
16. Hardiman, O., Van Den Berg, L. H., and Kiernan, M. C. (2011). Clinical diagnosis and management of amy- otrophic lateral sclerosis. *Nat. Rev. Neurol.* 7, 639–649.
17. Henkel, J. S., Beers, D. R., Zhao, W., and Appel, S. H. (2009). Microglia in ALS: the good, the bad, and the resting. *J. Neuroimmune Pharmacol.* 4, 389–398.
18. Hensley, K., Abdel-Moaty, H., Hunter, J., Mhatre, M., Mou, S., Nguyen, K., Potapova, T., Pye, Q. N., Qi, M., Rice, H., Stewart, C., Stroukoff, K., and West, M. (2006a). Primary glia expressing the G93A-SOD1 muta- tion present a neuroinflammatory phenotype and provide a cellular system for studies of glial inflamma- tion. *J. Neuroinflammation* 3, 2.
19. Hensley, K., Mhatre, M., Mou, S., Pye, Q. N., Stewart, C., West, M., and Williamson, K. S. (2006b). On the relation of oxidative stress to neuroinflammation: lessons learned from the G93A-SOD1 mouse model of amyotrophic lateral sclerosis. *Antioxid. Redox Signal.* 8, 2075–2087.
20. Howland, D. S., Liu, J., She, Y., Goad, B., Maragakis, N. J., Kim, B., Erick- son, J., Kulik, J., Devito, L., Psaltis, G., Degennaro, L. J., Cleveland, D. W., and Rothstein, J. D. (2002). Focal loss of the glutamate transporter EAAT2 in a transgenic rat model of SOD1 mutant-mediated amyotrophic lat- eral sclerosis (ALS). *Proc. Natl. Acad. Sci. U.S.A.* 99, 1604–1609.
21. Ince, P. G., Highley, J. R., Kirby, J., Whar- ton, S. B., Takahashi, H., Strong, M. J., and Shaw, P. J. (2011). Molecu- lar pathology and genetic advances in amyotrophic lateral sclerosis: an emerging molecular pathway and the significance of glial pathology. *Acta Neuropathol.* 122, 657–671.
22. Jaarsma, D., Teuling, E., Haasdijk, E. D., De Zeeuw, C. I., and Hoogen- raad, C. C. (2008). Neuron-specific expression of mutant superoxide dismutase is sufficient to induce amyotrophic lateral sclerosis in transgenic mice. *J. Neurosci.* 28, 2075–2088.
23. Karlsson, J., Fong, K. S., Hansson, M. J., Elmer, E., Csiszar, K., and Keep, F. (2004). Life span extension and reduced neuronal death after weekly intraventricular cyclosporin injections in the G93A transgenic mouse model of amyotrophic lateral sclerosis. *J. Neurosurg.* 101, 128–137.
24. Kawamata, T., Akiyama, H., Yamada, T., and McGeer, P. L. (1992). Immunologic reactions in amyotrophic lat- eral sclerosis brain and spinal cord tissue. *Am. J. Pathol.* 140, 691–707.
25. Kiaei, M., Petri, S., Kipiani, K., Gardian, G., Choi, D. K., Chen, J., Calingasan,
26. Y., Schafer, P., Muller, G. W., Stew- art, C., Hensley, K., and Beal, M. F. (2006). Thalidomide and lenalido- mide extend survival in a transgenic mouse model of amyotrophic lateral sclerosis. *J. Neurosci.* 26, 2467–2473.
27. Kipnis, J., Avidan, H., Caspi, R. R., and Schwartz, M. (2004). Dual effect of CD4+CD25+ regulatory T cells in neurodegeneration: a dialogue with microglia. *Proc. Natl. Acad. Sci. U.S.A.* 101(Suppl. 2), 14663–14669.
28. Kriz, J., Nguyen, M. D., and Julien, J. P. (2002). Minocycline slows disease progression in a mouse model of amyotrophic lateral sclerosis. *Neuro- biol. Dis.* 10, 268–278.
29. Kwiatkowski, T. J. Jr., Bosco, D. A., Leclerc, A. L., Tamrazian, E., Van- derburg, C. R., Russ, C., Davis, A., Gilchrist, J., Kasarskis, E. J., Mun- sat, T., Valdmanis, P., Rouleau, G. A., Hosler, B. A., Cortelli, P., De Jong, P. J., Yoshinaga, Y., Haines, J. L., Pericak-Vance, M. A., Yan, J., Ticozzi, N., Siddique, T., McKenna-Yasek, D., Sapp, P. C., Horvitz, H. R., Landers, J. E., and Brown, R. H. Jr. (2009). Mutations in the FUS/TLS gene on chromosome 16 cause familial amyotrophic lateral sclerosis. *Science* 323, 1205–1208.

30. Lepore, A. C., Rauck, B., Dejea, C., Pardo, A. C., Rao, M. S., Roth- stein, J. D., and Maragakis, N. J. (2008). Focal transplantation- based astrocyte replacement is neu- roprotective in a model of motor neuron disease. *Nat. Neurosci.* 11, 1294–1301.
31. MacKenzie, I. R., Bigio, E. H., Ince, P. G., Geser, F., Neumann, M., Cairns, N. J., Kwong, L. K., Forman, M. S., Ravits, J., Stewart, H., Eisen, A., McClusky, L., Kretzschmar, H. A., Monoranu, C. M., Highley, J. R., Kirby, J., Sid- dique, T., Shaw, P. J., Lee, V. M., and Trojanowski, J. Q. (2007). Patholog- ical TDP-43 distinguishes sporadic amyotrophic lateral sclerosis from amyotrophic lateral sclerosis with SOD1 mutations. *Ann. Neurol.* 61, 427–434.
32. Mantovani, S., Garbelli, S., Pasini, A., Alimonti, D., Perotti, C., Melazz- ini, M., Bendotti, C., and Mora, G. (2009). Immune system alterations in sporadic amyotrophic lateral scle- rosis patients suggest an ongoing neuroinflammatory process. *J. Neu- roimmunol.* 210, 73–79.
33. Maragakis, N. J., Dietrich, J., Wong, V., Xue, H., Mayer-Proschel, M., Rao, M. S., and Rothstein, J. D. (2004). Glu- tamate transporter expression and function in human glial progenitors. *Glia* 45, 133–143.
34. Meininger, V., Drory, V. E., Leigh, P. N., Ludolph, A., Robberecht, W., and Silani, V. (2009). Glatiramer acetate has no impact on disease progression in ALS at 40 mg/day: a double- blind, randomized, multicentre, placebo- controlled trial. *Amyotroph. Lateral Scler.* 10, 378–383.
35. Moisse, K., and Strong, M. J. (2006). Innate immunity in amyotrophic lateral sclerosis. *Biochim. Biophys. Acta* 1762, 1083–1093.
36. Nagai, M., Re, D. B., Nagata, T., Chalazonitis, A., Jessell, T. M., Wichterle, H., and Przedborski, S. (2007). Astrocytes expressing ALS- linked mutated SOD1 release factors selectively toxic to motor neurons. *Nat. Neurosci.* 10, 615–622.
37. Napoli, I., and Neumann, H. (2009). Microglial clearance function in health and disease. *Neuroscience* 158, 1030–1038.
38. Okada, S., Nakamura, M., Katoh, H., Miyao, T., Shimazaki, T., Ishii, K., Yamane, J., Yoshimura, A., Iwamoto, Y., Toyama, Y., and Okano, H. (2006). Conditional ablation of Stat3 or Socs3 discloses a dual role for reactive astrocytes after spinal cord injury. *Nat. Med.* 12, 829–834.
39. Papadimitriou, D., Le Verche, V., Jacquier, A., Ikiz, B., Przedborski, S., and Re, D. B. (2010). Inflammation in ALS and SMA: sorting out the good from the evil. *Neurobiol. Dis.* 37, 493–502.
40. Pehar, M., Cassina, P., Vargas, M. R., Castellanos, R., Viera, L., Beckman, J. S., Estevez, A. G., and Barbeito, L. (2004). Astrocytic production of nerve growth factor in motor neu- ron apoptosis: implications for amy- otrophic lateral sclerosis. *J. Neu- rochem.* 89, 464–473.
41. Rothstein, J. D., Martin, L. J., and Kuncl, R. W. (1992). Decreased glu- tamate transport by the brain and spinal cord in amyotrophic lat- eral sclerosis. *N. Engl. J. Med.* 326, 1464–1468.
42. Sanagi, T., Yuasa, S., Nakamura, Y., Suzuki, E., Aoki, M., Warita, H., Itoyama, Y., Uchino, S., Kohsaka, S., and Ohsawa, K. (2010). Appear- ance of phagocytic microglia adja- cent to motoneurons in spinal cord tissue from a presymptomatic trans- genic rat model of amyotrophic lateral sclerosis. *J. Neurosci. Res.* 88, 2736–2746.
43. Sreedharan, J., Blair, I. P., Tripathi, V. B., Hu, X., Vance, C., Rogelj, B., Ackerley, S., Durnall, J. C., Williams, K. L., Buratti, E., Baralle, F., De Belleroche, J., Mitchell, J. D., Leigh, P. N., Al- Chalabi, A., Miller, C. C., Nicholson, G., and Shaw, C. E. (2008). TDP-43 mutations in familial and sporadic amyotrophic lateral sclerosis. *Science* 319, 1668–1672.
44. Sta, M., Sylva-Steenland, R. M., Casula, M., De Jong, J. M., Troost, D., Aronica, E., and Baas, F. (2011). Innate and adaptive immunity in amy- otrophic lateral sclerosis: evidence of complement activation. *Neurobiol. Dis.* 42, 211–220.
45. Tan, C. F., Eguchi, H., Tagawa, A., Onodera, O., Iwasaki, T., Tsu- jino, A., Nishizawa, M., Kakita, A., and Takahashi, H. (2007). TDP- 43 immunoreactivity in neuronal inclusions in familial amyotrophic lateral sclerosis with or without SOD1 gene mutation. *Acta Neu- ropathol.* 113, 535–542.
46. Turner, B. J., and Talbot, K. (2008). Transgenics, toxicity and therapeu- tics in rodent models of mutant SOD1-mediated familial ALS. *Prog. Neurobiol.* 85, 94–134.
47. Vance, C., Rogelj, B., Hortobagyi, T., De Vos, K. J., Nishimura, A. L., Sreedharan, J., Hu, X., Smith, B., Ruddy, D., Wright, P., Ganesalingam, J., Williams, K. L., Tripathi, V., Al- Saraj, S., Al-Chalabi, A., Leigh, P. N., Blair, I. P., Nicholson, G., De Belleroche, J., Gallo, J. M., Miller, C. C., and Shaw, C. E. (2009). Muta- tions in FUS, an RNA processing protein, cause familial amyotrophic lateral sclerosis type 6. *Science* 323, 1208–1211.
48. Wang, L., Sharma, K., Grisotti, G., and Roos, R. P. (2009). The effect of mutant SOD1 dismutase activity on non-cell autonomous degeneration in familial amyotrophic lateral scle- rosis. *Neurobiol. Dis.* 35, 234–240.
49. Wijesekera, L. C., and Leigh, P. N. (2009). Amyotrophic lateral sclero- sis. *Orphanet. J. Rare Dis.* 4, 3.
50. Wu, V. W., Nishiyama, N., and Schwartz, J. P. (1998). A culture model of reactive astrocytes: increased nerve growth factor synthesis and reex- pression of cytokine responsiveness. *J. Neurochem.* 71, 749–756.
51. Yang, W. W., Sidman, R. L., Taksir, T. V., Treleaven, C. M., Fidler, J. A., Cheng, S. H., Dodge, J. C., and Shihabuddin, L. S. (2011). Relationship between neuropathology and disease pro- gression in the SOD1(G93A) ALS mouse. *Exp. Neurol.* 227, 287–295.
52. Yrjanheikki, J., Tikka, T., Keina- nen, R., Goldsteins, G., Chan, P. H., and Koistinaho, J. (1999). A tetracycline derivative, minocycline, reduces inflammation and protects against focal cerebral ischemia with a wide therapeutic window. *Proc. Natl. Acad. Sci. U.S.A.* 96, 13496–13500.
53. Zhu, S., Stavrovskaya, I. G., Drozda, M., Kim, B. Y., Ona, V., Li, M., Sarang, S., Liu, A. S., Hartley, D. M., Wu, D. C., Gullans, S., Ferrante, R. J., Przedborski, S., Kristal, B. S., and Fried- lander, R. M. (2002). Minocycline inhibits cytochrome *c* release and delays progression of amyotrophic lateral sclerosis in mice. *Nature* 417, 74–78.

21

Mechanisms underlying CD4+ Treg immune regulation in the adult: from experiments to models

Marta Caridade[1,2], Luis Graca[1,2]*‡ and Ruy M. Ribeiro[3]*†‡

[1] Instituto de Medicina Molecular, Faculdade de Medicina da Universidade de Lisboa, Lisbon, Portugal
[2] Instituto Gulbenkian de Ciência, Oeiras, Portugal
[3] Theoretical Biology and Biophysics, Los Alamos National Laboratory, Los Alamos, NM, USA

Edited by:
Carmen Molina-Paris, University of Leeds, UK

Reviewed by:
Akihiko Yoshimura, Keio University, Japan
Fernando A. Arosa, University of Beira Interior, Portugal

****Correspondence:***
Luis Graca, Instituto de Medicina Molecular, Faculdade de Medicina, Universidade de Lisboa, Avenida Prof. Egas Moniz, 1649-028 Lisbon, Portugal
e-mail: lgraca@fm.ul.pt;
Ruy M. Ribeiro, Theoretical Biology and Biophysics, Los Alamos National Laboratory, Los Alamos, NM 87545, USA
e-mail: ruy@lanl.gov

To maintain immunological balance the organism has to be tolerant to self while remaining competent to mount an effective immune response against third-party antigens. An important mechanism of this immune regulation involves the action of regulatory T-cell (Tregs). In this mini-review, we discuss some of the known and proposed mechanisms by which Tregs exert their influence in the context of immune regulation, and the contribution of mathematical modeling for these mechanistic studies. These models explore the mechanisms of action of regulatory T cells, and include hypotheses of multiple signals, delivered through simultaneous antigen-presenting cell (APC) conjugation; interaction of feedback loops between APC, Tregs, and effector cells; or production of specific cytokines that act on effector cells. As the field matures, and competing models are winnowed out, it is likely that we will be able to quantify how tolerance-inducing strategies, such as CD4-blockade, affect T-cell dynamics and what mechanisms explain the observed behavior of T-cell based tolerance.

Keywords: Tregs, mathematical models, CD4-blockade, regulation, tolerance

INTRODUCTION

Immunological tolerance can be defined as the state of unresponsiveness to an antigen, following prior contact with that antigen, where the host remains competent to mount an effective immune response against third-party antigens. Accomplishing therapeutic induced tolerance has been one of the major goals of immunology ever since the pioneering work of Medawar and colleagues (1).

There is a need to keep a balance between aggressive cells and cells that maintain tolerance to self. On occasions this balance can be disrupted originating either autoimmunity, when mechanisms leading to self-tolerance fail, or immunodeficiency and susceptibility to infection when the immune system is not able to mount a proper immune response. Usually, however, the immune system shows a significant capacity for self-tolerance, in spite of its equally efficient performance in the protection from foreign microbes. The ability to orchestrate protective immune responses is also the major hurdle impeding successful transplantation therapies and hinders the efficacy of therapeutic administration of foreign proteins and genes.

Random rearrangement of T-cell receptors (TCR) during cellular maturation leads to T cells that will recognize self-antigens. It was a long held assumption that central tolerance, by means of negative selection of autoreactive lymphocyte clones, could on its own account for the establishment of self-tolerance. Without such a censoring mechanism these autoreactive cells could eventually lead to autoimmune disease. Indeed thymocytes must survive the process of negative selection, which eliminates cells whose TCRs bind too avidly to self-antigens (2–4). The apoptosis of these thymocytes will prevent migration of autoreactive T cells to the periphery and prevent autoimmunity. Conversely, absence of negative selecting self-peptide-MHC complexes in the thymic medulla leads to an increase in mature autoreactive T cells (5, 6).

However, not all self-antigens are presented in the thymus, and some developing autoreactive T cells never encounter their antigens, eventually migrating to the periphery. Thus, although central tolerance contributes to the deletion of a large number of potentially autoreactive T cells, some autoreactive clones can be found in the periphery of healthy individuals (7, 8). There are, therefore, mechanisms that operate in the periphery (i.e., outside the thymus) to establish self-tolerance toward autoreactive clones that escape thymic negative selection.

Initially, one such mechanism was thought to be mediated by T-cell anergy, described as the functional state in which T cells remain viable but unable to respond to optimal stimulation through the TCR and co-stimulatory ligands (9), i.e., unable to proliferate or to produce interleukin-2 (IL-2) (10, 11). The first observation of anergy was made with purified human CD4$^+$ T cells stimulated with large quantities of peptide antigens (10). It was noted that after antigen stimulation there was down-regulation of TCR and this was associated with the molecular mechanism for anergy (12). Subsequent studies with mouse CD4$^+$ T cells suggested that occupancy of the TCR without any other signals was responsible for the induction of this state (13, 14).

Interestingly, anergic T cells were capable of suppressing proliferation of naïve T cells *in vitro* (15) and *in vivo* (16). In addition, anergic T cells have been shown to inhibit the antigen-presenting function and survival of dendritic cells (17). These and other observations led to the proposal of the "civil service model" (18), postulating that antigen-specific unresponsive cells can interfere with the generation of help by co-localizing with other T cells and competing for elements in the microenvironment (such as adhesion molecules or cytokines).

However, it was not clear how T cells would become anergic *in vivo*, and whether such mechanism was enough to maintain tolerance. More recently, a specific T cell subset, termed regulatory T (Treg) cells, gained prominence as being a key mechanism maintaining peripheral self-tolerance (19, 20). With hindsight, it is likely that many of the features of anergic T cells are a consequence of Treg function.

REGULATORY T CELLS

In 1995 Sakaguchi et al. (19) showed that depletion of a minor population of CD4$^+$ T cells constitutively expressing CD25 [IL-2 receptor α-chain (IL-2Rα)] led to the generation of a spectrum of autoimmune diseases when transferred to immune-compromised recipients. In addition, the co-transfer of CD25$^+$ T cells prevented the pathology.

Based on this CD25 marker, a population of natural (thymus-derived) regulatory T cells was identified in the resting immune system, both in mice and in humans (21). Subsequent studies showed that these cells express forkhead box transcription factor 3 (Foxp3) and this finding led to the definite establishment of a Treg subset (22–24). There is now abundant evidence that these regulatory T cells are actively engaged in the maintenance of self-tolerance (25). Furthermore, depletion of Foxp3$^+$ Tregs originates fatal multi-organ autoimmunity. The phenotype of this disease is virtually indistinguishable from the IPEX syndrome, caused by Foxp3 mutations in humans and equivalent to the Scurfy phenotype in mice (26–28).

THYMIC TREG CELLS

The Treg cells that develop in the thymus, first described as naturally occurring regulatory T cells (nTregs) appear to be selected for self-antigen/MHC expressed by thymic epithelial cells (29, 30), in a process that requires TCR triggering in the presence of co-stimulation (31, 32), but dispenses TGF-β and IL-2 (33, 34). Early studies with Treg cells showed that these cells express CD25, CD5, and cytotoxic T lymphocyte antigen 4 (CTLA-4), which are all induced upon TCR stimulation (19).

In the periphery, nTregs represent around 6–10% of the overall CD4$^+$ T-cell population. In order to be sustained they need continuous TCR triggering and co-stimulation in the presence of IL-2 (35–37), making IL-2 essential for natural Treg pool maintenance in the periphery (38). Comparative analysis of polyclonal TCR repertoires showed that TCR sequences from Treg cells were of broader variety and only partially overlapping with the ones from non-Treg cells (39). Some studies have shown that antigen-specific Treg cells are more potent at suppressing the induction of autoimmune disease than polyclonal populations (40). However, other studies have also shown that polyclonal Tregs are able to suppress independently of their specificity (41). Thus, Tregs with one antigen-specificity can suppress effector cells with many other antigen-specificities by bystander suppression. Moreover, transplantation studies have shown that Tregs can display a phenomenon called "linked suppression," where they can be activated in an antigen-specific manner, and subsequently suppress responses to unrelated antigens presented by the same cells (42). Tregs show a third property called infectious tolerance by which one population of Treg cells creates a regulatory milieu that promotes the outgrowth of a new population of Treg cells with antigen-specificities distinct from those of the original population, as long as the new antigen is present in the same tissue as the antigen recognized by the original Treg cell (43–45).

PERIPHERAL TREG INDUCTION

Besides nTreg, of thymic origin, it has become apparent that induced regulatory T cells (iTreg) also exist in the periphery (46, 47). After the discovery of the key role for Foxp3 in Tregs, it was demonstrated that it was possible for non-Treg cells to acquire both Foxp3 and the regulatory functions associated with it, therefore becoming Treg cells themselves (46, 48, 49).

It is likely that peripheral induction of iTreg occurs in response to non-self antigens like food, allergens, and commensal bacteria (39). Early evidence for *in vivo* peripheral conversion was derived from adoptive cell transfer experiments in which polyclonal CD4$^+$ CD25$^-$ naïve T cells were injected into lymphopenic mice or mice containing a monoclonal T cell repertoire devoid of nTregs, or when tolerance was imposed on monoclonal populations without Treg cells (49–51). In these conditions, homeostatic proliferation of the donor cells could be observed and part of the donor cell population became CD25$^+$CTLA-4$^+$GITR$^+$Foxp3$^+$ and acquired suppressive activity. Additionally, when congenitally marked CD4$^+$ CD25$^-$ T cells were transferred to WT hosts, 10% of those converted into CD4$^+$ CD25$^+$ Foxp3$^+$ T cells, within 6 weeks (52).

It was first shown *in vitro* that TCR activation in the presence of TGF-β would lead to Treg conversion (53). Subsequent studies supported this observation and demonstrated that iTreg conversion could be greatly enhanced by suboptimal TCR signals or a combination of strong TCR signals with high doses of TGF-β (47, 53–57). *In vivo* it is possible to induce oral tolerance by giving the antigen in the drinking water (58), or to induce transplantation tolerance using non-depleting anti-CD4 at the time of transplantation (48, 59). In both cases, tolerance induction is accompanied by induction of Foxp3$^+$ cells, in a process that requires TGF-β. In addition to these, many other factors influence the induction of Tregs both *in vitro* and *in vivo*, such as the co-stimulation environment, the strength of TCR signaling, mTOR inhibition with rapamycin, and low levels of essential amino-acids (44, 57, 60–69).

MECHANISMS OF ACTION OF TREG CELLS

In spite of intensive study of Tregs and their properties, the specific mechanisms by which they control immune responses are still not fully understood. There are several proposed mechanisms with experimental support, but it is likely that no single mechanism is responsible for the full range of biological phenomena involving Tregs (70). And it is also likely that in different milieu distinct mechanisms and even alternative subsets of regulatory cells are involved in tuning the immune response (71).

In **Figure 1**, we summarize five putative mechanisms of Treg function: (i) modulation of antigen-presenting cell (APC) activity through Treg engagement of co-stimulatory receptors on the surface of APC, leading to weak or abrogated signals from APC to naive/effector cells; (ii) Treg secretion of cytokines, such as IL10 and TGFβ, suppressing the activity of effector cells and APC; (iii) under certain circumstances, Tregs could have a direct cytotoxic effect, through the production of perforin/granzyme and induction of apoptosis in effector cells; (iv) Tregs may also cause metabolic disruption, for example stimulating APCs to produce enzymes that consume essential amino-acids, preventing naive/effector cell proliferation, and in the presence of TGFβ may induce the expression of Foxp3 in naive cells (i.e., they become Tregs); (v) Tregs could also compete with effectors cells for APC signals or cytokines, such as IL2.

There is mounting evidence [reviewed in (72)] that Treg cells exert their effects on different cell types, including CD4$^+$ and CD8$^+$ T cells, B cells, natural killer T cells (NKT), and DCs (70). The action of Tregs can be mediated by secretion of immunosuppressive cytokines, such as IL-10, TGF-β, IL-35, and galectin-1 (72) or by cell-dependent mechanisms through molecules such as GITR, CTLA-4, CD39, CD73, and LAG-3 (70). The spectrum of effect of Tregs on their targets goes from modifying the functional properties of other immune cells, such as down-regulating transcription of IL-2 (70, 71, 73), and other important growth factors; to actually killing those cells through granzyme B and perforin (70, 73–77). For example, there is evidence that Tregs can kill both immature and mature DCs (74).

Furthermore, Tregs may convert APCs to become themselves immunosuppressive (78). It has also been proposed that Tregs act by competing with other cells for growth factors, particularly IL-2 (79, 80). One possible outcome of these interactions is that other cells become themselves Foxp3$^+$ regulatory cells (45).

These and other suppressive mechanisms may be operational depending on the microenvironment, biological context, and

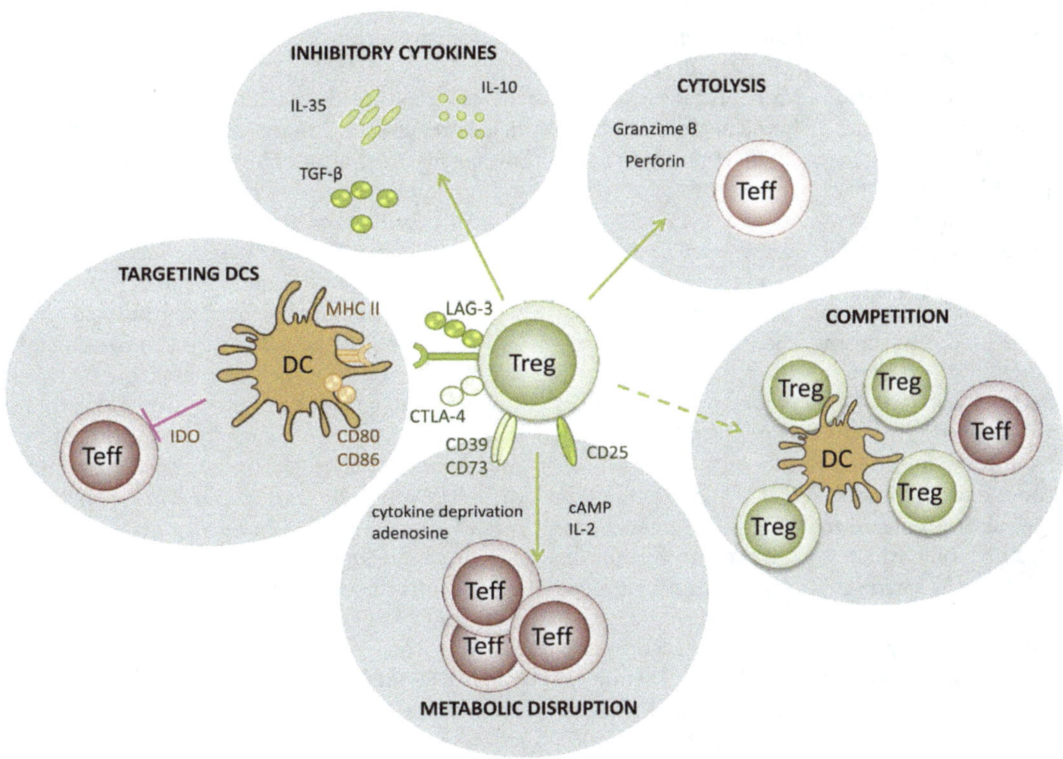

FIGURE 1 | Putative mechanisms used by regulatory T cells. (1) Targeting DCs – modulation of antigen-presenting cell activity through Treg engagement of co-stimulatory receptors on the DC surface, leading to weak or abrogated signals to naïve/effector T cells; (2) Metabolic disruption – includes cytokine deprivation, cyclic AMP-mediated inhibition, and adenosine receptor (A2A)-mediated immunosuppression; (3) Competition – for critical cytokines, such as IL-2, or direct disruption of effector cell engagement with APCs; (4) Cytolysis – direct cytotoxic effect through the production of Granzyme B and Perforin and consequent apoptosis of effector T cells or APCs; (5) Production of inhibitory cytokines – including IL-10, IL-35, and TGF-β.

immune response. For instance, IL-10 producing cells are more abundant in lamina propria (81, 82) and perforin or granzyme expressing Tregs are predominant in tumor environments (83).

MATHEMATICAL MODELING

Due to the complexity of the mechanisms and interactions involved in the processes of immune tolerance, mathematical modeling has been used as a tool to explore different conceptual frameworks of immunological tolerance. Many studies have analyzed the dynamics of thymocyte development, with positive and negative selection, as a mechanism of central tolerance (84–91).

Many other studies have focused on modeling the putative mechanisms of Treg suppression in the periphery. In these models, typically the dynamics of Tregs, effector cells, and APCs are studied to find the interaction mechanisms in the model that qualitatively reflect the experimental knowledge. For the purposes of this review, we can divide the models proposed in three categories, although there is overlap between these in some studies: (i) models that analyze different putative mechanisms of action of Tregs (**Table 1**); (ii) models that analyze the effects of Tregs on different processes, such as the immune response to pathogens and tumors, or in allergy; and (iii) models that study the maintenance of Tregs (homeostasis).

MODELS OF THE MECHANISMS OF TREG ACTION

An early model explicitly considering Tregs was developed by León and collaborators (92). They considered cross-regulation, where simultaneous conjugation of a Treg and an effector cell on the same APC can suppress effector function (92, 93). In this model, regulation could be due to competition for conjugation sites on the APC, or through inhibitory signals delivered to effector cells on the same APC, or by inducing conversion of effector cells to a regulatory phenotype. This model is developed and analyzed in detail in several subsequent publications (93–95), and it is reviewed in Carneiro et al. (96). Recently the model was expanded to study the dual effect of IL2 in promoting immunity and tolerance (97, 98). Some authors considered in more detail the dynamics of antigen and APCs, and compared mechanisms where regulatory T cells suppress APCs function or maturation with models where Tregs act directly on effector T cells (99). Other models along these lines included the processes of APC maturation and the differentiation of T cells into regulatory or effector phenotypes (100), following a previous proposal for this interaction (101). Interestingly, in these models, survival or proliferation of Tregs is dependent on feedback from effector T-cells, which is in part responsible for the bi-stability observed that is interpreted as states of tolerance or immunity.

Another mechanism of peripheral tolerance modeled by several authors involves anergy of effector cells (102, 103). This anergy can be achieved by tuning the threshold for activation, for example through repeated encounter with antigen or APC (102–106), or through modulation by Tregs. Carneiro et al. compared this mechanism with their previous model of cross-regulation discussed above (102). Another model that also explores thresholds for activation, but based on effector T-cell population response was studied by Burroughs et al. (107, 108). In this model the relative levels of Tregs and effector T cells depend on the respective strength of stimulation by antigen, which can be modulated by IL-2 – this model is reviewed in (109).

Typically these models consider a limited number of cell populations (3–6) and analyze one mechanism at a time. However, Kim et al. proposed a detailed model including dozens of cell populations, with a spatial component (tissue and lymph node), and considered multiple mechanisms of Treg action simultaneously (110). At the other end of the spectrum, Abreu et al. proposed a model where regulation of the immune system was simply based on cross-recognition of multiple antigens by the same cell, whether it is an effector, a regulatory, or an APC (111).

MODELS OF THE EFFECT OF TREGS ON THE IMMUNE RESPONSE

The studies discussed so far are mainly concerned with the mechanisms defining the interactions of Tregs and effector cells, often looking for steady states where one or the other population dominates, interpreted as tolerance or autoimmune states. Other models analyze the effects of the existence of Tregs on different processes.

Many of these models explore the system level effects of Treg failure and the potential development of autoimmunity. One of the first models to study this was by León et al. (112), where they analyzed the relationship between infections and autoimmunity in general. More recent studies analyzed specific autoimmune conditions, such as multiple sclerosis (113, 114) and inflammatory bowel disease (115). Grosse et al. analyzed the balance of Th1 vs. Th2 type responses and their control by Tregs in the context of allergies, with the objective of analyzing immunotherapy protocols (116). Another study looking at immunotherapy protocols, in this case modulation of IL2 therapy, used a mathematical model of helper, regulatory, and memory $CD4^+$ T cells (98). These studies are mostly theoretical. However, one report described an interesting experimental study of mice injected with tolerogenic or control peptides and followed for 16 days, with serial measurements of different T-cell subsets. These data were then analyzed with a mathematical model (117).

Some studies have analyzed the interplay between infections and regulation of the immune response. One of these modeled the immune decision between attacking or not a given antigen, based on the network of interactions between Tregs, Th17 cells, and growing levels of antigen (as in the case of a pathogen) (118). And a model analyzing the regulation of the immune response in early HIV infection, through the expansion of specific Tregs, was recently introduced (119). Finally, León et al. (120, 121) considered an expansion of their mechanistic model of Treg – T effector interactions to study the immune response against tumors, and their control or expansion.

MODELS OF TREG HOMEOSTASIS

An important question that has also been addressed by modeling studies is the maintenance of a healthy number of Tregs. Several studies included the possibility of the Treg population being maintained in the periphery in part by feedback from the effector cells (92, 99, 100). One such model (94) studied the effects of thymic output and positive/negative selection on proper balance between tolerance and immunity in the periphery, and concluded that repertoire selection plays an important role in maintaining

Table 1 | Summary of mechanistic models of Treg action.

Cell populations considered	Mechanisms of regulation of immune response	Some properties of the model	Reference
APC, Treg, Teff, and Treg, Teff conjugates on APC No explicit APC dynamics	Competition for activation on APC Tregs inhibit Teff on same conjugate Treg maintenance is dependent on Teff	Treg inhibit growth of Teff Treg induce Teff to become Treg	(92–94, 96)
As above plus IL2	Competition for IL2 Tregs condition APC	Non-local interactions Model used to study IL2-based therapies	(97, 98)
APC and Ag dynamics APC maturation T cells are activated into Treg or Teff by APC stimulation	Tregs directly suppress Teff (specifically and bystander) Tregs suppress APC maturation	Bystander effects are important Direct suppression was more effective	(99)
Antigen Immature APC, resting APC, activated APC Precursor T cells (Tp), Teff, Treg	Tp become Treg by interaction with resting APC Tp become Teff by interaction with activated APC Teff activates APC Treg induces activated APC to rest	Strength of antigen stimulus is crucial in defining whether system is in tolerant or non-tolerant state	(100)
Stochastic model of TCR triggering for T cells (both thymus and periphery)	Different thresholds for activation vs. anergy, with or without co-stimulation	Self-reactive cells in periphery are controlled by a mechanism of reversible anergy	(103)
T cells with tunable activation thresholds	Model for integration of signals in successive encounters with APC	Exhibits self-tolerance "More cells should lead to less anergy," which is not seen in adoptive transfer experiments	(102)
Inactive and active Treg and Teff IL2 for Teff proliferation, also helps Treg proliferate Cytokine (e.g., IL7) for Treg homeostasis	Tregs consume IL2 Treg inhibit Teff (from active to inactive) proportionally to Treg numbers	Strength of antigen stimulation (for Treg and Teff) defines relative levels of those two populations	(107–109)
APC with different antigens Teff of multiple specificities Tregs of multiple specificities	Cells interact with extensive cross-reactivity, but different avidities	Effector functions are the outcome of individual cellular decisions (based on cross-reactivity) A threshold of conjugation time can be identified that permits self/non-self discrimination	(111)

Comparison of some of the models for Treg action discussed in the text. The model by Kim et al. (110) is too complex to fit in this summary table.

that balance. Baltcheva et al. (122) developed a more detailed model to analyze the life-long dynamics of precursor and mature $CD25^{+}$ T cells (Tregs) in humans, including thymic production, density-dependent homeostasis, and effector T-cell conversion.

CONCLUSION

The field of regulatory T cells, although relatively recent, has had an explosion of knowledge driven by detailed experimental work (20, 65, 72, 123, 124). Indeed there are many more studies than we could possibly review or even allude to in this mini-review. However, the mechanistic details of this important function of the immune system are not completely elucidated (72). Many authors have developed mathematical models of the interactions between Tregs and effector cells to try to add to our understanding of these mechanisms. Still, there is a lack of true collaborations between experimental scientists and modelers in this field. Clearly, more progress would be possible if such integrated teams worked together, as has been the case in other areas of medicine, e.g., modeling of viral infections (125). As the field matures and competing models are winnowed out, it is likely that we will be able to quantify how tolerance-inducing strategies, such as CD4-blockade, affect T-cell dynamics, and what mechanisms explain the observed behavior of T-cell based tolerance.

ACKNOWLEDGMENTS

The authors thank Joana Duarte for assistance in preparing **Figure 1**. Luis Graca is funded by FCT/PTDC/SAU-TOX/114424/2009 and FCT/PTDC/SAU-IMU/120225/2010. Ruy M. Ribeiro received funding from the European Union 7th Framework Programme under grant n° PCOFUND-GA-2009-246542 and from Fundação para a Ciência e Tecnologia, Portugal.

REFERENCES

1. Medawar PB. The behaviour and fate of skin autografts and skin homografts in rabbits: a report to the War Wounds Committee of the Medical Research Council. *J Anat* (1944) **78**(Pt 5):176–99.Epub 1944/10/01
2. Kappler JW, Roehm N, Marrack P. T cell tolerance by clonal elimination in the thymus. *Cell* (1987) **49**(2):273–80. doi:10.1016/0092-8674(87)90568-X Epub 1987/04/24

3. MacDonald HR, Schneider R, Lees RK, Howe RC, Acha-Orbea H, Festenstein H, et al. T-cell receptor V beta use predicts reactivity and tolerance to Mlsa-encoded antigens. *Nature* (1988) **332**(6159):40–5. doi:10.1038/332040a0 Epub 1988/03/03
4. von Boehmer H, Teh HS, Kisielow P. The thymus selects the useful, neglects the useless and destroys the harmful. *Immunol Today* (1989) **10**(2):57–61. doi:10.1016/0167-5699(89)90307-1 Epub 1989/02/01
5. Laufer TM, DeKoning J, Markowitz JS, Lo D, Glimcher LH. Unopposed positive selection and autoreactivity in mice expressing class II MHC only on thymic cortex. *Nature* (1996) **383**(6595):81–5. doi:10.1038/383081a0 Epub 1996/09/05
6. Laufer TM, Fan L, Glimcher LH. Self-reactive T cells selected on thymic cortical epithelium are polyclonal and are pathogenic in vivo. *J Immunol* (1999) **162**(9):5078–84.Epub 1999/05/05
7. Ramsdell F, Lantz T, Fowlkes BJ. A nondeletional mechanism of thymic self tolerance. *Science* (1989) **246**(4933):1038–41. doi:10.1126/science.2511629 Epub 1989/11/24
8. Schonrich G, Momburg F, Hammerling GJ, Arnold B. Anergy induced by thymic medullary epithelium. *Eur J Immunol* (1992) **22**(7):1687–91. doi:10.1002/eji.1830220704 Epub 1992/07/01
9. Schwartz RH. Models of T cell anergy: is there a common molecular mechanism? *J Exp Med* (1996) **184**(1):1–8. doi:10.1084/jem.184.1.1 Epub 1996/07/01
10. Lamb JR, Skidmore BJ, Green N, Chiller JM, Feldmann M. Induction of tolerance in influenza virus-immune T lymphocyte clones with synthetic peptides of influenza hemagglutinin. *J Exp Med* (1983) **157**(5):1434–47. doi:10.1084/jem.157.5.1434 Epub 1983/05/01
11. Schwartz RH. A cell culture model for T lymphocyte clonal anergy. *Science* (1990) **248**(4961):1349–56. doi:10.1126/science.2113314 Epub 1990/06/15
12. Lamb JR, Feldmann M. Essential requirement for major histocompatibility complex recognition in T-cell tolerance induction. *Nature* (1984) **308**(5954):72–4. doi:10.1038/308072a0 Epub 1984/03/01
13. Jenkins MK, Schwartz RH. Antigen presentation by chemically modified splenocytes induces antigen-specific T cell unresponsiveness in vitro and in vivo. *J Exp Med* (1987) **165**(2):302–19. doi:10.1084/jem.165.2.302 Epub 1987/02/01
14. Quill H, Schwartz RH. Stimulation of normal inducer T cell clones with antigen presented by purified Ia molecules in planar lipid membranes: specific induction of a long-lived state of proliferative nonresponsiveness. *J Immunol* (1987) **138**(11):3704–12.Epub 1987/06/01
15. Lombardi G, Sidhu S, Batchelor R, Lechler R. Anergic T cells as suppressor cells in vitro. *Science* (1994) **264**(5165):1587–9. doi:10.1126/science.8202711 Epub 1994/06/10
16. Chai JG, Bartok I, Chandler P, Vendetti S, Antoniou A, Dyson J, et al. Anergic T cells act as suppressor cells in vitro and in vivo. *Eur J Immunol* (1999) **29**(2):686–92. doi:10.1002/(SICI)1521-4141(199902)29:02<686::AID-IMMU686>3.0.CO;2-N Epub 1999/03/04
17. Vendetti S, Chai JG, Dyson J, Simpson E, Lombardi G, Lechler R. Anergic T cells inhibit the antigen-presenting function of dendritic cells. *J Immunol* (2000) **165**(3):1175–81.Epub 2000/07/21
18. Waldmann H, Qin S, Cobbold S. Monoclonal antibodies as agents to reinduce tolerance in autoimmunity. *J Autoimmun* (1992) **5**(Suppl A):93–102. doi:10.1016/0896-8411(92)90024-K Epub 1992/04/01
19. Sakaguchi S, Sakaguchi N, Asano M, Itoh M, Toda M. Immunologic self-tolerance maintained by activated T cells expressing IL-2 receptor alpha-chains (CD25). Breakdown of a single mechanism of self-tolerance causes various autoimmune diseases. *J Immunol* (1995) **155**(3):1151–64.Epub 1995/08/01
20. Ohkura N, Kitagawa Y, Sakaguchi S. Development and maintenance of regulatory T cells. *Immunity* (2013) **38**(3):414–23. doi:10.1016/j.immuni.2013.03.002
21. Yagi H, Nomura T, Nakamura K, Yamazaki S, Kitawaki T, Hori S, et al. Crucial role of FOXP3 in the development and function of human CD25+CD4+ regulatory T cells. *Int Immunol* (2004) **16**(11):1643–56. doi:10.1093/intimm/dxh165
22. Fontenot JD, Gavin MA, Rudensky AY. Foxp3 programs the development and function of CD4+CD25+ regulatory T cells. *Nat Immunol* (2003) **4**(4):330–6. doi:10.1038/ni904
23. Hori S, Nomura T, Sakaguchi S. Control of regulatory T cell development by the transcription factor Foxp3. *Science* (2003) **299**(5609):1057–61. doi:10.1126/science.1079490 Epub 2003/01/11
24. Khattri R, Cox T, Yasayko SA, Ramsdell F. An essential role for Scurfin in CD4+CD25+ T regulatory cells. *Nat Immunol* (2003) **4**(4):337–42. doi:10.1038/ni909
25. Sakaguchi S. Naturally arising CD4+ regulatory t cells for immunologic self-tolerance and negative control of immune responses. *Annu Rev Immunol* (2004) **22**:531–62. doi:10.1146/annurev.immunol.21.120601.141122 Epub 2004/03/23
26. Bennett CL, Christie J, Ramsdell F, Brunkow ME, Ferguson PJ, Whitesell L, et al. The immune dysregulation, polyendocrinopathy, enteropathy, X-linked syndrome (IPEX) is caused by mutations of FOXP3. *Nat Genet* (2001) **27**(1):20–1. doi:10.1038/83713 Epub 2001/01/04
27. Wildin RS, Ramsdell F, Peake J, Faravelli F, Casanova JL, Buist N, et al. X-linked neonatal diabetes mellitus, enteropathy and endocrinopathy syndrome is the human equivalent of mouse scurfy. *Nat Genet* (2001) **27**(1):18–20. doi:10.1038/83707 Epub 2001/01/04
28. Brunkow ME, Jeffery EW, Hjerrild KA, Paeper B, Clark LB, Yasayko SA, et al. Disruption of a new forkhead/winged-helix protein, scurfin, results in the fatal lymphoproliferative disorder of the scurfy mouse. *Nat Genet* (2001) **27**(1):68–73. doi:10.1038/83784
29. Apostolou I, Sarukhan A, Klein L, von Boehmer H. Origin of regulatory T cells with known specificity for antigen. *Nat Immunol* (2002) **3**(8):756–63. doi:10.1038/ni816
30. Jordan MS, Boesteanu A, Reed AJ, Petrone AL, Holenbeck AE, Lerman MA, et al. Thymic selection of CD4+CD25+ regulatory T cells induced by an agonist self-peptide. *Nat Immunol* (2001) **2**(4):301–6. doi:10.1038/86302 Epub 2001/03/29
31. Tai X, Cowan M, Feigenbaum L, Singer A. CD28 costimulation of developing thymocytes induces Foxp3 expression and regulatory T cell differentiation independently of interleukin 2. *Nat Immunol* (2005) **6**(2):152–62. doi:10.1038/ni1160 Epub 2005/01/11
32. Fontenot JD, Rasmussen JP, Williams LM, Dooley JL, Farr AG, Rudensky AY. Regulatory T cell lineage specification by the forkhead transcription factor foxp3. *Immunity* (2005) **22**(3):329–41. doi:10.1016/j.immuni.2005.01.016
33. Fontenot JD, Rasmussen JP, Gavin MA, Rudensky AY. A function for interleukin 2 in Foxp3-expressing regulatory T cells. *Nat Immunol* (2005) **6**(11):1142–51. doi:10.1038/ni1263
34. Marie JC, Letterio JJ, Gavin M, Rudensky AY. TGF-beta1 maintains suppressor function and Foxp3 expression in CD4+CD25+ regulatory T cells. *J Exp Med* (2005) **201**(7):1061–7. doi:10.1084/jem.20042276
35. Gavin MA, Clarke SR, Negrou E, Gallegos A, Rudensky A. Homeostasis and anergy of CD4(+)CD25(+) suppressor T cells in vivo. *Nat Immunol* (2002) **3**(1):33–41. doi:10.1038/ni743
36. Knoechel B, Lohr J, Kahn E, Bluestone JA, Abbas AK. Sequential development of interleukin 2-dependent effector and regulatory T cells in response to endogenous systemic antigen. *J Exp Med* (2005) **202**(10):1375–86. doi:10.1084/jem.20050855
37. Lohr J, Knoechel B, Jiang S, Sharpe AH, Abbas AK. The inhibitory function of B7 costimulators in T cell responses to foreign and self-antigens. *Nat Immunol* (2003) **4**(7):664–9. doi:10.1038/ni939
38. Malek TR. The main function of IL-2 is to promote the development of T regulatory cells. *J Leukoc Biol* (2003) **74**(6):961–5. doi:10.1189/jlb.0603272
39. Josefowicz SZ, Lu LF, Rudensky AY. Regulatory T cells: mechanisms of differentiation and function. *Annu Rev Immunol* (2012) **30**:531–64. doi:10.1146/annurev.immunol.25.022106.141623 Epub 2012/01/10
40. Salomon B, Lenschow DJ, Rhee L, Ashourian N, Singh B, Sharpe A, et al. B7/CD28 costimulation is essential for the homeostasis of the CD4+CD25+ immunoregulatory T cells that control autoimmune diabetes. *Immunity* (2000) **12**(4):431–40. doi:10.1016/S1074-7613(00)80195-8 Epub 2000/05/05
41. Graca L, Le Moine A, Lin CY, Fairchild PJ, Cobbold SP, Waldmann H. Donor-specific transplantation tolerance: the paradoxical behavior of CD4+CD25+ T cells. *Proc Natl Acad Sci U S A* (2004) **101**(27):10122–6. doi:10.1073/pnas.0400084101 Epub 2004/06/26
42. Davies JD, Leong LY, Mellor A, Cobbold SP, Waldmann H. T cell suppression in transplantation tolerance through linked recognition. *J Immunol* (1996) **156**(10):3602–7.Epub 1996/05/15
43. Qin S, Cobbold SP, Pope H, Elliott J, Kioussis D, Davies J, et al. "Infectious" transplantation tolerance. *Science* (1993) **259**(5097):974–7.Epub 1993/02/12

44. Graca L, Honey K, Adams E, Cobbold SP, Waldmann H. Cutting edge: anti-CD154 therapeutic antibodies induce infectious transplantation tolerance. *J Immunol* (2000) **165**(9):4783–6.Epub 2000/10/25
45. Kendal AR, Chen Y, Regateiro FS, Ma J, Adams E, Cobbold SP, et al. Sustained suppression by Foxp3+ regulatory T cells is vital for infectious transplantation tolerance. *J Exp Med* (2011) **208**(10):2043–53. doi:10.1084/jem.20110767 Epub 2011/08/31
46. Apostolou I, von Boehmer H. In vivo instruction of suppressor commitment in naive T cells. *J Exp Med* (2004) **199**(10):1401–8. doi:10.1084/jem.20040249 Epub 2004/05/19
47. Kretschmer K, Apostolou I, Hawiger D, Khazaie K, Nussenzweig MC, von Boehmer H. Inducing and expanding regulatory T cell populations by foreign antigen. *Nat Immunol* (2005) **6**(12):1219–27. doi:10.1038/ni1265 Epub 2005/10/26
48. Cobbold SP, Castejon R, Adams E, Zelenika D, Graca L, Humm S, et al. Induction of foxP3+ regulatory T cells in the periphery of T cell receptor transgenic mice tolerized to transplants. *J Immunol* (2004) **172**(10):6003–10.Epub 2004/05/07
49. Curotto de Lafaille MA, Lino AC, Kutchukhidze N, Lafaille JJ. CD25− T cells generate CD25+Foxp3+ regulatory T cells by peripheral expansion. *J Immunol* (2004) **173**(12):7259–68.
50. Furtado GC, Curotto de Lafaille MA, Kutchukhidze N, Lafaille JJ. Interleukin 2 signaling is required for CD4(+) regulatory T cell function. *J Exp Med* (2002) **196**(6):851–7. doi:10.1084/jem.20020190
51. Cobbold SP, Graca L, Lin CY, Adams E, Waldmann H. Regulatory T cells in the induction and maintenance of peripheral transplantation tolerance. *Transpl Int* (2003) **16**(2):66–75. doi:10.1111/j.1432-2277.2003.tb00266.x Epub 2003/02/22
52. Liang S, Alard P, Zhao Y, Parnell S, Clark SL, Kosiewicz MM. Conversion of CD4+ CD25− cells into CD4+ CD25+ regulatory T cells in vivo requires B7 costimulation, but not the thymus. *J Exp Med* (2005) **201**(1):127–37. doi:10.1084/jem.20041201
53. Chen W, Jin W, Hardegen N, Lei KJ, Li L, Marinos N, et al. Conversion of peripheral CD4+CD25− naive T cells to CD4+CD25+ regulatory T cells by TGF-beta induction of transcription factor Foxp3. *J Exp Med* (2003) **198**(12):1875–86. doi:10.1084/jem.20030152
54. Selvaraj RK, Geiger TL. A kinetic and dynamic analysis of Foxp3 induced in T cells by TGF-beta. *J Immunol* (2007) **178**(12):7667–77.
55. Zheng SG, Wang JH, Gray JD, Soucier H, Horwitz DA. Natural and induced CD4+CD25+ cells educate CD4+CD25− cells to develop suppressive activity: the role of IL-2, TGF-beta, and IL-10. *J Immunol* (2004) **172**(9):5213–21.
56. Graca L, Chen TC, Le Moine A, Cobbold SP, Howie D, Waldmann H. Dominant tolerance: activation thresholds for peripheral generation of regulatory T cells. *Trends Immunol* (2005) **26**(3):130–5. doi:10.1016/j.it.2004.12.007 Epub 2005/03/05
57. Oliveira VG, Caridade M, Paiva RS, Demengeot J, Graca L. Sub-optimal CD4+ T-cell activation triggers autonomous TGF-beta-dependent conversion to Foxp3+ regulatory T cells. *Eur J Immunol* (2011) **41**(5):1249–55. doi:10.1002/eji.201040896 Epub 2011/04/07
58. Mucida D, Kutchukhidze N, Erazo A, Russo M, Lafaille JJ. Curotto de Lafaille MA. Oral tolerance in the absence of naturally occurring Tregs. *J Clin Invest* (2005) **115**(7):1923–33. doi:10.1172/JCI24487 Epub 2005/06/07
59. Lin CY, Graca L, Cobbold SP, Waldmann H. Dominant transplantation tolerance impairs CD8+ T cell function but not expansion. *Nat Immunol* (2002) **3**(12):1208–13. doi:10.1038/ni853 Epub 2002/11/05
60. Chen TC, Waldmann H, Fairchild PJ. Induction of dominant transplantation tolerance by an altered peptide ligand of the male antigen Dby. *J Clin Invest* (2004) **113**(12):1754–62. doi:10.1172/JCI20569 Epub 2004/06/17
61. Griffin MD, Lutz W, Phan VA, Bachman LA, McKean DJ, Kumar R. Dendritic cell modulation by 1alpha,25 dihydroxyvitamin D3 and its analogs: a vitamin D receptor-dependent pathway that promotes a persistent state of immaturity in vitro and in vivo. *Proc Natl Acad Sci U S A* (2001) **98**(12):6800–5. doi:10.1073/pnas.121172198 Epub 2001/05/24
62. Manicassamy S, Pulendran B. Dendritic cell control of tolerogenic responses. *Immunol Rev* (2011) **241**(1):206–27. doi:10.1111/j.1600-065X.2011.01015.x Epub 2011/04/15
63. Mucida D, Park Y, Kim G, Turovskaya O, Scott I, Kronenberg M, et al. Reciprocal TH17 and regulatory T cell differentiation mediated by retinoic acid. *Science* (2007) **317**(5835):256–60. doi:10.1126/science.1145697 Epub 2007/06/16
64. Steinbrink K, Wolfl M, Jonuleit H, Knop J, Enk AH. Induction of tolerance by IL-10-treated dendritic cells. *J Immunol* (1997) **159**(10):4772–80.Epub 1997/11/20
65. Waldmann H, Chen TC, Graca L, Adams E, Daley S, Cobbold S, et al. Regulatory T cells in transplantation. *Semin Immunol* (2006) **18**(2):111–9. doi:10.1016/j.smim.2006.01.010 Epub 2006/02/16
66. Yang J, Bernier SM, Ichim TE, Li M, Xia X, Zhou D, et al. LF15-0195 generates tolerogenic dendritic cells by suppression of NF-kappaB signaling through inhibition of IKK activity. *J Leukoc Biol* (2003) **74**(3):438–47. doi:10.1189/jlb.1102582 Epub 2003/09/02
67. Battaglia M, Stabilini A, Migliavacca B, Horejs-Hoeck J, Kaupper T, Roncarolo MG. Rapamycin promotes expansion of functional CD4+CD25+FOXP3+ regulatory T cells of both healthy subjects and type 1 diabetic patients. *J Immunol* (2006) **177**(12):8338–47.
68. Cobbold SP, Adams E, Farquhar CA, Nolan KF, Howie D, Lui KO, et al. Infectious tolerance via the consumption of essential amino acids and mTOR signaling. *Proc Natl Acad Sci U S A* (2009) **106**(29):12055–60. doi:10.1073/pnas.0903919106
69. Zhang R, Huynh A, Whitcher G, Chang J, Maltzman JS, Turka LA. An obligate cell-intrinsic function for CD28 in Tregs. *J Clin Invest* (2013) **123**(2):580–93. doi:10.1172/JCI65013
70. Miyara M, Sakaguchi S. Natural regulatory T cells: mechanisms of suppression. *Trends Mol Med* (2007) **13**(3):108–16. doi:10.1016/j.molmed.2007.01.003 Epub 2007/01/30
71. Toda A, Piccirillo CA. Development and function of naturally occurring CD4+CD25+ regulatory T cells. *J Leukoc Biol* (2006) **80**(3):458–70. doi:10.1189/jlb.0206095 Epub 2006/07/01
72. Shevach EM. Mechanisms of foxp3+ T regulatory cell-mediated suppression. *Immunity* (2009) **30**(5):636–45. doi:10.1016/j.immuni.2009.04.010
73. Wing K, Fehervari Z, Sakaguchi S. Emerging possibilities in the development and function of regulatory T cells. *Int Immunol* (2006) **18**(7):991–1000. doi:10.1093/intimm/dxl044 Epub 2006/05/25
74. Grossman WJ, Verbsky JW, Barchet W, Colonna M, Atkinson JP, Ley TJ. Human T regulatory cells can use the perforin pathway to cause autologous target cell death. *Immunity* (2004) **21**(4):589–601. doi:10.1016/j.immuni.2004.09.002 Epub 2004/10/16
75. Gondek DC, Lu LF, Quezada SA, Sakaguchi S, Noelle RJ. Cutting edge: contact-mediated suppression by CD4+CD25+ regulatory cells involves a granzyme B-dependent, perforin-independent mechanism. *J Immunol* (2005) **174**(4):1783–6.Epub 2005/02/09.
76. Sakaguchi S, Wing K, Onishi Y, Prieto-Martin P, Yamaguchi T. Regulatory T cells: how do they suppress immune responses? *Int Immunol* (2009) **21**(10):1105–11. doi:10.1093/intimm/dxp095 Epub 2009/09/10
77. Vignali DA, Collison LW, Workman CJ. How regulatory T cells work. *Nat Rev Immunol* (2008) **8**(7):523–32. doi:10.1038/nri2343
78. Kryczek I, Wei S, Zou L, Zhu G, Mottram P, Xu H, et al. Cutting edge: induction of B7-H4 on APCs through IL-10: novel suppressive mode for regulatory T cells. *J Immunol* (2006) **177**(1):40–4.Epub 2006/06/21
79. Scheffold A, Huhn J, Hofer T. Regulation of CD4+CD25+ regulatory T cell activity: it takes (IL-)two to tango. *Eur J Immunol* (2005) **35**(5):1336–41. doi:10.1002/eji.200425887 Epub 2005/04/14
80. Scheffold A, Murphy KM, Hofer T. Competition for cytokines: T(reg) cells take all. *Nat Immunol* (2007) **8**(12):1285–7. doi:10.1038/ni1207-1285 Epub 2007/11/21
81. Maynard CL, Harrington LE, Janowski KM, Oliver JR, Zindl CL, Rudensky AY, et al. Regulatory T cells expressing interleukin 10 develop from Foxp3+ and Foxp3− precursor cells in the absence of interleukin 10. *Nat Immunol* (2007) **8**(9):931–41. doi:10.1038/ni1504
82. Rubtsov YP, Rasmussen JP, Chi EY, Fontenot J, Castelli L, Ye X, et al. Regulatory T cell-derived interleukin-10 limits inflammation at environmental interfaces. *Immunity* (2008) **28**(4):546–58. doi:10.1016/j.immuni.2008.02.017
83. Cao X, Cai SF, Fehniger TA, Song J, Collins LI, Piwnica-Worms DR, et al. Granzyme B and perforin are important for regulatory T cell-mediated suppression of tumor clearance. *Immunity* (2007) **27**(4):635–46. doi:10.1016/j.immuni.2007.08.014
84. Faro J, Velasco S, Gonzalez-Fernandez A, Bandeira A. The impact of thymic antigen diversity on the size of the selected T cell repertoire. *J Immunol* (2004) **172**(4):2247–55.

85. Detours V, Mehr R, Perelson AS. Deriving quantitative constraints on T cell selection from data on the mature T cell repertoire. *J Immunol* (2000) **164**(1):121–8.
86. Detours V, Perelson AS. Explaining high alloreactivity as a quantitative consequence of affinity-driven thymocyte selection. *Proc Natl Acad Sci U S A* (1999) **96**(9):5153–8. doi:10.1073/pnas.96.9.5153
87. Mehr R, Globerson A, Perelson AS. Modeling positive and negative selection and differentiation processes in the thymus. *J Theor Biol* (1995) **175**(1):103–26. doi:10.1006/jtbi.1995.0124
88. Currie J, Castro M, Lythe G, Palmer E, Molina-Paris C. A stochastic T cell response criterion. *J R Soc Interface* (2012) **9**(76):2856–70. doi:10.1098/rsif.2012.0205
89. Castiglione F, Santoni D, Rapin N. CTLs' repertoire shaping in the thymus: a Monte Carlo simulation. *Autoimmunity* (2011) **44**(4):261–70. doi:10.3109/08916934.2011.523272
90. Muller V, Bonhoeffer S. Quantitative constraints on the scope of negative selection. *Trends Immunol* (2003) **24**(3):132–5. doi:10.1016/S1471-4906(03)00028-0
91. Sawicka ML, Reynolds J, Abourashchi N, Lythe G, Molina-Paris C, et al. Immunology and mathematics: a joint effort to estimate (murine) thymic selection rates. *Front Immunol* (in press).
92. Leon K, Perez R, Lage A, Carneiro J. Modelling T-cell-mediated suppression dependent on interactions in multicellular conjugates. *J Theor Biol* (2000) **207**(2):231–54. doi:10.1006/jtbi.2000.2169 Epub 2000/10/18
93. Leon K, Perez R, Lage A, Carneiro J. Three-cell interactions in T cell-mediated suppression? A mathematical analysis of its quantitative implications. *J Immunol* (2001) **166**(9):5356–65.Epub 2001/04/21
94. Leon K, Lage A, Carneiro J. Tolerance and immunity in a mathematical model of T-cell mediated suppression. *J Theor Biol* (2003) **225**(1):107–26. doi:10.1016/S0022-5193(03)00226-1 Epub 2003/10/16
95. Leon K, Faro J, Carneiro J. A general mathematical framework to model generation structure in a population of asynchronously dividing cells. *J Theor Biol* (2004) **229**(4):455–76. doi:10.1016/j.jtbi.2004.04.011 Epub 2004/07/13
96. Carneiro J, Leon K, Caramalho I, van den Dool C, Gardner R, Oliveira V, et al. When three is not a crowd: a crossregulation model of the dynamics and repertoire selection of regulatory CD4+ T cells. *Immunol Rev* (2007) **216**:48–68. doi:10.1111/j.1600-065X.2007.00487.x. Epub 2007/03/21
97. Garcia-Martinez K, Leon K. Modeling the role of IL-2 in the interplay between CD4+ helper and regulatory T cells: assessing general dynamical properties. *J Theor Biol* (2010) **262**(4):720–32. doi:10.1016/j.jtbi.2009.10.025 Epub 2009/11/03
98. Garcia-Martinez K, Leon K. Modeling the role of IL2 in the interplay between CD4+ helper and regulatory T cells: studying the impact of IL2 modulation therapies. *Int Immunol* (2012) **24**(7):427–46. doi:10.1093/intimm/dxr120
99. Alexander HK, Wahl LM. Self-tolerance and autoimmunity in a regulatory T cell model. *Bull Math Biol* (2011) **73**(1):33–71. doi:10.1007/s11538-010-9519-2 Epub 2010/03/03
100. Fouchet D, Regoes R. A population dynamics analysis of the interaction between adaptive regulatory T cells and antigen presenting cells. *PLoS One* (2008) **3**(5):e2306. doi:10.1371/journal.pone.0002306. Epub 2008/05/30
101. Powrie F, Maloy KJ. Immunology. regulating the regulators. *Science* (2003) **299**(5609):1030–1. doi:10.1126/science.1082031
102. Carneiro J, Paixao T, Milutinovic D, Sousa J, Leon K, Gardner R, et al. Immunological self-tolerance: Lessons from mathematical modeling. *J Comput Appl Math* (2005) **184**(1):77–100. doi:10.1016/j.cam.2004.10.025
103. Chan C, Stark J, George AJT. The impact of multiple T cell-APC encounters and the role of anergy. *J Comput Appl Math* (2005) **184**(1):101–20. doi:10.1016/j.cam.2004.07.036
104. Anderton SM, Wraith DC. Selection and fine-tuning of the autoimmune T-cell repertoire. *Nat Rev Immunol* (2002) **2**(7):487–98. doi:10.1038/nri842
105. Grossman Z, Paul WE. Adaptive cellular interactions in the immune system: the tunable activation threshold and the significance of subthreshold responses. *Proc Natl Acad Sci U S A* (1992) **89**(21):10365–9. doi:10.1073/pnas.89.21.10365
106. van den Berg HA, Rand DA. Quantitative theories of T-cell responsiveness. *Immunol Rev* (2007) **216**:81–92. doi:10.1111/j.1600-065X.2006.00491.x
107. Burroughs NJ, Miguel Paz Mendes de Oliveira B, Adrego Pinto A. Regulatory T cell adjustment of quorum growth thresholds and the control of local immune responses. *J Theor Biol* (2006) **241**(1):134–41. doi:10.1016/j.jtbi.2005.11.010 Epub 2006/01/13
108. Burroughs NJ, Oliveira BM, Pinto AA, Sequeira HJT. Sensibility of the quorum growth thresholds controlling local immune responses. *Math Comput Model* (2008) **47**(7–8):714–25. doi:10.1016/j.mcm.2007.06.007
109. Pinto AA, Burroughs NJ, Ferreira M, Oliveira BM. Dynamics of immunological models. *Acta Biotheor* (2010) **58**(4):391–404. doi:10.1007/s10441-010-9117-6
110. Kim PS, Lee PP, Levy D. Modeling regulation mechanisms in the immune system. *J Theor Biol* (2007) **246**(1):33–69. doi:10.1016/j.jtbi.2006.12.012 Epub 2007/02/03
111. de Abreu FV, Mostardinha P. Maximal frustration as an immunological principle. *J R Soc Interface* (2009) **6**(32):321–34. doi:10.1098/rsif.2008.0280
112. Leon K, Faro J, Lage A, Carneiro J. Inverse correlation between the incidences of autoimmune disease and infection predicted by a model of T cell mediated tolerance. *J Autoimmun* (2004) **22**(1):31–42. doi:10.1016/j.jaut.2003.10.002 Epub 2004/01/08
113. Martinez-Pasamar S, Abad E, Moreno B, Velez de Mendizabal N, Martinez-Forero I, Garcia-Ojalvo J, et al. Dynamic cross-regulation of antigen-specific effector and regulatory T cell subpopulations and microglia in brain autoimmunity. *BMC Syst Biol* (2013) **7**:34. doi:10.1186/1752-0509-7-34
114. Velez de Mendizabal N, Carneiro J, Sole RV, Goni J, Bragard J, Martinez-Forero I, et al. Modeling the effector – regulatory T cell cross-regulation reveals the intrinsic character of relapses in Multiple Sclerosis. *BMC Syst Biol* (2011) **5**:114. doi:10.1186/1752-0509-5-114
115. Lo WC, Arsenescu RI, Friedman A. Mathematical Model of the Roles of T Cells in Inflammatory Bowel Disease. *Bull Math Biol* (2013) **75**(9):1417–33. doi:10.1007/s11538-013-9853-2
116. Gross F, Metzner G, Behn U. Mathematical modeling of allergy and specific immunotherapy: Th1-Th2-Treg interactions. *J Theor Biol* (2011) **269**(1):70–8. doi:10.1016/j.jtbi.2010.10.013
117. Arazi A, Sharabi A, Zinger H, Mozes E, Neumann AU. In vivo dynamical interactions between CD4 Tregs, CD8 Tregs and CD4+ CD25− cells in mice. *PLoS One* (2009) **4**(12):e8447. doi:10.1371/journal.pone.0008447
118. Bewick S, Yang R, Zhang M. The danger is growing! A new paradigm for immune system activation and peripheral tolerance. *PLoS One* (2009) **4**(12):e8112. doi:10.1371/journal.pone.0008112
119. Simonov M, Rawlings RA, Comment N, Reed SE, Shi X, Nelson PW. Modeling adaptive regulatory T-cell dynamics during early HIV infection. *PLoS One* (2012) **7**(4):e33924. doi:10.1371/journal.pone.0033924
120. Leon K, Garcia K, Carneiro J, Lage A. How regulatory CD25+CD4+ T cells impinge on tumor immunobiology: the differential response of tumors to therapies. *J Immunol* (2007) **179**(9):5659–68.
121. Leon K, Garcia K, Carneiro J, Lage A. How regulatory CD25(+)CD4(+) T cells impinge on tumor immunobiology? On the existence of two alternative dynamical classes of tumors. *J Theor Biol* (2007) **247**(1):122–37. doi:10.1016/j.jtbi.2007.01.029
122. Baltcheva I, Codarri L, Pantaleo G, Le Boudec JY. Lifelong dynamics of human CD4+CD25+ regulatory T cells: insights from in vivo data and mathematical modeling. *J Theor Biol* (2010) **266**(2):307–22. doi:10.1016/j.jtbi.2010.06.024
123. Agua-Doce A, Graca L. Regulatory T cells and the control of the allergic response. *J Allergy* (2012) **2012**:948901. doi:10.1155/2012/948901 Epub 2012/10/12
124. Gratz IK, Rosenblum MD, Abbas AK. The life of regulatory T cells. *Ann N Y Acad Sci* (2013) **1283**:8–12. doi:10.1111/nyas.12011
125. Perelson AS. Modelling viral and immune system dynamics. *Nat Rev Immunol* (2002) **2**(1):28–36. doi:10.1038/nri700

The anti-inflammatory mechanisms of Hsp70

Thiago J. Borges[1†], Lotte Wieten[2†], Martijn J. C. van Herwijnen[2], Femke Broere[2], Ruurd van der Zee[2], Cristina Bonorino[1]* and Willem van Eden[2]

[1] Faculdade de Biociências e Instituto de Pesquisas Biomédicas, Pontifícia Universidade Católica do Rio Grande do Sul, Porto Alegre, Rio Grande do Sul, Brazil

[2] Department of Infectious Diseases and Immunology, Faculty of Veterinary Medicine, Utrecht University, Utrecht, Netherlands

Edited by:
Alexander Rudensky, Memorial Sloan-Kettering Cancer Center, USA

Reviewed by:
Francesco Annunziato, University of Florence, Italy
Miriam Wittmann, University of Leeds, UK

Correspondence:
Cristina Bonorino, Departamento de Biologia Celular e Molecular e Instituto de Pesquisas Biomédicas, Pontifícia Universidade Católica do Rio Grande do Sul, Av. Ipiranga, 6690 2° andar, 90680-001 Porto Alegre, Rio Grande do Sul, Brazil.
e-mail: cbonorino@pucrs.br;
Willem van Eden, Department of Infectious Diseases and Immunology, Faculty of Veterinary Medicine, Utrecht University, Yalelaan 1, 3584 CL Utrecht, Netherlands.
e-mail: w.vaneden@uu.nl

†Thiago J. Borges and Lotte Wieten have contributed equally to this work.

Immune responses to heat shock proteins (Hsp) develop in virtually all inflammatory diseases; however, the significance of such responses is only now becoming clear. In experimental disease models, Hsp administration can prevent or arrest inflammatory damage, and in initial clinical trials in patients with chronic inflammatory diseases, Hsp peptides have been shown to promote the production of anti-inflammatory cytokines, indicating immunoregulatory potential of Hsp. Therefore, the presence of immune responses to Hsp in inflammatory diseases can be seen as an attempt of the immune system to correct the inflammatory condition. Hsp70 can modulate inflammatory responses in models of arthritis, colitis and graft rejection, and the mechanisms underlying this effect are now being elucidated. Incubation with microbial Hsp70 was seen to induce tolerogenic dendritic cells (DCs) and to promote a suppressive phenotype in myeloid-derived suppressor cells and monocytes. These DC could induce regulatory T cells (Tregs), independently of the antigens they presented. Some Hsp70 family members are associated with autophagy, leading to a preferential uploading of Hsp70 peptides in MHC class II molecules of stressed cells. Henceforth, conserved Hsp70 peptides may be presented in these situations and constitute targets of Tregs, contributing to downregulation of inflammation. Finally, an interfering effect in multiple intracellular inflammatory signaling pathways is also known for Hsp70. Altogether it seems attractive to use Hsp70, or its derivative peptides, for modulation of inflammation. This is a physiological immunotherapy approach, without the immediate necessity of defining disease-specific auto-antigens. In this article, we present the evidence on anti-inflammatory effects of Hsp70 and discuss the need for experiments that will be crucial for the further exploration of the immunosuppressive potential of this protein.

Keywords: Hsp70, stress proteins, immunomodulation, adaptive immunity, innate immunity

Hsps ARE IMMUNODOMINANT PROTEINS

Heat shock proteins (Hsp) are highly conserved proteins, from microbes through mammals. They are preferentially induced in response to cell stresses including heat shock, oxidative stress, ultraviolet radiation, ischemia-reperfusion injury, viral infections, nutrient deprivation, and chemicals (Lindquist, 1986), protecting cells from injury and promoting refolding of denatured proteins. Hsp are grouped in families according to their molecular weight, and constitutive members of each family can be found in different cell compartments under non-stress conditions, performing chaperone functions (Lindquist and Craig, 1988).

Hsp70 is the most highly conserved protein known to date (Lindquist and Craig, 1988; Ellis, 1990; Feder and Hofmann, 1999). It was therefore surprising when Hsp, including Hsp70, were found to be immunodominant antigens. Early studies demonstrated that 10–20% of the T cells recognized Hsp60 of *Mycobacterium tuberculosis* after experimental mycobacterial immunization (Kaufmann et al., 1987). Hsp70 of *M. leprae* was shown to be a prominent antigen in humans infected with *M. leprae* (Kaufmann et al., 1987; Janson et al., 1991). Such mycobacterial-Hsp-specific T cell responses have also been observed in healthy individuals, not previously exposed to mycobacterial infections (Munk et al., 1989) and in cord blood (Fischer et al., 1992; Aalberse et al., 2011). Immunization with Hsp70 of *M. tuberculosis* (TB-Hsp70) led to a strong IgG response in 7 days without evidence of IgM production (Bonorino et al., 1998), suggesting that antigen-specific T cells able to provide help were already available in naïve mice. Interestingly, a detailed analysis of the peptides recognized by T cells, both in healthy and infected individuals, revealed that some of them were highly conserved (Quayle et al., 1992; Anderton et al., 1995).

Hsp70 AS AN IMMUNOMODULATORY AGENT

It was then hypothesized that, because of their homology with self, bacterial-Hsp would provoke autoimmunity through molecular mimicry with self-proteins. This idea was refuted by the finding that pre-immunization with bacterial-Hsp protected Lewis rats from adjuvant-induced arthritis (van Eden et al., 1988). Subsequently, immunoregulatory features of Hsp were demonstrated in various inflammatory diseases. The literature on immunomodulatory properties of Hsp is vast. In this review, we will focus on Hsp70. Although it may be tempting to generalize observations on different Hsp, it is important to consider that the different families of Hsp show no homology of sequence or structure, and are encoded by different genes, transcribed under the control of different transcription factors, that are not always activated in coordinate manner. Rather, Hsp are grouped under the same banner because they are commonly induced in similar situations of stress, cooperating to promote cell recovery and protection from injury.

Hsp70 was demonstrated to have a disease suppressive role in experimental models of autoimmunity. One study demonstrated that T cells reactive to peptide 234–252 of TB-Hsp70 suppressed inflammatory responses against *Listeria monocytogenes* via production of IL-10 (Kimura et al., 1998). The same group later showed that pretreatment with peptide 234–252 of TB-Hsp70 suppressed the development of adjuvant-induced arthritis in Lewis rats, generating T cells that were specific for this peptide, and produced high levels of IL-10, but not IFN-g (Tanaka et al., 1999). Also the treatment with anti-IL-10 antibody abrogated protection. This peptide showed 58% amino acid identity between rat and mycobacterial Hsp70. Another study revealed that a different peptide of Hsp70, conserved between rat and mycobacteria, protected Lewis rats from development of arthritis when given intra-nasally (Wendling et al., 2000), preventing disease development by the induction of IL-10 producing T cells. Endogenous Hsp70 presence in the mouse, guaranteed by the presence of heat shock factor 1 (HSF1), its transcription factor, was found to protect from induced colitis (Tanaka et al., 2007). More recently, treatment with whole endotoxin-free TB-Hsp70 inhibited acute rejection of skin and tumor allografts (Borges et al., 2010). Consequently, disease suppressive effects have been observed in the case of both microbial and self (mammalian) Hsp70, some studies using whole protein, some studies using just the peptide, and IL-10 was always important.

How could the conservation of Hsp be reconciled with this apparent predisposition for recognition by the immune system? One idea was that the protective effects of microbial Hsp were related, at least in part, to their capacity to induce T cell responses which were cross-reactive with self-Hsp. Cohen proposed that, to avoid excessive immune responses to both self- and foreign-antigens, the immune system would be selective in its responsiveness and focus on particular immunodominant proteins: the so-called immunological homunculus (Cohen and Young, 1991; Cohen, 2007). Hsp were thus postulated to be such proteins. However, the regulatory capacity of Hsp could not be completely explained by immunodominance and homology between bacterial- and self-Hsp. This was demonstrated in studies using the adjuvant-induced arthritis model, in which Hsps, but not other highly immunogenic and conserved proteins of bacterial origin, were found to suppress disease development (Prakken et al., 2001). So, which additional features of Hsp would endow them with the capacity to suppress inflammatory responses? Along the years, different groups have collected evidence on Hsp70 involvement in innate and adaptive immune responses.

INNATE IMMUNE CELL MODULATION BY Hsp70 – EXTRACELLULAR Hsp70

The idea that Hsp70 could modulate innate cell function comes from studies that analyzed the interaction of Hsp70, either delivered extracellularly or present in the outer cell membrane/exosomes, with receptors on cells such as monocytes, dendritic cells (DCs) and myeloid-derived suppressor cells (MDSCs). This notion was surprising initially, because Hsp70 was then believed to be an intracellular chaperone. However, studies by Hightower and Guidon Jr. (1989) revealed that Hsp70 could be released from cells, in a mechanism that was independent of blockage of secretory pathways. A series of studies followed, revealing that soluble Hsp70 could be measured in the serum of both healthy and diseased individuals (Pockley et al., 1998); and that this extracellular Hsp70 could be either actively secreted by a non-classical pathway, or released from dying cells, review in De Maio (2011).

Two new functions were then reported for extracellular Hsp70. One study demonstrated that (mammalian) Hsp70–peptide complexes purified from MethA sarcomas could lead to priming of cytotoxic T cell (CTL) responses against these tumors (Udono and Srivastava, 1993). That meant that Hsp70 could probably bind to a membrane receptor in antigen-presenting cells (APCs), and get access to the endogenous route of antigen processing and presentation in MHC class I – i.e., cross-priming. A different group later reported that human Hsp70 could bind to and activate human monocytes, promoting the secretion of inflammatory cytokines, such as TNF-α, IL-1β, and IL-6 (Asea et al., 2000a). Different groups went on to corroborate the findings of the cross-priming abilities of Hsp70 (Delneste et al., 2002; Kammerer et al., 2002; Ueda et al., 2004). However, the findings on the induction of pro-inflammatory cytokines were disputed (Gao and Tsan, 2004) when the removal of contaminating endotoxin of the recombinant preparations of human Hsp70 abrogated the induction of TNF-α by this protein. Hsp70 is a molecule with high affinity for hydrophobic moieties (Tsan and Gao, 2009) and the efficient removal of LPS and lipid-like contaminants from preparations of Hsp70 proved to be a challenge for those working with this protein. It is thus very likely that the ability of Hsp70 to bind cell surface receptors (see below) and be internalized, activating antigen presentation, which has been verified by independent groups, is independent of the induction of inflammatory cytokines by this protein, which, to this date, is still disputed.

The removal of contaminating endotoxin and lipopeptides by treatment with Triton X-114, a detergent, revealed that soluble Hsp70 had, in fact, anti-inflammatory properties. It was demonstrated that TB-Hsp70 could modulate cytokine production in blood and synovial cells of arthritis patients. *In vitro* treatment with endotoxin-free TB-Hsp70 for 48 h induced IL-10 production in peripheral blood mononuclear cells (PBMCs) from rheumatoid arthritis (RA) and reactive arthritis (ReA) patients as well as in normal controls PBMCs (Detanico et al., 2004). Concomitantly, PBMCs from these patients downregulated IFN-γ production (900-fold for RA patients and 750-fold for ReA patients when compared with untreated cells) and up-regulated IL-10 production (900-fold for RA patients and 500-fold for ReA patients). In addition, synovial cells incubated with TB-Hsp70 for 48 h showed a reversal of the inflammatory profile, with an induction of IL-10 [a 4.9-fold increase when compared with cells treated with bovine serum albumin (BSA) and LPS], correlating with a decrease in TNF-α and IFN-γ production. Synovial monocytes from the arthritis patients were the major source of IL-10 induced by TB-Hsp70. In accordance with these findings,

Luo et al. (2008) demonstrated that human Hsp70 downregulated in a concentration-dependent manner the TNF-α-induced production of pro-inflammatory mediators IL-6, IL-8, and MCP-1 in RA fibroblast-like synoviocytes when compared with OVA-treated cells. Thus, Hsp70, both bacterial and human, were shown to be associated with a protective phenotype in arthritis, corroborating the initial findings in adjuvant arthritis.

TB-Hsp70 could also modulate cytokine production in DCs. These cells provide a link between innate and adaptive responses, by presenting antigen to T cells, activating them, and shaping their differentiation into effector phenotypes (Heath and Carbone, 2009; Watowich and Liu, 2010). Production of IL-12 by DCs leads to a Th1 program of differentiation for the antigen-specific $CD4^+$ T cells, while IL-4 production induces a Th2 phenotype. Tolerogenic DCs, however, are characterized by low production of pro-inflammatory cytokines and high production of anti-inflammatory cytokines. It has been shown that cells expressing low levels of both MHC class II and T cell co-stimulatory molecules – such as CD80 and CD86, and that do or do not produce IL-10 and TGF-β, can be tolerogenic (Steinman et al., 2003; Rutella et al., 2006; Morelli and Thomson, 2007).

LPS-free TB-Hsp70 blocked the *in vitro* differentiation of DCs from bone marrow precursors. When murine bone marrow DCs (BMDCs) were treated with TB-Hsp70 for 24 or 48 h, an inhibition of maturation characterized by a failure to acquire MHC class II and CD86 expression was observed. TB-Hsp70-treated BMDCs had an eightfold increase in IL-10 production when compared with dexamethasone treated cells and produced 1,200-fold less TNF-α than LPS stimulated cells after 48 h of culture (Motta et al., 2007), suggesting not all transcription was inhibited in the treated BMDCs. More recently, a different group demonstrated that soluble inducible human Hsp70 (now known as HSPA1A) can also induce a regulatory phenotype in monocyte-derived DCs (MoDCs; Stocki et al., 2012). They tested three preparations of Hsp70, two commercial ones, with high or medium endotoxin levels, and one other with very low endotoxin levels. Only the Hsp70 preparations with high and medium endotoxin levels induced maturation of MoDCs in culture. The very low endotoxin level Hsp70, however, inhibited the maturation of MoDCs and reduced the capacity of those cells of stimulating allogeneic T cell proliferation. Together, these results indicated that both TB-Hsp70 and human Hsp70 produced a tolerogenic phenotype in DCs, provided that LPS contamination was eliminated.

These findings in DC have an important implication for a regulatory role of soluble forms of Hsp70. Tolerogenic DCs are known to contribute to the creation of a "suppressive environment" facilitating the peripheral generation of peripheral Tregs. Tregs play a crucial role in suppressing the excessive effector immune response that is harmful to the host (Sakaguchi et al., 2008). These cells can be divided into two subphenotypes. The first one is the Foxp3-expressing Tregs that develop in the thymus (nTregs; Feuerer et al., 2009). The second are the cells that can be induced in peripheral sites when given appropriate signals by the APCs (iTregs; Shevach, 2006). Tregs produce IL-10 or TGF-β, sometimes both, and actively suppress non-Treg proliferation (Vignali et al., 2008). Low levels of antigen presentation coupled to low co-stimulation have been linked to the differentiation of induced Tregs (iTregs; Jenkins et al., 1990; Steinman et al., 2000; Long et al., 2011). Thus, it was possible that, by modulating the APCs, Hsp70 could lead to the induction of Tregs in the periphery.

Confirming this prediction, soluble TB-Hsp70 was demonstrated to inhibit acute allograft rejection (Borges et al., 2010). When C57Bl/6 tumor cells or skin sections were pre-incubated in a solution with endotoxin-free TB-Hsp70 and then grafted onto a BALB/c host, the tumor cells formed a solid tumor, and skin rejection was delayed for 7–10 days, compared to controls. This effect was abrogated by depletion of Tregs, which were shown to infiltrate the accepted grafts. Interestingly, when soluble TB-Hsp70 was injected subcutaneously, this led to an increase in $CD4^+CD25^+Foxp3^+$ cells in the draining lymph node, which correlated to a diminished proliferation of lymph node cells in response to a T cell mitogen. The conclusion was that one single pretreatment with TB-Hsp70 could inhibit a powerful *in vivo* inflammatory process, and this correlated with the presence of Tregs.

The possibility that Hsp70 and Tregs are intimately linked is discussed in detail in the second part of this article (adaptive immunity). In the meantime, we wish discuss one more evidence that Hsp70 can act as an immunosuppressant – and this is related to another discovery, namely that Hsp70 could localize in membranes.

It was shown that Hsp70 (Vega et al., 2008), similarly to Hsc70 (Arispe and De Maio, 2000) could integrate into an artificial lipid bilayer, opening cationic conductance channels, and this ability was associated with the presence of phosphatidylserine (PS; Arispe et al., 2004). Other sphingolipids, such as globotriaosylceramide, have also been reported to enhance Hsp70 insertion into membranes (Gehrmann et al., 2008). This supported previous reports that Hsp70 could be found in the membrane of tumors (Ferrarini et al., 1992; Multhoff et al., 1995). Hsp70 was not simply associated with a receptor in the membrane, but rather inserted, because it could not be eluted by acid washes, or Triton X-1000 (Vega et al., 2008) and because only one antibody, recognizing a part of the C-terminus, but not antibodies that would recognize the N-terminus, would detect it (Botzler et al., 1998). The presence of Hsp70 in membranes of cells or exosomes of tumors presented one more way of extracellular interactions of Hsp70.

Myeloid-derived suppressor cells are a different, heterogeneous population of cells that are expanded during cancer, inflammation, and infection, with a remarkable ability to suppress T cell responses (Gabrilovich and Nagaraj, 2009). Chalmin et al. (2010) demonstrated, in mice and humans, that membrane-associated Hsp70 found in tumor-derived exosomes (TDEs) restrained tumor immune surveillance by promoting MDSCs suppressive functions. It was demonstrated that TDEs, contained in the tumor cell supernatant of three tumor cell lines, could mediate T cell-dependent immunosuppressive functions of MDSCs. The authors identified that the factor present on the TDEs that induced MDSCs activation was the inducible Hsp70 (HSPA1A) expressed on TDE cell surface. Hsp70 was only present on exosomal fractions, not in other microparticles. These findings indicated that immunomodulatory effects of tumor cells include their potential of inducing functional MDSCs by releasing exosomes expressing Hsp70.

Hsp70 PUTATIVE RECEPTORS AND RESPECTIVE SIGNALING PATHWAYS

Many studies asked the question of how would cells perceive the presence of extracellular Hsp. CD14 (Asea et al., 2000b), and Toll-like receptors (TLRs) 2 and 4 (Asea et al., 2002) were first proposed to be receptors for soluble extracellular human Hsp70 – and this was, as discussed above, disputed due to the contamination issue. CD40 (Wang et al., 2001) was then proposed as a receptor for mammalian Hsp70, however a different study (Binder, 2009) refuted this idea, demonstrating that Hsp70 would still bind to cells in CD40 knockout mice. CD91 (Basu et al., 2001) and LOX-1 (Delneste et al., 2002), two scavenger receptors, were shown to bind Hsp70–antigen complexes, increasing cross-presentation and eliciting a protective immune response against antigen-expressing tumor cells *in vivo*. Floto et al. (2006) suggested that TB-Hsp70 promoted DC aggregation, immune synapse formation between DCs and T cells, and an effector immune response the signaling through the CCR5 chemokine receptor. All these different results generated great confusion. A consistent finding among studies was the ability of extracellular Hsp70 to be internalized and interact with antigen presentation routes, inducing T cell responses to the peptides that associated with this protein. TLRs and CD40 are signaling receptors, rather than endocytic receptors. Scavenger receptors and lectin-like receptors are endocytic receptors, and the signaling events downstream binding and internalization that follows binding are not fully characterized.

A thorough study transfected Chinese hamster ovary (CHO) cells with cDNAs expressing each of these putative receptors, as well as other scavenger receptors and lectins, and studied their interaction with mammalian extracellular Hsp70 (Theriault et al., 2005). The authors verified no binding or internalization of Hsp70 with cells expressing TLR2, TLR4, CD40, or CD91. In a follow-up study, they used the same approach focusing on scavenger receptors (Theriault et al., 2006). They demonstrated that LOX-1, SREC-1, and FEEL-1 bind and internalize Hsp70. However, different forms of Hsp70 (peptide bound or ATP bound) interacted with each of these receptors with different affinities. In summary, while binding to signaling receptors was refuted by more than one study, different groups provided evidence for scavenger receptors as the likely receptors for extracellular Hsp70.

SIGNALING ROUTES ACTIVATED BY Hsp70

If extracellular Hsp70 indeed interacts with membrane-bound receptors, will it activate signaling pathways associated with these receptors? Few studies approached this issue.

Mitogen-activated protein (MAP) kinase cascade is one of the most ancient and evolutionarily conserved signaling pathways, which is also important for many processes in immune responses (Dong et al., 2002). TDE-associated Hsp70 was found to mediate the suppressive activity of the MDSCs via activation of STAT3 and ERK (Chalmin et al., 2010). An ERK-dependent route for IL-10 production by different immune system cells upon TLR stimulation has been described (Saraiva and O'Garra, 2010). It has been suggested that some TLR2 agonists are good inducers of IL-10 production (Dillon et al., 2006; Manicassamy et al., 2009; Saraiva and O'Garra, 2010; Yamazaki et al., 2011). It is an interesting feature of TLR2 that, depending on the nature of the ligand and the population of target cells, it can mediate either inflammatory or anti-inflammatory responses to the same infectious organism (Dillon et al., 2006; Frodermann et al., 2011), and the anti-inflammatory response is mediated by IL-10.

IL-10 is the main anti-inflammatory and immunosuppressive cytokine (Moore et al., 2001). However, depending on the situation, it can exert a pro-inflammatory role like in lupus erythematosus (Bussolati et al., 2000; Sharif et al., 2004). It has been suggested that type I interferons regulate the balance between anti- and pro-inflammatory role of IL-10 (Sharif et al., 2004). In monocytes of patients with systemic lupus erythematosus (SLE), it was demonstrated that IL-10 can stimulate production of platelet-activating factor (PAF) and this production was correlated with disease severity (Bussolati et al., 2000).

IL-10 production of by DCs stimulated via TLRs is diminished in presence of selective ERK inhibitors (Yi et al., 2002; Dillon et al., 2004; Kaiser et al., 2009) or in ERK-deficient cells (Agrawal et al., 2006). Besides, differences in IL-10 production by macrophages, myeloid DCs, and plasmacytoid DCs are correlated with different levels of ERK activation in these cells (Saraiva and O'Garra, 2010). Borges et al. (in preparation) observed that BMDCs treated with TB-Hsp70 showed a higher expression of phospho-ERK when compared with unstimulated cells, and inhibition of ERK expression with the specific ERK inhibitor PD98059 blocked IL-10 production upon incubation with Hsp70.

STAT3 is associated with IL-10 production and tolerance (Barton, 2006; Dhingra et al., 2011). Also, IL-10R recruits and activates JNK1-STAT3 pathway (Murray, 2006). In contrast, STAT3 can be activated by pro-inflammatory cytokines like IL-6, through IL-6R (Murray, 2007) and Oncostatin M (Halfter et al., 1999). Despite this duality in STAT3 activation, this transcription factor may be activated after IL-10 release induced by TB-Hsp70.

Based on this, we propose a model in which extracellular Hsp70 could regulate innate immune cell function, binding to cell surface receptors (a scavenger or lectin-like receptor), signaling through TLR2 via ERK to induce IL-10 production, resulting in an anti-inflammatory response. This model is depicted in **Figure 1**.

Is it possible to reconcile this model with what has been observed for the cross-priming and pro-inflammatory roles described for this protein? We believe that the next studies should test the possibility that extracellular Hsp70, upon binding to lectin-like or scavenger receptors, uses associated receptors to signal. It is possible that depending on the form of Hsp70 (associated with peptide; with membranes; with nucleotides; peptide-free) it will associate with a different receptor. Another issue that has to be considered is that, while in bacteria, Hsp70 comes from one gene, in mammals, there may be at least eight genes that code for Hsp70 (Kampinga et al., 2009). Bulk preparations of mammalian Hsp70 from cells contain not only the inducible, HSPA1A, but products from other genes as well. And this may also influence the outcome of the experiment. Finally, binding and internalization, followed by antigen presentation, may lead to inflammatory as well as to regulatory responses, depending on which receptor is engaged, as demonstrated in a recent study (Li et al., 2012). The authors verified that targeting an antigen to LOX-1 or DC-ASGPR on the surface of DCs led to internalization and cross-presentation of

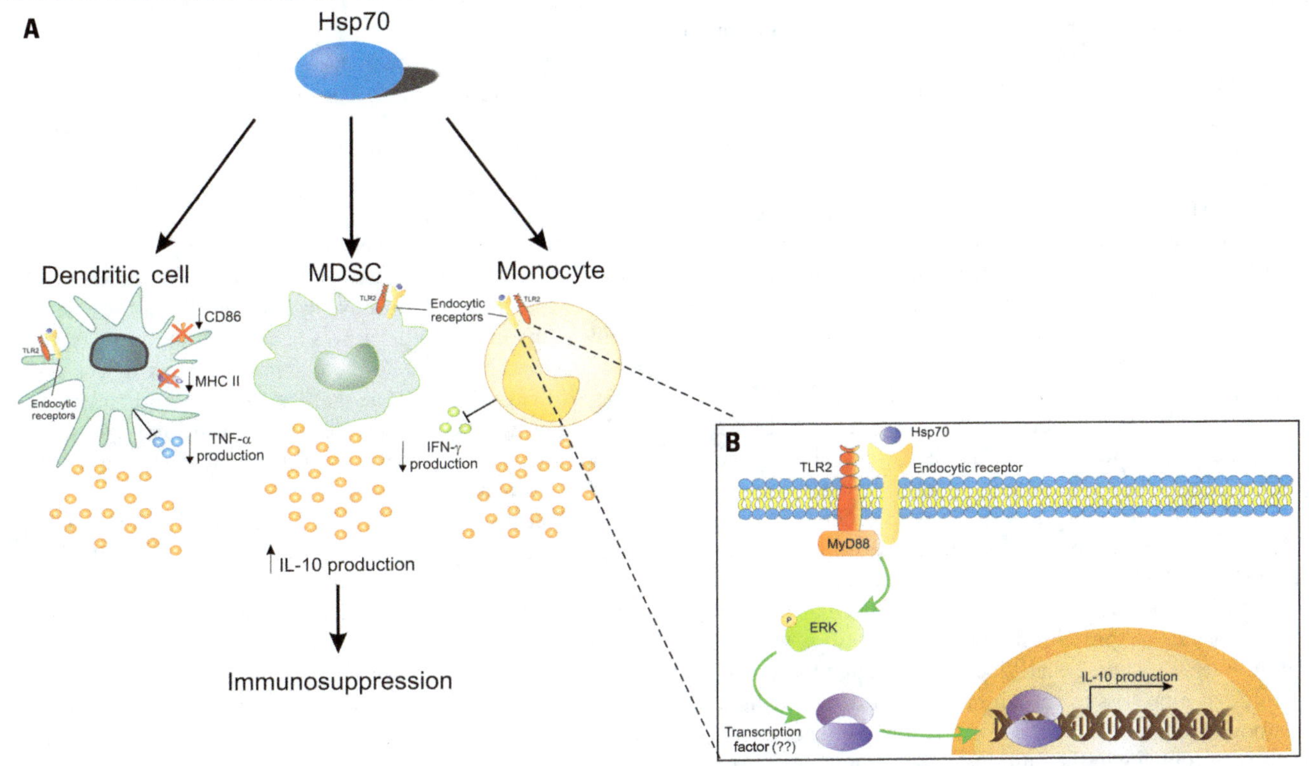

FIGURE 1 | Hsp70 can interact directly with innate immune cells. **(A)** A possible mechanism of the Hsp70 action is its interaction with dendritic cells (DCs), myeloid-derived suppressor cells (MDSCs), and monocytes. Hsp70 would bind to endocytic receptors, and be endocytosed, gaining access to routes of antigen presentation, modulating the cell phenotype toward a tolerogenic one, leading to the production of the anti-inflammatory cytokine IL-10 and consequently to immunosuppression. In DCs, Hsp70 downregulates CD86 and MHC class II expression, and inhibits TNF-α production. Also, Hsp70 can inhibit IFN-γ by monocytes. **(B)** Upon binding to an endocytic, Hsp70 signals through TLR2, resulting in MyD88 activation. The subsequent phosphorylation of ERK can trigger the activation of an undetermined transcription factor that will bind the *il-10* gene promoter leading to IL-10 production.

the antigen. However, while targeting to LOX-1 resulted in INF-gamma producing T cells, targeting to DC-ASGPR resulted in IL-10 producing CD4 T cells. Thus, it is possible that, depending on the form of extracellular Hsp70 and the target cell/tissue microenvironment, different outcomes may ensue. If this possibility is verified experimentally, that would in part explain some of the conflicting results previously discussed here. We are now left with the challenge to test these possibilities in order to elucidate the whole potential of Hsp70 as an immunomodulatory agent.

ADAPTIVE IMMUNITY REGULATION BY Hsp70

Besides the innate effects discussed above, several adaptive immunity associated mechanisms have been proposed for induction of Hsp-specific Tregs under physiological conditions.

The role of Hsp70 in adaptive immunity to mediate suppression through Tregs could be related to presentation of Hsp70 peptides, or to the modulation of the innate environment as described in the previous section, leading to the induction of Tregs.

The presentation of Hsp70 peptides in MHC molecules could result either from overexpression of endogenous Hsp70 in situations of physiological stress, or from endocytosis of extracellular Hsp; In response to physiological stress, intracellular levels of Hsp70 will rise in the stressed cells which can lead to presentation of Hsp peptides on MHC class I via the default MHC loading route for cytosolic proteins. This pathway includes degradation of the protein by the proteasome, transporter associated with antigen presentation (TAP) mediated translocation to the endoplasmic reticulum and subsequent loading of the peptides on MHC class I molecules (Neefjes et al., 2011). As will be discussed in more detail below, it is now becoming clear that via autophagy, intracellular Hsp can also be loaded on MHC class II molecules. Peptides derived from extracellular Hsp (pathogen-associated or secreted endogenous Hsp) can be presented via endocytic pathways by MHC class II molecules on APCs or on non-APCs upon stimulation with factors like IFNγ.

The mechanisms leading to production of Hsp-specific Treg can be manifold. Continuous encounter of bacterial-Hsp, in mucosal surfaces such as the gut can be a way to induce bacterial-Hsp-specific Treg, contributing to Hsp-specific mucosal tolerance (van Eden et al., 2005, 2007). Another possibility is the up-regulation of self-Hsp on non-professional APCs in response to various forms of stress in tissues. In the gut lamina propria of many species, MHC class II is also found to be present on non-professional APCs (Stokes et al., 1996). In addition, the inflammatory mediator IFN-γ is known to induce MHC class II in various cell types. Thus, MHC class II presentation of Hsp fragments in the absence of proper co-stimulation may add to the production of tolerogenic or regulatory T cell responses. In addition, presentation of self-Hsp70 conserved peptides in presence of TGF-β (Sela et al., 2011) could lead to Treg induction and/or expansion (Rosenblum et al., 2011). Also, because some self-Hsp70 peptides are not completely identical to their bacterial homolog peptides, such presented self-peptides could function as altered peptide ligands for bacterial-Hsp-specific cells leading to induction of a partially agonistic and therefore downmodulated T cell response (Wauben et al., 1993). Finally, induction of Treg might be reinforced by the increased levels of the immunoregulatory cytokine IL-10, induced upon stress in multiple tissues (Stordeur and Goldman, 1998).

AUTOPHAGY, LOADING Hsp PEPTIDES ON MHC CLASS II

To activate $CD4^+$ T cells, peptides should be presented by MHC class II molecules. Cytosolic proteins, like Hsp70, are by default loaded on MHC class I molecules while extracellular proteins will be presented on MHC class II. Thus, another fundamental question can be raised; how do Hsp peptides end up to become presented by MHC class II? The distinct localization between MHC class I and MHC class II loading pathways has been proven incorrect because cytosolic proteins have been eluted from MHC class II and vice versa (Schmid et al., 2007). Autophagy has been initially found as a process to sustain metabolic fitness during food deprivation through bulk protein degradation (Kuma et al., 2004). The role of autophagy in the immune system is only now becoming clear (Schmid and Munz, 2007; Munz, 2009). Two pathways can result in loading of intracellular peptides on MHC class II. First, intracellular proteins can be incorporated in autophagosomes that subsequently fuse with lysosomes for degradation of their cargo (macroautophagy). In addition, cytosolic proteins can be transported via LAMP2a directly into the lysosome (chaperone mediated autophagy; Munz, 2006; Schmid et al., 2007; Strawbridge and Blum, 2007). Recently, the role of autophagy in loading Hsp70 peptides has been described; in human HLA-$DR4^+$ B cells a striking increase of especially Hsp70 peptides was eluted from HLA-DR4 upon induction of autophagy by amino acid deprivation (Dengjel et al., 2005). Autophagy induction coincided with elevated Hsp70 mRNA levels. In other words, especially under conditions of cell stress, fragments of Hsp70 will be presented on APCs to T cells, possibly initiating a regulatory T cell response.

PHENOTYPE OF Hsp-SPECIFIC Treg

The phenotype of Hsp-specific Treg has not been studied in detail. However, since Hsp-specific T cells have been observed in cord blood, some of them will probably be thymus derived $CD4^+CD25^+Foxp3^+$ natural Treg (Sakaguchi et al., 1995; Tang and Bluestone, 2008). Also, Hsp-specific Treg can be induced in the periphery, which potentially leads to induction of several induced Treg subsets. For example, $Foxp3^-$ Tr1 cells, which are induced by repetitive stimulation with antigen in the presence of IL-10 (Groux et al., 1997; Roncarolo and Battaglia, 2007). Alternatively, mucosal exposure of Hsp can produce iTregs, expressing a $CD4^+CD25^+Foxp3^+$ phenotype (Chen et al., 1994; Weiner, 2001). Or, conversion of naïve $CD4^+CD25\text{-}Foxp3^-$ cells into induced $CD4^+CD25^+Foxp3^+$ can occur in the presence of IL-2 and TGF-β at low levels of pro-inflammatory cytokines (Horwitz et al., 2008).

The phenotype of the Hsp-specific Treg may depend on the exposure route. Intraperitoneal (i.p.) immunization with endotoxin-free TB-Hsp70 or OVA as a control resulted in $CD4^+CD25^+$ T cells from Hsp70 immunized mice expressing slightly enhanced levels of regulatory cytokine IL-10, but not increasingly expression of Foxp3 (Wieten et al., 2009a). In contrast, in a study in a mouse atherosclerosis model, oral Hsp administration increased Foxp3 expression (van Puijvelde et al., 2007). Enhanced Foxp3 expression, both systemically in the spleen and locally in the inflamed joint, was also found upon up-regulation of endogenous Hsp70 in Peyer's patches of carvacrol (a co-inducer of Hsp70) fed mice (Wieten et al., 2010). The finding that Foxp3 levels were increased in cells obtained from joint synovial fluid suggested that induced Treg could have actually migrated to the site of inflammation.

In a recent study, after local injection of whole TB-Hsp70, a higher percentage of $CD4^+CD25^+Foxp3^+$ cells in draining lymph nodes compared with local injection with OVA was observed. Moreover, TB-Hsp70 inhibition of lymph node cell proliferation was superior to the inhibition induced by dexamethasone after PHA stimulation. The authors also observed that inhibition of acute rejection induced by TB-Hsp70 was dependent on $CD4^+CD25^+$ T cells in a skin allograft model (Borges et al., 2010).

To study the phenotype of Hsp-specific Treg in more detail, the expression of the transcription factor Helios in Tregs elicited by Hsp70 treatment, to verify if they are nTregs or iTregs (Thornton et al., 2010), since peripherally induced Tregs do not usually express this molecule. It will also be interesting to see if T cells found at the site of inflammation are Hsp70 specific, and if they indeed express special homing receptors. Future studies should tell us the relative proportions of nTregs and iTregs in Hsp70-specific Tregs, as well as what are the mechanisms by which they can mediate suppression in each of these models.

SUPPRESSIVE MECHANISM OF Hsp-SPECIFIC Treg

Hsp-specific Treg will probably use similar suppressive mechanisms as other antigen-specific Treg, like the production of anti-inflammatory cytokines, cell contact dependent suppression or killing of effector T cells and conversion of APC into a tolerogenic state (Vignali et al., 2008). Most Treg subsets use IL-10 for suppression (Bluestone, 2005). It has been recently demonstrated that Treg IL-10 is important for local responses, and not for the systemic suppression of inflammation (Rubtsov et al., 2008). In previous studies, we showed that cross-reactive Hsp-specific T cell responses coincided with the production of IL-10 (Anderton et al., 1995; Wendling et al., 2000; Prakken et al., 2001). Subcutaneous injection of soluble TB-Hsp70 increased IL-10 production and the number of Tregs in draining lymph nodes when compared with OVA injection (Borges et al., 2010). Moreover, while addressing the role of IL-10 in modulation of Proteoglycan-induced arthritis (PGIA) upon i.p. immunization with TB-Hsp70 and after nasal administration of Hsp70 peptides, it was observed that both treatment strategies enhanced Hsp70-specific T cell proliferation and IL-10 production. TB-Hsp70 immunization failed to rescue IL-10 deficient mice from PGIA development. In both wild type and IL-10 deficient mice, Hsp70-specific T cell responses were found, but only in wild type mice these responses suppressed arthritis (Wieten et al., 2009a). In addition, increased PG-specific T cell proliferation, IFN-γ and IL-10 production were found in wild type, but not in IL-10 deficient mice. This illustrates that Hsp70 immunization also modified the PG response to a more anti-inflammatory response. It is therefore possible that Hsp70-induced Tregs generated a tolerogenic micro-milieu by their cytokine production that enabled the outgrowth of new Tregs with antigen specificities beyond Hsp and that IL-10 was required for this effect.

These findings emphasize that Hsp-specific Tregs use mechanisms of infectious tolerance for modulation of inflammation. This has been shown before in transplantation (Qin et al., 1993; Borges et al., 2010), type-1 diabetes (Tarbell et al., 2007), and experimental autoimmune encephalomyelitis (EAE; Mekala et al., 2005) models. Besides IL-10, the role of other cytokines associated with Tregs, like IL-35 has not been addressed but might be relevant.

HOW IMPORTANT IS STRESS-INDUCED Hsp EXPRESSION?

Hsp expression is up-regulated in virtually every inflammatory condition. Also in autoimmune disease this has been reported; enhanced expression of Hsp60 has been shown in synovial and mononuclear cells of juvenile idiopathic arthritis (JIA) patients (Boog et al., 1992; de Graeff-Meeder et al., 1995). In addition, increased expression of inducible Hsp70 and HSF1 has been shown in the inflamed joint of RA patients (Schett et al., 1998). This has also been seen for BiP, an ER restricted Hsp70 family member (Blass et al., 2001) and interestingly enhanced expression in RA synovium was also seen for the constitutive Hsc70 (Schick et al., 2004).

As mentioned before, stress-induced Hsp expression has been proposed to be important for induction, maintenance, and activation of Hsp-specific Treg. If indeed so, reduced expression of Hsp – like with aging, as also depicted in **Figure 2**, where a reduced HSF activity leads to a relatively poor capacity to up-regulate Hsp (Rao et al., 1999; Njemini et al., 2003) – can be expected to influence Hsp mediated immune homeostasis and therefore might contribute to development of chronic inflammatory diseases. In fact, Hsp70 polymorphisms have been associated with inflammatory or autoimmune diseases such as Crohn's disease (Debler et al., 2003), Alzheimer's disease (Clarimon et al., 2003), pancreatitis (Balog et al., 2005) and with development of graft versus host disease upon allogeneic hematopoietic stem cell transplantation (Bogunia-Kubik and Lange, 2005).

Decreased Hsp expression has been observed in several immune disorders. A low Hsp70 response has also been described in a subtype of Biobreeding (BB) rats with a high susceptibility for development of autoimmune (Bellmann et al., 1997). Similar results have been found in human PBMC from patients with newly diagnosed type-1 diabetes. In that study, stress responses were found to become re-established again in patients with longstanding diabetes, more than 8 months after disease manifestation. So, defective Hsp70 induction coincided with beta cell directed inflammatory activity, and seemed modulated by pro-inflammatory cytokines rather than metabolic factors (Burkart et al., 2008).

To amplify stress-induced Hsp70 expression, a study tested multiple food-derived compounds for their effect on Hsp70 expression (Wieten et al., 2009b). One of the compounds, carvacrol, was identified as a potent enhancer of stress-induced Hsp70 both *in vitro* and *in vivo*. Also *in vivo*, intragastric (i.g.) gavage of carvacrol enhanced Hsp70 expression in Peyer's patches (Wieten et al., 2010). Carvacrol was used to boost Hsp levels in APCs and this enhanced Hsp-specific T cell hybridoma activation. We also addressed the immunomodulatory potential of carvacrol *in vivo* and found that i.g. carvacrol treatment specifically boosted Hsp70-specific T cell responses. The finding that adoptive transfer of T cells, isolated from carvacrol treated donor mice, suppressed PGIA, were indicative of the induction of Treg.

The above mentioned findings suggested that the immune system can recognize and react on altered expression of these proteins.

PERSPECTIVES

Hsp expression or Hsp-specific T cell responses have been positively associated with a better disease prognosis in several inflammatory conditions (de Graeff-Meeder et al., 1991; de Kleer et al., 2003). In addition, the immunosuppressive action of Hsp has been demonstrated in multiple rodent disease models. So, it is attractive to speculate that simply enhancing Hsp mediated immunoregulation in either way could be used as therapy.

Apparently, this is oversimplified. Depending on multiple factors such as disease etiology and inflammatory status, patient age and genetic background, difficulties will be encountered. In general, defects in for example positive or negative selection in the thymus, IL-2 production by effector T cells or IL-10 or TGF-β production by Tregs can lead to loss of peripheral tolerance as a result of decreased T cell numbers or functioning (Brusko et al., 2008). Some of these defects might also influence Hsp-specific Treg. For example, the findings that Hsp70-induced suppression of arthritis failed in the absence of IL-10 (Wieten et al., 2009a), illustrated that defects in IL-10 production will also influence Hsp-specific Treg. Furthermore, as disease progresses, severe ongoing inflammation has been described to obstruct the effectiveness of antigen-specific Tregs (Valencia et al., 2006; Peluso et al., 2007). It is currently not known if Hsp-specific Treg can also be hampered by ongoing inflammation. Recent experiments performed by us (Lotte Wieten, Martijn J. C. van Herwijnen, Femke Broere, Ruurd van der Zee, and Willem van Eden) have indicated that this is not the case, however. Transfer of Hsp70 peptide-induced Tregs were found to suppress ongoing experimental arthritis (van Herwijnen et al., in preparation). Recently, it has been reported that iTreg but not natural Treg can convert into Th17 cells after exposure to IL-6 and TGF-β (Horwitz et al., 2008). Besides Th1 cells, Th17 cells are major pathogenic effector cells in many autoimmune diseases. Whether Hsp-specific Treg can convert into Th17 cells has not been studied, but if so, timing and route of boosting the Hsp response could be important to avoid exacerbation of disease instead of induction of regulation.

Earlier studies have emphasized the pro-inflammatory nature of stress proteins such as the Hsp70 family members. In this

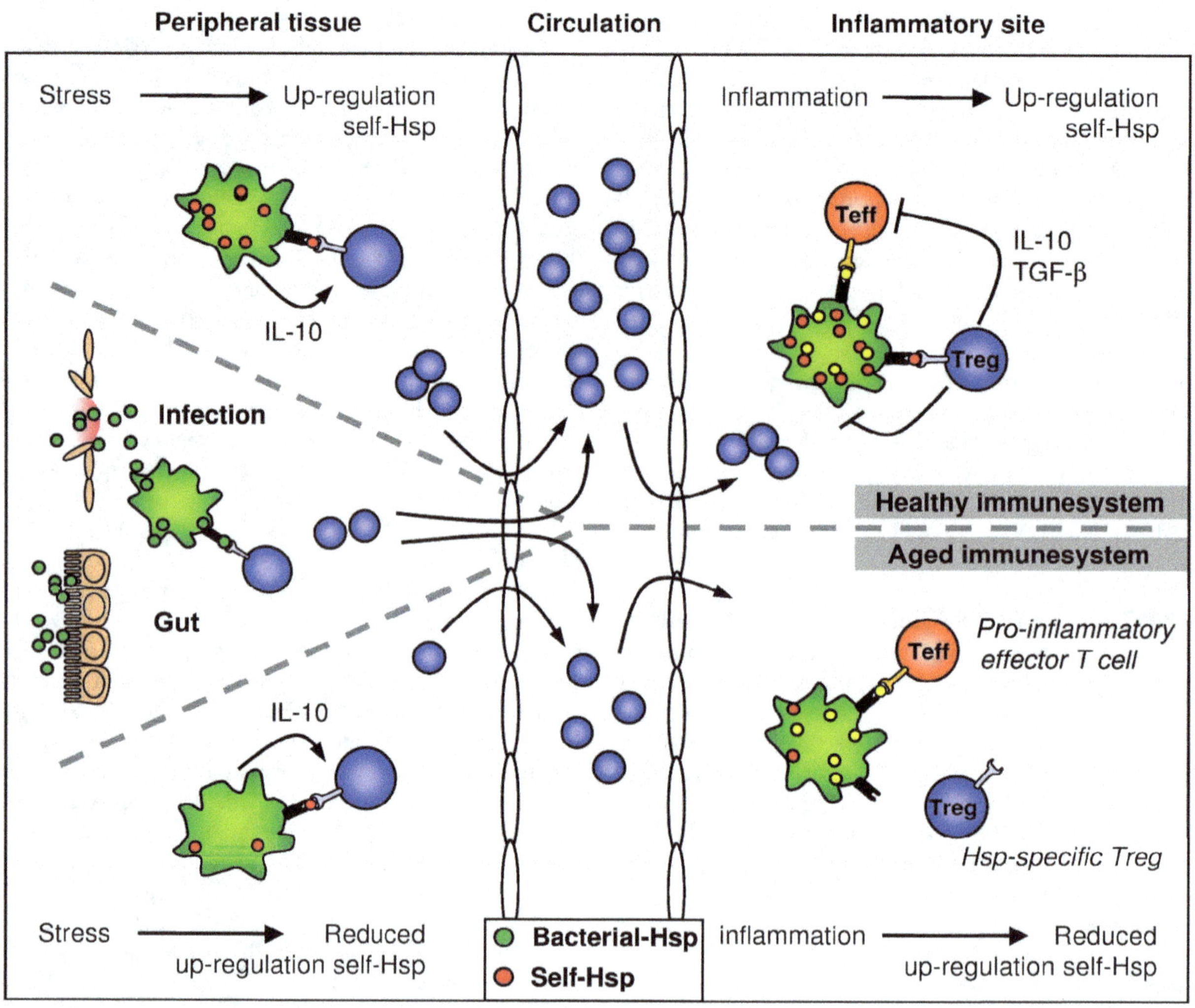

FIGURE 2 | Hsp-specific immunoregulation in the healthy and aged immune system. Self-Hsp-specific T cells reside in the circulation after escape from central tolerance in the thymus. Since Hsp are highly conserved, these self-Hsp-specific T cells can cross-recognize bacterial-Hsp. This T cell population can be expanded after exposure to bacterial-Hsp at mucosal surfaces like the gut or during infection. At mucosal surfaces, these T cells will be directed toward a regulatory phenotype through mechanisms of mucosal tolerance. In addition, Treg induction and maintenance will be promoted by stress-induced Hsp expression in peripheral tissues, because up-regulation of self-Hsp and presentation of Hsp peptides by MHC class II can occur in the absence of co-stimulation. Treg induction will be enhanced by IL-10 produced in response to stress. Furthermore, self-Hsp peptides can function as altered peptide ligands for bacterial-Hsp-specific T cells. During inflammation, Hsp will be induced and presented on professional APCs at the inflammatory site, leading to full activation of Hsp-specific Treg and local dampening ongoing inflammation. In the aged immune system, stress-induced Hsp expression is decreased. Therefore, reduced Hsp inducibility will probably influence both the induction of Hsp-specific Treg in the periphery and their activation during inflammation. Ultimately, this could result in reduced Treg numbers and function.

sense, they were often mentioned as prime examples of so-called DAMPs or damage-associated molecular patterns. It is possible that contaminating microbial components present in partially purified recombinant proteins used in the experiments have contributed to this (Bausinger et al., 2002; Gao and Tsan, 2004; Motta et al., 2007). Besides this, there are other arguments to make against a pro-inflammatory role of Hsp (Broere et al., 2011). As discussed here above, experimental evidence in favor of an immunomodulatory role for Hsp70 is accumulating and therefore Hsp70's immunosuppressive potential seems to constitute a real phenomenon. A more detailed characterization of the molecular pathways activated by Hsp70 in different cell subpopulations is needed. Such studies will allow us to understand and maximize the use of Hsp70 as an anti-inflammatory agent.

ACKNOWLEDGMENTS

Thiago J. Borges and Cristina Bonorino want to thank Dr. Bruno Paim for his support with the figures and CNPq and FINEP for the financial support. This work of Lotte Wieten, Martijn J. C. van Herwijnen, Femke Broere, Ruurd van der Zee, and Willem van Eden was supported by grants of IOP Genomics project nr IGE07004, the European Union FP7 TOLERAGE: HEALTH-F4-2008-20215 and the Dutch Arthritis Association.

REFERENCES

Aalberse, J. A., Kapitein, B., de Roock, S., Klein, M. R., de Jager, W., van der Zee, R., Hoekstra, M. O., van Wijk, F., and Prakken, B. J. (2011). Cord blood CD4 T cells respond to self heat shock protein 60 (HSP60). *PLoS ONE* 6, e24119. doi: 10.1371/journal. pone.0024119

Agrawal, A., Dillon, S., Denning, T. L., and Pulendran, B. (2006). ERK1−/− mice exhibit Th1 cell polarization and increased suscepti- bility to experimental autoimmune encephalomyelitis. *J. Immunol.* 176, 5788–5796.

Anderton, S. M., van der Zee, R., Prakken, B., Noordzij, A., and van Eden, W. (1995). Activation of T cells recognizing self 60-kD heat shock protein can protect against experi- mental arthritis. *J. Exp. Med.* 181, 943–952.

Arispe, N., and De Maio, A. (2000). ATP and ADP modulate a cation channel formed by Hsc70 in acidic phospho- lipid membranes. *J. Biol. Chem.* 275, 30839–30843.

Arispe, N., Doh, M., Simakova, O., Kurganov, B., and De Maio, A. (2004). Hsc70 and Hsp70 interact with phos- phatidylserine on the surface of PC12 cells resulting in a decrease of viabil- ity. *FASEB J.* 18, 1636–1645.

Asea, A., Kabingu, E., Stevenson, M. A., and Calderwood, S. K. (2000a). HSP70 peptidembearing and peptide-negative preparations act as chaperokines. *Cell Stress Chap- erones* 5, 425–431.

Asea, A., Kraeft, S. K., Kurt-Jones, E. A., Stevenson, M. A., Chen, L. B., Finberg, R. W., Koo, G. C., and Calderwood, S. K. (2000b). HSP70 stimulates cytokine production through a CD14-dependant pathway, demonstrating its dual role as a chaperone and cytokine. *Nat. Med.* 6, 435–442.

Asea, A., Rehli, M., Kabingu, E., Boch, J. A., Bare, O., Auron, P. E., Stevenson, M. A., and Calderwood, S. K. (2002). Novel signal transduction pathway utilized by extracellular HSP70: role of toll-like receptor (TLR) 2 and TLR4. *J. Biol. Chem.* 277, 15028– 15034.

Balog, A., Gyulai, Z., Boros, L. G., Farkas, G., Takacs, T., Lonovics, J., and Mandi, Y. (2005). Polymorphism of the TNF-alpha, HSP70-2, and CD14 genes increases susceptibility to severe acute pancreatitis. *Pancreas* 30, e46–e50.

Barton, B. E. (2006). STAT3: a potential therapeutic target in dendritic cells for the induction of transplant tol- erance. *Expert Opin. Ther. Targets* 10, 459–470.

Basu, S., Binder, R. J., Ramalingam, T., and Srivastava, P. K. (2001). CD91 is a common receptor for heat shock proteins gp96, hsp90, hsp70, and calreticulin. *Immunity* 14, 303–313.

Bausinger, H., Lipsker, D., Ziylan, U., Manie, S., Briand, J. P., Cazenave, J. P., Muller, S., Haeuw, J. F., Ravanat, C., de la Salle, H., and Hanau, D. (2002). Endotoxin-free heat-shock protein 70 fails to induce APC activa- tion. *Eur. J. Immunol.* 32, 3708–3713. Bellmann, K., Hui, L., Radons, J., Burkart, V., and Kolb, H. (1997). Low stress response enhances vulnerabil- ity of islet cells in diabetes-prone BB rats. *Diabetes* 46, 232–236.

Binder, R. J. (2009). CD40-independent engagement of mammalian hsp70 by antigen-presenting cells. *J. Immunol.* 182, 6844–6850.

Blass, S., Union, A., Raymackers, J., Schumann, F., Ungethum, U., Muller- Steinbach, S., de Keyser, F., Engel, J. M., and Burmester, G. R. (2001). The stress protein BiP is overexpressed and is a major B and T cell tar- get in rheumatoid arthritis. *Arthritis Rheum.* 44, 761–771.

Bluestone, J. A. (2005). Regulatory T-cell therapy: is it ready for the clinic? *Nat. Rev. Immunol.* 5, 343–349. Bogunia-Kubik, K., and Lange, A. (2005). HSP70-hom gene polymor- phism in allogeneic hematopoietic stem-cell transplant recipients correlates with the development of acute graft-versus-host disease. *Transplan- tation* 79, 815–820.

Bonorino, C., Nardi, N. B., Zhang, X., and Wysocki, L. J. (1998). Character- istics of the strong antibody response to mycobacterial Hsp70: a primary, T cell-dependent IgG response with no evidence of natural priming or gamma delta T cell involvement. *J. Immunol.* 161, 5210–5216.

Boog, C. J., de Graeff-Meeder, E. R., Lucassen, M. A., van der Zee, R., Voorhorst-Ogink, M. M., van Kooten, P. J., Geuze, H. J., and van Eden, W. (1992). Two monoclonal antibodies generated against human hsp60 show reactivity with synovial membranes of patients with juvenile chronic arthritis. *J. Exp. Med.* 175, 1805–1810.

Borges, T. J., Porto, B. N., Teixeira, C. A., Rodrigues, M., Machado, F. D., Ornaghi, A. P., de Souza, A. P., Maito, F., Pavanelli, W. R., Silva, J. S., and Bonorino, C. (2010). Pro- longed survival of allografts induced by mycobacterial Hsp70 is depen- dent on CD4+CD25+ regulatory T cells. *PLoS ONE* 5, e14264. doi: 10.1371/journal.pone.0014264

Botzler, C., Li, G., Issels, R. D., and Multhoff, G. (1998). Definition of extracellular localized epitopes of Hsp70 involved in an NK immune response. *Cell Stress Chaperones* 3, 6–11.

Broere, F., van der Zee, R., and van Eden, W. (2011). Heat shock proteins are no DAMPs, rather 'DAMPERs'. *Nat. Rev. Immunol.* 11, 565; author reply 565.

Brusko, T. M., Putnam, A. L., and Blue-stone, J. A. (2008). Human regulatory T cells: role in autoimmune dis- ease and therapeutic opportunities. *Immunol. Rev.* 223, 371–390.

Burkart, V., Germaschewski, L., Schloot, N. C., Bellmann, K., and Kolb, H. (2008). Deficient heat shock pro- tein 70 response to stress in leuko- cytes at onset of type 1 diabetes. *Biochem. Biophys. Res. Commun.* 369, 421–425.

Bussolati, B., Rollino, C., Mari- ano, F., Quarello, F., and Camussi, G. (2000). IL-10 stimulates pro- duction of platelet-activating fac- tor by monocytes of patients with active systemic lupus erythematosus (SLE). *Clin. Exp. Immunol.* 122, 471–476.

Chalmin, F., Ladoire, S., Mignot, G., Vincent, J., Bruchard, M., Remy- Martin, J. P., Boireau, W., Rouleau, A., Simon, B., Lanneau, D., de Thonel, A., Multhoff, G., Ham- man, A., Martin, F., Chauffert, B., Solary, E., Zitvogel, L., Garrido, C., Ryffel, B., Borg, C., Apetoh, L., Rebe, C., and Ghiringhelli, F. (2010). Membrane-associated Hsp72 from tumor-derived exosomes mediates STAT3-dependent immunosuppres- sive function of mouse and human myeloid-derived suppressor cells. *J. Clin. Invest.* 120, 457–471.

Chen, Y., Kuchroo, V. K., Inobe, J., Hafler, D. A., and Weiner, H. L. (1994). Regulatory T cell clones induced by oral tolerance: suppres- sion of autoimmune encephalomyeli- tis. *Science* 265, 1237–1240.

Clarimon, J., Bertranpetit, J., Boada, M., Tarraga, L., and Comas, D. (2003). HSP70-2 (HSPA1B) is associated with noncognitive symptoms in late-onset Alzheimer's disease. *J. Geriatr. Psychiatry Neurol.* 16, 146–150.

Cohen, I. R. (2007). Biomarkers, self-antigens and the immunologi- cal homunculus. *J. Autoimmun.* 29, 246–249.

Cohen, I. R., and Young, D. B. (1991). Autoimmunity, microbial immunity and the immunological homunculus. *Immunol. Today* 12, 105–110.

Debler, J., Schiemann, U., Seybold, U., Mussack, T., Landauer, N., Ladurner, R., and Gross, M. (2003). Heat- shock protein HSP70-2 genotypes in patients with Crohn's disease: a more severe clinical course with intestinal complications in presence of the PstI- polymorphism. *Eur. J. Med. Res.* 8, 120–124.

de Graeff-Meeder, E. R., van der Zee, R., Rijkers, G. T., Schuurman, H. J., Kuis, W., Bijlsma, J. W., Zegers, B. J., and van Eden, W. (1991). Recognition of human 60 kD heat shock protein by mononuclear cells from patients with juvenile chronic arthritis. *Lancet* 337, 1368–1372.

de Graeff-Meeder, E. R., van Eden, W., Rijkers, G. T., Prakken, B. J., Kuis, W., Voorhorst-Ogink, M. M., van der Zee, R., Schuurman, H. J., Helders, P. J., and Zegers, B. J. (1995). Juve- nile chronic arthritis: T cell reactivity to human HSP60 in patients with a favorable course of arthritis. *J. Clin. Invest.* 95, 934–940.

de Kleer, I. M., Kamphuis, S. M., Rijkers, G. T., Scholtens, L., Gor- don, G., de Jager, W., Hafner, R., van de Zee, R., van Eden, W., Kuis, W., and Prakken, B. J. (2003). The spontaneous remission of juve- nile idiopathic arthritis is character- ized by CD30+ T cells directed to human heat-shock protein 60 capable of producing the regulatory cytokine interleukin-10. *Arthritis Rheum.* 48, 2001–2010.

Delneste, Y., Magistrelli, G., Gauchat, J., Haeuw, J., Aubry, J., Nakamura, K., Kawakami-Honda, N., Goetsch, L., Sawamura, T., Bonnefoy, J., and Jean- nin, P. (2002). Involvement of LOX-in dendritic cell-mediated anti- gen cross-presentation. *Immunity* 17, 353–362.

De Maio, A. (2011). Extracellular heat shock proteins, cellular export vesi- cles, and the Stress Observation Sys- tem: a form of communication dur- ing injury, infection, and cell damage. It is never known how far a controver- sial finding will go! Dedicated to Fer- ruccio Ritossa. *Cell Stress Chaperones* 16, 235–249.

Dengjel, J., Schoor, O., Fischer, R., Reich, M., Kraus, M., Muller, M., Kreym- borg, K., Altenberend, F., Branden- burg, J., Kalbacher, H., Brock, R., Driessen, C., Rammensee, H. G., and Stevanovic, S. (2005). Autophagy promotes MHC class II presentation of peptides from intracellular source proteins. *Proc. Natl. Acad. Sci. U.S.A.* 102, 7922–7927.

Detanico, T., Rodrigues, L., Sabritto, A. C., Keisermann, M., Bauer, M. E., Zwickey, H., and Bonorino, C. (2004). Mycobacterial heat shock protein 70 induces interleukin-10 production: immunomodulation of synovial cell cytokine profile and den- dritic cell maturation. *Clin. Exp. Immunol.* 135, 336–342.

Dhingra, S., Bagchi, A. K., Ludke, A. L., Sharma, A. K., and Singal, P. K. (2011). Akt regulates IL-10 medi- ated suppression of TNFα-induced cardiomyocyte apoptosis by upreg- ulating Stat3 phosphorylation. *PLoS ONE* 6, e25009. doi: 10.1371/journal. pone.0025009

Dillon, S., Agrawal, A., van Dyke, T., Landreth, G., Mccauley, L., Koh, A., Maliszewski, C., Akira, S., and Pulen- dran, B. (2004). A Toll-like receptor ligand stimulates Th2 responses *in vivo*, via induction of extracellu- lar signal-regulated kinase mitogen- activated protein kinase and c-Fos in dendritic cells. *J. Immunol.* 172, 4733–4743.

Dillon, S., Agrawal, S., Banerjee, K., Letterio, J., Denning, T. L., Oswald- Richter, K., Kasprowicz, D. J., Kellar, K., Pare, J., van Dyke, T., Ziegler, S., Unutmaz, D., and Pulendran, B. (2006). Yeast zymosan, a stimulus for TLR2 and dectin-1, induces reg- ulatory antigen-presenting cells and immunological tolerance. *J. Clin. Invest.* 116,916–928.

Dong, C., Davis, R. J., and Flavell, R. A. (2002). MAP kinases in the immune response. *Annu. Rev. Immunol.* 20, 55–72.

Ellis, R. J. (1990). The molecular chap- erone concept. *Semin. Cell Biol.* 1, 1–9.

Feder, M. E., and Hofmann, G. E. (1999). Heat-shock proteins, molecular chaperones, and the stress response: evolutionary and ecologi- cal physiology. *Annu. Rev. Physiol.* 61, 243–282.

Ferrarini, M., Heltai, S., Zocchi, M. R., and Rugarli, C. (1992). Unusual expression and localization of heat- shock proteins in human tumor cells. *Int. J. Cancer* 51, 613–619.

Feuerer, M., Hill, J. A., Mathis, D., and Benoist, C. (2009). Foxp3+ regula- tory T cells: differentiation, specification, subphenotypes. *Nat. Immunol.* 10, 689–695.

Fischer, H. P., Sharrock, C. E., and Panayi, G. S. (1992). High fre- quency of cord blood lymphocytes against mycobacterial 65-kDa heat- shock protein. *Eur. J. Immunol.* 22, 1667–1669.

Floto, R. A., Macary, P. A., Boname, J. M., Mien, T. S., Kampmann, B., Hair, J. R., Huey, O. S., Houben, E. N., Pieters, J., Day, C., Oehlmann, W., Singh, M., Smith, K. G., and Lehner, P. J. (2006). Dendritic cell stim- ulation by mycobacterial Hsp70 is mediated through CCR5. *Science* 314, 454–458.

Frodermann, V., Chau, T. A., Sayedya- hossein, S., Toth, J. M., Heinrichs, D. E., and Madrenas, J. (2011). A modulatory interleukin-10 response to staphylococcal peptidoglycan pre- vents Th1/Th17 adaptive immunity to *Staphylococcus aureus*. *J. Infect. Dis.* 204, 253–262.

Gabrilovich, D. I., and Nagaraj, S. (2009). Myeloid-derived suppressor cells as regulators of the immune system. *Nat. Rev. Immunol.* 9, 162–174.

Gao, B. C., and Tsan, M. F. (2004). Induction of cytokines by heat shock proteins and endotoxin in murine macrophages. *Biochem. Biophys. Res. Commun.* 317, 1149–1154.

Gehrmann, M., Radons, J., Molls, M., and Multhoff, G. (2008). The therapeutic implications of clini- cally applied modifiers of heat shock protein 70 (Hsp70) expression by tumor cells. *Cell Stress Chaperones* 13, 1–10.

Groux, H., O'Garra, A., Bigler, M., Rouleau, M., Antonenko, S., de Vries, J. E., and Roncarolo, M. G. (1997). A CD4+ T-cell subset inhibits antigen- specific T-cell responses and prevents colitis. *Nature* 389, 737–742.

Halfter, H., Friedrich, M., Postert, C., Ringelstein, E. B., and Stogbauer, F. (1999). Activation of Jak-Stat and MAPK2 pathways by oncostatin M leads to growth inhibition of human glioma cells. *Mol. Cell Biol. Res. Commun.* 1, 109–116.

Heath, W. R., and Carbone, F. R. (2009). Dendritic cell subsets in pri- mary and secondary T cell responses at body surfaces. *Nat. Immunol.* 10, 1237–1244.

Hightower, L. E., and Guidon, P. T. Jr. (1989). Selective release from cultured mammalian cells of heat-shock (stress) proteins that resemble glia- axon transfer proteins. *J. Cell. Physiol.* 138, 257–266.

Horwitz, D. A., Zheng, S. G., and Gray, J. D. (2008). Natural and TGF- beta-induced Foxp3(+)CD4(+) CD25(+) regulatory T cells are not mirror images of each other. *Trends Immunol.* 29, 429–435.

Janson, A. A., Klatser, P. R., van der Zee, R., Cornelisse, Y. E., de Vries, R. R., Thole, J. E., and Ottenhoff, T. H. (1991). A systematic molecular analysis of the T cell-stimulating anti- gens from *Mycobacterium leprae* with T cell clones of leprosy patients. Iden- tification of a novel *M. leprae* HSP 70 fragment by *M. leprae*-specific T cells. *J. Immunol.* 147, 3530–3537.

Jenkins, M. K., Chen, C. A., Jung, G., Mueller, D. L., and Schwartz, R. H. (1990). Inhibition of antigen-specific proliferation of type 1 murine T cell clones after stimulation with immo- bilized anti-CD3 monoclonal anti- body. *J. Immunol.* 144, 16–22.

Kaiser, F., Cook, D., Papoutsopoulou, S., Rajsbaum, R., Wu, X., Yang, H. T., Grant, S., Ricciardi-Castagnoli, P., Tsichlis, P. N., Ley, S. C., and O'Garra, A. (2009). TPL-2 negatively regulates interferon-beta pro- duction in macrophages and myeloid dendritic cells. *J. Exp. Med.* 206, 1863–1871.

Kammerer, R., Stober, D., Riedl, P., Oehninger, C., Schirmbeck, R., and Reimann, J. (2002). Noncovalent association with stress protein facilitates cross-priming of CD8+ T cells to tumor cell antigens by dendritic cells. *J. Immunol.* 168, 108–117.

Kampinga, H. H., Hageman, J., Vos, M. J., Kubota, H., Tanguay, R. M., Bruford, E. A., Cheetham, M. E., Chen, B., and Hightower, L. E. (2009). Guidelines for the nomen- clature of the human heat shock proteins. *Cell Stress Chaperones* 14, 105–111.

Kaufmann, S. H., Vath, U., Thole, J. E., van Embden, J. D., and Emm- rich, F. (1987). Enumeration of T cells reactive with *Mycobacterium tuber- culosis* organisms and specific for the recombinant mycobacterial 64- kDa protein. *Eur. J. Immunol.* 17, 351–357.

Kimura, Y., Yamada, K., Sakai, T., Mishima, K., Nishimura, H., Mat- sumoto, Y., Singh, M., and Yoshikai, Y. (1998). The regulatory role of heat shock protein 70-reactive CD4+ T cells during rat listeriosis. *Int. Immunol.* 10, 117–130.

Kuma, A., Hatano, M., Matsui, M., Yamamoto, A., Nakaya, H., Yoshi- mori, T., Ohsumi, Y., Tokuhisa, T., and Mizushima, N. (2004). The role of autophagy during the early neona- tal starvation period. *Nature* 432, 1032–1036.

Li, D., Romain, G., Flamar, A. L., Duluc, D., Dullaers, M., Li, X. H., Zurawski, S., Bosquet, N., Palucka, A. K., Le Grand, R., O'Garra, A., Zurawski, G., Banchereau, J., and Oh, S. (2012). Targeting self- and foreign antigens to dendritic cells via DC-ASGPRgen- erates IL-10-producing suppressive CD4+ T cells. *J. Exp. Med.* 209, 109–121.

Lindquist, S. (1986). The heat-shock response. *Annu. Rev. Biochem.* 55, 1151–1191.

Lindquist, S., and Craig, E. A. (1988). The heat-shock proteins. *Annu. Rev. Genet.* 22, 631–677.

Long, S. A., Rieck, M., Tatum, M., Bollyky, P. L., Wu, R. P., Muller, I., Ho, J. C., Shilling, H. G., and Buckner, J. H. (2011). Low-dose antigen pro- motes induction of FOXP3 in human CD4+ T cells. *J. Immunol.* 187, 3511–3520.

Luo, X., Zuo, X., Zhou, Y., Zhang, B., Shi, Y., Liu, M., Wang, K., Mcmillian, D. R., and Xiao, X. (2008). Extracellular heat shock protein 70 inhibits tumour necrosis factor-alpha induced proin- flammatory mediator production in fibroblast-like synoviocytes. *Arthritis Res. Ther.* 10, R41.

Manicassamy, S., Ravindran, R., Deng, J., Oluoch, H., Denning, T. L., Kas- turi, S. P., Rosenthal, K. M., Evavold, B. D., and Pulendran, B. (2009). Toll- like receptor 2-dependent induction of vitamin A-metabolizing enzymes in dendritic cells promotes T regula- tory responses and inhibits autoim- munity. *Nat. Med.* 15, 401–409.

Mekala, D. J., Alli, R. S., and Geiger, T. L. (2005). IL-10-dependent infectious tolerance after the treat- ment of experimental allergic encephalomyelitis with redirected CD4+CD25+ T lymphocytes. *Proc. Natl. Acad. Sci. USA* 102, 11817–11822.

Moore, K. W., de Waal Malefyt, R., Coff- man, R. L., and O'Garra, A. (2001). Interleukin-10 and the interleukin- 10 receptor. *Annu. Rev. Immunol.* 19, 683–765.

Morelli, A. E., and Thomson, A. W. (2007). Tolerogenic dendritic cells and the quest for transplant toler- ance. *Nat. Rev. Immunol.* 7, 610–621.

Motta, A., Schmitz, C., Rodrigues, L., Ribeiro, F., Teixeira, C., Detan- ico, T., Bonan, C., Zwickey, H., and Bonorino, C. (2007). Mycobac- terium tuberculosis heat-shock pro- tein 70 impairs maturation of den- dritic cells from bone marrow precur- sors, induces interleukin-10 produc- tion and inhibits T-cell proliferation *in vitro*. *Immunology* 121, 462–472. Multhoff, G., Botzler, C., Wiesnet, M.,

Muller, E., Meier, T., Wilmanns, W., and Issels, R. D. (1995). A stress- inducible 72-kDa heat-shock protein (HSP72) is expressed on the sur- face of human tumor cells, but not on normal cells. *Int. J. Cancer* 61, 272–279.

Munk, M. E., Schoel, B., Modrow, S., Karr, R. W., Young, R. A., and Kaufmann, S. H. (1989). T lympho- cytes from healthy individuals with specificity to self-epitopes shared by the mycobacterial and human 65- kilodalton heat shock protein. *J. Immunol.* 143, 2844–2849.

Munz, C. (2006). Autophagy and antigen presentation. *Cell. Microbiol.* 8, 891–898.

Munz, C. (2009). Enhancing immu- nity through autophagy. *Annu. Rev. Immunol.* 27, 423–449.

Murray, P. J. (2006). Understanding and exploiting the endogenous interleukin-10/STAT3-mediated anti-inflammatory response. *Curr. Opin. Pharmacol.* 6, 379–386.

Murray, P. J. (2007). The JAK-STAT signaling pathway: input and out- put integration. *J. Immunol.* 178, 2623–2629.

Neefjes, J., Jongsma, M. L., Paul, P., and Bakke, O. (2011). Towards a systems understanding of MHC class I and MHC class II antigen presentation. *Nat. Rev. Immunol.* 11, 823–836.

Njemini, R., Lambert, M., Demanet, C., Vanden Abeele, M., Vandebosch, S., and Mets, T. (2003). The induc- tion of heat shock protein 70 in peripheral mononuclear blood cells in elderly patients: a role for inflam- matory markers. *Hum. Immunol.* 64, 575–585.

Peluso, I., Fantini, M. C., Fina, D., Caruso, R., Boirivant, M., Macdon- ald, T. T., Pallone, F., and Monteleone, G. (2007). IL-21 counteracts the reg- ulatory T cell-mediated suppression of human CD4+ T lymphocytes. *J. Immunol.* 178, 732–739.

Pockley, A. G., Shepherd, J., and Cor- ton, J. M. (1998). Detection of heat shock protein 70 (Hsp70) and anti- Hsp70 antibodies in the serum of normal individuals. *Immunol. Invest.* 27, 367–377.

Prakken, B. J., Wendling, U., van der Zee, R., Rutten, V. P., Kuis, W., and van Eden, W. (2001). Induction of IL-10 and inhibition of experimen- tal arthritis are specific features of microbial heat shock proteins that are absent for other evolutionarily con- served immunodominant proteins. *J. Immunol.* 167, 4147–4153.

Qin, S., Cobbold, S. P., Pope, H., Elliott, J., Kioussis, D., Davies, J., and Waldmann, H. (1993). "Infec- tious" transplantation tolerance. *Sci- ence* 259, 974–977.

Quayle, A. J., Wilson, K. B., Li, S. G., Kjeldsen-Kragh, J., Oftung, F., Shinnick, T., Sioud, M., Forre, O., Capra, J. D., and Natvig, J. B. (1992). Peptide recognition, T cell receptor usage and HLA restriction elements of human heat-shock protein (hsp) 60 and mycobacterial 65-kDa hsp- reactive T cell clones from rheumatoid synovial fluid. *Eur. J. Immunol.* 22, 1315–1322.

Rao, D. V., Watson, K., and Jones, G. L. (1999). Age-related attenuation in the expression of the major heat shock proteins in human peripheral lym- phocytes. *Mech. Ageing Dev.* 107, 105–118.

Roncarolo, M. G., and Battaglia, M. (2007). Regulatory T-cell immunotherapy for tolerance to self antigens and alloantigens in humans. *Nat. Rev. Immunol.* 7, 585–598.

Rosenblum, M. D., Gratz, I. K., Paw, J. S., Lee, K., Marshak-Rothstein, A., and Abbas, A. K. (2011). Response to self antigen imprints regulatory memory in tissues. *Nature* 480, 538–542.

Rubtsov, Y. P., Rasmussen, J. P., Chi, E. Y., Fontenot, J., Castelli, L., Ye, X., Treuting, P., Siewe, L., Roers, A., Henderson, W. R. Jr., Muller, W., and Rudensky, A. Y. (2008). Reg- ulatory T cell-derived interleukin 10 limits inflammation at envi- ronmental interfaces. *Immunity* 28, 546–558.

Rutella, S., Danese, S., and Leone, G. (2006). Tolerogenic dendritic cells: cytokine modulation comes of age. *Blood* 108, 1435–1440.

Sakaguchi, S., Sakaguchi, N., Asano, M., Itoh, M., and Toda, M. (1995). Immunologic self-tolerance main- tained by activated T cells expressing IL-2 receptor alpha-chains (CD25). Breakdown of a single mechanism of self-tolerance causes various autoim- mune diseases. *J. Immunol.* 155, 1151–1164.

Sakaguchi, S., Yamaguchi, T., Nomura, T., and Ono, M. (2008). Regulatory T cells and immune tolerance. *Cell* 133, 775–787.

Saraiva, M., and O'Garra, A. (2010). The regulation of IL-10 production by immune cells. *Nat. Rev. Immunol.* 10, 170–181.

Schett, G., Redlich, K., Xu, Q., Bizan, P., Groger, M., Tohidast-Akrad, M., Kiener, H., Smolen, J., and Steiner, G. (1998). Enhanced expression of heat shock protein 70 (hsp70) and heat shock factor 1 (HSF1) activation in rheumatoid arthritis synovial tis- sue. Differential regulation of hsp70 expression and hsf1 activation in syn- ovial fibroblasts by proinflammatory cytokines, shear stress, and antiin- flammatory drugs. *J. Clin. Invest.* 102, 302–311.

Schick, C., Arbogast, M., Lowka, K., Rzepka, R., and Melchers, I. (2004). Continuous enhanced expression of Hsc70 but not Hsp70 in rheuma- toid arthritis synovial tissue. *Arthritis Rheum.* 50, 88–93.

Schmid, D., and Munz, C. (2007). Immune surveillance via self diges- tion. *Autophagy* 3, 133–135.

Schmid, D., Pypaert, M., and Munz, C. (2007). Antigen-loading compart- ments for major histocompatibility complex class II molecules continu- ously receive input from autophago- somes. *Immunity* 26, 79–92.

Sela, U., Olds, P., Park, A., Schlesinger, S. J., and Steinman, R. M. (2011). Dendritic cells induce antigen-specific regulatory T cells that prevent graft versus host disease and persist in mice. *J. Exp. Med.* 208, 2489–2496.

Sharif, M. N., Tassiulas, I., Hu, Y., Mecklenbrauker, I., Tarakhovsky, A., and Ivashkiv, L. B. (2004). IFN- alpha priming results in a gain of proinflammatory function by IL- 10: implications for systemic lupus erythematosus pathogenesis. *J. Immunol.* 172, 6476–6481.

Shevach, E. M. (2006). From vanilla to 28 flavors: multiple varieties of T regulatory cells. *Immunity* 25, 195–201.

Steinman, R. M., Hawiger, D., and Nussenzweig, M. C. (2003). Tolero- genic dendritic cells. *Annu. Rev. Immunol.* 21, 685–711.

Steinman, R. M., Turley, S., Mellman, I., and Inaba, K. (2000). The induc- tion of tolerance by dendritic cells that have captured apoptotic cells. *J. Exp. Med.* 191, 411–416.

Stocki, P., Wang, X. N., and Dickin son, A. M. (2012). Inducible Hsp70 reduces T cell responses and stimu- latory capacity of monocyte-derived dendritic cells. *J. Biol. Chem.* 287, 12387–12394.

Stokes, C. R., Haverson, K., and Bai- ley, M. (1996). Antigen presenting cells in the porcine gut. *Vet. Immunol. Immunopathol.* 54, 171–177.

Stordeur, P., and Goldman, M. (1998). Interleukin-10 as a regulatory cytokine induced by cellular stress: molecular aspects. *Int. Rev. Immunol.* 16, 501–522.

Strawbridge, A. B., and Blum, J. S. (2007). Autophagy in MHC class II antigen processing. *Curr. Opin. Immunol.* 19, 87–92.

Tanaka, K., Namba, T., Arai, Y., Fujimoto, M., Adachi, H., Sobue, G., Takeuchi, K., Nakai, A., and Mizushima, T. (2007). Genetic evi- dence for a protective role for heat shock factor 1 and heat shock protein 70 against colitis. *J. Biol. Chem.* 282, 23240–23252.

Tanaka, S., Kimura, Y., Mitani, A., Yamamoto, G., Nishimura, H., Spallek, R., Singh, M., Noguchi, T., and Yoshikai, Y. (1999). Activation of T cells recognizing an epitope of heat- shock protein 70 can protect against rat adjuvant arthritis. *J. Immunol.* 163, 5560–5565.

Tang, Q., and Bluestone, J. A. (2008). The Foxp3+ regulatory T cell: a jack of all trades, master of regulation. *Nat. Immunol.* 9, 239–244.

Tarbell, K. V., Petit, L., Zuo, X., Toy, P., Luo, X., Mqadmi, A., Yang, H., Suthanthiran, M., Mojsov, S., and Steinman, R. M. (2007). Dendritic cell-expanded, islet-specific CD4+ CD25+ CD62L+ regulatory T cells restore normoglycemia in diabetic NOD mice. *J. Exp. Med.* 204, 191–201.

Theriault, J. R., Adachi, H., and Calder- wood, S. K. (2006). Role of scavenger receptors in the binding and internal- ization of heat shock protein 70. *J. Immunol.* 177, 8604–8611.

Theriault, J. R., Mambula, S. S., Sawamura, T., Stevenson, M. A., and Calderwood, S. K. (2005). Extracellu- lar HSP70 binding to surface recep- tors present on antigen presenting cells and endothelial/epithelial cells. *FEBS Lett.* 579, 1951–1960.

Thornton, A. M., Korty, P. E., Tran, Q., Wohlfert, E. A., Mur- ray, P. E., Belkaid, Y., and She- vach, E. M. (2010). Expression of Helios, an Ikaros transcription factor family member, differenti- ates thymic-derived from peripher- ally induced Foxp3+ T regulatory cells. *J. Immunol.* 184, 3433–3441.

Tsan, M. F., and Gao, B. (2009). Heat shock proteins and immune system. *J. Leukoc. Biol.* 85, 905–910.

Udono, H., and Srivastava, P. K. (1993). Heat shock protein 70-associated peptides elicit specific cancer immu- nity. *J. Exp. Med.* 178, 1391–1396.

Ueda, G., Tamura, Y., Hirai, I., Kamiguchi, K., Ichimiya, S., Tori- goe, T., Hiratsuka, H., Sunakawa, H., and Sato, N. (2004). Tumor- derived heat shock protein 70-pulsed dendritic cells elicit tumor-specific cytotoxic T lymphocytes (CTLs) and tumor immunity. *Cancer Sci.* 95, 248–253.

Valencia, X., Stephens, G., Goldbach- Mansky, R., Wilson, M., Shevach, M., and Lipsky, P. E. (2006). TNF downmodulates the function of human CD4+CD25hi T-regulatory cells. *Blood* 108, 253–261.

van Eden, W., Thole, J. E., van der Zee, R., Noordzij, A., van Embden, J. D., Hensen, E. J., and Cohen, I. R. (1988). Cloning of the mycobac- terial epitope recognized by T lym- phocytes in adjuvant arthritis. *Nature* 331, 171–173.

van Eden, W., van der Zee, R., and Prakken, B. (2005). Heat-shock pro- teins induce T-cell regulation of chronic inflammation. *Nat. Rev. Immunol.* 5, 318–330.

van Eden, W., Wick, G., Albani, S., and Cohen, I. (2007). Stress, heat shock proteins, and autoimmunity: how immune responses to heat shock proteins are to be used for the con- trol of chronic inflammatory dis- eases. *Ann. NY Acad. Sci.* 1113, 217–237.

van Puijvelde, G. H., van Es, T., van Wanrooij, E. J., Habets, K. L., de Vos, P., van der Zee, R., van Eden, W., van Berkel, T. J., and Kuiper, J. (2007). Induction of oral tolerance to HSP60 or an HSP60-peptide activates T cell regulation and reduces atheroscler o- sis. *Arterioscler. Thromb. Vasc. Biol.* 27, 2677–2683.

Vega, V. L., Rodriguez-Silva, M., Frey, T., Gehrmann, M., Diaz, J. C., Steinem, C., Multhoff, G., Arispe, N., and de Maio, A. (2008). Hsp70 translocates into the plasma membrane after stress and is released into the extracellular environment in a membrane-associated form that activates macrophages. *J. Immunol.* 180, 4299–4307.

Vignali, D. A., Collison, L. W., and Workman, C. J. (2008). How regulatory T cells work. *Nat. Rev. Immunol.* 8, 523–532.

Wang, Y., Kelly, C. G., Karttunen, J. T., Whittall, T., Lehner, P. J., Duncan, L., Macary, P., Younson, J. S., Singh, M., Oehlmann, W., Cheng, G., Bergmeier, L., and Lehner, T. (2001). CD40 is a cellular receptor mediating mycobacterial heat shock protein 70 stimulation of CC-chemokines. *Immunity* 15, 971–983.

Watowich, S. S., and Liu, Y. J. (2010). Mechanisms regulating dendritic cell specification and development. *Immunol. Rev.* 238, 76–92.

Wauben, M. H., van der Zee, R., Joosten, I., Boog, C. J., van Dijk, A. M., Holewijn, M. C., Meloen, R. H., and van Eden, W. (1993). A peptide variant of an arthritis-related T cell epitope induces T cells that recognize this epitope as a synthetic peptide but not in its naturally processed form. *J. Immunol.* 150, 5722–5730.

Weiner, H. L. (2001). Induction and mechanism of action of transforming growth factor-beta-secreting Th3 regulatory cells. *Immunol. Rev.* 182, 207–214.

Wendling, U., Paul, L., van der Zee, R., Prakken, B., Singh, M., and van Eden, W. (2000). A conserved mycobacterial heat shock protein (hsp) 70 sequence prevents adjuvant arthritis upon nasal administration and induces IL-10-producing T cells that cross-react with the mammalian self-hsp70 homologue. *J. Immunol.* 164, 2711–2717.

Wieten, L., Berlo, S. E., Ten Brink, C. B., van Kooten, P. J., Singh, M., vander Zee, R., Glant, T. T., Broere, F., and van Eden, W. (2009a). IL-10 is critically involved in mycobacterial HSP70 induced suppression of proteoglycan-induced arthritis. *PLoS ONE* 4, e4186. doi: 10.1371/journal. pone.0004186

Wieten, L., van der Zee, R., Goedemans, R., Sijtsma, J., Serafini, M., Lubsen, N. H., van Eden, W., and Broere, F. (2009b). Hsp70 expression and induction as a readout for detection of immune modulatory components in food. *Cell Stress Chaperones* 15, 25–37.

Wieten, L., van der Zee, R., Spiering, R., Wagenaar-Hilbers, J., van Kooten, P., Broere, F., and van Eden, W. (2010). A novel heat-shock protein coinducer boosts stress protein Hsp70 to activate T cell regulation of inflammation in autoimmune arthritis. *Arthritis Rheum.* 62, 1026–1035.

Yamazaki, S., Okada, K., Maruyama, A., Matsumoto, M., Yagita, H., and Seya, T. (2011). TLR2-dependent induction of IL-10 and Foxp3+ CD25+ CD4+ regulatory T cells prevents effective anti-tumor immunity induced by Pam2 lipopeptides *in vivo*. *PLoS ONE* 6, e18833. doi: 10.1371/journal.pone.0018833

Yi, A. K., Yoon, J. G., Yeo, S. J., Hong, S. C., English, B. K., and Krieg, A. M. (2002). Role of mitogen-activated protein kinases in CpG DNA-mediated IL-10 and IL-12 production: central role of extra cellular signal-regulated kinase in the negative feedback loop of the CpG DNA-mediated Th1 response. *J. Immunol.* 168, 4711–4720..

23

Models of somatic hypermutation targeting and substitution based on synonymous mutations from high-throughput immunoglobulin sequencing data

Gur Yaari[1,2], Jason A. Vander Heiden[3], Mohamed Uduman[2], Daniel Gadala-Maria[3], Namita Gupta[3], Joel N. H. Stern[4,5], Kevin C. O'Connor[4,6], David A. Hafler[4,7], Uri Laserson[8], Francois Vigneault[9] and Steven H. Kleinstein[2,3]*

[1] Bioengineering Program, Faculty of Engineering, Bar Ilan University, Ramat Gan, Israel
[2] Department of Pathology, Yale School of Medicine, New Haven, CT, USA
[3] Interdepartmental Program in Computational Biology and Bioinformatics, Yale University, New Haven, CT, USA
[4] Department of Neurology, Yale School of Medicine, New Haven, CT, USA
[5] Department of Science Education, Hofstra North Shore-LIJ School of Medicine, Hempstead, NY, USA
[6] Human and Translational Immunology Program, Yale School of Medicine, New Haven, CT, USA
[7] Department of Immunobiology, Yale School of Medicine, New Haven, CT, USA
[8] Department of Genetics, Harvard Medical School, Boston, MA, USA
[9] AbVitro, Inc., Boston, MA, USA

Edited by:
Ramit Mehr, Bar-Ilan University, Israel

Reviewed by:
Ronald B. Corley, Boston University School of Medicine, USA
Masaki Hikida, Kyoto University, Japan

***Correspondence:**
Steven H. Kleinstein, Department of Pathology, Yale School of Medicine, Suite 505, 300 George Street, New Haven, CT 06511, USA
e-mail: steven.kleinstein@yale.edu

Analyses of somatic hypermutation (SHM) patterns in B cell immunoglobulin (Ig) sequences contribute to our basic understanding of adaptive immunity, and have broad applications not only for understanding the immune response to pathogens, but also to determining the role of SHM in autoimmunity and B cell cancers. Although stochastic, SHM displays intrinsic biases that can confound statistical analysis, especially when combined with the particular codon usage and base composition in Ig sequences. Analysis of B cell clonal expansion, diversification, and selection processes thus critically depends on an accurate background model for SHM micro-sequence targeting (i.e., hot/cold-spots) and nucleotide substitution. Existing models are based on small numbers of sequences/mutations, in part because they depend on data from non-coding regions or non-functional sequences to remove the confounding influences of selection. Here, we combine high-throughput Ig sequencing with new computational analysis methods to produce improved models of SHM targeting and substitution that are based only on synonymous mutations, and are thus independent of selection. The resulting "S5F" models are based on 806,860 Synonymous mutations in 5-mer motifs from 1,145,182 Functional sequences and account for dependencies on the adjacent four nucleotides (two bases upstream and downstream of the mutation). The estimated profiles can explain almost half of the variance in observed mutation patterns, and clearly show that both mutation targeting and substitution are significantly influenced by neighboring bases. While mutability and substitution profiles were highly conserved across individuals, the variability across motifs was found to be much larger than previously estimated. The model and method source code are made available at http://clip.med.yale.edu/SHM

Keywords: immunoglobulin, B cell, somatic hypermutation, mutability, substitution, targeting, AID, affinity maturation

1. INTRODUCTION

During the course of an immune response, B cells that initially bind antigen with low affinity through their immunoglobulin (Ig) receptor are modified through cycles of proliferation, somatic hypermutation (SHM), and affinity-dependent selection to produce high-affinity memory and plasma cells. Current models of SHM recognize activation-induced deaminase (AID), along with several DNA repair pathways, as critical to the mutation process (1). AID initiates SHM by converting cytosines (Cs) to uracils (Us), thus creating U:G mismatches in the Ig V(D)J sequence. If not repaired before cell replication, these mismatches produce C → T (thymine) transition mutations (2). The AID-induced mismatches can alternatively be recognized by UNG or MSH2/MSH6 to initiate base excision or mismatch repair pathways, respectively. These pathways operate in an error-prone manner to introduce the full spectrum of mutations at the initial lesion, as well as spreading mutations to the surrounding bases. Overall, SHM introduces point mutations into the Ig locus at a rate of $\sim 10^{-3}$ per base-pair per division (3, 4). While the process of SHM appears to be stochastic, there are clear intrinsic biases, both in the bases that are targeted (5, 6) as well as the substitutions that are introduced (7, 8). Accurate background models for SHM micro-sequence targeting (i.e., hot/cold-spots) and nucleotide substitution would greatly aid the analysis of B cell clonal expansion, diversification, and selection processes. In addition, targeting and substitution models could provide important insights into the relative contributions of the various error-prone DNA repair pathways that mediate SHM.

Computational models and analyses of SHM have separated the process into two independent components (7–11): (1) a targeting model that defines where mutations occur (by specifying the relative rates at which positions in the Ig sequence are mutated), and (2) a nucleotide substitution model that defines the resulting mutation (by specifying the probability of each base mutating to each of the other three possibilities). In experimentally derived Ig sequences, observed mutation patterns are influenced by selection. The affinity maturation process selects for affinity-increasing mutations, while many mutations at structurally important positions in the framework regions are selected against (12). To avoid the confounding influences of selection, most existing models are built using mutation data from intronic regions flanking the V gene (13) and non-productively rearranged Ig genes (6–10, 14). These works have identified several specific motifs as being "hot" or "cold" spots of SHM. Hot-spots include WR$\underline{C}$Y/R$\underline{G}$YW and W$\underline{A}$/$\underline{T}$W (where W = {A, T}, Y = {C, T} R = {G, A}, and the mutated position is underlined, see for example (5, 6)). Although it has been argued that WR$\underline{C}$H/D$\underline{G}$YW (where $H = \{A, C, T\}$ and $D = \{A, G, T\}$) is a better predictor of mutability at C:G bases (15). A single cold-spot motif has also been recognized: SY$\underline{C}$/$\underline{G}$RS (where $S = \{C, G\}$) (16). Despite the wide recognition of these specific hot-spot and cold-spot motifs, it is clear that a hierarchy of mutabilities exists that is highly dependent on the surrounding bases (7, 10). More recently, it has been recognized that the profile of nucleotide substitutions may also be dependent on the surrounding bases (8, 17). Modeling SHM targeting and substitution is important for the analysis of mutation patterns since these intrinsic biases can give the appearance of selection due to the particular codon usage and base composition in Ig sequences (17, 18). Moreover, having such a model could shed light on the molecular mechanisms underlying SHM, which are not fully understood.

Previous work has attempted to model the dependencies on surrounding bases, but has been limited to (at most) the targeted base and three surrounding bases (19), mainly due to the relatively small data sets available. The use of intronic regions has also limited the number of motifs that can be modeled (because of the limited diversity of these regions), and non-productively rearranged Ig genes may still be influenced by selection (e.g., if the event rendering the sequence non-productive happened in the course of affinity maturation). In this study, we take advantage of the wealth of data available from high-throughput Ig sequencing technologies to build improved targeting and substitution models for SHM. To avoid the biasing effects of selection, we have developed a new methodology for constructing models from synonymous mutations only, thus avoiding the need to limit analysis to non-productive Ig sequences. The increased data set size allows modeling of dependencies on the surrounding four bases (two bases upstream and downstream of the mutation). These "S5F" (Synonymous, 5-mer, Functional) models confirm the existence of proposed hot- and cold-spots of SHM, but also show much more extreme difference between hot- and cold-spots compared with previous models. We also find that the nucleotide substitution profiles at all bases are dependent on the surrounding nucleotides. The S5F targeting and substitution models can be employed as background distributions for mutation analysis, such as the detection and quantification of affinity-dependent selection in Ig sequences (11, 20). These models improve dramatically the ability to analyze mutation patterns in Ig sequences, and provide insights into the SHM process.

2. RESULTS

To develop models for SHM targeting and substitution preferences, we curated a large database of mutations from high-throughput sequencing studies (**Table 1**). These data were derived from 7 human blood and lymph node samples, and Ig sequencing was carried out using both Roche 454 and Illumina MiSeq next-generation sequencing technologies. In total, the data contained 42,122,509 raw reads, which were processed (see Materials and Methods) to arrive at 1,145,182 "high-fidelity" Ig sequences, which were each supported by a minimum of two independent reads in a sample. These high-fidelity sequences were clustered to identify clones (sequences related by a common ancestor) and one effective sequence was constructed per clone so that each observed mutation corresponded to an independent event. Overall, this process produced a set of 806,860 synonymous mutations that were used to model somatic hypermutation targeting and substitution.

2.1. THE NUCLEOTIDE SUBSTITUTION SPECTRUM IS AFFECTED BY ADJACENT NUCLEOTIDES

A nucleotide substitution model specifies the probability of each base (A, T, G, or C) mutating to each of the other three possibilities. For example, when a C is mutated, we might find that 50% of the time it is replaced by T, while 30% of the substitutions are to G, and the remaining 20% lead to A. These probabilities may depend on the surrounding bases (i.e., the micro-sequence context), as was previously suggested for mutations at A (17) and more generally (8). To derive a nucleotide substitution model, the set of mutations was filtered to include only those that occurred in positions where none of the possible base substitutions lead to amino acid exchanges. Focusing on positions where only synonymous mutations were possible removes the confounding influence of selection. The resulting 408,422 mutations were analyzed and grouped into "5-mers" according to the germline sequence of the mutated position and surrounding bases (two base-pairs upstream and two base-pairs downstream of the mutated position). For each of the 1024 possible 5-mers (M), a substitution model was derived by calculating S_B^M, the probability that the central base in the 5-mer motif (M) mutates to base B. For example, in the 5-mer CCATC mutations at A are always synonymous whenever this motif starts a reading frame, in which case it codes for a Proline (CCA) followed by a Serine (TCN). In this case, the number of observed mutations that led to each of the other three possible nucleotides (C, G, or T) was recorded: N_C^{CCATC}, N_G^{CCATC}, N_T^{CCATC}. The maximum likelihood value for the probability that A is substituted by base B is then calculated as:

$$S_B^{CCATC} = \frac{N_B^{CCATC}}{N_C^{CCATC} + N_G^{CCATC} + N_T^{CCATC}}$$

Table 1 | Next-generation sequencing data sets used to construct the "S5F" targeting and substitution models.

Study	Sample	Subject	Tissue	Tech.	Raw reads	Processed reads	Clones	# Mutations (substitution)	# Mutations (targeting)
1	3931LN	1	LN	MiSeq	3,641,633	79,777	16,272	25,307	53,840
1	4014LN	2	LN	MiSeq	3,714,152	106,006	32,972	57,215	106,265
1	4106LN	3	LN	MiSeq	10,917,517	231,387	54,400	108,591	208,338
1	3928LN	4	LN	MiSeq	7,691,509	99,519	76,375	68,051	132,795
2	PGP1-1	5	PBMC	MiSeq	3,851,658	55,606	50,514	23,939	48,558
2	PGP1-2	5	PBMC	MiSeq	3,946,514	59,611	54,374	24,971	50,117
2	PGP1-3	5	PBMC	MiSeq	4,543,353	48,971	45,788	20,865	42,737
2	PGP1-4	5	PBMC	MiSeq	3,121,884	52,844	49,054	23,243	47,049
3	hu420143	6	PBMC	454	178,584	92,055	14,956	23,260	48,838
3	420IV	7	PBMC	454	398,517	248,363	39,047	24,771	50,899
3	PGP1-5	5	PBMC	454	117,188	71,043	12,275	8,209	17,424
Total	–	–	–	–	42,122,509	1,145,182	446,027	408,422	806,860

Tissue types are lymph node (LN) or peripheral blood mononuclear cell (PBMC). The different filters applied to arrive at the number of (synonymous) mutations used for the targeting and substitution models are described in the text. All three studies relate to manuscripts in preparation.

A bootstrapping procedure was used to estimate 95% confidence intervals (21).

Comparison of the substitution profiles for different 5-mer motifs with the same central base clearly showed the significant influence of surrounding bases. As an example, **Figure 1A** shows how the profile of substitutions at G changes for several different 5-mers (AC<u>G</u>AT, GC<u>G</u>AG, GT<u>G</u>TA, and GG<u>G</u>AA). Such dependencies were identified for every base (A, T, G, and C) (**Figure 1B** and Figure S1 in Supplementary Material). The importance of including two bases upstream and downstream was confirmed by comparing these profiles with analogous profiles that only account for the immediately adjacent bases (3-mer motifs) (**Figure 1A**). For the 3-mer C<u>G</u>A, G → C and G → A substitutions were equally likely (45% and 43% of substitutions, respectively), while G → C substitutions were significantly more likely than G → A in the context of the GC<u>G</u>AG motif (51% and 35% of substitutions, respectively). If one ignores neighboring nucleotides, the substitution profiles were qualitatively similar to previous estimates (7), although significant quantitative differences were apparent (presumably due to the much larger size of the dataset compiled here). Thus, nucleotide substitution profiles at every base are significantly affected by adjacent nucleotides, including at least two bases on either side of the mutating base.

2.1.1. *The complete substitution model for somatic hypermutation is not strand-symmetric*

It is not possible to estimate substitution profiles for all 5-mer motifs using the above methodology because: (1) not all 5-mers appear within the set of Ig sequences, and (2) some 5-mers (such as NA<u>N</u>NN) can never appear in a context where all substitutions at the central (underlined) base are synonymous. Among the 11 datasets used here, these issues prevent estimation of the substitution profiles for 717 of the 1024 5-mers. For the profiles that could be directly estimated, there was a high correlation (on average Pearson R = 0.63) between different individuals (Figures S2 and S3 in Supplementary Material), and so all the samples were combined to estimate a single substitution model. To infer values for the missing motifs, four methods were evaluated. In the first method ("inner 3-mer"), the substitution profile for each missing 5-mer was inferred by averaging over profiles for all 5-mers with the same 3-mer core (i.e., for which the middle three bases were shared). In the second and third methods, missing values were replaced by averaging over motifs sharing the two bases upstream and downstream of the mutated base, respectively. In the fourth method ("hot-spot"), the missing substitution profile was inferred by averaging over 5-mers sharing the two upstream bases when the mutated position was "C" or "A," and two downstream bases when the mutated position was "G" or "T." This final option was motivated by the dependencies of known "hot" and "cold" spots for SHM targeting (5, 6). To choose between these four methods, we compared their performance on 5-mers that could be directly estimated from the data. Specifically, we calculated the correlation between the inferred and directly estimated ratios for the parameter *R*, which was defined as the ratio between the highest substitution probability with the next highest one for a given 5-mer (**Table 2**). Pearson and Spearman coefficients were both used in order to be robust to the linear dependency assumption, and they yielded comparable results. While the "hot-spot" method clearly had the worst performance, the other three methods resulted in very similar models. The "inner 3-mer" method produced the highest Pearson correlation (0.4, see **Table 2**) and was chosen as the basis to infer missing values. We refer to the resulting substitution model as a "S5F" model since it is based on Synonymous mutations at 5-mers in Functional Ig sequences. In contrast to previous studies (8), there was no significant correlation between substitution values of 5-mers and their reverse complements (Pearson correlation of 0.005, Spearman correlation of 0.087), suggesting that at least one component of the substitution mechanism is not strand-symmetric.

2.2. THE HIERARCHY OF MOTIF MUTABILITIES IS CONSERVED ACROSS INDIVIDUALS

The mutability of a motif is defined here as the (non-normalized) probability of the central base in the motif being targeted for SHM relative to all other motifs. Similar to the substitution model, the targeting model was based on 5-mer motifs, including the

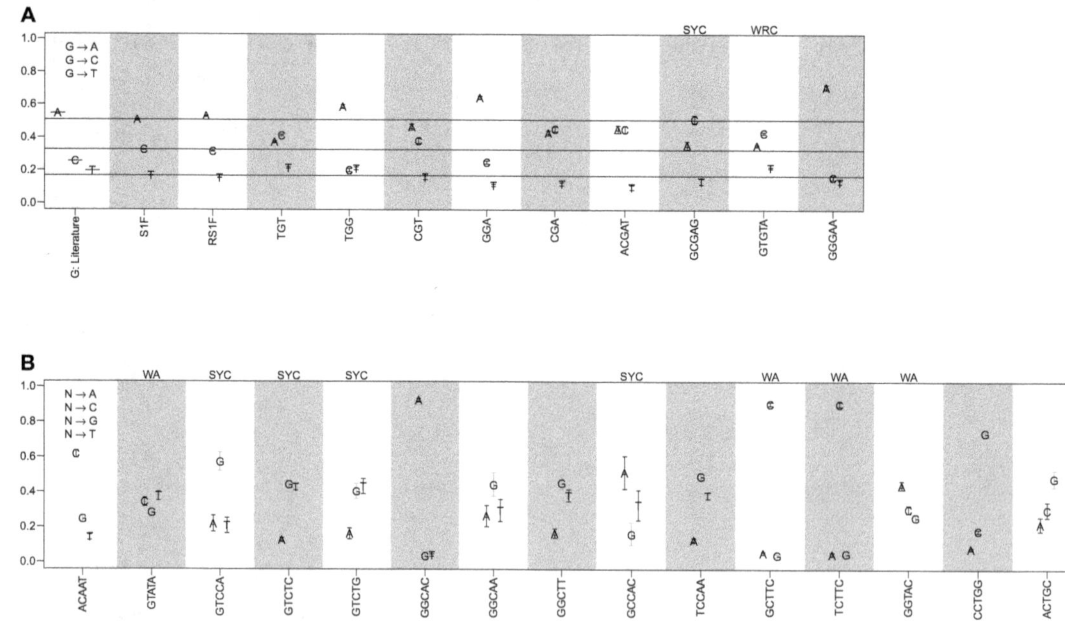

FIGURE 1 | The substitution profile is significantly influenced by surrounding bases. Substitution profiles for various micro-sequence contexts are shown for substitutions at **(A)** guanine and **(B)** adenosine, cytidine, and thymidine. G: literature indicates values estimated by Smith et al. (7), while S1F and RS1F refer to models estimated using the methods proposed here using all (replacement and silent) or only silent mutations, respectively, and averaging over surrounding bases. 3-mer motifs were estimated using silent mutations and dependencies on the immediately adjacent bases (S3F), while 5-mer motifs refer to the complete S5F model. Horizontal lines in **(A)** indicate the substitution values for the S1F model following the color scheme shown in the legend. Motifs that fall into one of the standard hot or cold-spots categories are indicated by the motif above the column.

Table 2 | Correlation coefficients for inferring missing mutability/substitution values.

Model	Correlation	Middle	Upstream	Downstream	Hot spots
Substitution	Pearson	0.40	0.37	0.15	0.04
	Spearman	0.20	0.24	0.23	0.09
Mutability	Pearson	0.58	0.57	0.61	0.73
	Spearman	0.61	0.58	0.64	0.79

two nucleotides immediately upstream and downstream of the mutated base. The use of a 5-mer model is motivated by the well-known WRC̲Y hot-spot (where the underlined C is targeted for mutation), and its reverse-complement (RG̲YW) which, when taken together, create dependencies with the two bases on either side of the mutating base.

When estimating the mutability (μ) for a motif (M), it is critical to account for the background frequency of M. To see why this is the case, consider the extreme example of a sequence composed of all C nucleotides. Since all mutations will occur at CCC̲CC motifs, one might consider this motif a hot-spot, except that its background frequency is 100% so it is actually targeted at the expected frequency. When calculating mutabilities it is also important to avoid statistical artifacts due to heterogeneity (e.g., the Simpson paradox (22)). Thus, Ig sequences were first analyzed individually since each has a different background 5-mer distribution. These individual-sequence targeting models were then combined into a single aggregated targeting model for each data set. Estimating the relative mutabilities of 5-mer motifs for an individual Ig sequence involves two steps: (1) Calculating the background frequency of the different 5-mers based on the germline (unmutated) version of the sequence, and (2) creating a table of the 5-mers that were mutated in the sequence. To avoid the confounding influence of selection, only mutations that were synonymous (i.e., that do not produce an amino acid exchange in the germline context) were included in the analysis. Note that these criteria are slightly different from those used in the substitution model. In the substitution model, mutations were used only where all possible mutations at that position had to be synonymous, while all synonymous mutations were considered for mutabilities (see **Table 1**).

For each of the 1024 possible 5-mers motifs (M) in each Ig sequence, the background frequency (B_M) was calculated as follows:

$$B_M = \sum_i \sum_b S_b^M I_{\overrightarrow{GL}}(i, M, b) \quad (1)$$

where i is summed over all (non-N) positions in the Ig sequence, M is the 5-mer nucleotide sequence centered at position i and b includes all possible nucleotides ({A, C, T, G}). In this equation GL is a vector containing the nucleic content of each position in the germline sequence, S_b^M is the relative rate at which the center nucleotide in M ($GL[i]$) mutates to b (as estimated in the previous section, and where $S_{GL[i]}^M = 0$) and $I_{\overrightarrow{GL}}(i, M, b)$ is an indicator function that is 1 in cases where the 5-mer surrounding $GL[i]$

is M and a mutation in position i from $GL[i]$ to b results in a synonymous mutation (and 0 otherwise). A similar array was also calculated for the mutated positions:

$$C_{\mathrm{M}} = \sum_{i} I_{\overrightarrow{GL},\overrightarrow{OS}}(i, \mathrm{M}) \tag{2}$$

where i is summed over all (non-N) positions in the observed Ig sequence (OS), and the indicator function $I_{\overrightarrow{GL},\overrightarrow{OS}}$ (i, M) is 1 in cases where the 5-mer surrounding $GL[i]$ is M and a mutation in position i from $GL[i]$ to $OS[i]$ is synonymous and 0 otherwise. After calculating the arrays $\vec{C}$ and $\vec{B}$, a mutability score, μ, was defined for each motif M in the vector (for sequence j) as:

$$\mu_{\mathrm{M}}^{j} = C_{\mathrm{M}}^{j} / B_{\mathrm{M}}^{j} \tag{3}$$

which was then normalized to one:

$$\bar{\mu}_{\mathrm{M}}^{j} = \mu_{\mathrm{M}}^{j} / \sum_{\mathrm{m}} \mu_{\mathrm{m}}^{j} \tag{4}$$

where m is an index spanning all positions in $\vec{\mu}^{j}$. Note that μ_{M}^{j} is not defined wherever $B_{\mathrm{M}}^{j} = 0$ (i.e., the motif M does not appear in the Ig sequence, or can not admit any synonymous mutations). Finally, a single mutability score is generated for each 5-mer motif (M) as the weighted average of the mutabilities scores for each sequence j ($\bar{\mu}_{\mathrm{M}}^{j}$), where weights correspond to the number of synonymous mutations in the sequence ($\sum_{\mathrm{M}} C_{\mathrm{M}}^{j}$). This process resulted in an array of (relative) mutabilities, μ_{M} for each of the 5-mers observed in the dataset. The resulting vector was renormalized so that the mean mutability was one.

2.2.1. *Inference of missing values to complete targeting model*

It was not possible to estimate mutabilities for 468 of the 1024 possible 5-mer motifs because not all 5-mers appeared within the set of Ig sequences. The same four methods tested for inferring missing values in the substitution model were also tested to infer these mutabilities (see 2.1.1 and **Table 2**). The "inner 3-mer" method produced a Pearson correlation of 0.58 (0.61 for Spearman), while the "hot-spot" method had a correlation of 0.73 (0.79 for Spearman). Thus, in contrast to the nucleotide substitution model, mutabilities were best predicted by averaging over 5-mers which shared the two upstream bases when the mutated position was "C" or "A," and two downstream bases when the mutated position was "G" or "T." This result is consistent with the expected influence of the classic SHM hot-spot (WRCY/RGYW).

2.2.2. *Targeting is conserved across individuals*

To test whether the micro-sequence specificity of SHM was conserved across individuals, separate targeting models were constructed for each of the 11 samples in our study (**Table 1**). Comparison of the motif mutabilities between pairs of samples showed that the models were highly consistent, with Pearson correlation ~0.9 (**Figure 2** and Figure S4 in Supplementary Material). Thus, we combined the data from all of the samples and generated a single targeting model, with confidence intervals based on the middle 50% quantiles of the mutability across samples. As with the substitution model, we refer to this targeting model as a "S5F" model. In order to visualize this model, we created "hedgehog" plots to display the directly estimated mutability values and the complete S5F model (**Figures 3A,B**, respectively).

2.2.3. *The true "hotness" of SHM hot-spots*

Visual inspection of the "hedgehog" plots (**Figure 3B**) shows clearly that the S5F model is consistent with known micro-sequence preferences for SHM (5, 6). WRC/GYW and WA/TW hot-spot motifs are generally more mutable, while SYC/GRS cold-spot motifs generally show the lowest mutability. However, the mutability of "hot-spot" motifs was observed to be highly variable. There is a 62.7-fold difference between the most mutable (GGGCA, mutability = 9.56) and least mutable (TGCGA, mutability = 0.15) WRC/GYW hot-spot motif. Indeed, ~10% of so-called "hot-spots" had mutabilities that were lower than the mean mutability for "neutral" motifs (**Figure 4A**). This high variance was especially obvious when looking at the subset of WRCA/TGYW hot-spot motifs, and may help explain why WRCH/DGYW has been proposed to be a better predictor of mutation at C:G compared with WRCY/RGYW (15). The mutabilities estimated by the S5F approach paint a qualitatively different picture of SHM when compared with those estimated by the existing tri-nucleotide model of Shapiro et al. (10). In the S5F model, the average mutability of motifs that correspond to the WRC/GYW SHM hot-spot was 3.2-fold higher than neutral motifs, and 9.6-fold higher than the mutability of motifs corresponding to the cold-spot SYC/GRS (**Figure 4A**). Using the tri-nucleotide model, hot-spots were only 1.3-fold and 1.6-fold more mutable than neutral and cold-spots, respectively (**Figure 4B**). In addition, in direct opposition to the S5F model, the tri-nucleotide method predicted that A/T hot-spots (WA/TW) were more mutable than C/G hot-spots (WRC/GYW). The mutabilities estimated by the S5F model better predicted the positional-distribution of *in vivo* mutations. The Pearson correlation between the expected mutability and observed mutation frequency calculated over IMGT-numbered positions in 12,000 sequences derived from a variety of germline segments was 0.67 and 0.47 for the S5F and tri-nucleotide models, respectively (**Figure 5** and Figure S5 in Supplementary Material). In both methods, deviations from the expected frequencies that likely reflect both positive and negative selection were observed (**Figure 5**). The observation of position-specific signals suggests that there is something generic about the Ig structure at these positions, and may help refine traditional definitions of the complementarity determining regions (CDR) and framework regions (FWR) (see also (23)). Consistent with previous studies (24), the S5F model displayed significant strand-bias at A/T hot-spots, but not C/G hot-spots (**Figure 6**). Overall, the S5F targeting model provides a new view of SHM with hot-spots being significantly more targeted (and significantly more variable) than previously thought.

3. MATERIALS AND METHODS

3.1. HIGH-THROUGHPUT IG SEQUENCING DATA SETS

A total of 11 human Ig repertoires were sequenced from blood and lymph node samples from 7 different individuals. Next-generation sequencing was carried out using Illumina MiSeq 250

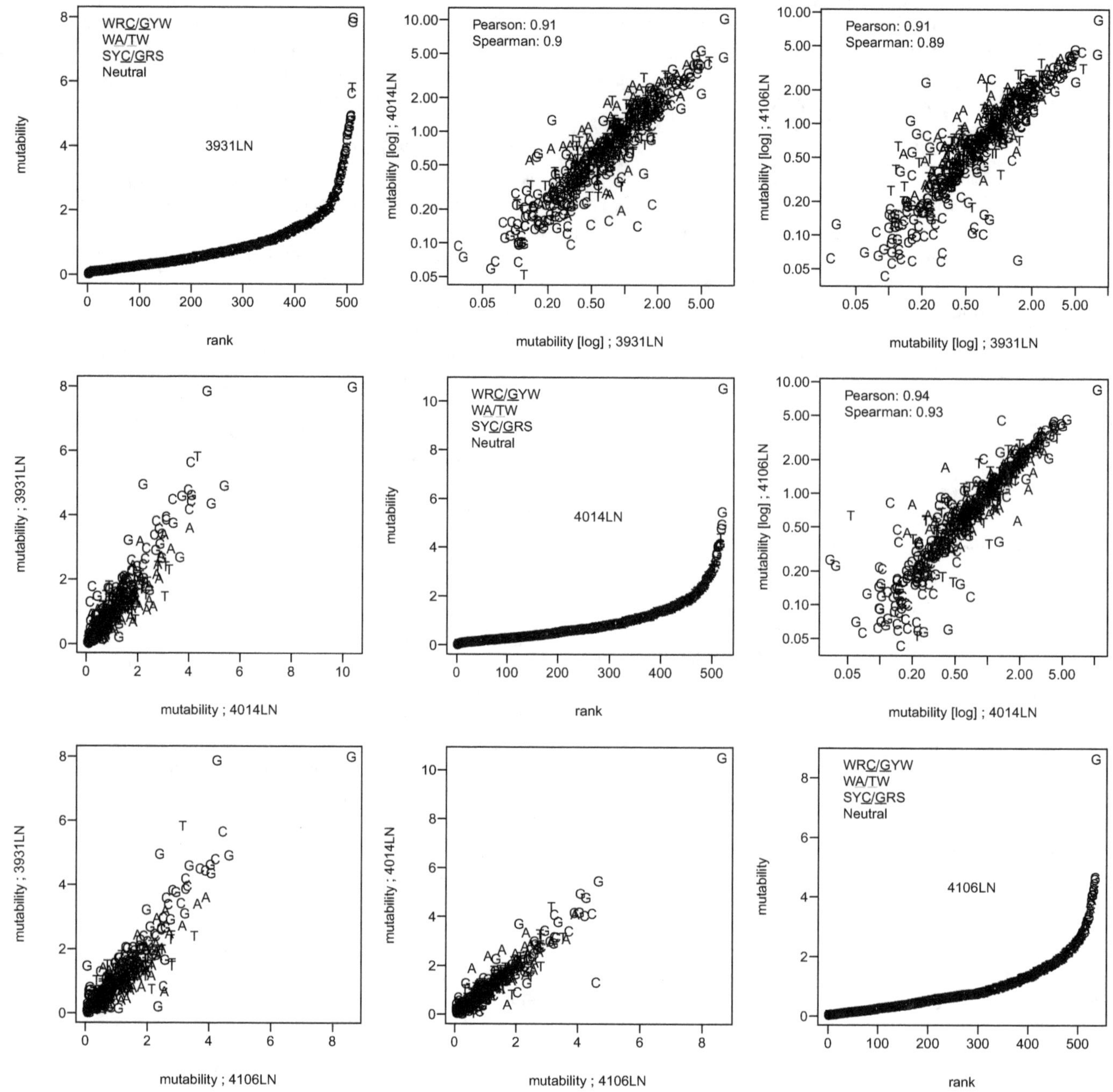

FIGURE 2 | The S5F targeting model is consistent across individuals. Targeting models were constructed independently for each of the samples listed in **Table 1**. Estimated values for all 5-mer motifs derived using lymph node samples from three individuals (3931LN, 4014LN, and 4106LN) are shown along the diagonal. Mutability values are ranked (from lowest to highest) and color coded by their category (WRC/GYW are red, SYC/GRS are blue, WA/TW are green, and the rest are gray). Symbols indicate the mutated nucleotide (in the center of the 5-mer). Correlations between the mutabilities for all 5-mer motifs across individuals are shown in the upper (log-log scale) and lower (linear scale) triangles.

base-pair paired-end reads (8 samples) and Roche/454 GS FLX (3 samples). Details are provided in **Table 1**. These samples were originally collected and sequenced as part of three ongoing studies (manuscripts in preparation).

3.1.1. Illumina MiSeq data

Human lymph node specimens were collected under an exempt protocol approved by the Human Research Protection Program at Yale School of Medicine. Tissues were processed and RNA isolated as previously described (25). Blood samples were collected under the approval of the Personal Genome Project (26). Total RNA was immediately extracted from each blood sample and stored at −80°C until use. To carry out sequencing, mRNA was reverse transcribed into cDNA using gene-specific primers mapping to the constant region of the Ig heavy chain. Resultant cDNA was tagged with 17 nucleotide single-molecule barcodes and amplified

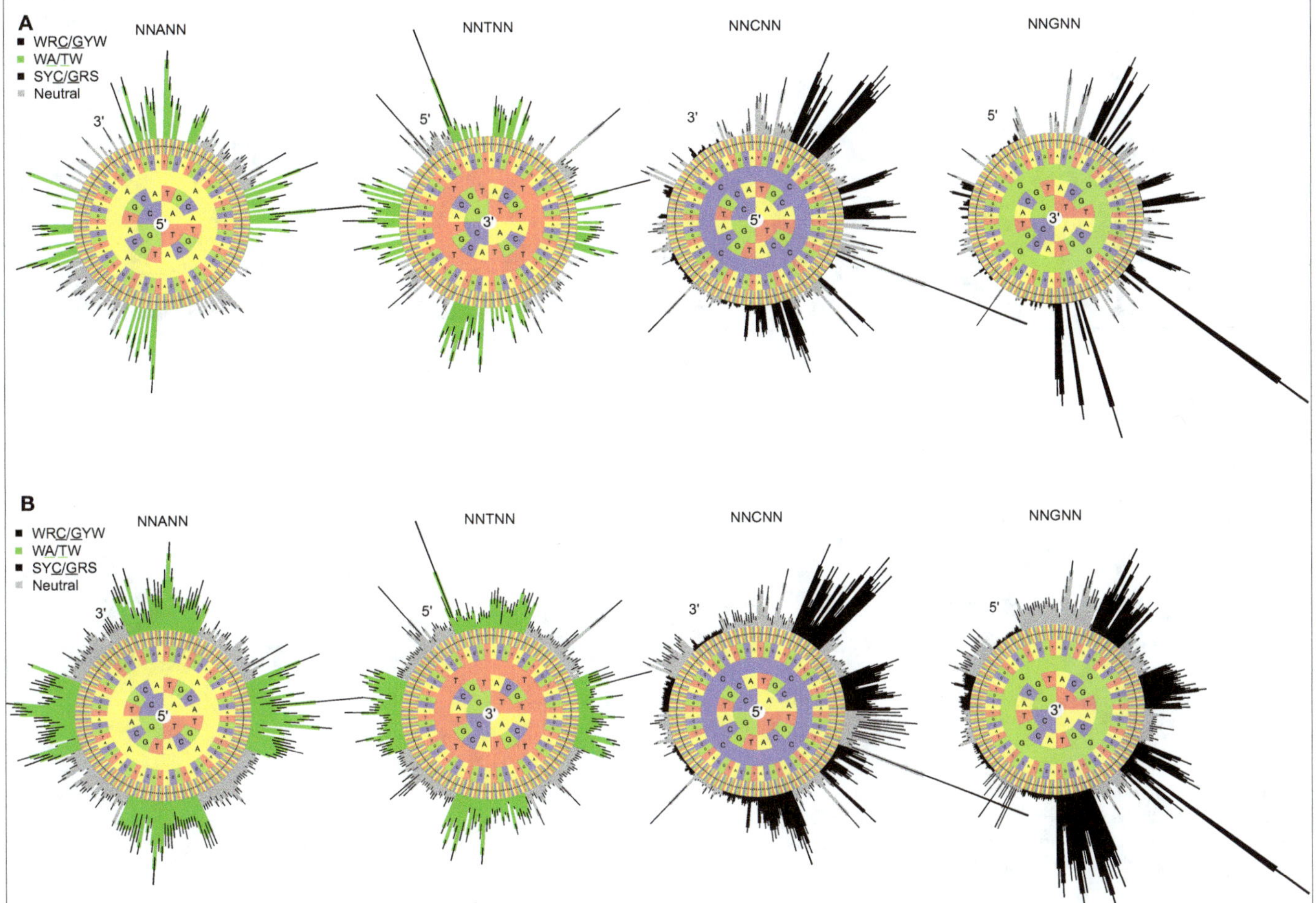

FIGURE 3 | "Hedgehog" plots for the S5F targeting model for somatic hypermutation targeting A, T, C, and G nucleotides (individual circles). **(A)** 5-mer mutabilities estimated directly from the Ig sequencing data. **(B)** The complete S5F targeting model after inferring values for missing 5-mer motifs. Bars radiating from each circle depict the mutability as a function of surrounding bases. The inner-most ring in the circle corresponds to two positions upstream (5′) of the mutated base for A and C, and two positions downstream (3′) of the mutated base for T and G. Bar colors indicate known hot/cold-spot motifs (WRC/GYW are red, WA/TW are green, SYC/GRS are blue, and "neutral" are gray). Each plot corresponds to a different mutated nucleotide. Error bars indicate confidence intervals based on the middle 50% quantiles of the mutability value distribution across the set of samples.

by PCR in a multiplex reaction using primer sets for all possible V-regions ($n = 45$) and isotype/J-regions ($n = 6$) to generate heavy chain transcripts. The amplified library was tagged with barcodes for sample multiplexing, PCR enriched, and annealed to the required Illumina clustering adapters. High-throughput 250 base-pair paired-end sequencing was performed using the Illumina MiSeq platform. Raw reads were exported without the sample barcodes and Illumina clustering adapters.

3.1.2. *Roche/454 GS FLX data*

Blood samples were collected under the approval of the Personal Genome Project (26). Total RNA was immediately extracted from each blood sample and stored at −80°C until use. Ig heavy chain mRNA were reverse-transcribed using a pool of 6 primers specific to the Ig constant regions and cDNA was amplified using 16 cycles of PCR with a pool of 46 V-region-specific primers and 6 nested constant region primers. Following ligation of 454-compatible sequencing adapters, the expected heavy chain V gene fragments were purified using PAGE. Each sample was uniquely barcoded during the ligation process, allowing subsequent mixing of all the samples into one common reaction sample (performed independently for each replicate run). Emulsion PCR and 454 GS FLX sequencing were performed directly at the 454 Life Sciences facility according to the manufacturer's standard protocols.

3.2. SEQUENCING DATA PRE-PROCESSING

Raw sequencing reads were filtered in several steps to identify and remove low-quality sequences. Conservative thresholds were applied in all cases to increase the reliability of the resulting mutation calls, at the potential expense of excluding some real mutations. Pre-processing was carried out using the Repertoire

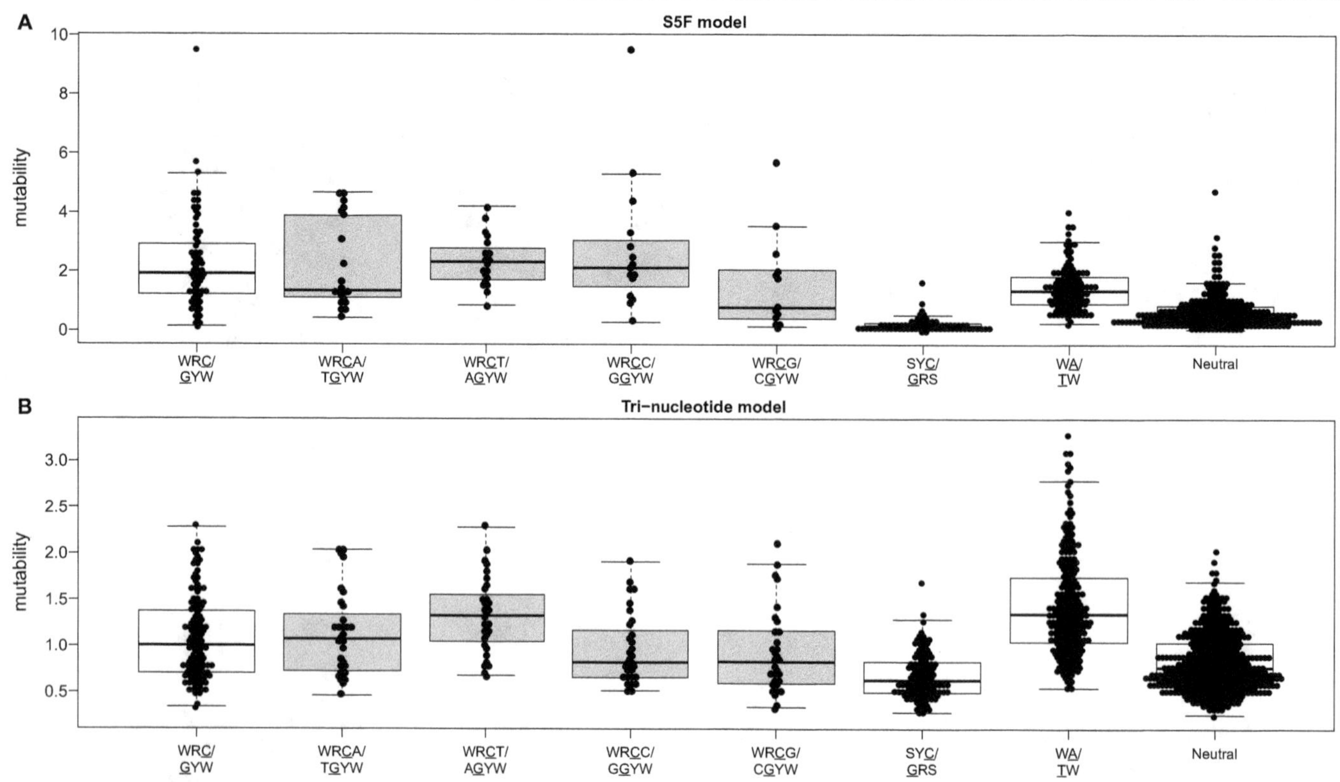

FIGURE 4 | The hierarchy of hot/cold-spot motifs. Mutability values predicted by the **(A)** S5F model or **(B)** the tri-nucleotide model of Shapiro et al. were grouped by the type of motif. Boxes borders correspond to the first and fourth quartiles while the horizontal bar inside the box corresponds to the median of the distribution. Hot/cold spot motif groups are plotted using the same colors as in **Figure 3B** with open boxes. WRCN/NGYW motifs are plotted using filled boxes.

Sequencing Toolkit (pRESTO) (http://clip.med.yale.edu/pRESTO, manuscript in preparation), and involved:

- Quality control
  1. Removal of low-quality reads (mean Phred quality score <20).
  2. Removal of reads where the primer could not be identified or had a poor alignment score (mismatch rate greater than 0.1).
  3. For the MiSeq data, sets of sequences with identical molecular IDs (corresponding to the same mRNA molecule) were identified. Sets were collapsed into one consensus sequence per set, after discarding those having a mean mismatch rate across all positions >0.2.
  4. For the MiSeq data, the two paired-end reads were assembled into a complete Ig sequence.
  5. Removal of sequences that do not appear in a single sample at least twice.
- Assignment of germline V(D)J segments for each of the Ig sequences: initial V(D)J assignments for each sequence were obtained using IMGT/HighV-QUEST (27). Using these assignments, non-mutated sequences were identified and a V segment germline repertoire for each individual was determined as the set of: (1) V genes that composed at least 0.1% of the sequences, and (2) V gene alleles that composed at least 10% of the assignments to that V gene. Ig sequences that were initially assigned V segments not included in this germline repertoire were then re-assigned to the closest present V segment based on the Hamming distance.
- Removal of non-functional sequences due to the occurrence of a stop codon or/and a reading frame shift between the V gene and the J gene.
- Removal of sequences with more than 30 mutations and masking (replacement with Ns) of positions with Phred quality scores <20.
- Removal of mutations in codons that had more than one mutation, as it is usually not possible to infer the order in which the mutations occurred (and thus the micro-sequence context of the mutations is unknown).
- Identification of clonally related sequences: a two-step approach was applied to identify sequences that were part of a B cell clone (i.e., related through descent from a common ancestor). First, the sequences were divided into groups based on equivalence of their V-gene assignment, J-gene assignment, and the number of nucleotides in their junction. Second, clones were defined within each of these groups as the collection of sequences with junction regions that differed from one sequence to any of the others by no more than three point mutations.

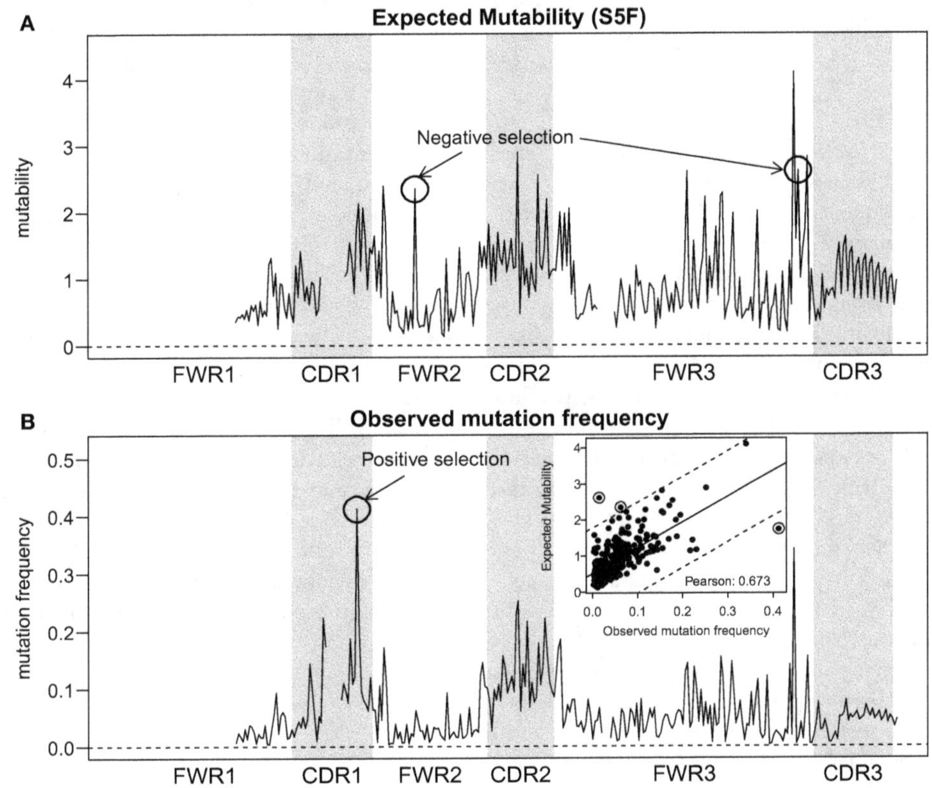

FIGURE 5 | Comparison between expected and observed somatic hypermutation targeting. (A) The predicted mutability from the S5F model and **(B)** the observed mutation frequency from sample 3931LN (averaged over all clones) for each position in the Ig sequence (IMGT-aligned along the *x*-axis). The correlation across positions (points) is shown in the inset of **(B)**. Two positions with evidence of negative selection (red circles) and one position with positive selection (blue circles) are indicated. The threshold for calling a position with significant selection was set to 3 SD away from the linear regression line (shown as a solid line in the inset, with thresholds plotted as dashed lines).

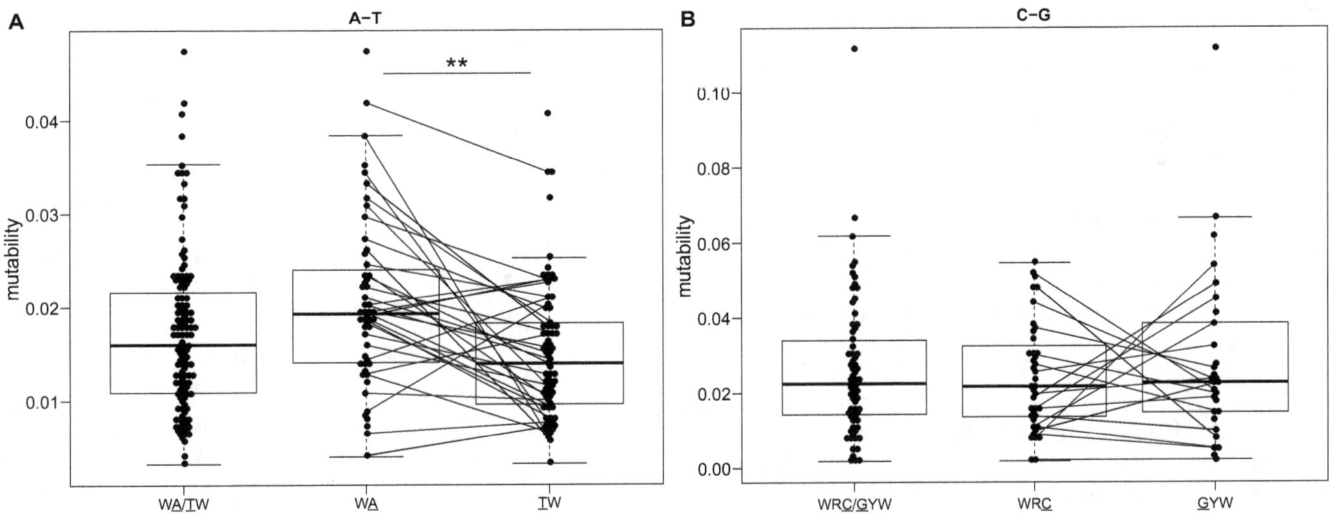

FIGURE 6 | Somatic hypermutation targeting at C/G, but not A/T, hot-spots is strand symmetric. Mutability values directly estimated by the S5F model (**Figure 3**) for **(A)** WA and **(B)** WRC "hot-spot" motifs are compared between different strands. Lines connect reverse-complement motifs for cases where both could be directly estimated from the data. $^{**}P < 5 \times 10^{-4}$ by a paired Mann–Whitney–Wilcoxon test.

The threshold of three was determined after manual inspection of the mutation patterns in resulting clones identified through building lineage trees.

4. DISCUSSION

We have constructed new SHM targeting and substitution models using a collection of more than 800,000 synonymous mutations from next-generation Ig sequencing studies. The exclusive use of synonymous mutations allowed us to include mutations from functional Ig sequences without the biasing influence of selection. The large size of the resulting mutation data set allowed us to model targeting and substitution dependencies on the mutating base as well as on two bases upstream and downstream of the mutation. The resulting "S5F" models validate, and also help refine, previously defined SHM hot and cold spots. **Figure 4** shows how the classic WRCY/RGYW hot-spot excludes some highly mutable WRCA/TGYW motifs, implying that, as proposed by Rogozin and Diaz (15), WRCH/DGYW could be a better predictor of mutation. However, while the most mutable WRCA/TGYW motifs are even hotter than WRCY/RGYW, others are comparable to neutral motifs. This high variance demonstrates the importance of including higher order dependencies, as we have done.

It has been suggested that nucleotide substitution profiles are also dependent on the micro-sequence context of the mutating base (8, 17). We confirm that the substitution profiles at all nucleotides are highly dependent on neighboring bases and these dependencies are conserved across individuals. Interestingly, the fact that substitution rates depend on surrounding bases may resemble the situation in meiotic mutations as was suggested in the past (9). The ability of the S5F models to estimate mutability and substitution at each of the 1024 DNA 5-mer motifs will allow for detailed, quantitative comparison of SHM with other mutation processes.

A potential source of error in the approach taken here is the existence of novel polymorphisms among the seven individuals studied (**Table 1**). Since mutation detection depends on comparison with known V and J segments that are part of the IMGT repertoire, undetected polymorphisms will look like mutations. However, any effect on the S5F model is expected to be small relative to the estimated confidence intervals. Based on a new statistical tool to detect novel germline alleles from high-throughput sequencing data (manuscript in preparation), the magnitude of this effect was estimated to be less than ~1% of the sequences and less than ~0.1% of the mutations used for the current analysis. The S5F mutability and substitution models presented here were developed using human heavy chain data, and thus may not be valid for light chains or mouse sequences. Given the large amount of sequencing data becoming available, it may be possible to extend the proposed approach to model 7-mers instead of 5-mers. However, even with 5-mers, the values for some motifs had to be inferred because of the limited diversity in germline repertoires. It will be important to estimate the quality of these inferences experimentally. Future experiments might be designed to enrich for non-productively rearranged Ig sequences which could then be sequenced using high-throughput technologies. Since mutations in these sequences are (presumably) not subject to selection, they provide a way to independently estimate substitution profiles and mutabilities for at least some of the motifs inferred in the S5F model. It will be important to confirm that the mutation process operating on these non-productive sequences is equivalent to the process at the productive alleles. This uncertainty is one reason why only productively rearranged Ig sequences were included in the current model.

The targeting and substitution models developed here provide a quantitative description of SHM in the absence of selection, and thus provide an important background for statistical analysis of SHM patterns in experimental data. For example, such models play an important role in quantifying antigen-driven selection in Ig sequences (11, 20), and we have now made the S5F model available as an option on our website for quantifying selection (http://clip.med.yale.edu/baseline). When combined with high-throughput sequencing, it should now be possible to quantify selection for each position of the Ig sequence independently and link these values back to the physical structure of the protein. Following the approach of Brard and Guguen (28), these models could also be incorporated into methods for building lineage trees of B cell clones (29), thus helping to provide insight into the underlying population dynamics of adaptive immunity. The model and method source code are made available at http://clip.med.yale.edu/SHM.

ACKNOWLEDGMENTS

We thank the Yale High Performance Computing Center (funded by NIH grant: RR19895) for use of their computing resources. Funding: this work was partially supported by NIH R03AI092379. The work of Jason A. Vander Heiden, Daniel Gadala-Maria and Namita Gupta were supported in part by NIH Grant T15 LM07056 from the National Library of Medicine.

REFERENCES

1. Chahwan R, Edelmann W, Scharff MD, Roa S. AIDing antibody diversity by error-prone mismatch repair. *Semin Immunol* (2012) **24**(4):293–300. doi:10.1016/j.smim.2012.05.005
2. Peled JU, Kuang FL, Iglesias-Ussel MD, Roa S, Kalis SL, Goodman MF, et al. The biochemistry of somatic hypermutation. *Annu Rev Immunol* (2008) **26**(1):481–511. doi:10.1146/annurev.immunol.26.021607.090236
3. McKean D, Huppi K, Bell M, Staudt L, Gerhard W, Weigert M. Generation of antibody diversity in the immune response of BALB/c mice to influenza virus hemagglutinin. *Proc Natl Acad Sci U S A* (1984) **81**(10):3180–4. doi:10.1073/pnas.81.10.3180
4. Kleinstein SH, Louzoun Y, Shlomchik MJ. Estimating hypermutation rates from clonal tree data. *J Immunol* (2003) **171**(9):4639–49.
5. Betz AG, Rada C, Pannell R, Milstein C, Neuberger MS. Passenger transgenes reveal intrinsic specificity of the antibody hypermutation mechanism: clustering, polarity, and specific hot spots. *Proc Natl Acad Sci U S A* (1993) **90**(6):2385–8. doi:10.1073/pnas.90.6.2385
6. Shapiro GS, Aviszus K, Ikle D, Wysocki LJ. Predicting regional mutability in antibody v genes based solely on di- and trinucleotide sequence composition. *J Immunol* (1999) **163**(1):259–68.
7. Smith DS, Creadon G, Jena PK, Portanova JP, Kotzin BL, Wysocki LJ. Di- and trinucleotide target preferences of somatic mutagenesis in normal and autoreactive b cells. *J Immunol* (1996) **156**:2642–52.
8. Cowell LG, Kepler TB. The nucleotide-replacement spectrum under somatic hypermutation exhibits microsequence dependence that is strand-symmetric

and distinct from that under germline mutation. *J Immunol* (2000) **164**(4):1971–6.

9. Oprea M, Cowell LG, Kepler TB. The targeting of somatic hypermutation closely resembles that of meiotic mutation. *J Immunol* (2001) **166**(2):892–9.
10. Shapiro GS, Ellison MC, Wysocki LJ. Sequence-specific targeting of two bases on both DNA strands by the somatic hypermutation mechanism. *Mol Immunol* (2003) **40**(5):287–95. doi:10.1016/S0161-5890(03)00101-9
11. Uduman M, Yaari G, Hershberg U, Stern JA, Shlomchik MJ, Kleinstein SH. Detecting selection in immunoglobulin sequences. *Nucleic Acids Res* (2011) **39**(Suppl 2):W499–504. doi:10.1093/nar/gkr413
12. Shlomchik MJ, Watts P, Weigert MG, Litwin S. Clone: a Monte-Carlo computer simulation of b cell clonal expansion, somatic mutation, and antigen-driven selection. *Curr Top Microbiol Immunol* (1998) **229**:173–97. doi:10.1007/978-3-642-71984-4_13
13. MacCarthy T, Kalis SL, Roa S, Pham P, Goodman MF, Scharff MD, et al. V-region mutation in vitro, in vivo, and in silico reveal the importance of the enzymatic properties of AID and the sequence environment. *Proc Natl Acad Sci U S A* (2009) **106**(21):8629–34. doi:10.1073/pnas.0903803106
14. Spencer J, Dunn M, Dunn-Walters DK. Characteristics of sequences around individual nucleotide substitutions in IgVH genes suggest different GC and AT mutators. *J Immunol* (1999) **162**(11):6596–601.
15. Rogozin IB, Diaz M. Cutting edge: DGYW/WRCH is a better predictor of mutability at G:C bases in ig hypermutation than the widely accepted RGYW/WRCY motif and probably reflects a two-step activation-induced cytidine deaminase-triggered process. *J Immunol* (2004) **172**(6):3382–4.
16. Bransteitter R, Pham P, Calabrese P, Goodman MF. Biochemical analysis of hypermutational targeting by wild type and mutant activation-induced cytidine deaminase. *J Biol Chem* (2004) **279**(49):51612–21. doi:10.1074/jbc.M408135200
17. Spencer J, Dunn-Walters DK. Hypermutation at A-T base pairs: the A nucleotide replacement spectrum is affected by adjacent nucleotides and there is no reverse complementarity of sequences flanking mutated A and T nucleotides. *J Immunol* (2005) **175**(8):5170–7.
18. Bose B, Sinha S. Problems in using statistical analysis of replacement and silent mutations in antibody genes for determining antigen-driven affinity selection. *Immunology* (2005) **116**(2):172–83. doi:10.1111/j.1365-2567.2005.02208.x
19. Cohen RM, Kleinstein SH, Louzoun Y. Somatic hypermutation targeting is influenced by location within the immunoglobulin Z region. *Mol Immunol* (2011) **48**(12-13):1477–83. doi:10.1016/j.molimm.2011.04.002
20. Yaari G, Uduman M, Kleinstein SH. Quantifying selection in high-throughput immunoglobulin sequencing data sets. *Nucleic Acids Res* (2012) **40**(17):e134. doi:10.1093/nar/gks457
21. Correa J. *Interval Estimation of the Parameters of the Multinomial Distribution*. Statistics on the Internet (2001). Available from: inter-stat.statjournals.net.
22. Simpson EH. The interpretation of interaction in contingency tables. *J R Stat Soc B* (1951) **13**(2):238–41.
23. Kunik V, Ashkenazi S, Ofran Y. Paratome: an online tool for systematic identification of antigen-binding regions in antibodies based on sequence or structure. *Nucleic Acids Res* (2012) **40**:W521–4. doi:10.1093/nar/gks480
24. Rogozin IB, Pavlov YI, Bebenek K, Matsuda T, Kunkel TA. Somatic mutation hotspots correlate with DNA polymerase error spectrum. *Nat Immunol* (2001) **2**(6):530–6. doi:10.1038/88732
25. Willis SN, Mallozzi SS, Rodig SJ, Cronk KM, McArdel SL, Caron T, et al. The microenvironment of germ cell tumors harbors a prominent antigen-driven humoral response. *J Immunol* (2009) **182**(5):3310–7. doi:10.4049/jimmunol.0803424
26. Nirantar SR, Ghadessy FJ. Compartmentalized linkage of genes encoding interacting protein pairs. *Proteomics* (2011) **11**(7):1335–9. doi:10.1002/pmic.201000643
27. Lefranc M-P, Pommi C, Ruiz M, Giudicelli V, Foulquier E, Truong L, et al. IMGT unique numbering for immunoglobulin and t cell receptor variable domains and ig superfamily v-like domains. *Dev Comp Immunol* (2003) **27**(1):55–77. doi:10.1016/S0145-305X(02)00039-3
28. Brard J, Guguen L. Accurate estimation of substitution rates with neighbor-dependent models in a phylogenetic context. *Syst Biol* (2012) **61**(3):510–21. doi:10.1093/sysbio/sys024
29. Barak M, Zuckerman NS, Edelman H, Unger R, Mehr R. IgTree: creating immunoglobulin variable region gene lineage trees. *J Immunol Methods* (2008) **338**(12):67–74. doi:10.1016/j.jim.2008.06.006

24

Small and long regulatory RNAs in the immune system and immune diseases

Anna Stachurska[†], Maria M. Zorro[†], Marijke R. van der Sijde[†] and Sebo Withoff *

Department of Genetics, University Medical Center Groningen, University of Groningen, Groningen, Netherlands

Edited by:
Susan Carpenter, University of Massachusetts Medical School, USA

Reviewed by:
Carlo Pucillo, University of Udine, Italy
Behdad Afzali, King's College London, UK

***Correspondence:**
Sebo Withoff, University Medical Center Groningen, Hanzeplein 1, 9713 GZ, Groningen, Netherlands
e-mail: s.withoff@umcg.nl

[†]Anna Stachurska, Maria M. Zorro and Marijke R. van der Sijde have contributed equally to this work.

Cellular differentiation is regulated on the level of gene expression, and it is known that dysregulation of gene expression can lead to deficiencies in differentiation that contribute to a variety of diseases, particularly of the immune system. Until recently, it was thought that the dysregulation was governed by changes in the binding or activity of a class of proteins called transcription factors. However, the discovery of micro-RNAs and recent descriptions of long non-coding RNAs (lncRNAs) have given enormous momentum to a whole new field of biology: the regulatory RNAs. In this review, we describe these two classes of regulatory RNAs and summarize what is known about how they regulate aspects of the adaptive and innate immune systems. Finally, we describe what is known about the involvement of micro-RNAs and lncRNAs in three different autoimmune diseases (celiac disease, inflammatory bowel disease, and multiple sclerosis).

Keywords: regulatory RNAs, miRNAs, long non-coding RNAs, immune system, autoimmune diseases

INTRODUCTION

The discovery of the first micro-RNA (miRNA) in 1993 (1, 2) was the start of research that has led to the understanding that gene regulation is not only controlled by proteins (transcription factors) but also RNA molecules. Since then, thousands of novel non-coding RNAs, which can be subdivided into dozens of families (3), have been identified. Two of the most widely studied classes of non-coding RNAs, miRNAs and long non-coding RNAs (lncRNAs), are now recognized as important regulators of gene expression. These molecules are also designated as (small or long) regulatory RNAs. At the time of writing this review, the authorative miRNA database miRBase (release 21) describes 1,881 human miRNA precursors and 2,588 human mature miRNA sequences (4), whereas the GENCODE compendium (V19) mentions 13,870 human lncRNA genes (5). MiRNAs are thought to affect gene expression by inhibiting target mRNA translation (which leads indirectly to degradation of the target) or they can directly induce target mRNA degradation. Many lncRNAs are thought to be involved in chromatin modification processes that, in turn, affect gene expression levels (**Figure 1**). The role of miRNAs in homeostasis and the deregulation of miRNAs in human disease have been well established, but the role of lncRNAs in these processes is not yet fully appreciated. Here, we will review what is known about the role of miRNAs and lncRNAs in the development and activation of the adaptive and innate immune systems in health and disease.

Abbreviations: 3′-UTR, 3′-untranslated region; Aicda, activation-induced cytidine deaminase; BACE1, gene encoding β-secretase-1; AGO, Argonaute; AP-1, activator protein-1; APAF1, apoptotic protease activating factor 1; APC, antigen-presenting cell; Bak1, Bcl-2 homologus antagonist/killer 1; BBB, blood–brain barrier; Bcl-2, B-cell lymphoma-2; BDNF, brain-derived neurothrophic factor; Bim, pro-apoptotic factor; BLIMP-1, B lymphocyte-induced maturation protein-1; BM, bone marrow; CaMKII, calcium/calmodulin-dependent protein kinase II; Cepba, CCAAT/enhancer binding protein-α; CCL1, chemokine (C-C motif) ligand 1; CD, Crohn's disease; CDK, cyclin-dependent kinase; CeD, celiac disease; C-ETS, c-E26 transformation specific transcription factor; CLP, common lymphoid progenitor; CMP, common myeloid progenitor; CRC, colorectal carcinoma; CREB, cyclic AMP-responsive element binding protein; CSF, cerebrospinal fluid; CSF1, colony stimulating factor 1; CXCL10, C-X-C motif chemokine 10; DC, dendritic cell; DGCR8, DiGeorge syndrome critical region gene 8; DN, double negative; DOCK-1, dedicator of cytokinesis-1; DP, double positive (CD4+CD8+); DSS, dextran sulfate sodium; EAE, autoimmune encephalomyelitis; EBV, Epstein–Barr virus; eQTL, expression quantitative trait locus; FADD, Fas-associated death domain; Fo, follicular B-cell; Foxp3, forkhead box P3; GC, germinal center; GWAS, genome-wide association study; hnRNP, heterogeneous nuclear ribonucleoprotein; HOX, homeobox; HSC, hematopoietic stem cell; IBD, inflammatory bowel disease; IFN, interferon; IGF-1, insulin-like growth factor 1; Ikzf4, Ikaros family zinc finger 4; IL, interleukin; IPA, ingenuity pathway analysis; IRAK1, interleukin-1 receptor-associated kinase 1; IRF4, IFN regulatory factor 4; IRS-1, insulin regulatory subunit-1; iTreg, induced regulatory T-cell; JNK, JUN N-terminal kinase; KO, knockout; lincRNA, long intergenic ncRNA; LLRK2, leucine-rich repeat kinase-2; lncRNA, long non-coding RNA; LPS, lipopolysaccharide; Lt-α, lymphotoxin-α; MAPK, mitogen-activated protein kinase; MBP, oligodendrogial myelin basic protein; MEK, MAPK kinase; miRNA, micro-RNA; mirtron, intron-derived splicing-dependent miRNA; MS, multiple sclerosis; mTOR, mammalian target of rapamycin; MZ, marginal zone; MZF-1, myeloid zinc finger-1; NATs, natural antisense transcripts; ncRNA, non-coding RNA; NEAT1, nuclear enriched abundant transcript 1; NF-κB, nuclear factor-κB; NK, natural killer; PBMC, peripheral blood mononuclear cell; Phlpp2, PH domain and leucine-rich repeat protein phosphatase 2; PI3K, phosphoinositide 3-kinase; PP-MS, primary-progressive multiple sclerosis; PMN, polymorphonuclear cells; PRDM1, PR domain zinc finger protein 1; pre-miRNA, precursor-miRNA; pri-miRNA, primary miRNA; PTEN, phosphatase and tensin homolog; RISC, RNA-induced silencing complex; RR-MS, relapsing-remitting multiple sclerosis; RUNX-1, runt-related transcription factor 1; siRNA, small interference RNA; SFPQ, splicing factor proline/glutamine-rich; SOCS1, suppressor of cytokine signaling-1; simtron, intron-derived splicing-independent miRNA; sncRNA715, small non-coding RNA 715; SNP, single nucleotide polymorphism; SOD2, superoxide dismutase 2; SP-MS, secondary progressive multiple sclerosis; STAT, signal transducer and activator of transcription; T-bet, T-box expressed in T-cells; TCR, T-cell receptor; TGFβ, transforming growth factor β; TGFβR, TGFβ-receptor; Th, T helper; THRIL, TNFα- and hnRNPL-related immunoregulatory lincRNA; TLR, Toll-like receptor; TNF, tumor necrosis factor; TRAF, TNF receptor-associated factor; Treg, regulatory T-cell; UC, ulcerative colitis; VE-cadherin, vascular endothelial-cadherin; XPO5, exportin 5.

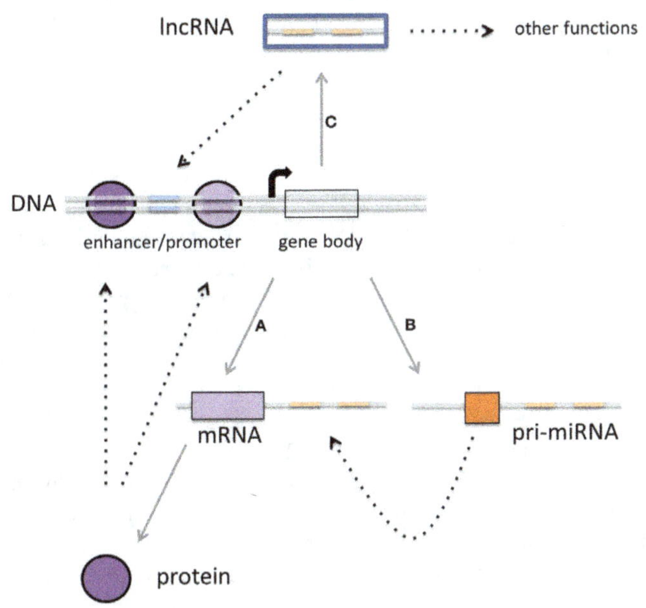

FIGURE 1 | Multiple layers of gene expression controlled by transcription factors, miRNAs, and lncRNAs. **(A)** Protein-coding genes are transcribed into mRNA, which subsequently are translated into proteins. These proteins can function as the classical transcription factors. **(B)** There is a second class of RNAs that is not translated into protein but rather is regulating the expression of other transcripts. The third class of transcripts described in this review **(C)** is the long non-coding RNAs that can regulate gene expression as well, although other functions for these transcripts have been described (see **Figure 3**). It is becoming clear that there is interaction within each class, but also between these three classes, which can converge on transcriptional outcome (see text for details).

MiRNAs

Micro-RNAs are short (19–24 nt), single-stranded, RNAs that are involved in the post-transcriptional regulation of gene expression. Their sequences are evolutionary strongly conserved. miRNA expression profiles and target mRNA sites are also conserved, allowing the translation of findings in mouse models to human physiology.

Micro-RNAs are transcribed by RNA polymerase II into longer (several hundred to several thousand nucleotides) primary miRNAs (pri-miRNAs), containing a cap as well as a poly-A tail. The pri-miRNA is processed in the nucleus by a *microprocessor*, a complex composed of Drosha (a class III RNase) and the DiGeorge syndrome critical region gene 8 (DGCR8), into a ~60 nt precursor-miRNA (pre-miRNA). In this step, the double-stranded stem-loop structures are specifically recognized by the microprocessor, which catalyzes the cleavage of the pri-miRNA near the base of the stem (6, 7). Then, the double-stranded pre-miRNA stem-loop structure is transported into the cytoplasm by a complex containing exportin 5 (XPO5), where it is recognized and further processed by a class III RNase named Dicer into a double-stranded RNA duplex of ~19–24 nt in length. Next, only one of the strands is incorporated into the RNA-induced silencing complex (RISC) composed of Argonaute (AGO) and GW182. The RISC complex is guided to the 3′-untranslated region (3′-UTR) of target mRNA molecules. This leads successively to a decrease in target stability, resulting in accelerated uncapping and deadenylation (8) and/or inhibition of translation (9) (**Figure 2**). It has been suggested that the translational repression of mRNAs takes place in specialized compartments called processing bodies (P-bodies), compartments in the cytoplasm involved in the storage, and degradation of repressed mRNAs (10). To make things more complex, miRNAs were shown to be transported to the nucleus, where they can affect their own expression or the expression of other miRNAs (11). Moreover, lncRNAs can act as sponges for miRNAs. It was demonstrated that the lncRNA phosphatase and tensin homolog *(PTEN)* pseudogene1 (*PTENpg1*) sequesters various *PTEN*-targeting miRNAs, thereby indirectly regulating the PTEN mRNA level (12).

Reports describing that miRNAs can originate from other regulatory RNAs, like tRNAs (13) or pre-ribosomal RNAs (14), complicate the "canonical pathway of miRNA production." MiRNAs can also be derived from introns, which mimic the structural features of pre-miRNAs and these miRNAs can, therefore, enter the miRNA processing pathway independent of Drosha (15). This group of miRNAs can even be subdivided into two groups: (a) splicing-dependent miRNAs (mirtrons, e.g., human *miR-877* and *miR-1226*) or (b) splicing-independent simtrons (human *miR-1225* and *miR-1228*). The processing of mirtrons requires the spliceosome but not Drosha or DGCR8, whereas the generation of simtrons depends on Drosha (but not on DGCR8). Mirtrons are exported from the nucleus by XPO5, cleaved by Dicer, and subsequently enter the RISC complex, similarly to canonical miRNAs. We do not yet know what factors regulate simtron export from the nucleus, but simtrons also enter the RISC complex in the cytoplasm (16).

Interest in miRNAs grew when it was found that miRNAs can be detected in many body fluids such as serum, cerebrospinal fluid (CSF), saliva, and urine (17) and that miRNA profiles are remarkably stable (e.g., resistant to RNases, freeze-thaw cycles). This protection from degradation is probably conferred by one or more mechanisms: (1) miRNAs can be bound to protein components of the RISC complex (AGO2), (2) they can be bound to high density lipoproteins, or (3) they can be packaged in exosomes (18). It was exciting to discover that miRNA profiles in circulation can be disease or even disease stage specific (19). Moreover, they can be useful in predicting treatment response (20). Research into the biological role of circulating miRNAs is still in its infancy, but recent papers describe the intriguing possibility that miRNA can be secreted by one cell type and can then exert its function on or in other cell types (21–23). Exosomes have been shown to participate in various processes that are crucial for immune system function and they can be released by various immune cell types, e.g., T-cells, B-cells, and dendritic cells (DCs). Importantly, these exosomes contain miRNAs, some of which are cell-type specific, while others are present in exosomes of various cell types. Moreover, some miRNAs are more highly expressed in exosomes than in the cells that excrete them, implying that a subset of miRNAs is specifically packaged (24). The selection of miRNA for packaging into exosomes has been described based on two specific motifs in the miRNA sequence; these are recognized by sumoylated heterogeneous nuclear ribonucleoprotein A2/B1 (hnRNPA2B1), a protein controlling miRNA loading into exosomes (25).

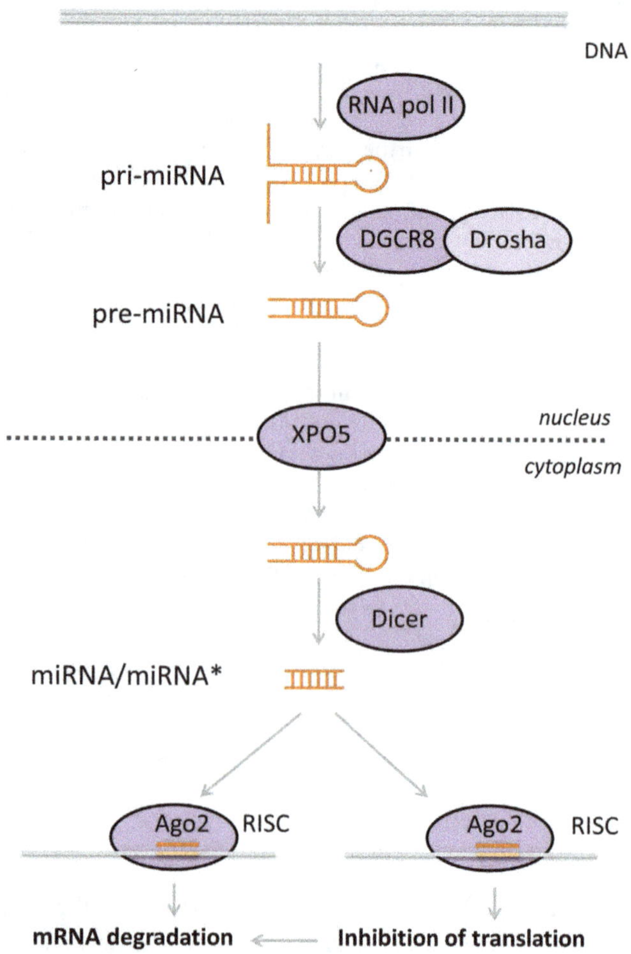

FIGURE 2 | Biogenesis of miRNAs. MiRNAs are transcribed by RNA pol II in the nucleus. Double-stranded miRNA hairpins in the pri-miRNA transcript are recognized and cleaved by the microprocessor complex, composed of Drosha and DGCR8, producing the pre-miRNA. These are subsequently exported into the cytoplasm by XPO5, where they are recognized by Dicer, which cuts off the loop of the hairpin yielding a small double-stranded RNA molecule. One of these strands, the mature miRNA, is loaded into the RISC complex that contains AGO2. This complex is guided to the target mRNA, based on sequence homology between the miRNA and the target. Ultimately, this leads to diminished mRNA translation and/or degradation of the target.

LONG NON-CODING RNAs

Long non-coding RNAs are a heterogeneous group of non-coding transcripts longer than 200 nucleotides (26, 27) and they constitute the major class of regulatory RNA genes (28, 29). Thousands of mammalian lncRNAs have been identified since the first genome-wide discovery studies in the early 2000s and it has become clear that they play important roles in regulating several biological processes, such as gene expression, chromatin remodeling, and protein transport. Although many lncRNAs have been identified, little is known about either their general characteristics or their possible mechanisms of action in health and disease. They can be detected both in the nucleus and in the cytosol, and can be polyadenylated or not. Compared to protein-coding genes, lncRNAs have fewer but longer exons, which are poorly conserved across species (26, 30). In general, the expression of lncRNAs is lower than that of protein-coding genes, although in a cell-type-specific context the expression can be just as high (26). There is growing evidence pointing to changes in lncRNA expression being associated with the etiopathology of diseases, for instance in cancer and autoimmune disease (18, 31). Expression profiling of specific immune cell subsets has revealed an enrichment of long intergenic non-coding RNAs (lincRNAs) that are expressed in immune cells in autoimmune disease-associated loci, thereby implying that these non-coding RNAs play a role in the etiology of autoimmune disease (Barbara Hrdlickova, personal communication). Furthermore, expression quantitative trait locus (eQTL) analysis has demonstrated that disease-associated single nucleotide polymorphisms (SNPs) can affect the expression of lncRNAs, relating lncRNAs to disease susceptibility (32).

Long non-coding RNAs are a structurally and functionally heterogeneous group of transcripts. One approach classifies them into four different subclasses based on their location with respect to the closest protein-coding gene (5, 18). The largest subclass consists of the lincRNAs, which do not overlap with protein-coding genes. Of the remaining "genic" lncRNAs (the second largest subclass), the antisense lncRNA group contains transcripts that overlap with exons of protein-coding genes on the opposite strand (natural antisense transcripts, or NATs) or transcripts that reside in an intron of the protein-coding gene on the opposite strand (antisense intronic transcripts). The antisense and sense transcripts are often co-expressed. The third subclass of lncRNAs encompasses the sense lncRNAs. These transcripts can contain coding genes within an intron on the same strand (sense overlapping transcripts), or they can be located within an intron of a protein-coding gene on the same strand (sense intronic transcripts). The fourth subclass comprises the bi-directional or divergent lncRNA transcripts. These are antisense transcripts that co-transcribe in the opposite direction to the protein-coding gene.

The GENCODE (V7) compendium has annotated over 13,000 human lncRNAs, of which only a fraction, however, has a known function (26). LncRNAs can have diverse molecular functions relayed by the molecules they interact with: mRNA, protein, miRNAs, or DNA (**Figure 3**) (33). These interactions can affect processes like transcription, translation, splicing, translation, or RNA degradation (34, 35). Chang and Rinn classified lncRNAs into four subclasses by their different functions (34). For example, lncRNAs can function as molecular scaffolds to bring proteins together in a complex, but they can also act as a signal for a specific biological condition or state, for instance cellular stress or temperature. The signal can subsequently activate or repress the expression of other genes. Another function lncRNAs can exhibit is that of being a decoy, in which they bind to other RNAs or proteins and interfere with their function. Finally, lncRNAs can guide protein complexes to targets, where they can act as activators or repressors of other genes. In addition to these four main functions, some lncRNAs can inhibit the function of miRNAs, thereby alleviating the downregulating effect of the miRNA on the gene expression (36–38). Note that it is also possible for lncRNAs to exert multiple of these functions.

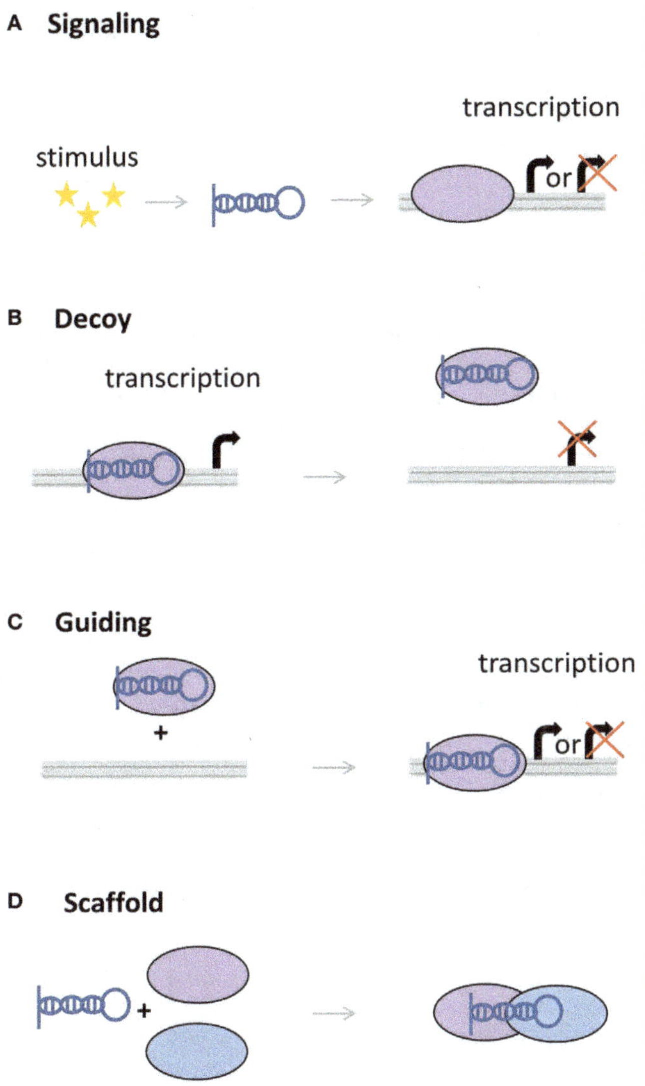

FIGURE 3 | Molecular functions of lncRNAs. (A) LncRNAs can act as signaling molecules, affecting the expression of genes in response to a stimulus. **(B)** LncRNAs can divert transcription factors or other proteins away from the DNA. **(C)** Other lncRNAs can recruit proteins, bringing them closer to target genes. **(D)** As scaffolds, lncRNAs can bring together multiple proteins to form complexes.

THE ROLE OF miRNAs AND lncRNAs IN THE IMMUNE SYSTEM

It has been proposed that miRNA emerged as a primitive immune response against viral infection. The fact that they show remarkable conservation in animals and plants suggests they hold important biological functions. MiRNAs play important roles in cell physiology, as clearly demonstrated by the fact that Dicer knockout in mouse embryos is incompatible with life. Deleting or overexpressing individual miRNAs in mice offers the opportunity to study their roles in the immune response (39). Lineage-specific knockout (KO) of miRNAs in specific immune cell types results in severe perturbation of immune cell numbers, their composition, and function. These all points to miRNAs being essential for immune cell development, differentiation, function, and homeostasis (39–43).

Dicer1 deletion in granulocyte-macrophage progenitors (derived from a myeloid-specific *CCAAT/enhancer binding protein-α (Cebpa)-Cre*-driven *Dicer1*-deleter mouse strain) resulted in changes in gene expression profiles, increased self-renewal ability of precursors in the bone marrow (BM), monocyte depletion, and myeloid dysplasia, underlining the essential contribution of miRNAs to myeloid development (44). The role of Dicer and miRNAs has also been demonstrated in natural killer (NK) cells. By using mice with conditional deletion of *Dicer1* or *Dgcr8* in NK cells, a reduced cellularity in the spleen was observed with a concomitant reduced frequency of splenic NK cells, but without alterations in T- and B-cell frequencies. *Dicer* and *Dgcr8* deficiency was associated with an increase in NK apoptosis and an impairment in NK activation, suggesting that miRNAs are required for NK homeostasis and function (45).

As discussed above, miRNAs can be packaged into exosomes that are subsequently secreted from the cell. It has been suggested that circulating miRNAs could act in intercellular communication, also in the immune system. For example, it was suggested that T-cells communicate with antigen-presenting cells (APCs) by a unidirectional transfer of exosomal miRNA. Another example is the transfer of miR-335 (downregulating SOX4, a progenitor cell transcription factor), which was correlated with the transfer of CD63 upon formation of the immune synapse (24). Furthermore, exosomes released from mature BM-derived DCs contain more *miR-125-5p*, *miR-146a*, and *miR-148*, which are negative regulators of pro-inflammatory factors in myeloid cells and DCs. Exosomes released by both immature and by mature BM-derived DCs contain *miR-34a* and *miR-21* (known to regulate the differentiation of hematopoietic precursors into myeloid DCs), as well as *miR-221* and *miR-222* (that prevent differentiation into plasmacytoid DCs). Such exosomes can be taken up by recipient DCs, and the packaged miRNAs can then be released to target known binding sites, as shown by 3′-UTR-luciferase experiments (46). Exosome-derived miRNAs have also been implicated in the progression of Epstein–Barr virus (EBV) infection. Exosomes containing EBV-derived miRNAs are released from infected B-cells and taken up by DCs, where the miRNAs can then downregulate the expression of genes encoding immune-stimulation factors (47). Together, these limited but suggestive data point to a role for miRNA-based intercellular communication, mediated by exosomes, in the immune system, which has implications for health and disease.

Because lncRNAs are not produced via a lncRNA-specific biochemical pathway, it is not feasible to generate general or lineage-specific lncRNA-knockout mice. The lack of evolutionary conservation of lncRNAs across species further complicates the study of their individual function. Nevertheless, several mouse knockouts have been generated for single lncRNAs. A landmark study described the generation of 18 mouse strains, all with one lncRNA deleted (48). Although the lncRNA candidates were not selected for immune cell specificity, the study revealed key roles for several individual lincRNAs in the viability and developmental processes of the mice and it also highlighted the importance of using *in vivo* models to reveal the biological significance and functional diversity of lncRNAs (48).

In the next section, we give examples of how key miRNAs play regulatory roles in the development and activation of the immune system and we summarize the much smaller body of evidence implicating lncRNAs in these processes.

THE ROLE OF miRNAs IN THE DEVELOPMENT OF INNATE IMMUNE CELLS

The innate immune system includes myeloid cells derived from hematopoietic stem cells (HSCs) and myeloid progenitors. These cells give rise to monocytes, which can develop into macrophages and DCs, and to granulocytes (neutrophils, eosinophils, basophils) through a series of developmental stages (myeloblast, promyelocyte, myelocyte, metamyelocyte, band cell or monoblast, and promonocyte) (**Figure 4**). One of the first studies of miRNA expression in normal human granulocytes reported sets of miRNAs that were subject to upregulation or downregulation at discrete maturation stages in neutrophil development. Although the majority of miRNA family members showed coordinated expression patterns, the expression of some miRNAs in the same cluster is not always synchronized. For example, the *miR-17-92/oncomir-1* cluster encompasses six miRNAs (*miR-17, -18a, -19a, -20a, -19b-1, -92a-1*). Among the cluster's targets are antitumor, pro-apoptotic, and tumor suppressor proteins. HSCs and early progenitors in the BM express high levels of miRNAs from this cluster, whereas their expression is reduced during myeloid and lymphoid differentiation (49, 50). Of this cluster, *miR-20a* and *miR-92* are downregulated in metamyelocytes, *miR-18a, miR-19a* and *miR-19b* are downregulated in neutrophils, while *miR17-5p* gradually decreased from myeloblasts in the subsequent stages of development (51). In *miR-223* KO mice, it was shown that *miR-223* deletion leads to an increase in the number of granulocyte progenitors and neutrophil hyperactivity, suggesting that *miR-223* acts as a crucial regulator of granulocyte production and the inflammatory response (52).

In vitro overexpression or knockdown experiments of *miR-29a* or *miR-142-3p* in human leukemia cell lines showed that the miRNA overexpression promoted monocytic and myelocytic maturation, while blockage with antisense inhibitors promoted not only the expression of early progenitor markers but also reduced cell maturation, indicating these miRNAs play roles as regulators of normal myeloid differentiation. *MiR-29a* and *miR-142-3p* were both shown to target cyclin T2 (*CCNT2*), while they were also specifically targeting the cyclin-dependent kinase 6 (*CDK6*) gene (*miR-29a*) and the transforming growth factor β (*TGF*β) activated kinase 1/MAP3K7 binding protein 2 (*TAB2*) gene (*miR-142-3p*) (41).

An important group of miRNAs in myeloid biology is the *miR-125* family, consisting of *miR-125a, -125b1,* and *-125b2.* The family members target crucial factors involved in HSC survival and apoptosis (42). *MiR-125b* overexpression, instigated by transplanting fetal liver cells ectopically expressing *miR-125b* in mice, caused a lethal myeloproliferative disorder (43). In addition, enforced expression of *miR-125b* in BM chimeric mice promoted myelopoiesis. B-cell lymphoma-2 (Bcl-2) homologous antagonist/killer 1 (*Bak1*) and the signal transducer and activator of transcription 3 (*Stat3*) were proposed as possible target genes (53). Moreover, using a miRNA-sponge approach, it was shown that *miR-125b* can also regulate myelopoiesis in mice by targeting *Lin28A*, an important regulator of hematopoiesis (54).

In PU.1-deficient mice, the development of macrophages, granulocytes, and B-lymphocytes is impaired, revealing that the PU.1 transcription factor is involved in myeloid and lymphoid development (55). Several miRNAs, including the *miR-17-92* cluster, are activated by PU.1 to modulate macrophage development. In PUER cells (murine myeloid progenitors in which macrophage development can be supported on inducing a tamoxifen-inducible PU.1 transgene), it was demonstrated that macrophage differentiation requires downregulation of *miR-17-92* (49). Moreover, PU.1 may also regulate macrophage development by inducing *miR-146a, miR-342, miR-338,* and *miR-155* (56). *miR-142* is another miRNA involved in myeloid development. In *miR-142*-deficient mice, a reduction of $CD4^+$ DCs is accompanied by a severe defect in their ability to prime $CD4^+$ T-cells (57). MiRNA expression profiling during human monocyte differentiation has shown a decrease in levels of miRNAs, the *miR-17-92* cluster (*miR-17-5p* and *miR-20a*), as well as of *miR-106a* (a member of *miR-106a-363*, a paralog of the *miR-17-92* cluster), compared to early progenitors. One of the shared targets of *miR-17-5p, miR-20a,* and *miR-106a* is the runt-related transcription factor 1 (*RUNX-1*) gene, an important regulator of hematopoiesis (58).

Analysis of miRNA profiles in human BM precursors and neutrophils revealed that 135 miRNAs were differentially expressed between the myeloid developmental stages. For instance, high levels of *miR-130a, miR-155,* and *miR-146a* were observed in myeloblasts and promyelocytes, followed by a decrease in expression in more mature cells. Potential targets for these miRNAs include transcripts encoding members of the TGFβ signaling pathway, such as *TGF*β*-receptor 1 (TGF*β*R1)* and *TGF*β*R2, SMAD2, SMAD4,* and *SMAD5 (miR-130)*. Some miRNAs clustered with the intermediate stages of development (*miR-222, miR-200, miR 29a*), while others were associated with mature neutrophils (*miR-132, miR-212*). Among the predicted targets of the miRNAs listed above are transcripts encoding cell cycle regulators, such as *CDK2* (*miR-155*), or proteins associated with apoptosis such as apoptotic protease activating factor 1 (*APAF1*), *CASP8*, and Fas-associated death domain (*FADD*), which are targeted by *miR-132, miR-212* (59).

Another miRNA important in the development of the innate immune system is *miR-21*. It has been identified as one of the most highly upregulated miRNAs in allergic diseases and this is associated with high numbers of eosinophils, the main effector cells in allergic responses. In a report by Lu et al. (60), the role of *miR-21* was evaluated in a murine *ex vivo* culture system. By using RT-PCR, it was shown that during eosinophil differentiation *miR-21* was upregulated threefold from day 4 to day 14 in culture. Cultures derived from $miR\text{-}21^{-/-}$ eosinophil progenitor cells showed higher apoptosis than cultures from $miR\text{-}21^{+/+}$ progenitor cells, suggesting that *miR-21* regulates the development of eosinophils by modulating eosinophil progenitor cell growth. In agreement with these findings, $miR\text{-}21^{-/-}$ mice showed reduced blood eosinophil levels, concomitant with a reduced capacity to produce eosinophils in the BM. Microarray analysis revealed the

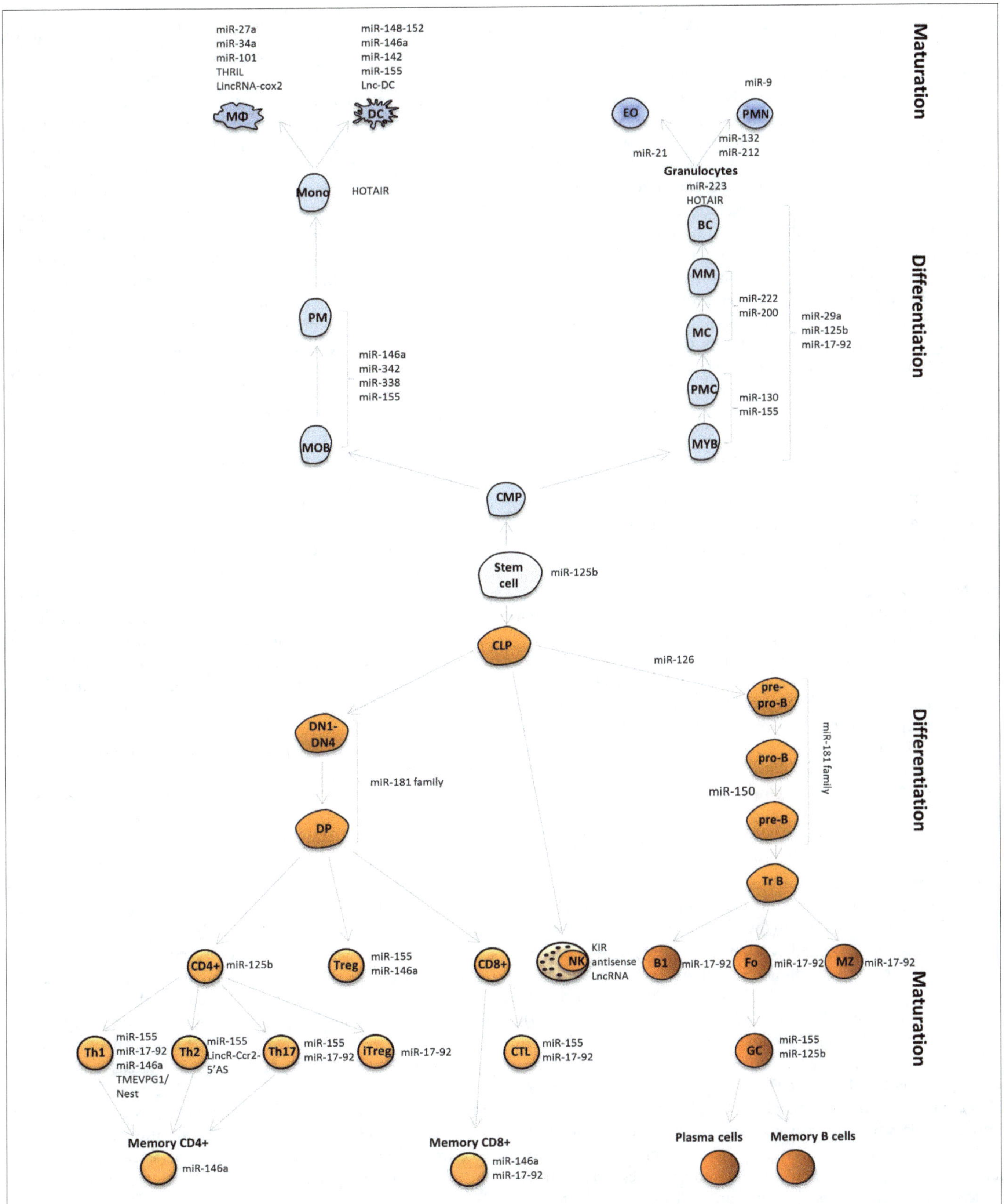

FIGURE 4 | MiRNAs and lncRNAs influence immune cell fate and function. MiRNAs and lncRNAs were shown to modulate development and function the immune system. LncRNAs and selected miRNAs that are discussed in this review are depicted.

differential expression of genes involved in cell proliferation, cell cycle control, and the immune response (60).

MiRNAs INVOLVED IN INNATE IMMUNE CELL ACTIVATION

The best-known example of a miRNA involved in the activation of innate and adaptive immune cells is *miR-155*. It has also been implicated as a general and conserved feature of mouse and human DC activation by various Toll-like receptor (TLR) ligands (61, 62). Analyses of *miR-155*-deficient mice demonstrated that although the development of DCs was unaffected, *miR-155* is required for DC maturation and the ability to promote antigen-specific T-cell activation (61). DC maturation is also affected by *miR-150*, *miR-34a*, and *let-7i* by mechanisms that involve silencing c-Fos (*miR-155*), *Csf1r* (which controls M-CSF receptor expression; *miR-34a*), and suppressor of cytokine signaling-1 (SOCS1) (*let-7i*) expression (61–64). Another group of miRNAs, including *miR-146a*, *miR-148*, and *miR-142*, have been associated with downregulation of inflammatory pathways and modulation of DC maturation (65–67). *MiR-146a* controls DC cross-priming (by suppressing Notch1 expression and IL-12p70 production) and DC activation (by targeting TLR9, TLR2, interleukin-1 receptor-associated kinase 1 (IRAK1), and tumor necrosis factor (TNF) receptor-associated factor 6 (TRAF6) signaling) (65–68). Another important regulator of DC maturation is calcium/calmodulin-dependent protein kinase II (CaMKII), which is a target of three members of the *miR-148/152* family (*miR-148a*, *miR-148b*, and *miR-152*). These miRNAs downregulate CaMKII leading to reduced expression of MHCII, reduced cytokine production (IL-12, IL-6, TNF-α), and a reduced antigen-presenting capacity of DCs (66).

Micro-RNA profiling of macrophages stimulated with TLR ligands and cytokines has shown the involvement of several miRNAs in inflammation. After incubation of murine macrophages with lipopolysaccharide (LPS), poly I:C, or interferon β (IFN-β), the expression of *miR-9*, *miR-101*, *miR-155* was upregulated, while *miR-34* and *miR-27a* were downregulated to modulate the levels of important regulators of inflammation. The upregulated miRNAs target nuclear factor-κB1 (NFκB1, *miR-9*), mitogen-activated protein kinase 1 (MAPK1, *miR-101*), and JUN N-terminal kinase (JNK, *miR-155*), while the downregulated miRNAs target NOTCH1 (*miR-34a*) and STAT3 (*miR-27a*), and the production of pro-inflammatory cytokines such as TNF-α, interleukin-6 (IL-6), and IL-10 (69–73).

MiR-9 was also associated with the response of polymorphonuclear cells (PMN) to TLR stimulation. It was interesting that out of the 365 miRNAs tested, *miR-9* was the only one upregulated in both human macrophages and PMN after LPS activation (69). In contrast, *miR-155*, *miR-146a*, *miR-146b*, *miR-187*, *miR-125a*, *miR-99b*, and *let-7e* appeared to be macrophage-specific, while *miR-196a* was PMN-specific. This underscores how some miRNAs are involved in the activation of multiple lineages of innate immune cells, while others play a more lineage-specific role (69).

Recent studies have shown that microorganisms can modulate miRNA expression and thus the immune response during infection, as a mechanism of immune evasion. *Mycobacterium tuberculosis* induces *miR-21* expression in macrophages and DCs. It was suggested that by targeting IL-12, *miR-21* modulates the Th1 immune response (74). *Leishmania* has also developed strategies to subvert the host macrophage response. On *Leishmania* infection of human macrophages *in vitro*, approximately 64 out of 365 analyzed miRNAs were found to be modulated. Enrichment analyses have revealed that several of these differentially expressed miRNAs are involved in the regulation of TLR and pro-apoptotic pathways (75). By using the murine model of *Toxoplasma* infection, an increase in the levels of the immune-miRNAs *miR-146a* and *miR-155* was observed in the brain of chronically infected mice compared with non-infected controls. Further assays in *miR-146* KO mice demonstrated that *miR-146* ablation promotes parasite control, resulting in long-term survival (76). MiRNA profile expression analyses of human macrophages infected with *Toxoplasma* showed that the *miR-17-92* cluster expression was significantly upregulated and that the levels of *miR-17-92* were closely related with a decrease in expression of the pro-apoptotic regulator Bim. Interestingly, the Bim 3'-UTR contains predicted binding sites for multiple miRNAs derived from the *miR-17-92* family. All the above evidence suggests miRNAs are involved in parasite persistence and modulation of apoptosis (77).

LONG NON-CODING RNAs IN INNATE IMMUNITY

So far, most lncRNA studies have been performed in normal cellular development or in cancer (78–82), although the role of lncRNAs in hematopoiesis and the immune system is slowly starting to emerge. The lncRNA *HOTAIRM1*, located antisense to homeobox A1 (HOXA1) and HOXA2 of the HOXA gene cluster, is expressed specifically in the myeloid lineage (83). *HOTAIRM1* is upregulated during retinoic acid-driven granulocytic differentiation in NB4 promyelocytic leukemia cells, which are a model for granulocytic differentiation. Knockdown of *HOTAIRM1* prevents the expression of HOXA1, HOXA4, CD11b, and CD18, but not of the more distal HOXA genes and decreased myeloid differentiation.

The *KIR antisense lncRNA* was found to be expressed only in human embryonic stem cells and other cell types with stem cell properties (84). KIR genes encode class-I MHC receptors expressed on human NK cells. *KIR antisense lncRNA* overlaps with exons 1 and 2 of the protein-coding KIR gene, as well as with an upstream proximal promoter region of the KIR genes. Overexpression of the lncRNA in NK cells was found to decrease the expression of the KIR protein-coding gene. Wright et al. speculated that the KIR genes are silenced in NK progenitors so that they are not able to influence the process of NK cell differentiation (84). As the KIR distal antisense promoter contains myeloid zinc finger-1 (MZF-1)-binding sites, it is assumed that this transcription factor regulates the expression of the *KIR antisense lncRNA*. MZF-1 is a transcriptional regulator that is able to activate transcription in cells of hematopoietic origins, whereas it can repress transcription in other cell types. However, the precise mechanism of the regulation of *KIR antisense lncRNA* expression is unknown.

Lnc-DC, exclusively expressed in conventional human DCs (85), was found to induce the nuclear translocation of STAT3. The proposed mechanism of action for this lncRNA is to prevent SHP1 from binding to phosphorylated STAT3 and dephosphorylating it, thereby preventing its dimerization and translocation to the nucleus. This is an example of a lncRNA affecting cellular differentiation by a mechanism that takes place in the cytoplasm.

In another study, 54 mouse pseudogene lncRNAs were found to be induced by TNF-α (86). One of these, *Lethe*, functions as a negative feedback signal that inhibits NF-κB. Its expression is increased when TNF-α activates NF-κB, after which *Lethe* binds to NF-κB and prevents it from binding to DNA, thereby inhibiting the expression of inflammatory proteins, such as IL-6, IL-8, and superoxide dismutase 2 (SOD2).

A whole-transcriptome profiling of mouse macrophages stimulated with different TLR ligands uncovered dozens of expressed lncRNAs (87). Activation by the synthetic bacterial lipopeptide Pam3CSK4, a TLR2 ligand, resulted in the expression of 62 lncRNAs. One of them, *lincRNA-Cox2,* acts as a key regulator of the inflammatory response by mediating both activation and repression of several immune genes. In response to TLR2-stimulation, *lincRNA-Cox2* induces the expression of hundreds of genes, including Tlr1, Il-6, and Il-23a. *LincRNA-Cox2*-mediated repression of target gene expression was found to require the interaction of *lincRNA-Cox2* with hnRNPA/B and hnRNPA2/B1, repressing the transcription of immune cells.

Stimulation of human THP1 macrophage cells by a synthetic lipopeptide ligand of TLR2 induced 159 lincRNAs (88). One of these, TNFα and hnRNPL-related immunoregulatory lincRNA (*THRIL*), form a complex with hnRNPL. This complex can bind the promoter of TNFα and regulate its transcription. Microarray analysis showed that *THRIL* is required for the expression of various immune genes, including cytokines and other regulators of TNFα expression, including IL-8, C-X-C motif chemokine 10 (CXCL10), chemokine (C-C motif) ligand 1 (CCL1), and the colony stimulating factor 1 (CSF1). *THRIL* expression was also reported to be correlated with the severity of symptoms in patients with Kawasaki disease, an autoimmune disease mostly seen in children.

NEAT1 (nuclear enriched abundant transcript 1) is a lncRNA that was shown to be essential for the formation of paraspeckles. Paraspeckles are nuclear bodies found in mammalian cell nuclei and it has been proposed that they play a role in several biological processes, including cellular differentiation and the stress response (89). It has been shown that *NEAT1* is induced by viral infection as well as by poly I:C stimulation and that, in response to such a stimulus, *NEAT1* binds to paraspeckle protein splicing factor proline/glutamine-rich (SFPQ). This complex binds to and regulates the expression of several antiviral genes, including *IL-8,* which induces the formation of paraspeckles (90).

THE ROLE OF miRNA IN THE DEVELOPMENT OF CELLS OF THE ADAPTIVE IMMUNE SYSTEM

miRNAs IN T-CELL DEVELOPMENT AND ACTIVATION

Micro-RNAs have been shown to be crucial for both immune system development and its functioning. MiRNAs that are characteristically enriched in HSCs and progenitor cells are *miR-125a-5p, miR-125b-5p, miR-155, miR-130a, miR-196b, miR-99a, miR-126-3p, miR-181c, miR-193b, miR-542-5p,* and *let-7e* (91). Their expression changes during immune cell development.

Some miRNAs are selectively expressed in specific stages of immune cell development, whereas others are more broadly expressed. Profiling studies showed that there are miRNAs, which are preferentially upregulated in lymphocytes. The *miR-181* family is abundant expressed in developing BM B-cells and thymocytes.

The importance of miRNAs in T-cell biology has been extensively studied in mice with conditional *Dicer1* deletion. Conditional deletion of *Dicer1* in T-cell precursors using *Lck-Cre* demonstrated that Dicer is necessary for the generation and survival of normal numbers of αβ T-cells (92). *Cd4-Cre*-mediated deletion did not affect the viability of Cd4+ T-cells, but the numbers of Th1 and Th2 cells were significantly reduced, resulting from both decreased proliferation as well as from increased apoptosis. Dicer-deficient Cd4+ cells have been described as more prone to differentiate into Th1 cells and Dicer-deficient cells cannot repress Inf-γ upon Th2 stimulation (93).

Profiling of different stages of T-cell development, starting from the double negative 1 (DN1) thymocyte stage, reveals that miRNA profiles are similar for cells with similar developmental status (94). DN3 and DN4 populations cluster together based on their miRNA expression profiles, as do mature single positive Cd4+ and Cd8+ cells. DN1 cells are more similar to DN3 and DN4 cells. Nevertheless, expression of individual miRNAs changes depending on their developmental stage. Each of the stages is characterized by elevated expression of at least one miRNA or miRNA family. In DN1 cells, *miR-21, miR-29b, miR-342, miR-221,* and *miR-223* are elevated and *miR-16, miR-181a,* and *miR-15b* are decreased. *MiR-191* is upregulated and *miR-142-3p* is downregulated in DN3 cells. *MiR-142-5p, miR-20a, miR-16,* and *miR-128b* are increased, whereas *miR-150* is decreased in DN4 cells. In double positive (DP) cells, expression of *miR-92, miR-181a, miR-181b,* and *miR-350* are enhanced, while in Cd4+ cells, *miR-669c* and *miR-297* are elevated. In Cd4+ and Cd8+ cells, *miR-128* is abundant.

It is interesting that, on activation of Cd4+ T-cells, Ago2 ubiquitination and consequentially its proteosomal degradation is induced, leading to global miRNA downregulation. Moreover, naive T-cells display reduced levels of Ago2 and differentiate more rapidly. These findings led to the hypothesis that the decrease in the miRNA pool on T-cell activation allows the expression of genes regulating CD4+ T-cell differentiation and facilitates the gain of T-cell effector functions (95). Although these are global effects on the miRNA pool, some miRNAs can be picked out that play key roles in T-cell biology. For example, the *miR-181* family is upregulated in DP cells and its family member *miR-181a* decreases the expression of Cd69, T-cell receptor α (Tcrα), and Bcl-2 (94).

Another key player is *miR-125b*. This miRNA is part of the *miR-99a/100~125b* tricistrons, located on human chromosomes 11, 19, and 21. The tricistron on chromosome 21, encompassing *miR-99a/let-7c/miR-125b-2,* is highly expressed in HSCs and is responsible for maintaining stem cell properties (96). In human naive CD4+ T-cells, *miR-125b* downregulates proteins that are critically involved in T-cell differentiation: *IFN-γ, IL-2RB, IL-10RA,* and *PR domain zinc finger protein 1* (*PRDM1,* encoding B lymphocyte-induced maturation protein-1, BLIMP-1). Overexpression of *miR-125b* inhibits the differentiation of naive T-cells into effector cells (97). This miRNA is an example of one that affects various stages of immune cell differentiation in different immune cell lineages.

T-cell activation leads to highly elevated expression of *miR-155* (98). Experiments conducted on Cd4+ T-cells isolated from mice deficient for *Bic*, the primary transcript encoding *miR-155*, uncovered elevated Th2 polarization, and Th2 cytokine production (Il-4, Il-5, and Il-10) in these cells. This effect is mediated by upregulation of c-Maf, a Th2-specific transcription factor known to induce the expression of Il-4/5/10 (99). Th1 and Th17 responses are also regulated by *miR-155*. Transfection with *miR-155* promotes, whereas *miR-155* inhibition decreases, the number of Th1 and Th17 cells in mice with experimental autoimmune encephalomyelitis (EAE) (100). Mice lacking *Bic* also display decreased levels of regulatory T-cells (Tregs) in the thymus and in the periphery while the function of these cells *in vitro* is not affected. This indicates that *miR-155* is required for Treg development (101). Characteristically, *miR-155* expression is induced in Tregs by forkhead box P3 (Foxp3), while one of the main targets of *miR-155* in Tregs is Socs1. When *miR-155* is high, Socs1 is low, which contributes to maintaining the competitive fitness and proliferative potential of Tregs (102).

The *miR-17-92* cluster is a master switch involved in the differentiation into Th1 and Th17 cells. Experiments conducted in *cd4-cre*-driven *miR-17-92* conditional KO mice demonstrated that Th1 development is critically controlled by *miR-17* and *miR-19b*, which target *TgfβrII* and *cyclic AMP-responsive element binding protein 1 (Creb1, miR-17)*, and *Pten* (*miR-19b*). Together, these two miRNAs enhance T-cell proliferation and Inf-γ production, protect from activation-induced cell death, and repress induced Treg (iTreg) differentiation. Interestingly, *miR-18a* of the same cluster antagonizes the pro-Th1 effect of *miR-17* and *miR-19b* through elevation of activation-induced cell death and inhibition of proliferation (103). Subsequent experiments conducted on T-cells isolated from conditional *miR-17-92*-depleted mice (that had been retrovirally transduced with selected miRNAs from the *miR-17-92* cluster), showed that *miR-17* and *miR-19b* were also the miRNAs promoting Th17 differentiation. This is mediated by *miR-17*-induced downregulation of Ikaros family zinc finger 4 (Ikzf4) and the downregulation of Pten by *miR-19b* (104).

Another miRNA regulating the adaptive response is *miR-146a*. Profiling studies in mice showed that *miR-146a* expression is high in Th1 cells and low in naive T-cells and Th2 cells (105), but very high in Tregs (106). Level of *miR-146a* is also elevated in human memory cells (both in CD4 and CD8 memory cells). *MiR-146* expression is induced on TCR stimulation and is regulated by NF-κB and the c-E26 transformation specific (c-ETS) transcription factor. It was suggested that *miR-146a* exerts its regulatory function by targeting FADD, leading to a decrease in apoptosis. On TCR stimulation, activator protein-1 (AP-1) activity and IL-2 production are induced, but *miR-146* targets both of them, thereby enabling *miR-146a* to affect the duration of T-cell activation phases (107).

As can be expected, the importance of miRNAs in CD8+ biology has been well studied. *Cd4-Cre*-induced Dicer deletion in mice leads to reduced development of peripheral Cd8+ cells due to decreased cell survival and defective migration out of the primary lymphoid compartment (93). As was also the case for CD4+ cells, a decrease in Dicer (and therefore in the miRNA pool) leads to differentiation, characterized by increased levels of perforin, granzymes, and effector cytokines that are usually targeted by *miR-139* (targets Eomes and perforin) and *miR-150* (targets Cd25) (108). Another study reported that *miR-15b*, *miR-150*, *miR-24*, and *miR-27a* were increased in Cd8+ cells (94).

MiR-155 expression also plays an important regulatory role in CD8+ cells. It is most highly expressed in primary effector Cd8+, shows intermediate expression in effector memory Cd8+ T-cells, and low expression in naive Cd8+ and central memory Cd8+ cells. Its role in the antiviral response of Cd8+ cells was demonstrated in *miR-155*-deficient mice, which are characterized by an attenuated antiviral response due to a diminished response of Cd8+ cells. On the contrary, overexpression of *miR-155* in mice enhanced the antiviral Cd8+ response (109).

In short-lived effector CD8+ cells, *miR-17-92* is upregulated in contrast to memory cells. Experiments on mice with a conditional gain or loss of *miR-17-92* expression in mature Cd8+ cells after activation (controlled by the human Granzyme B promoter) revealed that *miR-17-92* regulates Cd8+ expansion and the balance between effector and memory differentiation. *MiR-17-92* overexpression elevates the differentiation into terminal effector cells and concomitantly decreases the formation of polyfunctional lymphoid memory cells. As *miR-17-92* overexpression correlates with downregulation of Pten, and in consequence induces the PI3K (phosphoinositide 3-kinase)-Akt-mTor (mammalian target of rapamycin) pathway, here too it was suggested that this could be the main pathway involved in regulating cellular proliferation. In contrast, conditional deletion of *miR-17-92* leads to attenuated proliferation of antigen-specific cells, increased Il-7Rα and Bck-2 expression, and faster acquisition of memory cell properties (110).

miRNAs IN B-CELL BIOLOGY

Experiments with conditional Dicer-KO mice in early B-cell progenitors (*Mb1-Cre* drives deletion starting from the pro-B-cell stage) resulted in a block in B-cell development at the transition from pro- to pre-B-cell stage (111). Conditional deletion of *Dicer-1* in later stages of B-cell development showed that miRNAs are also critically important for the transition from transitional B-cells to germinal center (GC) or follicular (Fo) B-cells (112). Conditional deletion of Dicer in activated B-cells [*activation-induced cytidine deaminase (Aicda-cre)*] confirmed that Dicer is essential for GC B-cell generation. The ablation of Bim partially rescued this effect (113).

The analysis of different cell subtypes during B-cell development in mice underscored the highly regulated, developmental stage specific, expression of miRNAs. Hierarchical clustering of BM and spleen B populations leads to a perfect recapitulation of the B-cell developmental pathway. This study found the population with the most distinct miRNA profile was that of fraction A (FrA) B-cells, characterized by expression of *miR-2138*, *-542-3p*, *-500*, *-1959*, *-221*, *-1965*, *-1900*, *-1893*, *-501-5p*, and *let-7f**. FrA cells have been reported to still retain the capacity to differentiate into T-cells, while Pax5 and Cd19 expression is induced in the next developmental stage leading to FrB/C B-cells. Among the miRNAs not expressed in the BM are *miR-150* and *miR-155*. These miRNAs start to be expressed in transitional B-cells and are most highly expressed in mature B-cells in the spleen (50).

In this B-cell lineage, specific or more broadly expressed miRNAs also control the differentiation and activation. *MiR-126* expression decreases during B-cell maturation. Injecting *miR-126*-overexpressing HSC/progenitors cells into lethally irradiated mice showed that *miR-126* induces the differentiation of B-cell myeloid progenitors. One of the genes regulated by *miR-126* in this process is insulin regulatory subunit-1 (Irs-1) (114).

MiR-181 is preferentially expressed in the B-cells in the BM. Its overexpression in HSCs and progenitor cells leads to increased levels of B-cells. Moreover, ectopic expression of *miR-181* in Lin^- BM cells transplanted into sublethally irradiated mice leads to an increase in B-cells, with a concomitant decrease of T-lymphoid cells (115).

Mice without *miR-17-92* (a *Cre-deletor* mouse strain with *Cre* controlled by the human β-*actin* promoter) die shortly after birth. Analysis of fetal liver cells from these mice showed that the frequency of HSCs and the number of early progenitors was not affected, but that the number of pre-B-cells was significantly reduced. In *miR-17-92*-deficient adult mice, marginal zone (MZ), Fo, and newly formed B-cells in spleen (as well as peritoneal B1a and B1b cells) are reduced, whereas the relative number of transitional B-cells was not altered. Moreover, in these mice, the frequency of red blood cells, granulocytes, and monocytes was also not altered (116). In contrast, another study showed that B-cell-specific *miR-17-92* overexpressing mice develop B-cell lymphomas due to the downregulation of negative regulators of the PI3K pathway [Pten and PH domain and leucine-rich repeat protein phosphatase 2 (*Phlpp2*)] and the NF-κB pathway (*Cyld, A20, Itch, Rnfl1, and Tax1bp1*), as well as due to the downregulation proapoptotic protein Bim and cell cycle regulator E2F3. Together, this results in constitutive activation of pro-survival pathways (117).

MiR-150 is expressed in mature B-cells but not in BM B-cells. Premature overexpression of *miR-150* in HSCs showed that *miR-150* blocks the generation of mature B-cells by preventing the transition of pro-B-cells to pre-B-cells, but not the development of T-cells, granulocytes, or macrophages. The main target involved in this mechanism is c-Myb (118, 119).

MiR-155 controls the GC response at least partially via regulation of cytokine production. Mature *miR-155*$^{-/-}$ cells isolated from spleens are deficient in Tnf and lymphotoxin-α (Lt-α) production (120). *MiR-155* was also shown to be critically involved in isotype switching, as reduced extrafollicular and GC responses, and a concomitant lack of high-affinity IgG1, were observed in the absence of *miR-155* (121). *MiR-155* is often overexpressed in B-cell lymphomas including DLBCL (122), and *Eμ-enhancer* driven *miR-155* overexpression leads to lympho-proliferative disease followed by B-cell malignancy (123).

Finally, *miR-125b* appears to inhibit GC B-cell differentiation by targeting BLIMP-1 and IFN regulatory factor 4 (IRF4); it is essential for the post-GC plasma B-cell differentiation (124).

THE ROLE OF LONG NON-CODING RNA IN THE ADAPTIVE IMMUNE SYSTEM

Mouse CD8 + T-cells were found to specifically express hundreds of lncRNA genes. Many of these are specific for lymphoid cells and their expression was dynamically changed during lymphocyte differentiation or activation (125). A subset of 39 lncRNAs appear to be precursor transcripts to small regulatory RNAs (miRNAs and small interference RNAs, siRNAs), suggesting that some lncRNAs function via smaller RNA species.

The dynamic nature and cell-specific lncRNA expression during mouse T-cell differentiation was demonstrated by RNA-seq analysis of 42 T-cell subsets (from early T-cell progenitors to terminally differentiated T helper subsets, at multiple time points during differentiation) (126). This led to the identification of 1,524 lincRNAs, most of which are located adjacent to key proteins that regulate the immune system. Knockdown of one of these lncRNAs, *LincR-Ccr2-5'AS*, led to deregulation of its neighboring chemokine receptor genes and prevented Th2 migration into the lung tissue (126).

In 2003, the *Tmevpg1* gene was shown to control the persistence of Theiler's virus in the mouse central nervous system (127). Both the mouse gene and its human ortholog, *TMEVPG1/NeST*, encode a non-coding RNA located in a cluster of cytokine genes, including the IFN-γ gene, and it was suggested to be involved in controlling IFN-γ expression (128). Both the mouse and human lncRNAs are expressed in Th1 cells and depend on Stat4 and T-box expressed in T-cells (T-bet), two transcription factors regulating Th1 differentiation (128). Comparison of mouse strains with and without the capacity to clear Theiler's virus revealed that mice that cannot clear the infection express *Tmevpg1* to a higher level, concomitantly with increased IFN-γ synthesis and enhanced resistance to *Salmonella enterica* infection (129). These results indicate that lncRNA *TMEVPG1/NeST* regulates IFN-γ expression and plays an important role in the susceptibility to viral and bacterial infections.

THE ROLE OF miRNAs AND lncRNAs IN AUTOIMMUNE DISEASES

CELIAC DISEASE

Celiac disease (CeD) is characterized by a severe inflammatory reaction to gluten peptides derived from grain storage proteins; it occurs in patients with a susceptibility genotype. Besides sharing a number of phenotypic characteristics with inflammatory bowel disease (IBD), CeD also shares multiple genetic susceptibility loci with IBD (130). So far, there are limited data on the involvement of miRNAs in CeD and there are no publications on the role of lncRNAs in this autoimmune disease. The lack of a suitable animal model for CeD makes it impossible to study the role of specific miRNAs *in vivo*. However, profiling of miRNA expression in small intestinal biopsies from patients with active CeD versus controls showed that *miR-449, -492, -644, -503, -196a, -504, -500*, and *-330* were differentially expressed in CeD patients, with *miR-449* as the most upregulated miRNA. Putative targets of *miR-449* include mRNAs encoding proteins involved in the NOTCH signaling pathway. In agreement with this, the expression of the inflammation regulator, NOTCH1, was found to be decreased in the small intestine of CeD patients, suggesting that miRNAs can also control inflammation in CeD (131). Indirect evidence for the involvement of particular miRNAs in CeD was found by analyzing genome-wide association study (GWAS) data. Kumar et al. have described how CeD-associated SNPs may actually affect the 3'-UTR of *IRF4, PTPRK*, and *ICOSLG* and suggested that these might change miRNA-binding sites (132).

INFLAMMATORY BOWEL DISEASE

Inflammatory bowel disease includes Crohn's disease (CD) and ulcerative colitis (UC) (133). Recent GWAS and meta-analyses have identified 163 common risk loci for IBD and 47 unique risk loci associated with UC (134). Although the cause of IBD is unknown, there is evidence to suggest that an abnormal immune response to intestinal flora leads to this disease in genetically susceptible individuals. There have been various miRNA profiling studies published on IBD and the miRNA profiles in tissues or serum of UC and CD patients at different stages underscore the importance of miRNA as key regulators of the immune response in this disease (130, 131). Circulating miRNAs in serum were suggested as useful biomarkers for CD diagnosis. MiRNA RT-PCR revealed a set of 11 miRNAs that were significantly elevated in CD patients, but not in the serum of controls or in the serum of patients with active CeD (135).

The first report of miRNA expression in colonic mucosa samples from IBD patients identified 11 miRNA differentially expressed in active UC patients versus controls (136). Since then, the number of miRNAs linked with IBD has increased gradually (137). Several reports have demonstrated the alterations in expression of miRNAs involved in modulating different aspects of the innate and adaptive immunity, such as *miR-21*, *miR-29a*, *miR-150*, and *miR-155* (136, 138, 139). Recently, by using microarray-based miRNA profiling of colonic mucosal biopsies, five miRNAs were shown to be upregulated in patients with active UC compared to quiescent UC, CD patients, and controls. In addition, expression of two miRNAs, *miR-125b-1* and *let-7e**, was enhanced in patients with quiescent UC compared with active UC, CD patients, and controls, supporting the utility of miRNAs as biomarkers to distinguish the different IBD stages (140). An interesting point is that SNP rs2910164, which has been associated with susceptibility to CD, has also been linked to *miR-146a* (141). Subsequent reports have identified other miRNAs that may affect the control of inflammation during IBD. *MiRNA-155*, which has been associated with T-cell, B-cell, and innate cell function, was detected in the blood of CD and UC patients, but not in that of healthy controls (142). RT-PCR has revealed an upregulation in *miR-21* levels in mucosal tissue and serum and UC patients (143). Further, *in vitro* analyses demonstrated that overexpression of *miR-21* in mucosa from UC patients and in the Caco-2 cell model resulted in impaired tight junction formation and decreased barrier function, suggesting a pathogenic role for *miR-21* in UC (143). Using the murine model of dextran sulfate sodium (DSS)-induced colitis, it was found that overexpression of *miR-146b* (by expression vector) or ablation of *miR-21* (*miR-21* KO mice) reduces intestinal inflammation and restores epithelial barrier function by activating NF-κB (*miR-146b*) or by negatively regulating RhoB (*miR- 21*) (144, 145).

The involvement of other inflammatory pathways and processes regulated by miRNAs was also proven to be important in IBD pathogenesis. Several studies have shown that the pattern recognition receptor NOD 2 is upregulated by *miR-146* or downregulated by *miR-122*, while the colonic leukocytic trafficking is regulated by *miR-141* (146–148).

More studies have led to an understanding of the role of miRNAs on carcinogenesis, since IBD has been well established to be a predisposing condition for colorectal carcinoma (CRC). For instance, the levels of *miR-143* and *miR-145* were downregulated in UC patients compared with normal controls. Among the putative targets of these miRNAs are proteins associated with cell cycle regulation, such as K-RAS, API5, MAPK kinase-2 (MEK-2), and IRS-1 (149). A recent study identified *miR-224* as one of the most upregulated miRNAs during the transition from IBD to IBD-associated CRC. *In silico* analysis and functional assays confirmed that *miR-224* targets the cell cycle regulator p21, which could suggest the involvement of *miR-224* in IBD-associated carcinogenesis (150). Other studies have demonstrated a dysregulation of *miR-21* and *miR-155* during active IBD in IBD-dysplastic lesions (151, 152).

In conclusion, these inflammation-related miRNAs target important regulators of carcinogenesis, such as programed cell death 4 and mismatch repair elements, which could provide a biochemical link from IBD to cancer development (151, 152).

Because of their specific expression profiles, miRNAs are considered useful biomarkers for IBD diagnosis and as predictors of disease progression (153). *MiR-122*, *miR-17*, and *let-7e* were found to be altered during the progression of IBD (147), while a set of studies on immune-mediated diseases (including IBD) highlighted miRNAs as promising indicators of response to immunosuppressor treatment (20).

However, the role of lncRNA in the pathogenesis of CD remains elusive. A GWAS study identified *leucine-rich repeat kinase-2 (LLRK2)*, which is part of a complex including the large noncoding RNA repressor of NFAT, as associated with CD. In line with this, when wild-type mice were sublethally irradiated and reconstituted with *Lrrk2*-deficient hematopoietic cells, they were more susceptible to DSS-induced colitis. This suggests that *LLRK2* deficiency increases UC severity (154). In addition, high levels of lncRNA *DQ786243* were found in the blood of patients with CD. Subsequent overexpression of *DQ786243* in Jurkat cells showed a correlation between the lncRNA and the expression of the Foxp3 regulator, CREB, suggesting that *DQ786243* is involved in inflammation control and CD pathogenesis (155).

MULTIPLE SCLEROSIS

Multiple sclerosis (MS) is an autoimmune, demyelinating neurodegenerative disorder, mostly affecting adults. Most often, the disease first manifests itself as relapsing-remitting MS (RR-MS), which typically progresses into secondary progressive MS (SP-MS) after 10–25 years. It is thought that RR-MS is more pro-inflammatory in nature, while SP-MS is mostly associated with neurodegeneration, although there is a small percentage of patients who present with neurodegenerative symptoms, without any evidence for former pro-inflammatory episodes. They have an aggressive form of MS called primary-progressive MS (PP-MS) (156). Multiple studies suggest the involvement of miRNAs in MS and changes in miRNAs have been detected in circulation, in brain tissue, in immune cells, and in CSF. Several miRNAs associated with the immune response have also been linked with MS, including miRNAs regulating the Th1 response, such as *miR-155* (100) and *miR-29* (157), but also Th17-associated miRNAs [*miR-155* (100), *miR-17-92* (104), *miR-132* (158), and *miR-326* (159)]. Of interest is that the level of *miR-326* in peripheral blood lymphocytes was suggested to distinguish between the relapsing and remitting phases of MS (160).

One of the miRNAs important in MS pathology is *miR-155*, the expression of which is elevated in RR-MS patients during relapse, as well as in the murine EAE model. In EAE mice, delivery of *miR-155* stimulates the development of inflammatory Th17 and Th1 cells, whereas applying miR-155 inhibitors reduces these processes (100).

The immune response in MS in the brain may be also regulated indirectly by changes in the blood–brain barrier (BBB) permeability. Elevated levels of *miR-155* in the neurovascular part of the brain of MS patients as well as in EAE mice are linked with a decreased function of the BBB. The potential targets of *miR-155* suggested to be involved in BBB function are focal adhesion proteins (DOCK-1, dedicator of cytokinesis-1, and Syntenin-1) and proteins involved in cell–cell interaction (Annexin-2 and Claudin-1) (161).

Another miRNA that plays a crucial role in regulating the function of the BBB, and consequently in regulating the immune cell influx in the brain, is *miR-125a-5p*. Overexpression of this miRNA elevates barrier tightness, with thicker and more continuous tight junctions formed by vascular endothelial-cadherin (VE-cadherin) and zona-occludens-1 (162).

*MiR-92a-1** is reported to be increased specifically in the plasma of RR-MS patients compared to healthy controls or SP-MS patients. Furthermore, its level correlates negatively with disease duration and disability score. Elevated levels of *miR-92* can also distinguish RR-MS from another neuronal disease, amyotrophic lateral sclerosis. Using ingenuity pathway analysis (IPA), it was predicted that *miR-92* affects CD40 signaling by targeting CD40 directly (163).

Let-7a expression is diminished in SP-MS patients compared to healthy controls. IPA analysis led to the suggestion that *let-7a* targets TLR4 and TLR9, as well as IL-12RB2 and TGF-βR1 (163). *Let-7a* also regulates neuronal differentiation (164).

MiR-145 appears to decrease during the transition from RR-MS to SP-MS and is negatively correlated with disability score (163). This miRNA is known to regulate insulin-like growth factor 1 (IGF-1) signaling (IGF-1R, IRS1, and IRS2) (165).

Long non-coding RNAs have been shown to be involved in the development of neurodegenerative disorders, like *β-secretase-1 (BACE1)-AS*, the *brain cytoplasmic RNA* (*BC200 RNA*) in Alzheimer's disease, and the *brain-derived neurothrophic factor* (*BDNF*)*-AS* in Huntington's disease (166). *BACE1-AS* elevates the protein level of BACE1, an enzyme involved in generating β-amyloid, by binding and stabilizing BACE1 mRNA (167). The level of *BC200 RNA* is elevated in the brains of Alzheimer's patients (168) and this lncRNA was shown to interact with proteins participating in mRNA transport in neurons (166). *BDNF-AS* inhibits the expression of BDNF, a growth factor promoting neuron maturation and survival (169, 170). It is not yet known whether these lncRNAs are also involved in MS.

Impaired remyelination and neuron apoptosis are two hallmarks of the neurodegenerative phase of SP-MS. Interestingly, the level of *the small non-coding RNA 715 (sncRNA715)*, which inhibits oligodendrogial myelin basic protein (MBP) translation, is elevated in demyelinated chronic lesions in MS patients (171). In contrast, remyelination can be affected by exosomes released by DCs. Stimulating DCs with low levels of INF-γ causes the release of exosomes enriched in miRNA involved in the regulation of myelin production (*miR-219*) and anti-inflammatory response (*miR-181a*, *-451*, *-532-5p*, and *-665*) compared to exosomes released from unstimulated DCs. This, in turn, increases myelination and reduces oxidative stress in hippocampal slice cultures. Moreover, intranasal delivery of these exosomes elevates the central nervous system myelination *in vivo* (172). LncRNAs have also been implicated in the regulation of apoptosis, and because neuron apoptosis is important in MS, the role of lncRNA in apoptosis in MS should be investigated further (173).

Two MS SNPs are associated with miRNA genes (*miR-223*; rs1044165 and *miR-23*; rs3745453) and the expression of these miRNAs was investigated in MS patients (174). *MiR-223* is important for the innate immune system, e.g., affecting the non-canonical NF-κB pathway during macrophage differentiation (175), whereas *miR-23a* promotes myelination by elevating oligodendrocyte differentiation and myelin synthesis (176). Both *miR-223* and *miR-23a* are decreased in serum from RR-MS patients. However, the expression of *miR-233* is increased in peripheral blood mononuclear cells (PBMCs) from both RR-MS as well as PP-MS patients, whereas *miRNA-23a* is upregulated only in PBMCs from RR-MS patients (174). Thus far, no eQTL-effect of both SNPs on the respective miRNAs has been found.

Another study predicted that SNP rs28366, which is in moderate linkage disequilibrium ($r^2 = 0.4$) with MS risk variant rs17066096, might affect the binding of *miR-2278* and *miR-411-5p-* to the 3′-UTR of *IL22RA2*. However, although these miRNAs did indeed bind to the 3′-UTR in an *in vitro* assay, the SNP did not affect the binding (177).

PERSPECTIVES

Integration of autoimmune disease-associated SNPs with data on the functional regions in the genome shows that ~90% of these SNPs intersect with regulatory regions in the DNA (enhancers, promoters) rather than with protein-coding regions (exons) (29, 130). Autoimmune disease-associated loci often encompass genes known to play critical roles in immunological diseases. In these common illnesses, characteristically dozens of disease-associated SNPs have been identified, each predisposing moderately to disease. The general consensus for these immune-related diseases is that many SNPs with modest effects converge on a limited number of biological pathways and it is the sum of these effects that influences the phenotype to a large extent.

In the last two decades, thousands of regulatory RNA genes have been identified that also regulate gene expression. In fact, the total number of known miRNA genes plus lncRNA genes is now more than 15,000 and this is starting to approach the number of known protein-coding genes (~22,000). There is convincing evidence that autoimmune SNPs also affect miRNA and lncRNA biology. SNPs have been identified that locate to miRNA-binding sites and some SNPs appear to regulate the expression of lncRNAs (32, 132, 174, 177). This means that to fully understand the changes to transcriptional programs that contribute to disease, we need to take into account multiple gene-regulatory pathways, involving classical transcription factors, miRNAs, and lncRNAs. This situation is further complicated by the fact that these pathways, and the molecules involved in them, not only regulate other molecules within their own class, but also molecules of other classes. In the case of miRNAs and lncRNAs, for instance, it has already been reported that lncRNAs can be targeted by miRNAs, that lncRNAs can encode miRNAs, that lncRNAs and miRNAs can compete for targets, and that some lncRNAs can function as miRNA sponges (178).

With advances in next generation sequencing technology and the anticipated reduction in the cost of using these techniques, many more regulatory RNAs (and perhaps even novel classes of regulatory RNAs) are likely to be discovered. If we focus on discovering novel miRNAs and lncRNAs, we should take into account that the expression of both classes of regulatory RNAs is more cell-type- and stimulus-dependent than the expression of protein-coding genes. This has two consequences: (1) for regulatory RNAs affecting other RNA species, both the regulator and the target need to be expressed in the same cell type and (2) to better understand the molecular basis of human disease, it means that the tissues that specifically contribute to a disease need to be identified, isolated, and profiled. Subsequently, the targets of the known and novel regulatory RNAs need to be identified; this is currently a major challenge. It is known that miRNAs can bind dozens of targets and that single mRNAs can be regulated by multiple miRNAs. Canonical miRNA action is based on complementarity between the seed sequence of the miRNA and a binding sequence in the 3′-UTR of its target. This "rule" has been used to design algorithms that predict miRNA-binding sites in the 3′-UTRs of target mRNAs [see review by Hrdlickova et al. (18) for listing of web-based tools]. The field of lncRNA research is quite new and the functions of lncRNAs are still poorly understood. Although characteristics such as cell-type specificity and their role in epigenetic regulation also make lncRNAs interesting therapeutic targets, much more basic research is required to fully understand and appreciate the potential importance of lncRNAs in diagnostic work and treatment. There are currently no target prediction algorithms for lncRNAs, primarily because lncRNAs represent a heterogeneous group of regulatory RNAs that exhibit many different mechanisms of action. Moreover, their interaction with specific targets, which can be DNA or protein, appears to be determined by their structure rather than by their sequence. A factor that complicates lncRNA research is that they exhibit little sequence conservation throughout evolution. It is, therefore, not easy to identify mouse homologs of human lncRNAs for instance. However, it is possible that functional structures – independent of sequence – are more conserved, but there is not yet enough data available to prove definitely that this is a general feature. In contrast, miRNAs and their targets are well conserved throughout evolution, which makes it relatively easy to extrapolate mouse miRNA results to the human system.

Importantly, *in silico* predictions of targets and functions for regulatory RNAs need to be followed up by *in vitro* validation. Recently, advanced assays have been developed based on cross-linking of regulatory RNAs to their targets followed by analysis of their binding partners. By using such assays, miRNA targets can be identified by RNA sequencing [e.g., (179)] and lncRNA interacting partners can be determined by DNA sequencing or mass spectrometry [e.g., (180)]. These technically challenging assays are currently considered to be the state-of-the-art in pinpointing the targets of regulatory RNAs.

Much attention in the miRNA field is currently focused on the potential of using circulating miRNAs as biomarkers for disease. Tissue-specific expression profiles of miRNAs and lncRNAs are one of the features that make them attractive biomarker candidates. MiRNAs are of particular interest because it has been shown that they exhibit stability in plasma and serum, a feature that is not expected of lncRNAs. MiRNA (and lncRNA) levels can be measured by PCR, array technology, or by next generation sequencing applications, with each technique having its own advantages and disadvantages (181). Unfortunately, there are no simple tests (for instance dip-sticks) available to detect RNAs. Additionally, miRNAs are attractive targets for therapy. For instance, decoys can be applied to prevent miRNAs or lncRNAs from binding to their targets. Miravirsen, an inhibitor of miR-122, was shown to reduce HCV viremia in monkeys and is currently the most advanced miRNA-based drug in the clinical testing pipeline (Phase II). For more details on the potential of miRNAs or lncRNAs in the clinic and on the challenges associated with their delivery to target tissues, we recommend the reviews by Ling et al (182) and Li and Rana (183). It is clear, however, that the elucidation of more complete transcriptional networks, containing regulatory RNAs and protein-coding genes, will soon provide several more potential targets for therapeutic options.

ACKNOWLEDGMENTS

We thank Jackie Senior for editing the manuscript. The authors are supported by the European Research Council (ERC) under the European Union's Seventh Framework Program (FP/2007-2013; ERC Grant Agreement no. 2012-322698 to C. Wijmenga), the Dutch Multiple Sclerosis Foundation (11-752 to Sebo Withoff), NWO-VENI grant 863.09.007 to J. Fu, and the Systems Biology Centre for Metabolism and Ageing (SBC-EBA).

REFERENCES

1. Lee RC, Feinbaum RL, Ambros V. The C. elegans heterochronic gene lin-4 encodes small RNAs with antisense complementarity to lin-14. *Cell* (1993) **75**:843–54. doi:10.1016/0092-8674(93)90529-Y
2. Wightman B, Ha I, Ruvkun G. Posttranscriptional regulation of the heterochronic gene lin-14 by lin-4 mediates temporal pattern formation in *C. elegans. Cell* (1993) **75**:855–62. doi:10.1016/0092-8674(93)90530-4
3. Taft RJ, Pang KC, Mercer TR, Dinger M, Mattick JS. Non-coding RNAs: regulators of disease. *J Pathol* (2010) **220**:126–39. doi:10.1002/path.2638
4. Kozomara A, Griffiths-Jones S. miRBase: annotating high confidence microRNAs using deep sequencing data. *Nucleic Acids Res* (2014) **42**:D68–73. doi:10.1093/nar/gkt1181
5. Harrow J, Frankish A, Gonzalez JM, Tapanari E, Diekhans M, Kokocinski F, et al. GENCODE: the reference human genome annotation for the ENCODE project. *Genome Res* (2012) **22**:1760–74. doi:10.1101/gr.135350.111
6. Denli AM, Tops BBJ, Plasterk RHA, Ketting RF, Hannon GJ. Processing of primary microRNAs by the microprocessor complex. *Nature* (2004) **432**:231–5. doi:10.1038/nature03049
7. Lee Y, Ahn C, Han J, Choi H, Kim J, Yim J, et al. The nuclear RNase III Drosha initiates microRNA processing. *Nature* (2003) **425**:415–9. doi:10.1038/nature01957
8. Chen C-YA, Zheng D, Xia Z, Shyu A-B. Ago-TNRC6 triggers microRNA-mediated decay by promoting two deadenylation steps. *Nat Struct Mol Biol* (2009) **16**:1160–6. doi:10.1038/nsmb.1709
9. Takimoto K, Wakiyama M, Yokoyama S. Mammalian GW182 contains multiple argonaute-binding sites and functions in microRNA-mediated translational repression. *RNA* (2009) **15**:1078–89. doi:10.1261/rna.1363109
10. Liu J, Valencia-Sanchez MA, Hannon GJ, Parker R. MicroRNA-dependent localization of targeted mRNAs to mammalian P-bodies. *Nat Cell Biol* (2005) **7**:719–23. doi:10.1038/ncb1274
11. Wei Y, Li L, Wang D, Zhang C-Y, Zen K. Importin 8 regulates the transport of mature microRNAs into the cell nucleus. *J Biol Chem* (2014) **289**:10270–5. doi:10.1074/jbc.C113.541417

12. Johnsson P, Ackley A, Vidarsdottir L, Lui W-O, Corcoran M, Grandér D, et al. A pseudogene long-noncoding-RNA network regulates PTEN transcription and translation in human cells. *Nat Struct Mol Biol* (2013) **20**:440–6. doi:10.1038/nsmb.2516
13. Cole C, Sobala A, Lu C, Thatcher SR, Bowman A, Brown JWS, et al. Filtering of deep sequencing data reveals the existence of abundant dicer-dependent small RNAs derived from tRNAs. *RNA* (2009) **15**:2147–60. doi:10.1261/rna.1738409
14. Son DJ, Kumar S, Takabe W, Kim CW, Ni C-W, Alberts-Grill N, et al. The atypical mechanosensitive microRNA-712 derived from pre-ribosomal RNA induces endothelial inflammation and atherosclerosis. *Nat Commun* (2013) **4**:3000. doi:10.1038/ncomms4000
15. Ruby JG, Jan CH, Bartel DP. Intronic microRNA precursors that bypass Drosha processing. *Nature* (2007) **448**:83–6. doi:10.1038/nature05983
16. Havens MA, Reich AA, Duelli DM, Hastings ML. Biogenesis of mammalian microRNAs by a non-canonical processing pathway. *Nucleic Acids Res* (2012) **40**:4626–40. doi:10.1093/nar/gks026
17. Weber JA, Baxter DH, Zhang S, Huang DY, Huang KH, Lee MJ, et al. The microRNA spectrum in 12 body fluids. *Clin Chem* (2010) **56**:1733–41. doi:10.1373/clinchem.2010.147405
18. Hrdlickova B, de Almeida RC, Borek Z, Withoff S. Genetic variation in the non-coding genome: involvement of micro-RNAs and long non-coding RNAs in disease. *Biochim Biophys Acta* (2014) **1842**:1910–22. doi:10.1016/j.bbadis.2014.03.011
19. Iborra M, Bernuzzi F, Correale C, Vetrano S, Fiorino G, Beltrán B, et al. Identification of serum and tissue micro-RNA expression profiles in different stages of inflammatory bowel disease. *Clin Exp Immunol* (2013) **173**:250–8. doi:10.1111/cei.12104
20. De Iudicibus S, Lucafò M, Martelossi S, Pierobon C, Ventura A, Decorti G. MicroRNAs as tools to predict glucocorticoid response in inflammatory bowel diseases. *World J Gastroenterol* (2013) **19**:7947–54. doi:10.3748/wjg.v19.i44.7947
21. Liu Y, Zhao L, Li D, Yin Y, Zhang C-Y, Li J, et al. Microvesicle-delivery miR-150 promotes tumorigenesis by up-regulating VEGF, and the neutralization of miR-150 attenuate tumor development. *Protein Cell* (2013) **4**:932–41. doi:10.1007/s13238-013-3092-z
22. Lehmann SM, Krüger C, Park B, Derkow K, Rosenberger K, Baumgart J, et al. An unconventional role for miRNA: let-7 activates toll-like receptor 7 and causes neurodegeneration. *Nat Neurosci* (2012) **15**:827–35. doi:10.1038/nn.3113
23. Park C-K, Xu Z-Z, Berta T, Han Q, Chen G, Liu X-J, et al. Extracellular microRNAs activate nociceptor neurons to elicit pain via TLR7 and TRPA1. *Neuron* (2014) **82**:47–54. doi:10.1016/j.neuron.2014.02.011
24. Mittelbrunn M, Gutiérrez-Vázquez C, Villarroya-Beltri C, González S, Sánchez-Cabo F, González MÁ, et al. Unidirectional transfer of microRNA-loaded exosomes from T cells to antigen-presenting cells. *Nat Commun* (2011) **2**:282. doi:10.1038/ncomms1285
25. Villarroya-Beltri C, Gutiérrez-Vázquez C, Sánchez-Cabo F, Pérez-Hernández D, Vázquez J, Martin-Cofreces N, et al. Sumoylated hnRNPA2B1 controls the sorting of miRNAs into exosomes through binding to specific motifs. *Nat Commun* (2013) **4**:2980. doi:10.1038/ncomms3980
26. Derrien T, Johnson R, Bussotti G, Tanzer A, Djebali S, Tilgner H, et al. The GENCODE v7 catalog of human long noncoding RNAs: analysis of their gene structure, evolution, and expression. *Genome Res* (2012) **22**:1775–89. doi:10.1101/gr.132159.111
27. Guttman M, Russell P, Ingolia NT, Weissman JS, Lander ES. Ribosome profiling provides evidence that large noncoding RNAs do not encode proteins. *Cell* (2013) **154**:240–51. doi:10.1016/j.cell.2013.06.009
28. Djebali S, Davis CA, Merkel A, Dobin A, Lassmann T, Mortazavi A, et al. Landscape of transcription in human cells. *Nature* (2012) **489**:101–8. doi:10.1038/nature11233
29. Bernstein BE, Birney E, Dunham I, Green ED, Gunter C, Snyder M. An integrated encyclopedia of DNA elements in the human genome. *Nature* (2012) **489**:57–74. doi:10.1038/nature11247
30. Guttman M, Amit I, Garber M, French C, Lin MF, Feldser D, et al. Chromatin signature reveals over a thousand highly conserved large non-coding RNAs in mammals. *Nature* (2009) **458**:223–7. doi:10.1038/nature07672
31. Li J, Xuan Z, Liu C. Long non-coding RNAs and complex human diseases. *Int J Mol Sci* (2013) **14**:18790–808. doi:10.3390/ijms140918790
32. Kumar V, Westra H-J, Karjalainen J, Zhernakova DV, Esko T, Hrdlickova B, et al. Human disease-associated genetic variation impacts large intergenic non-noding RNA expression. *PLoS Genet* (2013) **9**:e1003201. doi:10.1371/journal.pgen.1003201
33. Wang KC, Chang HY. Molecular mechanisms of long noncoding RNAs. *Mol Cell* (2011) **43**:904–14. doi:10.1016/j.molcel.2011.08.018
34. Rinn JL, Chang HY. Genome regulation by long noncoding RNAs. *Annu Rev Biochem* (2012) **81**:145–66. doi:10.1146/annurev-biochem-051410-092902
35. Guttman M, Rinn JL. Modular regulatory principles of large non-coding RNAs. *Nature* (2012) **482**:339–46. doi:10.1038/nature10887
36. Salmena L, Poliseno L, Tay Y, Kats L, Pandolfi PP. A ceRNA hypothesis: the Rosetta Stone of a hidden RNA language? *Cell* (2011) **146**:353–8. doi:10.1016/j.cell.2011.07.014
37. Cesana M, Cacchiarelli D, Legnini I, Santini T, Sthandier O, Chinappi M, et al. A long noncoding RNA controls muscle differentiation by functioning as a competing endogenous RNA. *Cell* (2011) **147**:358–69. doi:10.1016/j.cell.2011.09.028
38. Karreth FA, Tay Y, Perna D, Ala U, Tan SM, Rust AG, et al. In vivo identification of tumor- suppressive PTEN ceRNAs in an oncogenic BRAF-induced mouse model of melanoma. *Cell* (2011) **147**:382–95. doi:10.1016/j.cell.2011.09.032
39. Contreras J, Rao DS. MicroRNAs in inflammation and immune responses. *Leukemia* (2012) **26**:404–13. doi:10.1038/leu.2011.356
40. O'Connell RM, Rao DS, Chaudhuri AA, Baltimore D. Physiological and pathological roles for microRNAs in the immune system. *Nat Rev Immunol* (2010) **10**:111–22. doi:10.1038/nri2708
41. Wang XS, Gong JN, Yu J, Wang F, Zhang XH, Yin XL, et al. MicroRNA-29a and microRNA-142-3p are regulators of myeloid differentiation and acute myeloid leukemia. *Blood* (2012) **119**:4992–5004. doi:10.1182/blood-2011-10-385716
42. O'Connell RM, Zhao JL, Rao DS. MicroRNA function in myeloid biology. *Blood* (2011) **118**:2960–9. doi:10.1182/blood-2011-03-291971
43. Bousquet M, Harris MH, Zhou B, Lodish HF. MicroRNA miR-125b causes leukemia. *Proc Natl Acad Sci U S A* (2010) **107**:21558–63. doi:10.1073/pnas.1016611107
44. Alemdehy MF, van Boxtel NGJA, de Looper HWJ, van den Berge IJ, Sanders MA, Cupedo T, et al. Dicer1 deletion in myeloid-committed progenitors causes neutrophil dysplasia and blocks macrophage/dendritic cell development in mice. *Blood* (2012) **119**:4723–30. doi:10.1182/blood-2011-10-386359
45. Bezman NA, Cedars E, Steiner DF, Blelloch R, Hesslein DGT, Lanier LL. Distinct requirements of microRNAs in NK cell activation, survival, and function. *J Immunol* (2010) **185**:3835–46. doi:10.4049/jimmunol.1000980
46. Montecalvo A, Larregina AT, Shufesky WJ, Stolz DB, Sullivan MLG, Karlsson JM, et al. Mechanism of transfer of functional microRNAs between mouse dendritic cells via exosomes. *Blood* (2012) **119**:756–66. doi:10.1182/blood-2011-02-338004
47. Pegtel DM, Cosmopoulos K, Thorley-Lawson DA, van Eijndhoven MAJ, Hopmans ES, Lindenberg JL, et al. Functional delivery of viral miRNAs via exosomes. *Proc Natl Acad Sci U S A* (2010) **107**:6328–33. doi:10.1073/pnas.0914843107
48. Sauvageau M, Goff LA, Lodato S, Bonev B, Groff AF, Gerhardinger C, et al. Multiple knockout mouse models reveal lincRNAs are required for life and brain development. *Elife* (2013) **2**:e01749. doi:10.7554/eLife.01749
49. Pospisil V, Vargova K, Kokavec J, Rybarova J, Savvulidi F, Jonasova A, et al. Epigenetic silencing of the oncogenic miR-17-92 cluster during PU.1-directed macrophage differentiation. *EMBO J* (2011) **30**:4450–64. doi:10.1038/emboj.2011.317
50. Spierings DC, McGoldrick D, Hamilton-Easton AM, Neale G, Murchison EP, Hannon GJ, et al. Ordered progression of stage-specific miRNA profiles in the mouse B2 B-cell lineage. *Blood* (2011) **117**:5340–9. doi:10.1182/blood-2010-10-316034
51. Sun SM, Dijkstra MK, Bijkerk AC, Brooimans RA, Valk PJM, Erkeland SJ, et al. Transition of highly specific microRNA expression patterns in association with discrete maturation stages of human granulopoiesis. *Br J Haematol* (2011) **155**:395–8. doi:10.1111/j.1365-2141.2011.08682.x
52. Johnnidis JB, Harris MH, Wheeler RT, Stehling-Sun S, Lam MH, Kirak O, et al. Regulation of progenitor cell proliferation and granulocyte function by microRNA-223. *Nature* (2008) **451**:1125–9. doi:10.1038/nature06607
53. Surdziel E, Cabanski M, Dallmann I, Lyszkiewicz M, Krueger A, Ganser A, et al. Enforced expression of miR-125b affects myelopoiesis by targeting multiple

signaling pathways. *Blood* (2011) **117**:4338–48. doi:10.1182/blood-2010-06-289058
54. Chaudhuri AA, So AY-L, Mehta A, Minisandram A, Sinha N, Jonsson VD, et al. Oncomir miR-125b regulates hematopoiesis by targeting the gene Lin28A. *Proc Natl Acad Sci U S A* (2012) **109**:4233–8. doi:10.1073/pnas.1200677109
55. Scott EW, Simon MC, Anastasi J, Singh H. Requirement of transcription factor PU.1 in the development of multiple hematopoietic lineages. *Science* (1994) **265**:1573–7. doi:10.1126/science.8079170
56. Ghani S, Riemke P, Schönheit J, Lenze D, Stumm J, Hoogenkamp M, et al. Macrophage development from HSCs requires PU.1-coordinated microRNA expression. *Blood* (2011) **118**:2275–84. doi:10.1182/blood-2011-02-335141
57. Mildner A, Chapnik E, Manor O, Yona S, Kim KW, Aychek T, et al. Mononuclear phagocyte miRNome analysis identifies miR-142 as critical regulator of murine dendritic cell homeostasis. *Blood* (2013) **121**:1016–27. doi:10.1182/blood-2012-07-445999
58. Fontana L, Pelosi E, Greco P, Racanicchi S, Testa U, Liuzzi F, et al. MicroRNAs 17-5p-20a-106a control monocytopoiesis through AML1 targeting and M-CSF receptor upregulation. *Nat Cell Biol* (2007) **9**:775–87. doi:10.1038/ncb1613
59. Larsen MT, Hother C, Häger M, Pedersen CC, Theilgaard-Mönch K, Borregaard N, et al. MicroRNA profiling in human neutrophils during bone marrow granulopoiesis and in vivo exudation. *PLoS One* (2013) **8**:e58454. doi:10.1371/journal.pone.0058454
60. Lu TX, Lim EJ, Itskovich S, Besse JA, Plassard AJ, Mingler MK, et al. Targeted ablation of miR-21 decreases murine eosinophil progenitor cell growth. *PLoS One* (2013) **8**:e59397. doi:10.1371/journal.pone.0059397
61. Dunand-Sauthier I, Santiago-Raber ML, Capponi L, Vejnar CE, Schaad O, Irla M, et al. Silencing of c-Fos expression by microRNA-155 is critical for dendritic cell maturation and function. *Blood* (2011) **117**:4490–500. doi:10.1182/blood-2010-09-308064
62. Riepsaame J, van Oudenaren A, den Broeder BJH, van Ijcken WFJ, Pothof J, Leenen PJM. MicroRNA-mediated down-regulation of M-CSF receptor contributes to maturation of mouse monocyte-derived dendritic cells. *Front Immunol* (2013) **4**:353. doi:10.3389/fimmu.2013.00353
63. Mi QS, Xu YP, Qi RQ, Shi YL, Zhou L. Lack of microRNA miR-150 reduces the capacity of epidermal langerhans cell cross-presentation. *Exp Dermatol* (2012) **21**:876–7. doi:10.1111/exd.12008
64. Zhang M, Liu F, Jia H, Zhang Q, Yin L, Liu W. Inhibition of microRNA let-7i depresses maturation and functional state of dendritic cells in response to lipopolysaccharide stimulation via targeting suppressor of cytokine signaling 1. *J Immunol* (2011) **187**:1674–83. doi:10.4049/jimmunol.1001937
65. Jurkin J, Schichl YM, Koeffel R, Bauer T, Richter S, Konradi S, et al. miR-146a is differentially expressed by myeloid dendritic cell subsets and desensitizes cells to TLR2-dependent activation. *J Immunol* (2010) **184**:4955–65. doi:10.4049/jimmunol.0903021
66. Liu X, Zhan Z, Xu L, Ma F, Li D, Guo Z, et al. MicroRNA-148/152 impair innate response and antigen presentation of TLR-triggered dendritic cells by targeting CaMKIIα. *J Immunol* (2010) **185**:7244–51. doi:10.4049/jimmunol.1001573
67. Bai Y, Qian C, Qian L, Ma F, Hou J, Chen Y, et al. Integrin CD11b negatively regulates TLR9-triggered dendritic cell cross-priming by upregulating microRNA-146a. *J Immunol* (2012) **188**:5293–302. doi:10.4049/jimmunol.1102371
68. Hua C, Sun L, Yang Y, Tan R, Hou Y. Mechanisms of CpG-induced CD40 expression on murine bone marrow-derived dendritic cells. *Autoimmunity* (2013) **46**:177–87. doi:10.3109/08916934.2012.751980
69. Bazzoni F, Rossato M, Fabbri M, Gaudiosi D, Mirolo M, Mori L, et al. Induction and regulatory function of miR-9 in human monocytes and neutrophils exposed to proinflammatory signals. *Proc Natl Acad Sci U S A* (2009) **106**:5282–7. doi:10.1073/pnas.0810909106
70. Jiang P, Liu R, Zheng Y, Liu X, Chang L, Xiong S, et al. MiR-34a inhibits lipopolysaccharide-induced inflammatory response through targeting notch1 in murine macrophages. *Exp Cell Res* (2012) **318**:1175–84. doi:10.1016/j.yexcr.2012.03.018
71. Zhu Q-Y, Liu Q, Chen J-X, Lan K, Ge B-X. MicroRNA-101 targets MAPK phosphatase-1 to regulate the activation of MAPKs in macrophages. *J Immunol* (2010) **185**:7435–42. doi:10.4049/jimmunol.1000798
72. O'Connell RM, Taganov KD, Boldin MP, Cheng G, Baltimore D. MicroRNA-155 is induced during the macrophage inflammatory response. *Proc Natl Acad Sci U S A* (2007) **104**:1604–9. doi:10.1073/pnas.0610731104
73. Xie N, Cui H, Banerjee S, Tan Z, Salomao R, Fu M, et al. miR-27a regulates inflammatory response of macrophages by targeting IL-10. *J Immunol* (2014) **193**:327–34. doi:10.4049/jimmunol.1400203
74. Wu Z, Lu H, Sheng J, Li L. Inductive microRNA-21 impairs anti-mycobacterial responses by targeting IL-12 and Bcl-2. *FEBS Lett* (2012) **586**:2459–67. doi:10.1016/j.febslet.2012.06.004
75. Lemaire J, Mkannez G, Guerfali FZ, Gustin C, Attia H, Sghaier RM, et al. MicroRNA expression profile in human macrophages in response to *Leishmania* major infection. *PLoS Negl Trop Dis* (2013) **7**:e2478. doi:10.1371/journal.pntd.0002478
76. Cannella D, Brenier-Pinchart M-P, Braun L, van Rooyen JM, Bougdour A, Bastien O, et al. miR-146a and miR-155 delineate a microRNA fingerprint associated with *Toxoplasma* persistence in the host brain. *Cell Rep* (2014) **6**:928–37. doi:10.1016/j.celrep.2014.02.002
77. Cai Y, Chen H, Mo X, Tang Y, Xu X, Zhang A, et al. Toxoplasma gondii inhibits apoptosis via a novel STAT3-miR-17-92-Bim pathway in macrophages. *Cell Signal* (2014) **26**:1204–12. doi:10.1016/j.cellsig.2014.02.013
78. Gibb EA, Vucic EA, Enfield KSS, Stewart GL, Lonergan KM, Kennett JY, et al. Human cancer long non-coding RNA transcriptomes. *PLoS One* (2011) **6**:e25915. doi:10.1371/journal.pone.0025915
79. Gutschner T, Hämmerle M, Diederichs S. MALAT1 – a paradigm for long noncoding RNA function in cancer. *J Mol Med (Berl)* (2013) **91**:791–801. doi:10.1007/s00109-013-1028-y
80. Kim K, Jutooru I, Chadalapaka G, Johnson G, Frank J, Burghardt R, et al. HOTAIR is a negative prognostic factor and exhibits pro-oncogenic activity in pancreatic cancer. *Oncogene* (2013) **32**:1616–25. doi:10.1038/onc.2012.193
81. Hu W, Alvarez-Dominguez JR, Lodish HF. Regulation of mammalian cell differentiation by long non-coding RNAs. *EMBO Rep* (2012) **13**:971–83. doi:10.1038/embor.2012.145
82. Fatica A, Bozzoni I. Long non-coding RNAs: new players in cell differentiation and development. *Nat Rev Genet* (2014) **15**:7–21. doi:10.1038/nrg3606
83. Zhang X, Lian Z, Padden C, Gerstein MB, Rozowsky J, Snyder M, et al. A myelopoiesis-associated regulatory intergenic noncoding RNA transcript within the human HOXA cluster. *Blood* (2009) **113**:2526–34. doi:10.1182/blood-2008-06-162164
84. Wright PW, Huehn A, Cichocki F, Li H, Sharma N, Dang H, et al. Identification of a KIR antisense lncRNA expressed by progenitor cells. *Genes Immun* (2013) **14**:427–33. doi:10.1038/gene.2013.36
85. Wang P, Xue Y, Han Y, Lin L, Wu C, Xu S, et al. The STAT3-binding long noncoding RNA lnc-DC controls human dendritic cell differentiation. *Science* (2014) **344**:310–3. doi:10.1126/science.1251456
86. Rapicavoli NA, Qu K, Zhang J, Mikhail M, Laberge R-M, Chang HY. A mammalian pseudogene lncRNA at the interface of inflammation and anti-inflammatory therapeutics. *Elife* (2013) **2**:e00762. doi:10.7554/eLife.00762
87. Carpenter S, Aiello D, Atianand MK, Ricci EP, Gandhi P, Hall LL, et al. A long noncoding RNA mediates both activation and repression of immune response genes. *Science* (2013) **341**:789–92. doi:10.1126/science.1240925
88. Li Z, Chao T-C, Chang K-Y, Lin N, Patil VS, Shimizu C, et al. The long noncoding RNA THRIL regulates TNFα expression through its interaction with hnRNPL. *Proc Natl Acad Sci U S A* (2014) **111**:1002–7. doi:10.1073/pnas.1313768111
89. Mao YS, Zhang B, Spector DL. Biogenesis and function of nuclear bodies. *Trends Genet* (2011) **27**:295–306. doi:10.1016/j.tig.2011.05.006
90. Imamura K, Imamachi N, Akizuki G, Kumakura M, Kawaguchi A, Nagata K, et al. Long noncoding RNA NEAT1-dependent SFPQ relocation from promoter region to paraspeckle mediates IL8 expression upon immune stimuli. *Mol Cell* (2014) **53**:393–406. doi:10.1016/j.molcel.2014.01.009
91. O'Connell RM, Chaudhuri AA, Rao DS, Gibson WSJ, Balazs AB, Baltimore D. MicroRNAs enriched in hematopoietic stem cells differentially regulate long-term hematopoietic output. *Proc Natl Acad Sci U S A* (2010) **107**:14235–40. doi:10.1073/pnas.1009798107
92. Cobb BS, Nesterova TB, Thompson E, Hertweck A, O'Connor E, Godwin J, et al. T cell lineage choice and differentiation in the absence of the RNase III enzyme Dicer. *J Exp Med* (2005) **201**:1367–73. doi:10.1084/jem.20050572
93. Muljo SA, Ansel KM, Kanellopoulou C, Livingston DM, Rao A, Rajewsky K. Aberrant T cell differentiation in the absence of Dicer. *J Exp Med* (2005) **202**:261–9. doi:10.1084/jem.20050678

94. Neilson JR, Zheng GXY, Burge CB, Sharp PA. Dynamic regulation of miRNA expression in ordered stages of cellular development. *Genes Dev* (2007) **21**:578–89. doi:10.1101/gad.1522907
95. Bronevetsky Y, Villarino AV, Eisley CJ, Barbeau R, Barczak AJ, Heinz GA, et al. T cell activation induces proteasomal degradation of argonaute and rapid remodeling of the microRNA repertoire. *J Exp Med* (2013) **210**:417–32. doi:10.1084/jem.20111717
96. Ooi AGL, Sahoo D, Adorno M, Wang Y, Weissman IL, Park CY. MicroRNA-125b expands hematopoietic stem cells and enriches for the lymphoid-balanced and lymphoid-biased subsets. *Proc Natl Acad Sci U S A* (2010) **107**:21505–10. doi:10.1073/pnas.1016218107
97. Rossi RL, Rossetti G, Wenandy L, Curti S, Ripamonti A, Bonnal RJP, et al. Distinct microRNA signatures in human lymphocyte subsets and enforcement of the naive state in CD4+ T cells by the microRNA miR-125b. *Nat Immunol* (2011) **12**:796–803. doi:10.1038/ni.2057
98. Kuchen S, Resch W, Yamane A, Kuo N, Li Z, Chakraborty T, et al. Regulation of microRNA expression and abundance during lymphopoiesis. *Immunity* (2010) **32**:828–39. doi:10.1016/j.immuni.2010.05.009
99. Rodriguez A, Vigorito E, Clare S, Warren MV, Couttet P, Soond DR, et al. Requirement of bic/microRNA-155 for normal immune function. *Science* (2007) **316**:608–11. doi:10.1126/science.1139253
100. Zhang J, Cheng Y, Cui W, Li M, Li B, Guo L. MicroRNA-155 modulates Th1 and Th17 cell differentiation and is associated with multiple sclerosis and experimental autoimmune encephalomyelitis. *J Neuroimmunol* (2014) **266**:56–63. doi:10.1016/j.jneuroim.2013.09.019
101. Kohlhaas S, Garden OA, Scudamore C, Turner M, Okkenhaug K, Vigorito E. Cutting edge: the Foxp3 target miR-155 contributes to the development of regulatory T cells. *J Immunol* (2009) **182**:2578–82. doi:10.4049/jimmunol.0803162
102. Lu L-F, Thai T-H, Calado DP, Chaudhry A, Kubo M, Tanaka K, et al. Foxp3-dependent microRNA155 confers competitive fitness to regulatory T cells by targeting SOCS1 protein. *Immunity* (2009) **30**:80–91. doi:10.1016/j.immuni.2008.11.010
103. Jiang S, Li C, Olive V, Lykken E, Feng F, Sevilla J, et al. Molecular dissection of the miR-17-92 cluster's critical dual roles in promoting Th1 responses and preventing inducible Treg differentiation. (2011). *Blood* (2011) **118**:5487–97. doi:10.1182/blood-2011-05-355644
104. Liu SQ, Jiang S, Li C, Zhang B, Li QJ. miR-17-92 cluster targets phosphatase and tensin homology and ikaros family zinc finger 4 to promote TH17-mediated inflammation. (2014). *J Biol Chem* (2014) **289**:12446–56. doi:10.1074/jbc.M114.550723
105. Monticelli S, Ansel KM, Xiao C, Socci ND, Krichevsky AM, Thai TH, et al. MicroRNA profiling of the murine hematopoietic system. *Genome Biol* (2005) **6**:R71. doi:10.1186/gb-2005-6-8-r71
106. Cobb BS, Hertweck A, Smith J, O'Connor E, Graf D, Cook T, et al. A role for dicer in immune regulation. *J Exp Med* (2006) **203**:2519–27. doi:10.1084/jem.20061692
107. Curtale G, Citarella F, Carissimi C, Goldoni M, Carucci N, Fulci V, et al. An emerging player in the adaptive immune response: microRNA-146a is a modulator of IL-2 expression and activation-induced cell death in T lymphocytes. *Blood* (2010) **115**:265–73. doi:10.1182/blood-2009-06-225987
108. Trifari S, Pipkin ME, Bandukwala HS, Äijö T, Bassein J, Chen R, et al. MicroRNA-directed program of cytotoxic CD8+ T-cell differentiation. *Proc Natl Acad Sci U S A* (2013) **110**:18608–13. doi:10.1073/pnas.1317191110
109. Gracias DT, Stelekati E, Hope JL, Boesteanu AC, Doering TA, Norton J, et al. The microRNA miR-155 controls CD8(+) T cell responses by regulating interferon signaling. *Nat Immunol* (2013) **14**:593–602. doi:10.1038/ni.2576
110. Khann AA, Penny LA, Yuzefpolskiy Y, Sarkar S, Kalia V. MicroRNA-17 92 regulates effector and memory CD8 T-cell fates by modulating proliferation in response to infections. (2013). *Blood* (2013) **121**:4473–83. doi:10.1182/blood-2012-06-435412
111. Koralov SB, Muljo SA, Galler GR, Krek A, Chakraborty T, Kanellopoulou C, et al. Dicer ablation affects antibody diversity and cell survival in the B lymphocyte lineage. *Cell* (2008) **132**:860–74. doi:10.1016/j.cell.2008.02.020
112. Belver L, de Yébenes VG, Ramiro AR. MicroRNAs prevent the generation of autoreactive antibodies. *Immunity* (2010) **33**:713–22. doi:10.1016/j.immuni.2010.11.010
113. Xu S, Guo K, Zeng Q, Huo J, Lam K-P. The RNase III enzyme dicer is essential for germinal center B-cell formation. *Blood* (2012) **119**:767–76. doi:10.1182/blood-2011-05-355412
114. Okuyama K, Ikawa T, Gentner B, Hozumi K, Harnprasopwat R, Lu J, et al. MicroRNA-126-mediated control of cell fate in B-cell myeloid progenitors as a potential alternative to transcriptional factors. *Proc Natl Acad Sci U S A* (2013) **110**:13410–5. doi:10.1073/pnas.1220710110
115. Chen C-Z, Li L, Lodish HF, Bartel DP. MicroRNAs modulate hematopoietic lineage differentiation. *Science* (2004) **303**:83–6. doi:10.1126/science.1091903
116. Ventura A, Young AG, Winslow MM, Lintault L, Meissner A, Erkeland SJ, et al. Targeted deletion reveals essential and overlapping functions of the miR-17 through 92 family of miRNA clusters. *Cell* (2008) **132**:875–86. doi:10.1016/j.cell.2008.02.019
117. Jin HY, Oda H, Lai M, Skalsky RL, Bethel K, Shepherd J, et al. MicroRNA-17 92 plays a causative role in lymphomagenesis by coordinating multiple oncogenic pathways. *EMBO J* (2013) **32**:2377–91. doi:10.1038/emboj.2013.178
118. Zhou B, Wang S, Mayr C, Bartel DP, Lodish HF. miR-150, a microRNA expressed in mature B and T cells, blocks early B cell development when expressed prematurely. *Proc Natl Acad Sci U S A* (2007) **104**:7080–5. doi:10.1073/pnas.0702409104
119. Xiao C, Calado DP, Galler G, Thai T-H, Patterson HC, Wang J, et al. MiR-150 controls B cell differentiation by targeting the transcription factor c-Myb. *Cell* (2007) **131**:146–59. doi:10.1016/j.cell.2007.07.021
120. Thai T-H, Calado DP, Casola S, Ansel KM, Xiao C, Xue Y, et al. Regulation of the germinal center response by microRNA-155. *Science* (2007) **316**:604–8. doi:10.1126/science.1141229
121. Vigorito E, Perks KL, Abreu-Goodger C, Bunting S, Xiang Z, Kohlhaas S, et al. microRNA-155 regulates the generation of immunoglobulin class-switched plasma cells. *Immunity* (2007) **27**:847–59. doi:10.1016/j.immuni.2007.10.009
122. Eis PS, Tam W, Sun L, Chadburn A, Li Z, Gomez MF, et al. Accumulation of miR-155 and BIC RNA in human B cell lymphomas. *Proc Natl Acad Sci U S A* (2005) **102**:3627–32. doi:10.1073/pnas.0500613102
123. Costinean S, Zanesi N, Pekarsky Y, Tili E, Volinia S, Heerema N, et al. Pre-B cell proliferation and lymphoblastic leukemia/high-grade lymphoma in E(mu)-miR155 transgenic mice. *Proc Natl Acad Sci U S A* (2006) **103**:7024–9. doi:10.1073/pnas.0602266103
124. Gururajan M, Haga CL, Das S, Leu C-M, Hodson D, Josson S, et al. MicroRNA 125b inhibition of B cell differentiation in germinal centers. *Int Immunol* (2010) **22**:583–92. doi:10.1093/intimm/dxq042
125. Pang KC, Dinger ME, Mercer TR, Malquori L, Grimmond SM, Chen W, et al. Genome-wide identification of long noncoding RNAs in CD8+ T cells. *J Immunol* (2009) **182**:7738–48. doi:10.4049/jimmunol.0900603
126. Hu G, Tang Q, Sharma S, Yu F, Escobar TM, Muljo SA. Expression and regulation of intergenic long noncoding RNAs during T cell development and differentiation. *Nat Immunol* (2013) **14**:1190–8. doi:10.1038/ni.2712
127. Vigneau S, Rohrlich P-S, Brahic M, Bureau J-F. Tmevpg1, a candidate gene for the control of Theiler's virus persistence, could be implicated in the regulation of gamma interferon. *J Virol* (2003) **77**:5632–8. doi:10.1128/JVI.77.10.5632-5638.2003
128. Collier SP, Collins PL, Williams CL, Boothby MR, Aune TM. Cutting edge: influence of Tmevpg1, a long intergenic noncoding RNA, on the expression of Ifng by Th1 cells. *J Immunol* (2012) **189**:2084–8. doi:10.4049/jimmunol.1200774
129. Gomez JA, Wapinski OL, Yang YW, Bureau J-F, Gopinath S, Monack DM, et al. The NeST long ncRNA controls microbial susceptibility and epigenetic activation of the interferon-γ locus. *Cell* (2013) **152**:743–54. doi:10.1016/j.cell.2013.01.015
130. Ricaño-Ponce I, Wijmenga C. Mapping of immune-mediated disease genes. *Annu Rev Genomics Hum Genet* (2013) **14**:325–53. doi:10.1146/annurev-genom-091212-153450
131. Capuano M, Iaffaldano L, Tinto N, Montanaro D, Capobianco V, Izzo V, et al. MicroRNA-449a overexpression, reduced NOTCH1 signals and scarce goblet cells characterize the small intestine of celiac patients. *PLoS One* (2011) **6**:e29094. doi:10.1371/journal.pone.0029094
132. Kumar V, Wijmenga C, Withoff S. From genome-wide association studies to disease mechanisms: celiac disease as a model for autoimmune diseases. *Semin Immunopathol* (2012) **34**:567–80. doi:10.1007/s00281-012-0312-1
133. Geremia A, Biancheri P, Allan P, Corazza GR, Di Sabatino A. Innate and adaptive immunity in inflammatory bowel disease. *Autoimmun Rev* (2014) **13**:3–10. doi:10.1016/j.autrev.2013.06.004
134. Beaudoin M, Goyette P, Boucher G, Lo KS, Rivas MA, Stevens C, et al. Deep resequencing of GWAS loci identifies rare variants in CARD9, IL23R and RNF186

that are associated with ulcerative colitis. *PLoS Genet* (2013) **9**:e1003723. doi:10.1371/journal.pgen.1003723
135. Zahm AM, Thayu M, Hand NJ, Horner A, Leonard MB, Friedman JR. Circulating MicroRNA is a biomarker of pediatric Crohn disease. *J Pediatr Gastroenterol Nutr* (2011) **53**:26–33. doi:10.1097/MPG.0b013e31822200cc
136. Wu F, Zikusoka M, Trindade A, Dassopoulos T, Harris ML, Bayless T, et al. MicroRNAs are differentially expressed in ulcerative colitis and alter expression of macrophage inflammatory peptide-2 alpha. *Gastroenterology* (2008) **135**:1624–35. doi:10.1053/j.gastro.2008.07.068
137. Coskun M, Bjerrum JT, Seidelin JB, Nielsen OH. MicroRNAs in inflammatory bowel disease – pathogenesis, diagnostics and therapeutics. *World J Gastroenterol* (2012) **18**:4629–34. doi:10.3748/wjg.v18.i34.4629
138. Takagi T, Naito Y, Mizushima K, Hirata I, Yagi N, Tomatsuri N, et al. Increased expression of microRNA in the inflamed colonic mucosa of patients with active ulcerative colitis. *J Gastroenterol Hepatol* (2010) **25**(Suppl 1):S129–33. doi:10.1111/j.1440-1746.2009.06216.x
139. Fasseu M, Tréton X, Guichard C, Pedruzzi E, Cazals-Hatem D, Richard C, et al. Identification of restricted subsets of mature microRNA abnormally expressed in inactive colonic mucosa of patients with inflammatory bowel disease. *PLoS One* (2010) **5**(pii):e13160. doi:10.1371/journal.pone.0013160
140. Coskun M, Bjerrum JT, Seidelin JB, Troelsen JT, Olsen J, Nielsen OH. miR-20b, miR-98, miR-125b-1*, and let-7e* as new potential diagnostic biomarkers in ulcerative colitis. *World J Gastroenterol* (2013) **19**:4289–99. doi:10.3748/wjg.v19.i27.4289
141. Gazouli M, Papaconstantinou I, Stamatis K, Vaiopoulou A, Zeglinas C, Vassiliou I, et al. Association study of genetic variants in miRNAs in patients with inflammatory bowel disease: preliminary results. *Dig Dis Sci* (2013) **58**:2324–8. doi:10.1007/s10620-013-2640-y
142. Paraskevi A, Theodoropoulos G, Papaconstantinou I, Mantzaris G, Nikiteas N, Gazouli M. Circulating microRNA in inflammatory bowel disease. *J Crohns Colitis* (2012) **6**:900–4. doi:10.1016/j.crohns.2012.02.006
143. Yang Y, Ma Y, Shi C, Chen H, Zhang H, Chen N, et al. Overexpression of miR-21 in patients with ulcerative colitis impairs intestinal epithelial barrier function through targeting the Rho GTPase RhoB. *Biochem Biophys Res Commun* (2013) **434**:746–52. doi:10.1016/j.bbrc.2013.03.122
144. Nata T, Fujiya M, Ueno N, Moriichi K, Konishi H, Tanabe H, et al. MicroRNA-146b improves intestinal injury in mouse colitis by activating nuclear factor-κB and improving epithelial barrier function. *J Gene Med* (2013) **15**:249–60. doi:10.1002/jgm.2717
145. Shi C, Liang Y, Yang J, Xia Y, Chen H, Han H, et al. MicroRNA-21 knockout improve the survival rate in DSS induced fatal colitis through protecting against inflammation and tissue injury. *PLoS One* (2013) **8**:e66814. doi:10.1371/journal.pone.0066814
146. Ghorpade DS, Sinha AY, Holla S, Singh V, Balaji KN. NOD2-nitric oxide-responsive microRNA-146a activates Sonic hedgehog signaling to orchestrate inflammatory responses in murine model of inflammatory bowel disease. *J Biol Chem* (2013) **288**:33037–48. doi:10.1074/jbc.M113.492496
147. Chen Y, Wang C, Liu Y, Tang L, Zheng M, Xu C, et al. MiR-122 targets NOD2 to decrease intestinal epithelial cell injury in Crohn's disease. *Biochem Biophys Res Commun* (2013) **438**:133–9. doi:10.1016/j.bbrc.2013.07.040
148. Huang Z, Shi T, Zhou Q, Shi S, Zhao R, Shi H, et al. miR-141 regulates colonic leukocytic trafficking by targeting CXCL12β during murine colitis and human Crohn's disease. *Gut* (2013):1–11. doi:10.1136/gutjnl-2012-304213
149. Pekow JR, Dougherty U, Mustafi R, Zhu H, Kocherginsky M, Rubin DT, et al. miR-143 and miR-145 are downregulated in ulcerative colitis: putative regulators of inflammation and protooncogenes. *Inflamm Bowel Dis* (2012) **18**:94–100. doi:10.1002/ibd.21742
150. Olaru AV, Yamanaka S, Vazquez C, Mori Y, Cheng Y, Abraham JM, et al. MicroRNA-224 negatively regulates p21 expression during late neoplastic progression in inflammatory bowel disease. *Inflamm Bowel Dis* (2013) **19**:471–80. doi:10.1097/MIB.0b013e31827e78eb
151. Ludwig K, Fassan M, Mescoli C, Pizzi M, Balistreri M, Albertoni L, et al. PDCD4/miR-21 dysregulation in inflammatory bowel disease-associated carcinogenesis. *Virchows Arch* (2013) **462**:57–63. doi:10.1007/s00428-012-1345-5
152. Svrcek M, El-Murr N, Wanherdrick K, Dumont S, Beaugerie L, Cosnes J, et al. Overexpression of microRNAs-155 and 21 targeting mismatch repair proteins in inflammatory bowel diseases. *Carcinogenesis* (2013) **34**:828–34. doi:10.1093/carcin/bgs408
153. Kanaan Z, Rai SN, Eichenberger MR, Barnes C, Dworkin AM, Weller C, et al. Differential microRNA expression tracks neoplastic progression in inflammatory bowel disease-associated colorectal cancer. *Hum Mutat* (2012) **33**:551–60. doi:10.1002/humu.22021
154. Liu Z, Lee J, Krummey S, Lu W, Cai H, Lenardo MJ. The kinase LRRK2 is a regulator of the transcription factor NFAT that modulates the severity of inflammatory bowel disease. *Nat Immunol* (2011) **12**:1063–70. doi:10.1038/ni.2113
155. Qiao YQ, Huang ML, Xu AT, Zhao D, Ran ZH, Shen J. LncRNA DQ786243 affects Treg related CREB and Foxp3 expression in Crohn's disease. *J Biomed Sci* (2013) **20**:87. doi:10.1186/1423-0127-20-87
156. Vukusic S, Confavreux C. Prognostic factors for progression of disability in the secondary progressive phase of multiple sclerosis. *J Neurol Sci* (2003) **206**:135–7. doi:10.1016/S0022-510X(02)00426-4
157. Smith KM, Guerau-de-Arellano M, Costinean S, Williams JL, Bottoni A, Mavrikis Cox G, et al. miR-29ab1 deficiency identifies a negative feedback loop controlling Th1 bias that is dysregulated in multiple sclerosis. *J Immunol* (2012) **189**:1567–76. doi:10.4049/jimmunol.1103171
158. Nakahama T, Hanieh H, Nquyen NT, Chinen I, Ripley B, Millrine D, et al. Aryl hydrocarbon receptor-mediated induction of the microRNA-132/212 cluster promotes interleukin-17-producing T-helper cell differentiation. (2013). *Proc Natl Acad Sci U S A* (2013) **110**:11964–9. doi:10.1073/pnas.1311087110
159. Du C, Liu C, Kang J, Zhao G, Ye Z, Huang S, et al. MicroRNA miR-326 regulates TH-17 differentiation and is associated with the pathogenesis of multiple sclerosis. (2009). *Nat Immunol* (2009) **10**:1252–9. doi:10.1038/ni.1798
160. Honardoost MA, Kiani-Esfahani A, Ghaedi K, Etemadifar M, Salehi M. miR-326 and miR-26a, two potential markers for diagnosis of relapse and remission phases in patient with relapsing-remitting multiple sclerosis. *Gene* (2014) **544**:128–33. doi:10.1016/j.gene.2014.04.069
161. Lopez-Ramirez MA, Wu D, Pryce G, Simpson JE, Reijerkerk A, King-Robson J, et al. MicroRNA-155 negatively affects blood-brain barrier function during neuroinflammation. *FASEB J* (2014) **28**:2551–65. doi:10.1096/fj.13-248880
162. Reijerkerk A, Lopez-Ramirez MA, van Het Hof B, Drexhage JAR, Kamphuis WW, Kooij G, et al. MicroRNAs regulate human brain endothelial cell-barrier function in inflammation: implications for multiple sclerosis. *J Neurosci* (2013) **33**:6857–63. doi:10.1523/JNEUROSCI.3965-12.2013
163. Gandhi R, Healy B, Gholipour T, Egorova S, Musallam A, Hussain MS, et al. Circulating microRNAs as biomarkers for disease staging in multiple sclerosis. *Ann Neurol* (2013) **73**:729–40. doi:10.1002/ana.23880
164. Schwamborn JC, Berezikov E, Knoblich JA. The TRIM-NHL protein TRIM32 activates microRNAs and prevents self-renewal in mouse neural progenitors. *Cell* (2009) **136**:913–25. doi:10.1016/j.cell.2008.12.024
165. Li JJ, Dolios G, Wang R, Liao F-F. Soluble beta-amyloid peptides, but not insoluble fibrils, have specific effect on neuronal microRNA expression. *PLoS One* (2014) **9**:e90770. doi:10.1371/journal.pone.0090770
166. Ng S-Y, Lin L, Soh BS, Stanton LW. Long noncoding RNAs in development and disease of the central nervous system. *Trends Genet* (2013) **29**:461–8. doi:10.1016/j.tig.2013.03.002
167. Faghihi MA, Modarresi F, Khalil AM, Wood DE, Sahagan BG, Morgan TE, et al. Expression of a noncoding RNA is elevated in Alzheimer's disease and drives rapid feed-forward regulation of beta-secretase. *Nat Med* (2008) **14**:723–30. doi:10.1038/nm1784
168. Mus E, Hof PR, Tiedge H. Dendritic BC200 RNA in aging and in Alzheimer's disease. *Proc Natl Acad Sci U S A* (2007) **104**:10679–84. doi:10.1073/pnas.0701532104
169. Modarresi F, Faghihi MA, Lopez-Toledano MA, Fatemi RP, Magistri M, Brothers SP, et al. Inhibition of natural antisense transcripts in vivo results in gene-specific transcriptional upregulation. *Nat Biotechnol* (2012) **30**:453–9. doi:10.1038/nbt.2158
170. Xie Y, Hayden MR, Xu B. BDNF overexpression in the forebrain rescues Huntington's disease phenotypes in YAC128 mice. *J Neurosci* (2010) **30**:14708–18. doi:10.1523/JNEUROSCI.1637-10.2010
171. Bauer NM, Moos C, van Horssen J, Witte M, van der Valk P, Altenhein B, et al. Myelin basic protein synthesis is regulated by small non-coding RNA 715. *EMBO Rep* (2012) **13**:827–34. doi:10.1038/embor.2012.97
172. Pusic AD, Pusic KM, Clayton BLL, Kraig RP. IFNγ-stimulated dendritic cell exosomes as a potential therapeutic for remyelination. *J Neuroimmunol* (2014) **266**:12–23. doi:10.1016/j.jneuroim.2013.10.014

173. Rossi MN, Antonangeli F. LncRNAs: new players in apoptosis control. *Int J Cell Biol* (2014) **2014**:473857. doi:10.1155/2014/473857
174. Ridolfi E, Fenoglio C, Cantoni C, Calvi A, De Riz M, Pietroboni A, et al. Expression and genetic analysis of microRNAs involved in multiple sclerosis. *Int J Mol Sci* (2013) **14**:4375–84. doi:10.3390/ijms14034375
175. Li T, Morgan MJ, Choksi S, Zhang Y, Kim Y-S, Liu Z. MicroRNAs modulate the noncanonical transcription factor NF-kappaB pathway by regulating expression of the kinase IKKalpha during macrophage differentiation. *Nat Immunol* (2010) **11**:799–805. doi:10.1038/ni.1918
176. Lin S-T, Huang Y, Zhang L, Heng MY, Ptácek LJ, Fu Y-H. MicroRNA-23a promotes myelination in the central nervous system. *Proc Natl Acad Sci U S A* (2013) **110**:17468–73. doi:10.1073/pnas.1317182110
177. Lill CM, Schilling M, Ansaloni S, Schröder J, Jaedicke M, Luessi F, et al. Assessment of microRNA-related SNP effects in the 3′ untranslated region of the IL22RA2 risk locus in multiple sclerosis. *Neurogenetics* (2014) **15**:129–34. doi:10.1007/s10048-014-0396-y
178. Yoon J-H, Abdelmohsen K, Gorospe M. Functional interactions among microRNAs and long noncoding RNAs. *Semin Cell Dev Biol* (2014) **34C**:9–14. doi:10.1016/j.semcdb.2014.05.015
179. Grosswendt S, Filipchyk A, Manzano M, Klironomos F, Schilling M, Herzog M, et al. Unambiguous identification of miRNA:target site interactions by different types of ligation reactions. *Mol Cell* (2014) **54**:1042–54. doi:10.1016/j.molcel.2014.03.049
180. Chu C, Qu K, Zhong FL, Artandi SE, Chang HY. Genomic maps of long noncoding RNA occupancy reveal principles of RNA-chromatin interactions. *Mol Cell* (2011) **44**:667–78. doi:10.1016/j.molcel.2011.08.027
181. Mestdagh P, Hartmann N, Baeriswyl L, Andreasen D, Bernard N, Chen C, et al. Evaluation of quantitative miRNA expression platforms in the microRNA quality control (miRQC) study. *Nat Methods* (2014) **11**:809–15. doi:10.1038/nmeth.3014
182. Ling H, Fabbri M, Calin GA. MicroRNAs and other non-coding RNAs as targets for anticancer drug development. *Nat Rev Drug Discov* (2013) **12**:847–65. doi:10.1038/nrd4140
183. Li Z, Rana TM. Therapeutic targeting of microRNAs: current status and future challenges. *Nat Rev Drug Discov* (2014) **13**:622–38. doi:10.1038/nrd4359

Permissions

All chapters in this book were first published in AATIUIRASA, by Frontiers; hereby published with permission under the Creative Commons Attribution License or equivalent. Every chapter published in this book has been scrutinized by our experts. Their significance has been extensively debated. The topics covered herein carry significant findings which will fuel the growth of the discipline. They may even be implemented as practical applications or may be referred to as a beginning point for another development.

The contributors of this book come from diverse backgrounds, making this book a truly international effort. This book will bring forth new frontiers with its revolutionizing research information and detailed analysis of the nascent developments around the world.

We would like to thank all the contributing authors for lending their expertise to make the book truly unique.

They have played a crucial role in the development of this book. Without their invaluable contributions this book wouldn't have been possible. They have made vital efforts to compile up to date information on the varied aspects of this subject to make this book a valuable addition to the collection of many professionals and students.

This book was conceptualized with the vision of imparting up-to-date information and advanced data in this field. To ensure the same, a matchless editorial board was set up. Every individual on the board went through rigorous rounds of assessment to prove their worth. After which they invested a large part of their time researching and compiling the most relevant data for our readers.

The editorial board has been involved in producing this book since its inception. They have spent rigorous hours researching and exploring the diverse topics which have resulted in the successful publishing of this book. They have passed on their knowledge of decades through this book. To expedite this challenging task, the publisher supported the team at every step. A small team of assistant editors was also appointed to further simplify the editing procedure and attain best results for the readers.

Apart from the editorial board, the designing team has also invested a significant amount of their time in understanding the subject and creating the most relevant covers. They scrutinized every image to scout for the most suitable representation of the subject and create an appropriate cover for the book.

The publishing team has been an ardent support to the editorial, designing and production team. Their endless efforts to recruit the best for this project, has resulted in the accomplishment of this book. They are a veteran in the field of academics and their pool of knowledge is as vast as their experience in printing. Their expertise and guidance has proved useful at every step. Their uncompromising quality standards have made this book an exceptional effort. Their encouragement from time to time has been an inspiration for everyone.

The publisher and the editorial board hope that this book will prove to be a valuable piece of knowledge for researchers, students, practitioners and scholars across the globe.

List of Contributors

Peter J. L. Lane, Fiona M. McConnell, Graham Anderson, Maher G. Nawaf, Fabrina M. Gaspal and David R. Withers
MRC Centre for immune Regulation, Birmingham Medical School, Birmingham, UK

Afnan Alagha
Nonlinear Analysis and Applied Mathematics Research Group (NAAM), Department of Mathematics, King Abdulaziz University, Jeddah, Saudi Arabia

Alexey Zaikin
Department of Mathematics and Institute for Women's Health, University College London, London, UK

Patty Sachamitr, Simon Hackett and Paul Jonathan Fairchild
Sir William Dunn School of Pathology, University of Oxford, Oxford, UK

Lu Chen and Kellsye L. Fabian
Department of Immunology, University of Pittsburgh School of Medicine, Pittsburgh, PA, USA

Jennifer L. Taylor
Department of Dermatology, University of Pittsburgh School of Medicine, Pittsburgh, PA, USA

Walter J. Storkus
Department of Immunology, University of Pittsburgh School of Medicine, Pittsburgh, PA, USA
Department of Dermatology, University of Pittsburgh School of Medicine, Pittsburgh, PA, USA
University of Pittsburgh Cancer Institute, Pittsburgh, PA, USA

Gina J. Fiala
Faculty of Biology, Department of Molecular Immunology, Albert Ludwigs University Freiburg, Freiburg, Germany
Spemann Graduate School of Biology and Medicine (SGBM), Albert Ludwigs University Freiburg, Freiburg, Germany
Centre for Biological Signalling Studies BIOSS, Albert Ludwigs University Freiburg, Freiburg, Germany

Daniel Kaschek
Institute of Physics, Albert Ludwigs University Freiburg, Freiburg, Germany

Britta Blumenthal
Faculty of Biology, Department of Molecular Immunology, Albert Ludwigs University Freiburg, Freiburg, Germany
Medical Faculty, Centre for Chronic Immunodeficiency CCI, University Clinics Freiburg, Albert Ludwigs University Freiburg, Freiburg, Germany

Michael Reth
Faculty of Biology, Department of Molecular Immunology, Albert Ludwigs University Freiburg, Freiburg, Germany
Centre for Biological Signalling Studies BIOSS, Albert Ludwigs University Freiburg, Freiburg, Germany
Max Planck-Institute of Immunobiology and Epigenetics, Freiburg, Germany

Jens Timmer
Centre for Biological Signalling Studies BIOSS, Albert Ludwigs University Freiburg, Freiburg, Germany
Institute of Physics, Albert Ludwigs University Freiburg, Freiburg, Germany

Wolfgang W. A. Schamel
Faculty of Biology, Department of Molecular Immunology, Albert Ludwigs University Freiburg, Freiburg, Germany
Centre for Biological Signalling Studies BIOSS, Albert Ludwigs University Freiburg, Freiburg, Germany
Medical Faculty, Centre for Chronic Immunodeficiency CCI, University Clinics Freiburg, Albert Ludwigs University Freiburg, Freiburg, Germany

Yue Huang and Glenda M. Halliday
Neuroscience Research Australia, Sydney, NSW, Australia
University of New South Wales, Sydney, NSW, Australia

Ilgar Z. Mamedov, IvanV. Zvyagin and Dmitriy M. Chudakov
Shemyakin-Ovchinnikov Institute of Bioorganic Chemistry, Russian Academy of Science, Moscow, Russia
CEITEC, Masaryk University, Brno, Czech Republic

Olga V. Britanova, Maria A. Turchaninova, Dmitriy A. Bolotin, Ekaterina V. Putintseva and Yuriy B. Lebedev
Shemyakin-Ovchinnikov Institute of Bioorganic Chemistry, Russian Academy of Science, Moscow, Russia

Inbal Sela-Culang, Vered Kunik and Yanay Ofran
The Goodman Faculty of Life Sciences, Bar Ilan University, Ramat Gan, Israel

Walter G. Land
German Academy of Transplantation Medicine, Munich, Germany

Tim Dalessandri and Jessica Strid
Division of Immunology and Inflammation, Department of Medicine, Imperial College London, London, UK

Mario Castro
Grupo de Dinámica No-Lineal and Grupo Interdisciplinar de Sistemas Complejos (GISC), Escuela Técnica Superior de Ingeniería (ICAI), Universidad Pontificia Comillas, Madrid, Spain

Hisse M. van Santen, María Férez and Balbino Alarcón
Departamento de Biología Celular e Inmunología, Centro de Biología Molecular Severo Ochoa, Consejo Superior de Investigaciones Científicas, Universidad Autónoma de Madrid, Madrid, Spain

Grant Lythe and Carmen Molina-París
Department of Applied Mathematics, School of Mathematics, University of Leeds, Leeds, UK

Francisco J. Pérez-Cano, Malen Massot-Cladera, Àngels Franch, Cristina Castellote and Margarida Castell
Departament de Fisiologia, Facultat de Farmàcia, Universitat de Barcelona, Barcelona, Spain
Institut de Recerca en Nutrició i Seguretat Alimentària, Universitat de Barcelona, Barcelona, Spain

Dawn Barge and Gavin Spickett
Clinical Immunology, Newcastle upon Tyne Hospitals NHS Foundation Trust, Newcastle upon Tyne, UK

Laura Jardine, Ashley Ames-Draycott, Sarah Pagan, Sharon Cookson, Muzlifah Haniffa, Matthew Collin and Venetia Bigley
Human Dendritic Cell Laboratory, Institute of Cellular Medicine, Newcastle University, Newcastle upon Tyne, UK

Sahamoddin Khailaie
Department of Systems Immunology, Helmholtz Centre for Infection Research, Braunschweig, Germany

Fariba Bahrami
CIPCE, School of Electrical and Computer Engineering, College of Engineering, University of Tehran, Tehran, Iran

Mahyar Janahmadi
Neuroscience Research Centre and Department of Physiology, Faculty of Medicine, Shahid Beheshti University of Medical Sciences, Tehran, Iran

Pedro Milanez-Almeida and Jochen Huehn
Department of Experimental Immunology, Helmholtz Centre for Infection Research, Braunschweig, Germany

Michael Meyer-Hermann
Department of Systems Immunology, Helmholtz Centre for Infection Research, Braunschweig, Germany
Bio Centre for Life Science, Technische Universität Braunschweig, Braunschweig, Germany

Katherine J. L. Jackson, Marie J. Kidd, Yan Wang and Andrew M. Collins
School of Biotechnology and Biomolecular Sciences, University of New South Wales, Sydney, NSW, Australia

Patrick L. McGeer and Edith G. McGeer
Kinsmen Laboratory of Neurological Research, University of British Columbia, Vancouver, BC, Canada

Xiangyu Rao, Rob J. De Boer and Can Kesmir
Theoretical Biology and Bioinformatics, Utrecht University, Utrecht, Netherlands

Debbie van Baarle
Immunology Department, Wilhelmina Children's Hospital, University Medical Center Utrecht, Utrecht, Netherlands

Martin Maiers
National Marrow Donor Program, Minneapolis, MN, USA

Chen-Ting Lee
Department of Radiation Oncology, Duke University Medical Center, Durham, NC, USA

Elizabeth A. Repasky
Department of Immunology, Roswell Park Cancer Institute, Buffalo, NY, USA

Jing Sun and Vladimir Brusic
Cancer Vaccine Center, Dana-Farber Cancer Institute, Harvard Medical School, Boston, MA, USA
Department of Medicine, Harvard Medical School, Boston, MA, USA

Ulrich J. Kudahl and Christian Simon
Cancer Vaccine Center, Dana-Farber Cancer Institute, Harvard Medical School, Boston, MA, USA
Center for Biological Sequence Analysis, Technical University of Denmark, Lyngby, Denmark

Zhiwei Cao
School of Life Sciences and Technology, Tongji University, Shanghai, China

Ellis L. Reinherz
Cancer Vaccine Center, Dana-Farber Cancer Institute, Harvard Medical School, Boston, MA, USA
Department of Medicine, Harvard Medical School, Boston, MA, USA
Laboratory of Immunobiology, Department of Medical Oncology, Dana-Farber Cancer Institute, Harvard Medical School, Boston, MA, USA

Sudarshan Phani, Diane Berengere Re and Serge Przedborski
Department of Pathology and Cell Biology, Columbia University, New York, NY, USA
Center for Motor Neuron Disease, Department of Neurology, Columbia University, New York, NY, USA

Marta Caridade and Luis Graca
Instituto de Medicina Molecular, Faculdade de Medicina da Universida de de Lisboa, Lisbon, Portugal
Instituto Gulbenkian de Ciência, Oeiras, Portugal

Ruy M. Ribeiro
Theoretical Biology and Biophysics, Los Alamos National Laboratory, Los Alamos, NM, USA

Thiago J. Borges and Cristina Bonorino
Faculdade de Biociências e Instituto de Pesquisas Biomédicas, Pontifícia Universidade Católica do Rio Grande do Sul, Porto Alegre, Rio Grande do Sul, Brazil

Lotte Wieten, Martijn J. C. van Herwijnen, Femke Broere, Ruurd van der Zee and Willem van Eden
Department of Infectious Diseases and Immunology, Faculty of Veterinary Medicine, Utrecht University, Utrecht, Netherlands

Gur Yaari
Bioengineering Program, Faculty of Engineering, Bar Ilan University, Ramat Gan, Israel
Department of Pathology, Yale School of Medicine, New Haven, CT, USA

Jason A. Vander Heiden, Daniel Gadala-Maria and Namita Gupta
Interdepartmental Program in Computational Biology and Bioinformatics, Yale University, New Haven, CT, USA

Mohamed Uduman
Department of Pathology, Yale School of Medicine, New Haven, CT, USA

Joel N. H. Stern
Department of Neurology, Yale School of Medicine, New Haven, CT, USA
Department of Science Education, Hofstra North Shore-LIJ School of Medicine, Hempstead, NY, USA

Kevin C. O'Connor
Department of Neurology, Yale School of Medicine, New Haven, CT, USA
Human and Translational Immunology Program, Yale School of Medicine, New Haven, CT, USA

David A. Hafler
Department of Neurology, Yale School of Medicine, New Haven, CT, USA
Department of Immunobiology, Yale School of Medicine, New Haven, CT, USA

Uri Laserson
Department of Genetics, Harvard Medical School, Boston, MA, USA

Francois Vigneault
AbVitro, Inc., Boston, MA, USA

Steven H. Kleinstein
Department of Pathology, Yale School of Medicine, New Haven, CT, USA
Interdepartmental Program in Computational Biology and Bioinformatics, Yale University, New Haven, CT, USA

Anna Stachurska, Maria M. Zorro, Marijke R. van der Sijde and Sebo Withoff
Department of Genetics, University Medical Center Groningen, University of Groningen, Groningen, Netherlands

Index

www.ingramcontent.com/pod-product-compliance
Lightning Source LLC
LaVergne TN
LVHW080929210926
848485LV00004B/760
* 9 7 8 1 6 3 9 8 7 1 1 3 1 *